Textbook of
Bone Metastases

Textbook of Bone Metastases

Editors

CLAUDE JASMIN
*Head of the Department of Haematology and Tumour Biology,
Paul Brousse Hospital, Villejuif, France*

ROBERT E. COLEMAN
*Head, Department of Clinical Oncology,
Weston Park Hospital, Sheffield, UK*

LAWRENCE R. COIA
*Chairman, Department of Radiation Oncology,
Community Medical Center, Toms River, NJ, USA*

RODOLFO CAPANNA
*Head of Department of Orthopaedic Oncology,
Centro Traumatologico Ortopedico, Firenze, Italy*

GÉRARD SAILLANT
*Head of Department of Orthopaedics and Traumatology,
University Hospital Pitié-Salpêtière, Paris, France*

John Wiley & Sons, Ltd

Other Wiley Editorial Offices

John Wiley & Sons Inc., 111 River Street, Hoboken, NJ 07030, USA

Jossey-Bass, 989 Market Street, San Francisco, CA 94103-1741, USA

Wiley-VCH Verlag GmbH, Boschstr. 12, D-69469 Weinheim, Germany

John Wiley & Sons Australia Ltd, 33 Park Road, Milton, Queensland 4064, Australia

John Wiley & Sons (Asia) Pte Ltd, 2 Clementi Loop #02-01, Jin Xing Distripark, Singapore 129809

John Wiley & Sons Canada Ltd, 22 Worcester Road, Etobicoke, Ontario, Canada M9W 1L1

Wiley also publishes its books in a variety of electronic formats. Some content that appears in print may
not be available in electronic books.

Library of Congress Cataloging-in-Publication Data

Textbook of bone metastases / editors, Claude Jasmin ... [et al.].
      p. ; cm.
   Includes bibliographical references and index.
   ISBN 0-471-87742-5 (alk. paper)
    1. Bone metastasis. I. Jasmin, Claude, 1938–
   [DNLM: 1. Bone Neoplasms – secondary. 2. Bone Neoplasms – therapy. WE 258 T355 2005]
   RC280.B6T445 2005
   616.99'471–dc22
                                                                                2004053705

British Library Cataloguing in Publication Data

A catalogue record for this book is available from the British Library

ISBN 0 471 87742 5

Typeset by Dobbie Typesetting Ltd, Tavistock, Devon
Printed and bound in Great Britain by Antony Rowe Ltd, Chippenham
This book is printed on acid-free paper responsibly manufactured from sustainable forestry
in which at least two trees are planted for each one used for paper production.

Contents

Contributors

MOHAMED E. ABDEL-WANIS *Department of Orthopaedic Surgery, School of Medicine, Kanazawa University, 13-1 Takaramachi, Kanazawa 920-8641, Japan*

C. ADEM *Department of Neuroradiology, Hôpital de la Pitié-Salpétrière, 47 Boulevard de l'Hôpital, 75013 Paris, France*

SOPHIA AGELAKI *Division of Clinical Oncology, University General Hospital of Heraklion, PO Box 1352, Heraklion, 71110 Crete, Greece*

TOMOYUKI AKAMARU *Department of Orthopaedic Surgery, School of Medicine, Kanazawa University, 13-1 Takaramachi, Kanazawa 920-8641, Japan*

PENNY R. ANDERSON *Department of Radiation Oncology, Fox Chase Cancer Center, 7701 Burholme Avenue, Philadelphia, PA 19111, USA*

ROBERT U. ASHFORD *WHO Collaborating Centre for Metabolic Bone Diseases, University of Sheffield Medical School, Beech Hill Road, Sheffield S10 2RX, UK*

LODOVICO BALDUCCI *H. Lee Moffitt Cancer Center and Research Institute, Division of Medical Oncology and Hematology, 12902 Magnolia Drive, Tampa, FL 33612, USA*

STEFANO BANDIERA *Ospedale Maggiori, Largo B. Nigrisoli, 2-40133 Bologna, Italy*

JAMES R. BERENSON *Institute for Myeloma and Bone Cancer Research, 9201 Sunset Blvd., West Hollywood, CA 90069, USA*

NICK BISHOP *Section of Reproductive and Developmental Medicine, The Sheffield Children's Hospital, University of Sheffield, Western Bank, Sheffield S10 2TH, UK*

FRANÇOISE BODÉRÉ *Department of Nuclear Medicine, Centre René Gauducheau, Boulevard Jacques Monod, Saint Herblain, Cedex 44805, France*

J. J. BODY *Institut J. Bordet, 1 Rue Héger-Bordet, 1000 Bruxelles, Belgium*

STEFANO BORIANI *Ospedale Maggiori, Largo B. Nigrisoli, 2-40133 Bologna, Italy*

GIOVANNI BARBANTI BRÒDANO *Ospedale Maggiori, Largo B. Nigrisoli, 2-40133 Bologna, Italy*

J. E. BROWN *Department of Clinical Oncology, Weston Park Hospital, Whitham Road, Sheffield S10 2SJ, UK*

DOMENICO A. CAMPANACCI *Department of Orthopaedic Oncology, Centro Traumatologico Ortopedico, Largo Palagi 1, 50139 Firenze, Italy*

RODOLPHO CAPANNA *Department of Orthopaedic Oncology, Centro Traumatologico Ortopedico, Largo Palagi 1, 50139 Firenze, Italy*

L. CEUGNART *Service de Radiologie, Centre Oscar Lambret 3, Rue Frédéric Combemale, 59000 Lille, France*

JEAN-FRANÇOIS CHATAL *Department of Nuclear Medicine, Centre René Gauducheau, Boulevard Jacques Monod, Saint Herblain, Cedex 44805, France*

J. CHIRAS *Department of Neuroradiology, Hôpital de la Pitié-Salpétrière, 47 Boulevard de l'Hôpital, 75013 Paris, France*

EDWARD CHOW *Department of Radiation Oncology, Toronto Sunnybrook Regional Cancer Center, 2075 Bayview Avenue, Toronto, Ontario M4N 3M5, Canada*

PHILIPPE CLÉZARDIN *INSERM Research Unit 403, Faculty of Medicine Laënnec, Rue Guilliaume Paradin, 69372 Lyon, Cedex 08, France*

LAWRENCE R. COIA *Department of Radiation Oncology, Community Medical Center, 99 Highway 37 West, Toms River, NJ 08755, USA*

ROBERT E. COLEMAN *Cancer Research Centre, Academic Unit of Clinical Oncology, Weston Park Hospital, Whitham Road, Sheffield S10 2SJ, UK*

GARY J. R. COOK *Department of Nuclear Medicine, Royal Marsden Hospital, Downs Road, Sutton, Surrey SM2 5PT, UK*

A. COTTEN *Service de Radiologie Ostéoarticulaire, Hôpital Roger Salengro, Boulevard du Pr. J. Leclerqu, 59000 Lille, France*

PETER I. CROUCHER *University of Sheffield Medical School, Beech Hill Road, Sheffield S10 2RX, UK*

JANINE A. DANKS *St Vincent's Institute for Medical Research, 41 Victoria Parade, Melbourne 3065, Australia*

HELENA DAVIES *Section of Reproductive and Developmental Medicine, The Sheffield Children's Hospital, University of Sheffield, Western Bank, Sheffield S10 2TH, UK*

P. D. S. DIJKSTRA *Department of Orthopaedic Oncology, Leiden University Medical Centre, Albinusdreef 2, PO Box 9600, 2300 RC Leiden, The Netherlands*

ISRAEL DUDKIEWICZ *Department of Orthopaedic Surgery "A", The Chaim Sheba Medical Centre, Tel Hashomer 52621, Israel*

COLIN R. DUNSTAN *Bone Biology Unit, ANZAC Research Institute, Concord, NSW 2139, Australia*

SUZANNE A. ECCLES *Cancer Research UK Centre for Cancer Therapeutics, Institute of Cancer Research, McElwain Laboratories, Cotswold Road, Belmont, Sutton, Surrey SM2 5NG, UK*

E. A. ENKAOUA *Department of Orthopaedic Surgery and Traumatology, Hôpital de la Pitié-Salpêtrière, 47 Boulevard de l'Hôpital, 75013 Paris, France*

IGNAC FOGELMAN *Department of Nuclear Medicine, Guy's Hospital, London SE1 9RT, UK*

BRUNO FUCHS *Mayo Clinic College of Medicine, Rochester, MN 55905, USA*

ALESSANDRO GASBARRINI *Ospedale Maggiori, Largo B. Nigrisoli, 2-40133 Bologna, Italy*

VASSILIS GEORGOULIAS *Division of Clinical Oncology, University General Hospital of Heraklion, PO Box 1352, Heraklion, 71110 Crete, Greece*

ORA GILBAR *School of Social Work, University of Haifa, Mount Carmel, Haifa 31905, Israel*

MARJORIE C. GREEN *Division of Medicine, University of Texas M. D. Anderson Cancer Center, 1515 Holcombe Boulevard, Box 56, Houston, TX 77030, USA*

J. F. GUEST *Catalyst Health Economics Consultants Ltd, Pinner, Middlesex, UK*

R. GUILLEVIN *Department of Neuroradiology, Hôpital de la Pitié-Salpêtrière, 47 Boulevard de l'Hôpital, 75013 Paris, France*

KARIN GWYN *M. D. Anderson Cancer Center, 1515 Holcombe Boulevard, Box 520, Houston, TX 77030, USA*

WILLIAM F. HARTSELL *Radiation Oncology, Adovcate Good Samaritan Cancer Center, 3815 Highland Avenue, Downers Grove, IL 60515, USA*

MICHAEL A. HENDERSON *Department of Surgery, University of Melbourne, St Vincent's Hospital, 41 Victoria Parade, Melbourne 3065, Australia*

GABRIEL N. HORTOBAGYI *Department of Breast Medical Oncology, University of Texas M. D. Anderson Cancer Center, 1515 Holcombe Boulevard, Box 56, Houston, TX 77030, USA*

PETER J. HOSKIN *Cancer Centre, Mount Vernon Hospital, Rickmansworth Road, Northwood HA6 2RN, UK*

DAVID J. JACOFSKY *Department of Orthopaedic Surgery, Mayo Clinic College of Medicine, 200 First Street SW, Rochester, MN 55905, USA*

CLAUDE JASMIN *Department of Haematology, Hôpital Paul Brousse, 14–16 Avenue Paul Vaillant Couturier, 94804 Villejuif Cedex, France*

JOHN A. KANIS *WHO Collaborating Centre for Metabolic Bone Diseases, University of Sheffield Medical School, Beech Hill Road, Sheffield S10 2RX, UK*

NORIO KAWAHARA *Department of Orthopaedic Surgery, School of Medicine, Kanazawa University, 13-1 Takaramachi, Kanazawa 920-8641, Japan*

ROBERT A. KYLE *Mayo Clinic, 200 First Street SW, Rochester, MN 55905, USA*

F. LAFITTE *Department of Neuroradiology, Hôpital de la Pitié-Salpêtrière, 47 Boulevard de l'Hôpital, 75013 Paris, France*

D. LO *Department of Neuroradiology, Hôpital de la Pitié-Salpêtrière, 47 Boulevard de l'Hôpital, 75013 Paris, France*

D. A. LOSSIGNOL *Institut Jules Bordet, Bruxelles, Belgium*

J. C. MAILLARD *Department of Neuroradiology, Hôpital de la Pitié-Salpêtrière, 47 Boulevard de l'Hôpital, 75013 Paris, France*

UZMA MALIK *Department of Radiation Medicine, University of Kentucky Medical Center, Room N-14, 800 Rose Street, Lexington, KY 40536, USA*

T. J. MARTIN *St Vincent's Institute for Medical Research, 41 Victoria Parade, Melbourne 3065, Australia*

N. MARTIN-DUVERNEUIL *Department of Neuroradiology, Hôpital de la Pitié-Salpêtrière, 47 Boulevard de l'Hôpital, 75013 Paris, France*

EUGENE V. McCLOSKEY *WHO Collaborating Centre for Metabolic Bone Diseases, University of Sheffield Medical School, Beech Hill Road, Sheffield S10 2RX, UK*

D. W. MILES *Guy's Hospital–Imperial Cancer Research Fund Breast Cancer Biology Group, 3rd Floor, Thomas Guy House, London SE1 9RT, UK*

MOHAMMED MOHIUDDIN *Department of Radiation Medicine, University of Kentucky Medical Center, Room N-14, 800 Rose Street, Lexington, KY 40536, USA*

MALCOLM J. MOORE *Department of Radiation Oncology, Princess Margaret Hospital, 610 University Avenue, Toronto, Ontario M5G 2M9, Canada*

HIDEKI MURAKAMI *Department of Orthopaedic Surgery, School of Medicine, Kanazawa University, 13-1 Takaramachi, Kanazawa 920-8641, Japan*

KOSHI NANBU *Department of Orthopaedic Surgery, School of Medicine, Kanazawa University, 13-1 Takaramachi, Kanazawa 920-8641, Japan*

H. L. NEVILLE-WEBBE *Cancer Research Centre, Academic Unit of Clinical Oncology, Weston Park Hospital, Whitham Road, Sheffield S10 2SJ, UK*

STEFANIA PADERNI *Ospedale Maggiori, Largo B. Nigrisoli, 2-40133 Bologna, Italy*

CARLOS A. PEREZ *Mallinckrodt Institute of Radiology, Radiation Oncology Center, 4511 Forest Park Boulevard Ste 200, St Louis, MO 63108, USA*

T. A. PLUNKETT *Academic Oncology Unit/Guy's Hospital–Imperial Cancer Research Fund Breast Cancer Biology Group, 3rd Floor, Thomas Guy House, London SE1 9RT, UK*

STUART H. RALSTON *Bone Research Group, Department of Medicine and Therapeutics, Aberdeen University Medical School, Polwarth Building, Foresterhill Hospital, Aberdeen AB25 2ZD, UK*

O. REMAN *Service d'Hématologie Clinique, CHU de Caen, 14000 Caen, France*

ISABELLE RESCHE *Department of Nuclear Medicine, Centre René Gauducheau, Boulevard Jacques Monod, Saint Herblain, Cedex 44805, France*

MICHAEL J. ROGERS *Bone Research Group, Department of Medicine and Therapeutics, Aberdeen University Medical School, Polwarth Building, Foresterhill Hospital, Aberdeen AB25 2ZD, UK*

DANIEL E. ROOS *Department of Radiation Oncology, Royal Adelaide Hospital, North Terrace, Adelaide, South Australia 5000, Australia*

M. ROSE *Department of Neuroradiology, Hôpital de la Pitié-Salpêtrière, 47 Boulevard de l'Hôpital, 75013 Paris, France*

CAROLINE ROUSSEAU *Department of Nuclear Medicine, Centre René Gauducheau, Boulevard Jacques Monod, Saint Herblain, Cedex 44805, France*

R. D. RUBENS *Academic Oncology Unit, Guy's Hospital, London SE1 9RT, UK*

MOSHE SALAI *Head of Orthopaedic Department, Rabin Medical Center, Beilinson Campus, Petah Tikva, Israel*

FRANKLIN H. SIM *Department of Orthopaedic Surgery, Mayo Clinic, 200 First Street SW, Rochester, MN 55905, USA*

A. H. M. TAMINIAU *Department of Orthopaedic Oncology, Leiden University Medical Centre, Albinusdreef 2, PO Box 9600, 2300 RC Leiden, The Netherlands*

SILVIA TERZI *Ospedale Maggiori, Largo B. Nigrisoli, 2-40133 Bologna, Italy*

RICHARD THERIAULT *M. D. Anderson Cancer Center, 1515 Holcombe Boulevard, Box 520, Houston, TX 77030, USA*

VALLO TILLMAN *Section of Reproductive and Developmental Medicine, The Sheffield Children's Hospital, University of Sheffield, Western Bank, Sheffield S10 2TH, UK*

KATSURO TOMITA *Department of Orthopaedic Surgery, School of Medicine, Kanazawa University, 13-1 Takaramachi, Kanazawa 920-8641, Japan*

YASUHIRO UEDA *Department of Orthopaedic Surgery, School of Medicine, Kanazawa University, 13-1 Takaramachi, Kanazawa 920-8641, Japan*

J. N. VALLÉE *Department of Neuroradiology, Hôpital de la Pitié-Salpêtrière, 17 Boulevard de l'Hôpital, 75013 Paris, France*

PADRAIG WARDE *Department of Radiation Oncology, Princess Margaret Hospital, 610 University Avenue, Toronto, Ontario M5G 2M9, Canada*

R. WINDHAGER *Department of Orthopaedic Surgery, University of Graz, Auenbruggerplatz 29, 8036 Graz, Austria*

JACKSON WU *Department of Radiation Oncology, Tom Baker Cancer Center, 1331 29th Street NW, Calgary, AB T2N 4N2, Canada*

Preface

Optimal treatment of cancer requires a wide-ranging, multi-disciplinary approach. Over the last 20 years, quite remarkable progress has been made in all fields of oncology: in the biology and physiopathology of cancers, the assessment of clinical and biological parameters in patients, evaluation and measurement of tumour growth and the development of new treatments.

Despite this, metastases have remained a major problem in managing patients with malignant tumours. Indeed, most metastatic cancers today are considered incurable. Questions may then be raised as to the usefulness of having an entire textbook devoted to one type of metastases, in the present case bone metastases.

The epidemiological and clinical importance of bone metastases has long been recognised. It is known, for example, that the incidence of metastatic breast and prostate cancers on bone sites is 70%, whereas it is only 30–40% in metastatic lung cancer. In clinical terms, these metastases can have substantial negative effects on the patient's quality of life.

For a long time now, any progress in treatments of bone metastases has been almost exclusively in the fields of surgery and chemotherapy, plus palliative treatment. Bone metastases have also been neglected because of the difficulty in quantifying them, which has left them outside the scope of therapeutic trials.

The only justification, therefore, for the decision to devote a textbook to the subject of bone metastases is the quite remarkable progress made recently in the understanding of bone molecular and cellular mechanisms involved in osteogenesis and osteolysis and their development for therapeutic purposes. The discovery of marker molecules and of the cytokines, which control bone resorption by osteoclasts, and specifically soluble osteoprotegerin receptors, has made it possible to understand how osteoblasts and osteoclasts communicate for bone remodelling homeostasis. The distinguished journal *Science* published a supplement in September 2000 entitled "Bone Remodelling and Repair", which in itself is proof of this recent revolution in the knowledge of bone physiology and physiopathology.

The two solid tumours which most often give rise to bone metastases are breast cancer in women and prostate cancer in men. This shows just how important these new discoveries are, as they may lead to an understanding of the reasons for prostate metastases being osteoblastic, while metastases from most other cancers are osteolytic. These scientific advances have already produced better therapeutic approaches for the treatment of certain cancers, in particular with the use of oestrogen receptor modulators and, more importantly, the major development of bisphosphonates. The treatment of malignant hypercalcaemia has also been revolutionised by the use of bisphosphonates.

The revival of interest from cancer specialists and, indeed, from all specialists treating patients with bone metastases, can easily be seen through the increasing number of sessions on bone metastases at major cancer conferences and with the establishment of international societies and associations devoted to the subject, e.g. the newly founded International Society for Bone Metastases. Such interest can also be measured by the increase in the number of articles on bone metastases found in publications on both basic research and clinical experience.

There would seem to be good reason for collecting information on these very recent and major advances in the understanding and treatment of bone metastases, and for presenting such information as a textbook of importance and use to the medical community.

The intention was to produce a book offering a broad approach to recent progress in all fields related to bone metastases, ranging from epidemiology to the physiopathology of bone metastases and therapeutic approaches. The book is intended to provide a better understanding of recent advances and, more importantly, to give clinical practitioners all the elements needed to help them in the clinical and therapeutic management of patients with bone metastases.

The presentation has been designed to offer both vertical and cross-disciplinary views on bone metastases. The first part focuses on metastatic disease, covering epidemiology, biology, physiopathology, clinical aspects, the assessment of patients and their disease, together with different types of therapy available: surgery, interventional radiology, external radiotherapy, chemotherapy, immunotherapy and hormone therapy.

The second part of the book presents a broad-ranging view with an overall approach to the patient, including the treatment of pain (a major issue, as bone metastases can be extremely painful), the psychological and social ramifications of these conditions, together with a special approach needed for elderly patients with bone metastases. One chapter is devoted to the specific features of bone metastases in child cancer patients. A third section covers an integrated approach to bone metastases occurring in the course of certain conditions with which they are frequently associated, and also includes practical advice for bone metastases developing with cancers which do not usually develop such metastases. Guidelines for the treatment of bone metastases have been drawn up in consultation with a multi-disciplinary group of doctors, surgeons, radio-therapists and interventional radiologists and are designed to establish simple and reproducible criteria for decision-making in a range of clinical siguations.

Articles have been contributed by leading specialists on each of the subjects and the textbook should stand as an international reference in the field of bone metastases. Given the rate at which the advances are being made in the field, it is obvious that further updated editions will have to be published. Our ambition is to see improved management of patients over the years to come, by making the very latest knowledge in the field widely available.

Claude Jasmin, MD FACP

1

Biology of Bone Metastases

Section Editor: **Robert E. Coleman**

General Mechanisms of Metastasis

Suzanne A. Eccles

Institute of Cancer Research, Sutton, UK

HISTORICAL BACKGROUND

Malignant tumours occur in all higher multicellular organisms and have done so throughout evolution. Non-human primates are susceptible to the same types of cancer as man, and the natural history (including the patterns of metastatic spread) is very similar. Osteolytic lesions typical of multiple myeloma are found in ancient Egyptian skeletons and malignant melanoma metastases in the long bones, skulls and preserved skin of Peruvian pre-Columbian Incas dating from about 400 BC [1,2]. As well as this fascinating but relatively scanty physical evidence of metastatic cancer in ancient times, illustrations and writings of many early civilisations describe lesions that are clearly malignant tumours. These sources provide unique insights into the attempts of our distant forebears to recognise, understand and treat those diseases which thousands of years later still constitute a formidable medical problem.

Giovanni Battista Morgagni, in his major work, *On the Sources and Causes of Diseases*, published in 1761, was able to distinguish malignant cancers from benign swellings, with descriptions so accurate that the diseases can be diagnosed today. However, in a case of gastric cancer with extensive dissemination to the liver, Morgagni failed to connect the two observations, indicating that the phenomenon of distant metastasis was not recognised at this time.

When the achromatic microscope was developed in the 1820s, the age of histopathology was born and Johannes Müller pioneered the study of tumours. He first used the term "cell" (*Zelle*) to describe the components of malignant tissue, but this defined a macroscopic rather than a microscopic structure—a membrane-bound cluster of true cells visible with the naked eye. The correct definition of a cell as the basic unit of living matter is credited to botanists. Although by then it was well known that plants were composed of aggregations of cells, their autonomy and replicative capacity were first fully described by Matthias Schleiden in 1838. Soon afterwards, one of Müller's pupils, Theodor Schwann, published papers suggesting an analogous situation in animal tissues.

Schwann's and Müller's ideas complemented each other and led to general acceptance of the hypothesis that both normal tissues and their pathological counterparts (including tumours) were composed of cellular aggregates. Thus, the concept of the cancer cell quietly evolved. In 1855, another of Müller's students, Rudolf Virchow, coined the now famous aphorism, *omnis cellula e cellula*. This crucial concept of every cell deriving from another cell was originally formulated from Virchow's studies on tuberculosis lesions. Later, both Virchow's further work and Müller's reassessment of his structural analysis of tumours led to the realisation that the theory also applied to cancer. From this period, the cell held a central position in analysis of both normal and pathological processes; however, it was some time before it was recognised to be the key feature of cancer dissemination.

In 1829, Joseph Recamier, a gynaecologist in Paris, published his seminal *Recherches sur le traitment du cancer*, in which for the first time the discontiguous dissemination of cancer was recognised and named "metastasis". The direct spread of cancers to surrounding tissues and draining lymph nodes had been well documented over preceding centuries, but

Textbook of Bone Metastases. Edited by C. Jasmin, R. E. Coleman, L. R. Coia, R. Capanna and G. Saillant
© 2005 John Wiley & Sons Ltd: ISBN 0 471 87742 5

Recamier described invasion of veins and distant secondary growth in the brain of a breast cancer patient. The term is of Greek origin, defined as a "change in the seat of a disease". It was originally used by the Hippocratic physicians to describe any shift in manifestation of morbidity, (or as they saw it, imbalances of humors) within the body.

In the same year that Schleiden and Schwann began to crystallise their cell theories (1838), the pathologist Robert Carswell was amongst the first to suggest that cancer may disseminate through the circulation [3]. It seems, with the value of hindsight, that it would be a small step (particularly following the acceptance of Virchow's views) to surmise that the agent of spread was the cancer cell. However, even Virchow himself did not subscribe to this view. While acknowledging that cells might serve to disseminate cancer, he felt that clinical evidence indicated otherwise. For example, he noted that the lungs were invaded more rarely than the liver in cases of gastric, uterine and mammary cancer. He concluded that this was inconsistent with the idea of the active principle being of a "corpuscular" nature (which would be expected to lodge in the lungs) but that metastasis was due rather to the transference of certain fluids or "morbid juices" [4]. This "humoral" theory of metastasis, perhaps because someone as venerable as Virchow had championed it, was relinquished only gradually.

James Paget also wrote that there was no need to invoke corpuscles or germs to explain the spread of cancer, and that "an unformed cancerous blastema" must be assumed where dissemination occurred in organs "downstream" of the lungs [4]. It is clear that the causes of metastasis could not be fully appreciated whilst the origins and nature of primary cancer remained a mystery. In a remarkably prescient statement in the Bradshaw lecture at the Royal College of Surgeons in 1884, Sir William Savory said: "Before we shall ever be able to answer the question of why or how do [malignant] tumours form... we must be able to solve the problem of normal growth and development".

The Berlin anatomist William Waldeyer published a significant paper in 1867. From his studies in breast cancer, he propounded a convincing (if then unproven) thesis that all epithelial cancers were derived from normal epithelium by proliferation. This fact had been contentious for years, with several illustrious protagonists, including Virchow, convinced that carcinomas evolved from connective tissue, and also that in the case of metastasis it was the latter cells which became transformed by fluids secreted by the primary tumour. More importantly, Waldeyer's paper implicitly proposed that the movement of cancer cells into adjacent tissues was responsible for regional spread; also, that metastasis resulted from the blood- or lymph-borne transfer of cancer cells to distant sites, where they proliferated to generate new lesions. This led to the formulation of the "mechanical" theory of cancer dissemination. This proposed simply that tumour cells released from the primary site circulated in the blood or lymph until they became lodged in the microvessels of draining nodes or distant organs, where they proliferated to form metastases.

However, both the pioneering cancer surgeon Theodor Billroth and his mentor Langenbeck were unconvinced that embolisation could account for all metastases, and posed the question, "What is it that decides what organ shall suffer in a case of disseminated cancer?". The challenge to provide an answer was taken up by Stephen Paget in a now famous article published in *The Lancet* in March 1889. Like his father before him, Paget studied at St Bartholomew's Hospital in London, and it is likely that Sir James Paget's close friendship with Virchow, and his own speculations on the nature of cancer spread, fuelled his son's interest. Although Paget senior agreed with Virchow's ideas on the inductive nature of the disseminating principle, his son found evidence to the contrary.

Paget reviewed the autopsies of 735 breast cancer patients at the Middlesex Hospital and noted (as had Virchow in 1860) the frequency with which liver metastases were present (33%) compared with lung (10%) and spleen (2%). This was similar to the patterns observed with uterine cancer, where liver metastases again predominated and splenic metastases were exceedingly rare, in spite of an apparently similar risk of embolism in their vessels. He also noted a higher than expected involvement of the ovaries, and the predilection for certain bones (femur, humerus, cranium) but not others (hands and feet) to support metastasis.

He was also familiar with the "astonishing frequency" with which thyroid cancer generated bone metastases, and their almost complete absence in cases of gastric carcinoma. He interpreted these findings to suggest that tissues receiving cancer emboli were not passive or "impartial", but could afford either a congenial or hostile environment for the further development of metastases [5]. His paper concluded with a paragraph praising the "scientific botanists" who study the seed, but tentatively suggested that those like him—the mere ploughmen—may provide useful observations on the properties of the soil. This has only recently been appreciated fully with increasing evidence of the importance of microenvironment on the expression of malignant potential.

Others continued to believe that patterns of metastasis were explicable purely by circulatory anatomy and the embolic properties of tumour cells. In 1928, in the third edition of his classic text *Neoplastic Diseases*, Ewing stated that there was no need to evoke special affinities of particular tumour cells for certain tissues to explain the distribution of metastases. However, it is noteworthy that he deleted this statement from the fourth edition of his book! The relative contributions of Ewing's stochastic (mechanical) and Paget's selective (seed–soil) elements to the metastatic process continued to stimulate debate until the present day. It is now generally accepted that both processes occur. About 50–60% of the sites of metastases are predictable from the lymphatic and/or haematogenous route followed by the disseminating cells. For the remainder (and this includes bone), we are beginning to appreciate how subtle interactions between tumour and host cells at the cellular and molecular level collectively determine the probabilities and patterns of metastasis.

CURRENT PERSPECTIVE

Metastasis essentially discriminates benign from malignant lesions. It is the ultimate step in the multistage process of tumour progression and the major cause of treatment failure and cancer deaths. The term "metastasis" is generally reserved for the dissemination of tumour cells via the blood or lymphatics, although spread in the cerebrospinal fluid and transcoelomic passage may also occur. About 30% of cancer patients present with secondary disease and a similar percentage have occult metastases which manifest later. The prognosis of the majority of these patients is poor. Bone metastases are common in advanced disease and are particularly associated with certain cancers, notably breast and prostate carcinomas and also malignant myeloma, thyroid cancer, lung cancer, renal cancer and certain lymphomas (Figure 1.1). Sporadic cases of bone metastases from other cancers are also seen, but it is the biology, diagnosis and treatment of so-called "osteotropic" cancers that is of major importance [6–8].

Problems of Detection of Metastases in the Clinic and Laboratory

There is a critical need for reliable and early indicators of metastatic potential, in order that preventive or therapeutic measures can be promptly applied and unnecessary treatment of disease-free patients avoided.

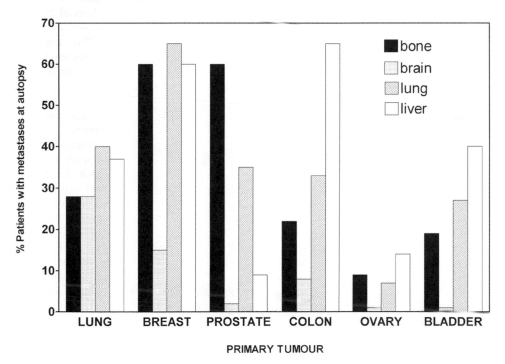

Figure 1.1. The relative distribution of metastases at autopsy for some common cancers

Current physical detection methods, such as computed tomography (CT), magnetic resonance imaging (MRI) or ultrasound, are too insensitive to pick up micrometastases. Similarly, measurement of circulating markers, such as carcinoembryonic antigen, prostate-specific antigen or CA125, may predict recurrence but do not give information on the site of relapse.

In some cases it is possible to sample regional nodes during surgery to test for the presence of disseminated cells. However, detection depending upon histological examination of a limited number of sections may miss small tumour deposits. Molecular techniques of detecting occult disease, e.g. using polymerase chain reaction (PCR) to pick up genetic abnormalities in biopsies or body fluids, are gaining ground, but there is as yet insufficient confidence in most cases to equate "positive" results with cellular clonogenic capacity or the unequivocal risk of developing overt metastases [9]. Similarly, when single viable tumour cells or small clusters are detected, there is no way of knowing whether they are capable of developing into a gross metastasis. Pantel et al. showed that colorectal cancer patients could harbour cytokeratin- and c-erbB-2 oncogene-positive cells in their bone marrow, yet rarely if ever developed overt metastases at this site [10]. In the laboratory, genetic "tags" such as green fluorescent protein (GFP) can be used to track disseminating cells, but again care is required, since loss of the label or immune recognition of the introduced foreign protein can lead to spurious results [11].

Haematogenous Metastasis

Blood-borne spread is the major route of dissemination of sarcomas and is also of clinical significance in carcinomas and haematopoietic malignancies. Many experimental models use the simple expedient of introducing tumour cells into the circulation to mimic haematogenous metastasis. Carcinoma or sarcoma cells injected into the peripheral circulation (unless pre-selected for specific dissemination patterns) yield predominantly or exclusively lung colonies (not strictly metastases) and liver colonies can be generated by injecting cells into the spleen, mesenteric veins or portal vein. Intravenously injected lymphoma cells frequently bypass the lungs to grow in liver, spleen and other sites—a simple illustration of "seed and soil" in action. Bone metastases can be modelled either by direct implantation into the tibia or by introduction into the left ventricle of the heart. Interestingly, systemically injected cells may colonise bone fragments

implanted subcutaneously in mice, again illustrating a degree of organ tropism.

It was generally assumed that tumour cells need to extravasate before establishing a colony in the target organ, but experimental observations suggest that embolisation and intravascular growth can precede this step [12] (Figure 1.2) It is likely that a bolus of intravenously injected cells (particularly if they have been released from tissue culture flasks by enzymes) are more "coagulogenic" than cells trickled into the circulation from a long-established primary tumour, and these assays must be treated with caution. However, there is clinical evidence of intravascular and intralymphatic proliferation of some cancers, albeit usually at a late stage in the disease.

Following initial mechanical contact and transient adhesion mediated primarily by endothelial (E)-selectins and their ligands (sialyl glycoproteins) on tumour cells, multiple pathways are activated which involve cytokines, bioactive lipids, growth factors, etc., similar to processes involved in vascular damage or embolisation [13]. Adhesion of tumour cells to platelets and leukocytes via P- and L-selectins also assist embolisation and arrest in the microvasculature. Engagement of integrin signalling pathways ensures that the anti-apoptotic machinery is enabled and proteolytic and chemotactic activity are activated, and tumour cells can then extravasate and invade the tissue. Their subsequent survival depends upon the sum of positive and negative interactions between tumour and host, and it is now thought that regulation of growth of disseminated cells at secondary sites is a major determinant of metastatic frequency [14].

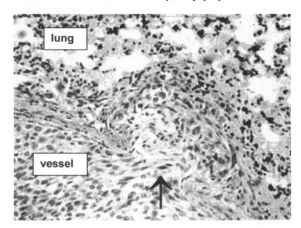

Figure 1.2. Histological section of experimental lung metastases of a human tumour xenograft. Note that a tumour colony has established intravascularly and also invaded across the vessel wall into the lung parenchyma (arrow)

Lymphatic Metastasis

The regional lymph nodes of primary tumours (especially carcinomas) are generally the first and most common site of metastasis and a major cause of morbidity. The number of involved nodes is a key prognostic factor for many cancers, and this has led to efforts to identify "sentinel" lymph nodes in order to improve predictions of cancer spread. Recently, specific lymphatic endothelial cell growth factors have been described (see section on Tumour Neoangiogenesis, below) the expression of which in some tumours correlates with nodal metastasis [15]. There is still debate as to whether patent lymphatic vessels exist *within* tumours, but the lymphangiogenic cytokines may stimulate proliferation of peritumoral vessels and thus aid lymphatic dissemination [16].

Lymphatic channels present less challenge to tumour cell entry than capillaries, since they have a scanty basement membrane (BM). Once in the lymphatics, tumour cells are carried to the subcapsular sinus of draining nodes, where they may arrest and grow, succumb to host defences, or leave the node via the efferent lymphatics (Figure 1.3). The propensity for a tumour cell to generate a lymphatic metastasis may depend upon its ability to adhere to reticular fibres in the subcapsular sinus. These fibres contain laminin, fibronectin and collagen IV, and different integrins expressed by different tumour cells may be responsible for adhesion to these structures and to the lymphatic endothelial cells [17]. Similarly, tumour cells may express CD44 variant adhesion molecules characteristic of recirculating lymphocytes, which may also contribute to lymph node tropism [18].

"Seed and Soil" and Organ Preference of Metastases

The organ distribution of metastases depends on the type and location of the primary tumour and many metastases occur in the first capillary bed or lymph node encountered. Sarcomas tend to metastasise to lungs because the venous drainage returns there; colon carcinoma cells enter the portal circulation, which delivers cells to the liver, and so on. However, a non-random element in metastatic patterns has long been recognised, with certain tumours tending to "favour" metastatic sites that are not explicable by circulatory anatomy (Table 1.1).

Experimental studies show that primary tumours are heterogeneous, and that cloned cells can vary in their ability to metastasise to different sites. It used to be thought that escape from the primary tumour and survival in the circulation were the major rate-limiting steps for successful metastasis. However, while there is a good deal of attrition at these stages in both experimental models and man, many tumour cells reach distant sites but may remain dormant, due either to lack of appropriate growth factors, their failure to induce neoangiogenesis [19] or control by host defences [20]. Interestingly, although few true metastasis-suppressor (as opposed to tumour-suppressor) genes have been described, two of these block proliferation of cells at secondary sites [21].

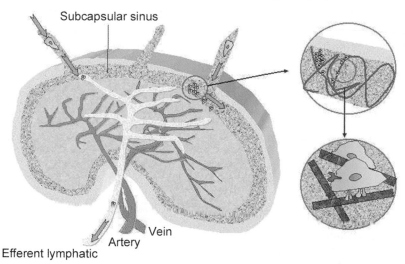

Figure 1.3. Routes of lymphatic metastasis. Cells gain access via the afferent lymphatic vessels and become localised in the subcapsular sinus. Adhesive interactions between integrins, CD44 and other molecules and the node medullary matrix assist tumour cell lodgement and establishment. Some cells leave via the efferent vessels

Table 1.1. "Seed and soil", examples of unusual sites of metastasis not explicable by circulatory anatomy

Primary tumour	Site of metastasis
Bronchial cancer	Adrenal (often bilateral)
Breast ductal carcinoma	Liver
Breast lobular carcinoma	Diffuse peritoneal seeding
Breast	Bone, ovary
Lung	Brain
Ocular melanoma	Liver
Prostate	Bone

Factors contributing to "organ preference" of metastasis are manifold (Table 1.2). First, differential adhesion of tumour cells to endothelial cells may be the first step in determining where tumour cells arrest. A very exciting initiative, the human vascular mapping project, using intravenously injected phage libraries, aims to identify the "zip codes" of different populations of endothelial cells, with a view to specifically targeting tumour neovasculature and other pathologies [22,23]. The selective adhesion of prostate cancer cells to bone marrow endothelium has been demonstrated [24], and this may also apply to other cancer types. When different labelled tumour cells are introduced into the arterial circulation, their tissue distribution patterns are distinct, but even greater variability in tumour outgrowth can be seen, suggesting that post-lodgement events are also rate-limiting. For example, tumour cells, which can modify their environment, may have an advantage, and cells expressing parathyroid hormone-related protein (PTHrP)—which activates osteoclast-mediated bone resorption—are especially able to colonise bone [25]. In addition, tumour cells that can take advantage of local growth factors (by expressing cognate receptors) will thrive in tissues in which these are abundant. Colon cancer cells that overexpress epidermal growth factor (EGFR) yield more metastases in the liver (a rich source of one of its major ligands, TGFα) than EGFR-negative cells [26]. Breast cancers overexpressing the related c-*erb*B receptors have increased risk of brain and visceral metastases [27], perhaps because these sites are rich in neuregulins, which bind directly to c-*erb*B-3 and B-4 and transactivate c-*erb*B-2.

Recently, it was found that breast tumour cells could mimic a process used in leukocyte trafficking. Chemokines are small proteins that interact with G protein-coupled receptors to mediate firm adhesion of leukocytes to endothelial cells, and to induce cytoskeletal alterations and motility. They act in concert with other cell surface proteins to direct the "homing" of

Table 1.2. Possible contributory factors to "organ selective" metastasis

ADHESION
    Interactions between tumour cells and vascular or lymphatic endothelia selectins/"addressins" zip codes
    Interactions between integrins/ BSP/osteopontin/ECM proteins/BM proteins (especially in tissues with fenestrated endothelium, e.g. liver, bone marrow)

CHEMOTAXIS
    Interactions between chemokine receptors on tumour cells and ligands in tissues
    Response to chemotactic gradients of motogenic ligands, e.g. HGF/c-met
    Response to chemotactic fragments released by proteases (e.g. laminin 5)

LOCAL GROWTH
    Interactions between tumour cell receptors and tissue growth factors
        EGFR/TGFα (e.g. liver)
        c-*erb*B receptors/HRGs (e.g. brain)
        c-met/HGF (e.g. liver)
        IGF1R/IGF, insulin (e.g. ovary)
        PDGFR/PDGF (e.g. lungs)

    "Modification" of local environment to potentiate favourable growth conditions
        PTHrP in bone
        Tissue damage/wounds (e.g. radiotherapy field, surgical anastomoses)

    Local inhibitory factors
        TIMPs (e.g. cartilage)
        a3 adenosine receptor antagonists (e.g. muscle)
        Immunological factors (spleen?)

BSP = bone sialo protein
TIMP = tissue inhibitor of metalloproteinase

haematopoietic cells to specific anatomical sites. High levels of CXCR4 (and CXCR7) receptor were found on malignant breast carcinoma cells recovered from metastases. In addition, the major CXCR4 and CXCR7 ligands (CXCL12 and CCL21) were preferentially expressed in lymph nodes, lungs, liver and bone marrow, the commonest sites of breast cancer metastasis [28]. Interestingly, CXCR4 is implicated in the homing of haematopoietic stem cells to marrow, and hence may be of particular significance to bone metastasis. Signalling through CXCR4 mediated pseudopodia formation, chemotaxis and invasion and was inhibited by CXCR4 blocking antibodies, as was lung colonisation and metastasis in xenografts.

These important observations indicate how a single ligand–receptor system could attract metastatic cells to specific sites and thence potentiate their invasion. It remains to be seen whether distinct chemokine receptor patterns can be defined for other cancers with different metastatic proclivities. In this regard the authors presented preliminary evidence that melanoma metastasis to skin may utilise the CCR10/CCL27 system, thought to represent a skin-specific homeostatic chemokine used by memory T cells. It is possible that antagonists of specific chemokine receptors could abort specific pathways of tumour cell dissemination, although this would need to be in a "chemoprevention" setting, since it would be unlikely to affect established metastases. Finally, we must consider the possible reasons for apparent resistance of certain tissues, such as cornea, cartilage and striated muscle to metastatic colonisation. The former contain several potent inhibitors of invasion and angiogenesis, e.g. tissue inhibitors of matrix metalloproteinase (TIMPs); in striated muscle the presence of natural antagonists to a3 adenosine (G protein associated) receptors has been implicated [29].

Genetic Determinants of Cancer Progression

It is evident that metastatic capacity may reflect both gain and loss of function, and indeed the search for "metastasis suppressor" genes has been more fruitful than identification of genes that specifically and reliably potentiate metastasis [30]. It is now possible, using laser capture microdissection and serial analysis of gene expression (SAGE) or proteomic techniques, to isolate invasive cancer cells and compare their gene or protein expression with non-invasive or normal cells from the same patient [31]. Prior to this, transfection of chromosomes or DNA from metastatic to non-metastatic cells (or vice versa), subtractive hybridisation/differential display PCR, cDNA array and other

strategies has resulted in identification of a handful of genes specifically linked to metastasis, although many others are also associated with cellular immortality, proliferation or developmental processes [30,32]. Examples of genes linked to suppression or potentiation of metastasis are shown in Table 1.3.

Tumour Progression, Heterogeneity and Clonal Dominance

Cancers generally arise from a single aberrant cell and their clonal origins have been demonstrated using genetic and biochemical markers. The progenitor cell may become transformed (perhaps by gene mutation or loss, or exposure to environmental carcinogens) and then proliferate to generate a clinically detectable tumour. Alternatively, many cells may undergo "initiation", but only one or a few "progress" to full malignancy. Certainly there are genetic traits in which individuals are at high risk of developing cancer in one or more organ systems, and in many instances this is due to functional loss of genes involved in regulation of cell division, repair of DNA damage or programmed cell death (apoptosis). In these individuals, certain tissues may be primed and require only a single further event to generate a tumour. In such cases, multiple primary tumours are not unusual.

Nowell, in his clonal evolution theory, proposed that the carcinogenic event induced "genetic lability", which permitted "stepwise selection of variant sublines". This model introduced the concept of progression from normal cells through pre-malignant lesions to fully malignant metastatic cancers (Figure 1.4). The cell population, as it expands, generates increasing heterogeneity from which subpopulations with relatively greater autonomy from host environmental controls will emerge by adaptation or selection. They may nevertheless retain the unique markers that identify their monoclonal origin. Recent work has begun to define the molecular genetic bases for some of these steps in tumours where pre-malignant lesions are identifiable and accessible, notably colorectal carcinoma, squamous cell carcinomas and, to a lesser extent, melanoma and breast carcinoma. It is clear that genes controlling tumour growth can be distinct from those controlling metastasis, since some tumours that are capable of indefinite growth fail to spread to distant organs (e.g. basal cell carcinoma) [33].

MICROENVIRONMENTAL INFLUENCES

Although tumour cells fail to respond appropriately to environmental cues, they are by no means fully

Table 1.3. Examples of genes linked to metastasis

Gene	Cancer type(s)	Reported role(s)in:
Putative metastasis suppressor genes		
nm23 H1 and H2	Breast (liver, ovary melanoma)	Cell migration?
Nucleoside diphosphate kinases		Signalling via G proteins microtubule assembly
PTEN	Prostate, glioma, breast	Migration, focal adhesions
KAI1/CD82	Prostate, stomach, colon, breast, pancreas, lung	Cell–cell adhesion, motility
E-cadherin	Many adenocarcinomas	Cell–cell adhesion, epithelial organisation
MKK4/SEK1	Prostate	Growth at secondary sites?
KiSS-1	Melanoma, breast	Downregulated MMP-9, growth at secondary sites?
DPC4	Colon, pancreas	?
BRMS1	Breast	Cell communication, motility
Genes linked to tumour progression		
c-erbB-2	Breast, ovary, stomach	Signal transduction with other type 1 RTK, cell proliferation, motility, drug resistance, angiogenesis
H-ras, K-ras	Sarcoma, colon	Cell cytoskeleton, deformability, invasion
c-fos/AP-1 transcription factor downstream of oncogenes	Sarcoma, squamous carcinoma	"Multigenic invasion programme"
MTA-1	Breast	Motility, regulation of gene expression?
rhoC	Melanoma	Migration
RHAMM	Breast, prostate	Motility
C-FABP	Breast, prostate	Angiogenesis?
Mts-1/S100A4/p9ka	Breast, colon	Binds calcium, associated with cytoskeleton, migration/motility
Osteopontin	Breast	Secreted phosphoprotein, binds calcium, interacts with integrins cellular adhesion and migration?

MKK4, mitogen-activated protein kinase kinase 4/stress activated protein/Erk kinase 1; RHAMM, receptor for hyaluronan-mediated motility; C-FABP, cutaneous fatty acid binding protein; S100A4, calvasculin.

autonomous and in some cases, the malignant phenotype can be apparently reversed, even in the face of major genetic abnormalities, by exposure to a "non-permissive" microenvironment. Such influences may contribute to the relative inefficiency of the metastatic process and some cases of dormancy.

Extracellular Matrix: Scaffolding and Repository of 'Growth' Factors

Normal tissue development, renewal and repair are regulated by a variety of factors providing both inhibitory and stimulatory messages. Ligand binding to cognate receptors transmits signals via a cascade of intracellular activation events that culminate in responses in the target cell, the most common of which is mitosis. However, the term "growth factor" is misleading, since pleiotropic responses are induced which affect differentiation status, cytoskeletal organisation, motility and other cellular functions. The transmembrane receptors therefore rather act as

relay stations through which, depending on intracellular and extracellular environmental conditions, a variety of different signals are transduced.

Further flexibility is provided by the fact that the same growth factor may produce different responses in different cell lineages, or in the same cell type at different stages of differentiation—again emphasising the importance of "context" in integrating cellular response decisions. For example, "scatter factor" is secreted by fibroblasts and induces epithelial cells to dissociate in culture; the cells also become dedifferentiated and more invasive. This molecule is identical to hepatocyte growth factor (HGF, a mitogen for liver cells) and induces diverse responses via a single receptor, c-met, in all cell types. HGF has been implicated in acquisition of an invasive phenotype in many types of carcinoma. Ligands may also evoke different responses, depending on the quantity available; fibroblasts respond to low concentrations of fibroblast growth factor 1 (FGF-1) by proliferation, and to high concentrations by movement towards it (chemotaxis).

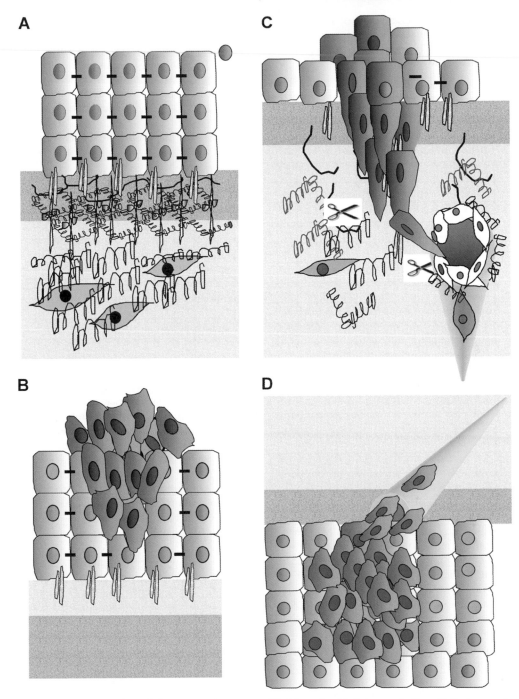

Figure 1.4. Simple representation of the metastatic process. (A) Normal epithelial organisation. Cells form cohesive sheets attached to each other by desmosomes, tight junctions, E-cadherin, etc., and to the underlying basement membrane (which separates them from the ECM) via integrins and other adhesion molecules. (B) Carcinoma *in situ*. A focus of abnormal cells has developed but has not breached the basement membrane. Neoangiogenesis may occur at this stage and assist the conversion to (C). Invasive cancer tumour cells have aberrant expression of adhesion molecules, increased motility and proteolytic activity. They can gain access to the ECM, blood capillaries and lymphatic channels. (D) Metastatic cancer. Cells that have survived in the circulation extravasate and form colonies in lymph node.

In the adult, growth and replacement of self-renewing tissues depends upon the proliferation of multipotent "stem" cells. These generate developmentally restricted progenitor cells whose progeny yield differentiated, fully functional, non-proliferative mature cells. This coordinated process must be closely regulated in order to maintain tissue integrity and function, and indeed it is the *imbalance* of proliferation and differentiation/cell death that is at the heart of malignant transformation. Many tumours secrete growth factors and/or overexpress their cognate receptors, and indeed oncogenes often encode these molecules or other components of the mitogenic signalling pathway. The potential of viruses to cause malignant transformation of cells in tissue culture and in animals is due to the integration of such oncogenes into their genomes.

Such observations led to the "autocrine" hypothesis of tumour development, i.e. the idea that a tumour cell survives because it is no longer dependent on exogenous growth factors. In the most extreme cases the receptor may be constitutively activated independently of ligand binding and hence constantly transmitting stimulatory signals to the cell. There is, however, compelling evidence that mutation or overexpression of growth factor receptors and/or their ligands not only provide a growth advantage for tumour cells but also stimulate neoangiogenesis, on which the continued expansion of the tumour mass depends, and potentiate invasion and dissemination.

Epidermal growth factor receptor (EGFR/c-*erb*B-1) and other oncogenic tyrosine kinases are overexpressed in many cancers and activation by autocrine or paracrine ligands triggers multiple downstream signalling cascades. These result in upregulation of angiogenic cytokines, specific MMPs and other genes involved in tumour progression [34]. c-*erb*B-2 is known to be involved in cell migration and angiogenesis [35]. So-called "platelet"-derived growth factors (PDGFs) promote angiogenic and desmoplastic responses in stromal cells and are reported to be pro-osteolytic [36], potentially contributing to bone metastasis. Antagonists such as monoclonal antibodies or kinase inhibitors may thus have both direct (antitumour) and indirect (antiangiogenic) effects [37–39].

Tumour Neoangiogenesis: a Necessary Prerequisite for Metastasis

Two themes replay again and again in invasion and metastasis and also in neoangiogenesis: (a) the binding of specific ligands to their receptors, followed by activation of pathways that affect cell proliferation, adhesion, migration and proteolysis; and (b) the importance of the balance of positive and negative signals. In each case, both tumour cells and host cells contribute to the eventual outcome. Neoangiogenesis in the adult is strictly controlled and most endothelial cells (except during wound healing and female reproductive processes) are quiescent. However, most tumours have the ability to induce their own blood supply, and there is now a growing appreciation of how this is linked to metastasis [40]. Nevertheless, some particularly aggressive tumours (e.g. melanomas) have been described which show "vasculogenic mimicry" and form channels capable of transporting blood without recruiting endothelial cells [41–43]. Also, the conventional notion that tumours induce neoangiogenesis from adjacent quiescent vessels has been challenged by the finding that at least a proportion of new vessels in certain types of tumours are derived from circulating bone marrow-derived precursor cells [44].

Tumours grown in avascular sites, such as cartilage, generally remain dormant and indeed this tissue has been found to contain a variety of angiogenesis inhibitors, some of which are now in clinical trial [45]. In tumours, the "angiogenic switch" [46] is triggered when the balance of positive signals outweighs the negative; this can be due to upregulation of the former, or downregulation of the latter, similar to the situation with proteolytic enzymes and their inhibitors (see below). The major angiogenic cytokines are the vascular endothelial growth factor (VEGF) family. VEGF-A binds to two tyrosine kinase receptors on endothelial cells, VEGFR-1 (Flt-1) and VEGFR-2 (Flk-1/KDR). VEGF-C and -D act as specific lymphangiogenic cytokines, since unlike VEGF-A they activate VEGFR-3 (Flt-4), which is preferentially expressed on lymphatic endothelial cells. In experimental xenograft tumours, transfection of VEGF-C and D genes has been shown to induce lymphangiogenesis and lymph node metastasis [47,48]. VEGFs, in addition to acting as potent survival factors, mitogens and chemotactic factors for endothelial cells, also enhance vessel permeability. Thus, activation of these signalling pathways may potentiate the opportunity for both vascular and lymphatic invasion and tumour spread.

One important regulatory pathway of VEGF-A expression is via hypoxia inducible factor 1 (HIF-1). The HIF-1α component of this heterodimeric transcription factor has a very short half-life when cells are well oxygenated, but is stabilised by hypoxia and hypoglycaemia, which are found in areas of tissue damage and are also common within growing tumours. VEGF can be produced by tumour cells and also host inflammatory cells (such as macrophages) and stromal cells. Interestingly, many genetic changes associated with malignant progression (mutation of H-ras, overexpression of c-erbB oncogenes, loss of p53) induce an angiogenic phenotype via upregulation of cytokines such as VEGF-A, bFGF and IL-8 [40,49], Induction of VEGF-A by oncogenes may be secondary to induction of HIF-1α, but activation of EGFR and other oncogenic signalling pathways can also upregulate VEGF-C, which is HIF-1-independent [50].

Fibroblast growth factors 1 and 2 (aFGF and bFGF) are further important angiogenic cytokines often upregulated in cancers [51], the latter particularly at the invasive edge, where tumour cells interact with host cells [52]. Although not specific endothelial cell mitogens, FGFs induce proteases in endothelial cells and their differentiation into capillary-like tubes in tissue cultures. Both FGFs and VEGFs are normally sequestered within the extracellular matrix, from which they are released by enzymes in tumour and/or host cells, an example of a cascade of events promoting several aspects of tumour progression. Finally, angiopoietins and ephrins play an important role in stabilising new vasculature, and again defects in their function and/or expression have been described in tumours [53]. Physiological negative regulators of angiogenesis include angiostatin and endostatin—paradoxically produced by tumour cells from proteolytic cleavage of plasminogen and collagen XVIII, respectively—and thrombospondin 1, which binds to CD36 on endothelial cells [6]. Other less specific inhibitors include TIMPs (tissue inhibitors of metalloproteinases), PEX (haemopexin-like domain of MMP-2), PAI-1 and interferon (IFN)α and β [40].

Cellular Mechanisms of Metastasis

Metastatic cells must be able to overcome regulatory processes which normally ensure maintenance of tissue structure and function and orderly cell proliferation. To recapitulate: events which contribute include changes in cell–cell and cell–matrix adhesion, alterations in cell shape, deformability and motility, induction of neovasculature, invasion of surrounding normal tissues, lymphatic or vascular channels, dissemination, survival of host defence mechanisms, extravasation and colonisation of secondary sites (see Figure 1.2).

Regulation of Tissue Structure and Function

Normal cellular organisation is regulated by positive and negative feedback loops, acting in concert to ensure that cell proliferation, differentiation and death (apoptosis) are strictly controlled in time and space. Genetic changes such as loss of suppressor genes, overexpression of growth factor receptors, production of autocrine ligands, etc., may lead to an imbalance in the cell "birth:death" ratios. However, this is insufficient for metastasis, and many experimental studies and clinical observations indicate that further genetic (and epigenetic) changes are required. These are perhaps harder to define than those involved in proliferation, since changes that enable cells to complete the entire metastatic process may be transient, or induced by the local microenvironment. For example, loss of adhesive interactions with neighbouring cells or stromal elements may favour cell detachment and release into the circulation, whereas ability to attach to platelets or endothelial cells may foster embolisation and extravasation. Similarly, an ability to survive (and thrive) in "ectopic" environments (which would drive a normal cell into apoptosis) may be aided by a variety of different mechanisms. One of the most important attributes of a metastatic cell may be the ability to adapt to changing environments (the primary site, the circulation, the secondary site) and this may be manifest in chameleon-like transient alterations in phenotype and even gene expression.

Homotypic Epithelial Adhesion Is Downregulated in Invasive Cells

Epithelial cells are normally polarised and firmly attached to each other via desmosomes, tight junctions and intercellular adhesion molecules and also bound to the basement membrane via integrins and other adhesion molecules. These allow cells to sense and respond to environmental cues using complex bidirectional signal transduction pathways. Several categories of cell–cell adhesion molecule (CAM) have been described, including intercellular adhesion molecules (ICAMs), selectins L, E and P (which bind carbohydrate moieties) and cadherins.

One of the most important molecules maintaining the integrity of epithelial structures is the calcium-dependent transmembrane glycoprotein E-cadherin [54]. Germline mutations in the E-cadherin gene are linked with predisposition to invasive gastric cancer, and in a transgenic mouse model of pancreatic oncogenesis, its loss is causally linked with malignant conversion. In many cases, the invasive ability of tumour cells is associated with a decrease in E-cadherin expression. In human squamous, gastric and hepatocellular carcinomas, E-cadherin expression is inversely correlated with the presence of lymph node metastases [55]. In some experimental studies, transfection of the E-cadherin gene to malignant cells resulted in loss of invasive potential and enhanced intercellular adhesion. However, invasive variants of MCF7 breast carcinoma continue to express high levels of E-cadherin, suggesting either that some function of the molecule was impaired, or alternatively that other "positive" invasion signals may override its influence in certain cell types [56].

The intracellular domains of cadherins associate with catenins and the actin cytoskeleton. The adenomatous polyposis coli (APC) gene (mutated in many inherited and sporadic colon cancers) normally regulates β-catenin expression and its interaction with E-cadherin. Mutations in APC (or β-catenin) increase cellular levels of the latter and facilitate interactions with transcription factors such as Tcf-Lef, which drive the expression of genes involved in inhibiting apoptosis and stimulating cell proliferation. Other genes commonly lost in cancers (e.g. DCC—deleted in colon carcinoma) also encode adhesion molecules. DCC is a member of the immunoglobulin superfamily, and another member, EMMPRIN, when expressed on cancer cell surfaces, is important in inducing collagenase expression in neighbouring host cells [57].

Although the mechanisms are not fully elucidated, circumstantial evidence in favour of an important regulatory role for E-cadherin and other adhesion molecules in tumour progression is compelling [58]. In developmental processes, migratory cells must first detach from their neighbours, and this involves changes in their adhesive status. The dynamic, orderly control of this process, when misregulated, can generate epithelial cells that have acquired properties more usually associated with mesenchymal cells, i.e. lack of polarisation, dedifferentiation and a motile, migratory phenotype—a process known as "epithelial–mesenchymal transition" (EMT).

Epithelial–Mesenchymal Transition (EMT) During Metastasis

The transient conversion of epithelial cells to a mesenchymal phenotype is a common event during embryonic development, but in the adult, epithelial cells normally only migrate during repair of tissue damage. In cancer progression, EMT involves dissociation of adherens junctions and desmosomes, accompanied by major cytoskeletal reorganisation involving rho family proteins. Several signalling pathways are implicated, with ras and TGFβ acting cooperatively and the transcription factors "slug" and "snail" playing a key role [59,60]. Specific phosphorylation sites in oncogenic c-erbB-2, which activate the Shc adapter protein, are associated with induction of EMT in epithelial cells via downregulation of E-cadherin, induction of motility and invasion [61]. Activation of other kinase receptors, such as c-met and EGFR, can also cause a similar phenotype. The mechanism is thought to involve phosphorylation of β-catenin, which releases E-cadherin, and induction of an E3-ubiquitin ligase (Hakai), which promotes its endocytosis [62]. In addition, in a rat bladder carcinoma model, EMT was induced by fibroblast growth factor FGF-1 (α-FGF) or by culturing the cells on collagen type 1 fibres; these and other observations indicate a key role for microenvironmental interactions [63]. Interestingly, an early response is the production of matrix metalloproteinases, illustrating how such a phenotypic shift could provide the range of abilities required for invasion by either embryonic or malignant cells.

The Importance of Mesenchymal–Epithelial Interactions and Cell Context

During organ development, many critical interactions between epithelia and mesenchyme occur. Mesenchymal factors are essential for growth and morphogenesis of epithelial cells in most tissue systems studied. The paracrine signals may be transmitted by three different modes: cell–cell contact, cell–matrix interactions or diffusion of soluble factors. Direct contact between epithelial and mesenchymal cells is important in the developing mammary gland and in the induction of new epithelia during kidney development. However, separation of the two cell types by filters has shown that mesenchymal induction of morphogenesis in other tissues (e.g. salivary gland) does not require direct contact.

Fibroblasts secrete a variety of ligands which interact in a paracrine (indirect) fashion with epithelial-specific receptors. In addition, several proteases can be produced by mesenchymal cells that bind to epithelial cells to mediate directed proteolysis, e.g. during capillary sprouting or ductal branching. Coordinated expression of matrix-degrading proteases and their inhibitors is also involved in involution of the mammary gland. Components of the extracellular matrix, such as collagens, can support branching of mammary epithelia, and soluble mediators such as HGF and a variety of growth factors also participate in morphogenesis. Many of these processes, albeit misregulated, also take place during invasion and metastasis. Malignant progression is not simply due to genetic abnormalities within the cancer genome, but also to aberrant interactions between the extracellular and intracellular microenvironment, the cell and the nucleus [64].

Changes in the Malignant Cell's Association with the Extracellular Matrix: the Multiple Functions of Integrins

Integrins are a family of heterodimeric proteins that mediate adhesion between cells and their surrounding matrices. Eighteen α- and eight β-subunits can combine to produce around 24 combinations of (generally non-exclusive) binding partners for most of the extracellular matrix (ECM) proteins, including laminin, fibronectin, collagen, etc. Far from being inert "glue", they are capable of transmitting important signals regulating cell survival, differentiation and migration [65]. These events are controlled by signals generated by ligand-occupied and clustered integrins activating pathways shared with many cell surface receptors. Integrins, however, uniquely provide an intersection where mechanical forces, cytoskeletal organisation and adhesion coincide [66].

Many differences in integrin expression between benign and malignant cells have been documented, but the patterns are complex. Both increases and decreases in abundance have been associated with invasion and/ or changes in the relative expression of different family members. In addition, their expression and binding affinity is influenced by the local microenvironment and soluble factors, enabling the tumour cell to respond to different conditions encountered throughout the metastatic cascade. Synthetic peptides containing sequences which compete with integrin binding to laminin (YIGSR) or fibronectin (RGD) can inhibit lung colonisation of intravenously injected cells in experimental models. Integrins may also mediate tissue-specific interactions, leading to selective tumour cell lodgement and growth. For example, the vitronectin receptor αvβ3 on breast carcinoma cells binds to bone sialoglycoprotein and potentiates cell migration, whereas adhesion and proliferation are mediated by αvβ5 [67]. Similarly, α3β1 can promote

adhesion and spreading of metastatic breast carcinoma cells on the lymph node stroma [68].

Integrins and their ligands are key collaborators with growth factors and, together with the cognate receptors and focal adhesion kinases, form active multimolecular complexes for signal transduction. α6β4 and α6β1 (laminin receptors), in addition to promoting survival via PI3 kinase, are mobilised by EGFR activation from hemidesmosomes to F-actin in lamellipodia and have been implicated in breast cancer progression [69]. Recently it was reported that certain integrins could directly phosphorylate tyrosine kinase growth factor receptors such as PDGF-R, c-met and VEGF-R via src. This process is ligand-independent, and results in different patterns of phosphorylation whose biological consequences are not yet clear [70]. Integrins such as αvβ3 and αvβ5 are also implicated in neoangiogenesis and are upregulated during endothelial cell migration. The former may be primarily involved in bFGF-induced angiogenesis and the latter in VEGF-induced angiogenesis. αvβ3 can also bind MMP-2 and potentiate proteolysis [71]. However, unligated integrins can induce apoptosis in endothelial cells, and soluble ligands can cause trans-dominant suppression of other integrins so, as with epithelial cells, their role is complex.

Dynamic Interactions during Cancer Cell Dissemination

Other adhesion molecules implicated in cancer progression include selectins such as sialyl Le^x and members of the immunoglobulin superfamily (ICAM-1, ICAM-2, VECAM and PECAM). The latter are upregulated on activated endothelial cells, and can interact with integrins on leukocytes and circulating tumour cells, assisting their arrest and extravasation [72]. Thrombospondin may mediate adhesion between circulating tumour cells, platelets and endothelial cells, promoting embolisation and arrest. Tumour cells gain access to the sub-endothelial basement membrane when endothelial cells retract in response to these emboli, and can then adhere to exposed proteins.

CD44 is another adhesion molecule utilised during lymphocyte "homing", and a change from the standard "epithelial" pattern to expression of splice variants associated with haematopoietic cells has been proposed to assist carcinoma cells in haematogenous dissemination. CD44 binds ECM components such as hyaluronic acid and the internal domain interacts with the cytoskeletal protein ankyrin and c-src, thus mediating cell migration. Specific isoforms of CD44 (e.g. v3, 8–10) may have an additional role in metastasis, since they are not only functionally coupled to rho GTPases, but also sequester heparin sulphate-binding growth factors such as bFGF and/or VEGF, which may potentiate tumour cell proliferation and angiogenesis. CD44 also co-associates with and potentiates activation of c-erbB-2 and MMP-9 on invadopodia [73].

Invasion

Epithelial cells are normally bounded by basement membrane (BM) which separates them from the underlying stroma and mesenchymal compartments. Breaching this barrier represents the transition from carcinoma in situ to invasive and potentially metastatic carcinoma. BM is composed of structural proteins, including collagen IV, laminin, entactin and also HSPGs. Interactions of tumour cells with BM have been considered to comprise three steps, which can readily be demonstrated in vitro: adhesion, matrix dissolution/proteolysis and migration [74]. The early steps in invasion may be very similar to those used by normal cells that "invade" or cross tissue boundaries, e.g. trophoblasts and activated lymphoid cells [75].

Reduced Dependence on Microenvironmental Pro-survival Signals

The first step in invasion (or, come to that, cell proliferation) involves cell detachment from the BM or extracellular matrix (ECM) and cells must overcome the loss of pro-survival signals normally provided by integrin signalling pathways, primarily through the PI3 kinase-Akt-GSK3β pathway. It is notable that many cancer cells, early in their evolution, develop means of activating this survival pathway independently, and of avoiding anoikis (apoptosis induced by disruption of cell–substrate connections). PTEN is a suppressor of PI3 kinase frequently lost in prostate carcinoma (including the early PIN stage) gliomas and other cancers [76].

Paweletz et al. [77], in an elegant longitudinal study using reverse phase protein microarrays in prostate carcinoma, found a sequential increase in phosphorylated Akt, phosphorylated (and hence inactivated) GSK3β and decreased apoptosis during progression from normal tissue (PIN)-invasive cancer. In parallel, levels of phosphorylated ERK (a key mediator of the ras-MAP kinase pathway) decreased. This example shows how coordinated regulation of different signalling pathways is required to evade apoptosis and promote mitosis—perhaps analogous for the need to both release the brake and apply the accelerator to move a car.

The cells in which these changes have taken place may also have an added advantage: PI3 kinase activation is associated not only with pro-survival signals but also with migration, one of the key components (together with increased proteolytic activity) of invasion. Again, these events are a caricature of normal processes. During development or wound healing, cell population expansion cannot occur without changes in adhesive interactions, (temporary) suspension of anoikis, and the ability of the daughter cells to move to their new position. The key difference in metastatic cells is that this process fails to "switch off" when it should.

Cell Motility, Migration and Chemotaxis

Motility, coupled with proteolysis, is the basis of tumour cell invasion, and is also important during intravasation and extravasation of blood and lymphatic vessels. Many motility factors have been described which may be tumour- or host-derived. Many "growth factors", such as transforming growth factor (TGFα), epidermal growth factor (EGF) and platelet-derived growth factor (PDGF), can induce chemotactic responses in tumour cells expressing the cognate receptors. "Scatter factor" (HGF) is a potent host-derived motogen, and tumour cells themselves secrete a variety of autocrine motility factors, including autotaxin and neuroleukin/phosphohexose isomerase. Autotaxin (NPP-2) is induced by bFGF and has also been implicated in several aspects of neoangiogenesis, such as endothelial differentiation into tubules and smooth muscle cell migration [78].

Cell migration is a highly organised and integrated process which requires the continuous assembly and disassembly of focal adhesions (to give "grip") coupled with a motor force—usually in response to a chemotactic gradient (to give directional motility). All of the components involved (including actin and its partners, signalling molecules, integrins, structural proteins, adaptor molecules, microtubules, etc.) must be coordinately regulated in both time and space (Figure 1.5). Understanding this complex interplay and piecing together the interdependent roles of all the key players is now a major research effort in both developmental biology and cancer [79]. C-src and members of the rho family of small GTPases are now recognised as

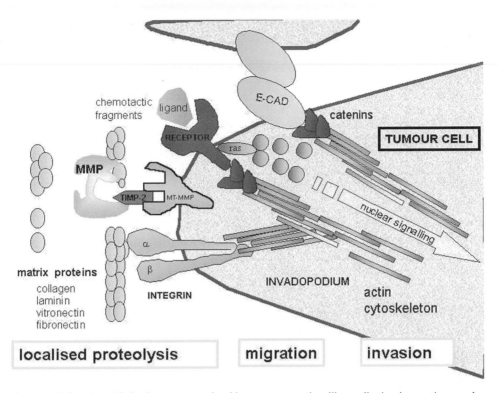

Figure 1.5. Integrated functional links between tyrosine kinase receptor signalling, adhesive interactions and proteolysis in tumour cell invasion, illustrated with reference to the c-*erb*B oncogene family (see text for mechanisms)

important regulators of cytokeletal organisation, cellular deformability and migration, linking both E-cadherin and integrin signalling pathways [80,81].

Enzyme Functions in Invasion and Metastasis

Invasive tumour cells show increased proteolytic activity due to upregulation of genes, enhanced activation of pro-enzymes or reduced expression of inhibitors. Tumour cells may also induce expression of enzymes by neighbouring host cells and "hijack" these to potentiate invasion. The major families of enzymes responsible for degrading the ECM are the matrix metalloproteinases (MMPs), adamalysin-related membrane proteinases, bone morphogenetic protein-1-type MMPs, serine proteases and also cysteine and aspartate proteases. Many clinical and experimental observations have correlated tumour invasion with enhanced degradative enzyme activity, although the relative contribution of different enzymes is complicated by the fact that proteolytic cascades involving co-activation of many enzymes is the norm. Proteolysis

of the ECM is again a physiological process that occurs during development, tissue repair/remodelling and angiogenesis, and it is imbalances in the system which potentiate pathological invasion.

Matrix Metalloproteinases

One of the most important groups of enzymes associated with invasion and angiogenesis are the matrix metalloproteinases. Different cancers may show different patterns of expression, e.g. squamous carcinomas frequently have high levels of MMP-9 (gelatinase B), MMP-3, MMP-10 and MMP-11 (stromelysins) and MMP-7 (matrilysin) [82]. Breast adenocarcinomas may have increased levels of MMP-2 (gelatinase A) and colon carcinomas commonly overexpress MMP-7. Metastatic prostate carcinomas overexpress MMP-11 and effectively degrade bone stroma-derived ECM. MMPs play a key role in bone metastasis from both breast and prostate cancers [83,84]. The prime substrate of the gelatinases is collagen IV, a major component of BM, whereas the stromelysins prefer laminin, fibronectin and proteoglycans, and can also activate pro-collagenase, (MMP-1), which in turn degrades the fibrillar collagens of the interstitial tissues. In addition, MT1-MMP, which activates MMP-2, is often upregulated in tumour and/or neighbouring host tissues. The overall balance between tumour- and host-derived MMPs and their natural inhibitors (TIMPs) determines the net proteolytic balance within a tumour, particularly at the invasive edge.

MMPs also contribute to tumour growth and metastasis by other means [85,86]. During angiogenesis, "invasion" of capillary sprouts requires local proteolysis (mediated in part by upregulated MMP-2 and MMP-9, together with uPA) and in addition MMP-9 has been implicated in the "angiogenic switch" by releasing VEGF from sequestration in the extracellular matrix [46]. MT1-MMP upregulates expression of VEGF, even in cells not expressing MMP-2, suggesting that this is independent of MMP-2 activation [87]. MMP-3 can cleave E-cadherin, and MMP-2 releases chemotactic fragments from laminin 5, contributing to reduced cell–cell adhesion and potentiation of migration (Table 1.4).

Cleavage of chemokines by diverse MMPs may influence the tissue distribution of metastasis [88]. Proteolytic release of tissue-specific growth factors may also play a role in organ selectivity of metastasis. For example, colorectal carcinoma cells overexpressing EGFR have a predilection for growth in the liver, where there are high concentrations of its ligands. All of these require proteolytic cleavage for activation, and this may be potentiated by the upregulation of certain MMPs by signalling via activated EGFR [89]. Furthermore, these proteases can contribute to the sustained growth of tumours in secondary sites by the ectodomain cleavage of membrane-bound pro-forms of growth factors, and the release of mitogenic peptides. TIMPs have multiple functions and in some cases potentiate cell proliferation and angiogenesis. TIMP-2 cooperates with MT1-MMP to activate MMP-2, so these molecules should more properly be considered regulators rather than simple inhibitors of MMP function [90].

Serine Proteases

Urokinase and tissue-type plasminogen activators (uPA and tPA) activate the zymogen plasminogen into its active form, plasmin. uPA is secreted in a latent pro-form that binds to a GPI-linked receptor uPAR, where it initiates a proteinase cascade that assists breakdown of the ECM and potentiates tumour and

Table 4. Functions of major enzymes implicated in invasion, angiogenesis and metastasis

Enzyme	Examples of substrates	Role in
Interstitial collagenase MMPs 1 and 13	Type I, II, III and VII collagens, perlecan	Stromal breakdown Release of bFGF, IGF, TNFα (1)
Stromelysins MMPs 3, 10 and 11	Type I, III, IV, V, IX collagens, laminin, fibronectin, gelatin, proteoglycans (perlecan, decorin)	Release of E-cadherin (3) Release of FGF (3) Release of TGFβ (3)
Gelatinases MMPs 2 and 9	Mainly Type IV collagen, fibronectin, fibrinogen laminin 5	Basement membrane breakdown, angiogenesis Release of VEGF, TGFβ Release of chemotactic fragments
Matrilysin MMP-7	Collagens III, IV, V, IX–XI HSPGs, laminin, fibronectin, decorin	Release of FasL Release of TGFβ
Metalloelastase MMP-12	Plasminogen and collagen XVIII	Generation of angiostatin and endostatin
MT MMPs MMPs 14,15,16,17, 24, 25	Gelatin, fibronectin, vitronectin, collagens, aggrecan	Activation of MMP-2 Upregulates VEGF Release of E-cadherin and CD44
ADAMs		Release of ligands and receptors
Serine proteases uPA, tPA, thrombin, plasmin	Plasminogen Pro MMP1, 7 and 9	Activation of MMPs Coagulation cascades
Cathepsins B, H, L, K (cysteine protease)	Collagen IV and laminin (B) tpA-plasminogen complex	Activation of MMPs (B) Activation of uPA (B)
Cathepsin D (aspartyl protease)		Binding annexin (B)
Heparanases	HSPG side chains	Release of angiogenic and tumorigenic cytokines Breakdown of PG scaffold

endothelial cell migration, partially by activation of MMPs including 1, 7 and 9 [91]. uPA and uPAR are frequently upregulated in cancer cells and/or stromal cells, and are independent prognostic indicators in several cancers [92]. Inhibition of uPA or uPAR can reduce tumour cell invasion *in vitro* and lung colonisation *in vivo*, and conversely transfection of uPA into cells potentiates these activities.

Plasminogen activator inhibitor type 1 (PAI-1) is the main natural antagonist of uPA and tPA. It regulates not only their proteolytic activity but also their level of receptor binding by promoting endocytosis of the trimolecular complex of uPA/uPAR/PAI-1. Again (similar to observations with TIMPs) there is an apparently paradoxical association between high levels of PAI-1 and poor prognosis in several cancers [93]. The reasons for these observations are not entirely clear. However, recent elegant experiments testing angiogenesis in tissues from mice deficient in one or more components of the PA system clearly showed that PAI-1 was critical for controlling plasmin-mediated proteolysis and microvessel formation. In addition, PAI-1 promoted angiogenesis at physiological concentrations, but was anti-angiogenic at higher concentrations [94]. These observations again show us that control of angiogenesis and metastasis is a complex balance of molecular messages [95]. Labelling entities "inhibitors" or "activators" may underestimate their full potential and the complexity of designing therapeutic intervention strategies.

Cysteine and Aspartyl Proteases

Other enzymes implicated in metastasis include the lysosomal cysteine proteinases (cathepsins B, H, L and K), some of which are released extracellularly. It has been suggested that exocytosis of cathepsin B may be regulated by the ras pathway [96]. Cathepsins B, H and L have been shown to participate in processes of tumour growth, vascularisation, invasion and metastasis. Their levels in tumour extracts can provide useful clinical information in breast, lung, colorectal, brain, and head and neck cancer patients. As with the MMPs, there is much debate as to whether tumour or host enzymes are the major contributors, and in colon cancer, cathepsin B was mainly expressed by macrophages at the invasive edge [97]. The aspartyl protease cathepsin D has been linked with poor prognosis in breast cancer [98]. Recently it was shown that serum levels of both cysteine cathepsins and their endogenous protein inhibitors (stefins and cystatin C) could also predict prognosis. In melanoma and colorectal cancer

patients, high serum levels of cathepsins B and H correlated with shorter survival [99].

Various cathepsins transfected into tumour cells or fibroblasts increase tumorigenicity and/or invasion, but studies with inhibitors have shown confusing results. In some systems tumour cell growth was inhibited, in others cell motility or invasion. Recently, van Noorden et al. [100] found that an inhibitor slowed the appearance of human pancreatic cancer xenografts, but once established the tumours grew at similar rates to controls. In other systems, spontaneous metastasis but not lung colonisation was inhibited. Many studies seem to show effects on growth and contact inhibition, rather than tumour cell extravasation. The mechanisms are not clear, but could relate to release of sequestered growth factors. Cathepsin B has been shown to affect cell motility, ECM breakdown, activation of other proteases (including uPA and MMPs) and degradation of TIMPs 1 and 2 [101]. Since cathepsin B has been detected in capillaries near the invading edge of gliomas and prostate carcinomas, and in activated endothelial cells *in vitro*, it may also contribute to angiogenesis [102].

Apart from a straightforward proteolytic/degradative function, it has been proposed that cathepsin B may be associated with the annexin II heterotetramer (AIIt) on the cell surface, providing a "proteolytic centre" for binding of tPA and plasmin for localised proteolysis and migration on ECM proteins [103]. Cathepsins can also bind to mannose 6-phosphate receptors on the cell surface, and may also displace IGFII from the IGFIIR to the IGFIR, with consequent changes in downstream signalling. Most studies indicate that the cathepsins play a role in *early* stages of tumour development. It seems that at later stages their role can be subsumed by other proteases, and they are then no longer critical for tumour progression.

Several cathepsins have been implicated in the process of osteolysis. Cathepsin D expression in breast cancer correlated with the presence of bone metastases but not lymph node metastases; however, this did not translate into prognostic information regarding survival [104]. When biopsies of aggressive bone metastases were assayed for proteinase activity, MMP-9 and cathepsins B and L were overexpressed [105]. In human oral squamous carcinoma xenografts with different patterns of invasion and metastasis, high levels of active MMP-2 were found in cells giving nodal metastases, and high cathepsin L in those that invaded the muscle and mandibular bone [106]. This observation was supported by a study in which 6/6 metastatic bone tumours (but only 3/6 primary bone tumours) were found to express cathepsin L [107]. The osteoclast-associated cathepsin K is expressed in bone-invading breast carcinoma cells, and in experimental studies antisense oligonucleotides inhibited bone resorption [108]. In addition, a specific inhibitor of cathepsin L prevented bone pit formation by activated osteoclasts *in vitro*, and reduced bone metastasis of A375 melanoma cells in mice [109]. These new findings offer the possibility of novel drugs specifically designed to combat proteolytic processes associated with bone metastasis.

Heparanases

Apart from structural proteins, the other major components of the BM and ECM are glycosaminoglycans, predominantly heparan sulphate proteoglycan (HSPG). HSPGs also coat cell surfaces, where they act as molecular sponges by binding and regulating numerous bioactive molecules [110]. Heparanases degrade the HS side chains of HSPGs and, like the proteases described above, not only assist in breakdown of ECM and BM, but also regulate growth factor and cytokine activity. Basic fibroblast growth factor (bFGF), and other heparin-binding growth factors are sequestered by HS, providing a localised depot available for release by heparanase. Similarly,

uPA and tPA can be released from HS, by heparanase, further potentiating proteolytic and mitogenic cascades. Recently, the gene encoding heparanase 1 has been cloned and shown to enhance metastasis when transfected into experimental tumour cell lines. Heparins and structurally similar polysaccharides can inhibit invasion and angiogenesis via multiple mechanisms [111–113].

Integrated Circuits and Microenvironmental Influences in Metastasis

An emerging theme in cancer cell biology, long appreciated in developmental biology, is the recognition that no cell (or molecule) is an island, and the old idea that cancer cells are autonomous entities which have dropped the shackles of social restraints to grow and spread at will within the body is far too simplistic. It is becoming clear that the cancer cell not only influences, but also is influenced by, the host microenvironment. At the molecular level, signals are less like linear "pathways" than integrated circuits, and it is now clear that multimolecular assemblies and reciprocal linkages regulate many key cellular processes in metastasis and angiogenesis [40,114,115].

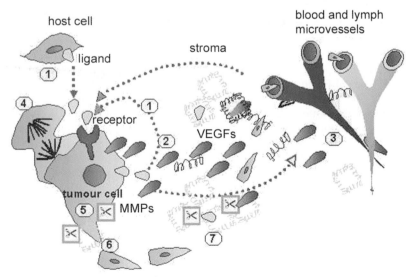

Figure 1.6. Some putative positive feedback loops in metastasis induced by a c-*erb*B receptor activation: (1) Autocrine or paracrine ligands activate receptors by either direct binding or trans-phosphorylation. (2) EGFR (and c-*erb*B-2) activation leads to enhanced production of VEGF-A and VEGF-C. (3) Capillary and lymphatic endothelial cells respond to VEGFs (<cell proliferation, migration, permeability). (4) Tumour growth and dissemination are potentiated by development of new vessels. (5) EGFR activation leads to upregulation of specific MMPs (predominantly MMP-9; also MMP-3 and MMP-7). (6) MMPs activate proteolytic cascade and potentiate tumour cell invasion through stroma and basement membranes, and also capillary sprouting. (7) MMPs release matrix-sequestered growth factors and process ligands, enhancing their availability to induce tumour and endothelial cell proliferation. Other oncogenic tyrosine kinases may also activate these pathways

Examples have been given above of cross-talk between receptor tyrosine kinases and the molecular machinery mediating motility, migration and invasion (Figure 1.6). Adhesion molecules respond to the environment and transmit signals between cells and from the cell surface to the nucleus. Enzymes are regulated at multiple levels, and influence both tumour cell and host cell behaviour; their interactions are key at the invading edge and in neoangiogenesis.

Connecting these notions is the demonstration that gene expression, even in malignant cells, is highly responsive to external cues [116]. Although the reductionist approach has been critically important in identifying individual genes or cellular traits which are linked to metastasis, the theme for the next decade will surely be the building of these isolated observations into an integrated and better understanding of the metastatic process.

THE FUTURE FOR METASTASIS THERAPY

"Do any of the current anti-cancer drugs in clinical use show any selectivity for metastatic cells?" Freije et al. used cells with low nm23 (which in several tumour types is associated with the metastatic phenotype) and tested a wide variety of drugs using the COMPARE computer algorithm. The outcome was that none of the standard cytotoxic agents showed any selectivity for these cells [117]. Nevertheless, they identified 40 new agents in the NCI repository of 30 000 compounds with the desired selectivity for metastatic cells, suggesting that such a strategy is viable. More effective therapeutics will emerge from a better understanding of the key differences between normal cells and metastatic cancer cells—cell proliferation (the original target for chemotherapeutic agents) does not give us that differential. Since tumour progression involves further genetic changes, an appreciation of the pathways that are misregulated in metastases will provide more opportunities for effectively targeting disseminated disease. For example, it is clear that the c-*erb*B oncogenes are overexpressed in cancers with high metastatic potential, and data show that their activation upregulates many components of the metastatic phenotype, including cell motility, invasion, protease production and angiogenesis. In addition, such cells are more likely to be refractory to conventional therapy. These observations not only explain some of

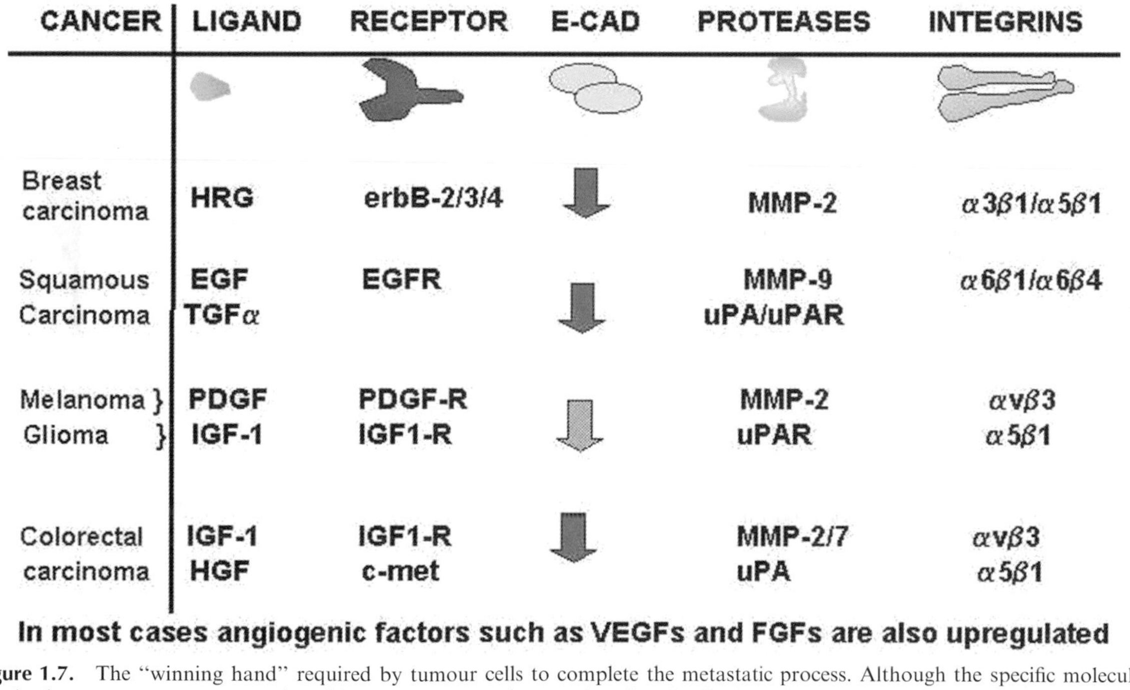

CANCER	LIGAND	RECEPTOR	E-CAD	PROTEASES	INTEGRINS
Breast carcinoma	HRG	erbB-2/3/4	⬇	MMP-2	$\alpha3\beta1/\alpha5\beta1$
Squamous Carcinoma	EGF TGFα	EGFR	⬇	MMP-9 uPA/uPAR	$\alpha6\beta1/\alpha6\beta4$
Melanoma } Glioma }	PDGF IGF-1	PDGF-R IGF1-R	⬇	MMP-2 uPAR	$\alpha v\beta3$ $\alpha5\beta1$
Colorectal carcinoma	IGF-1 HGF	IGF1-R c-met	⬇	MMP-2/7 uPA	$\alpha v\beta3$ $\alpha5\beta1$

In most cases angiogenic factors such as VEGFs and FGFs are also upregulated

Figure 1.7. The "winning hand" required by tumour cells to complete the metastatic process. Although the specific molecules involved may vary, most metastatic solid tumours show a decrease in cell–cell adhesion, changes in cell–substrate adhesion and an increase in proteolytic and angiogenic activity. These diverse processes may be coordinately regulated by oncogenic signalling pathways. HRG, heregulin; FGF (R), epidermal growth factor (receptor); TGFα, transforming growth factor alpha; IGF-1-(R), insulin-like growth factor 1 (receptor); PDGF(R), platelet-derived growth factor (receptor); MMP, matrix metalloproteinase, uPA (R), urokinase plasminogen activator (receptor); E-CAD, E (epithelial) cadherin

the failures of current drugs but also provide new, validated, molecular targets for intervention.

SUMMARY

The detection and treatment of micrometastatic disease remains a major challenge in oncology. With a greater understanding of the molecular mechanisms of metastasis, it is hoped that novel therapeutic strategies will emerge. Techniques enabling us to study populations of invasive or metastatic cells in comparison with primary tumours or normal cells from the same individual are revolutionising our understanding of tumour progression. Genomic and proteomic "fingerprints" of tumours, or indeed body fluids [118], may soon enable us to predict the likely probability (and possibly organ preference) of metastasis. Suspect genes identified in these profiles could be individually (or combinatorially) switched on or off in cells to validate their functions and survey the phenotypic changes they invoke [52]. Unravelling the complexity of oncogenic signalling pathways (and, more importantly, the ways in which these interact) is enabling us better to define key points for intervention with novel inhibitors [119–121]. Once a key target is validated, technical advances in screening, drug design and robust pre-clinical metastasis models are needed to turn this basic knowledge into improved survival statistics.

Metastasis requires a multigenic programme of coordinated gene expression, and different cancers may utilise different "winning hands" to succeed (Figure 1.7). Fortunately, evidence suggests that inhibiting single, pivotal points may be sufficient to subvert the process. However, it must be remembered that, since many cancers have already disseminated at presentation, interventions need to be focused primarily on control of existing micrometastases. There is much still to be discovered about the critical determinants of cancer dissemination in general and bone metastasis in particular, a common and debilitating problem in oncology. Nevertheless, our rate of progress is accelerating and there is reason for optimism.

REFERENCES

1. Urteaga O, Pack GT. The antiquity of melanoma. Cancer 1966; 19: 607–10.
2. Brothwell D. The evidence for neoplasms. In Brothwell D, Sandison AT (eds), Diseases in Antiquity. CC Thomas: Springfield, IL, 1967; 320–45.
3. Triollo VA. Nineteenth century foundations of cancer research: advances in tumor pathology, nomenclature, and theories of oncogenesis. Cancer Res 1965; 25: 75–106.
4. Onuigbo WIB. The paradox of Virchow's views on cancer metastasis. Bull Hist Med 1962; 36: 444–9.
5. Paget S. The distribution of secondary growths in cancer of the breast. Lancet 1889; 1: 9–11.
6. Hanahan D, Weinberg RA. The hallmarks of cancer. Cell 2000; 100: 57–70.
7. Yokota J. Tumor progression and metastasis. Carcinogenesis 2000; 21: 497–503.
8. Van der Pluijm G, Lowik C, Papapoulos S. Tumour progression and angiogenesis in bone metastasis from breast cancer: new approaches to an old problem. Cancer Treatment Rev 2000; 26: 11–27.
9. Bostick P et al. Limitations of specific reverse-transcriptase polymerase chain reaction markers in the detection of metastases in the lymph nodes and blood of cancer patients. J Clin Oncol 1998; 16: 2632–40.
10. Pantel K, Schlimok G, Braun S et al. Differential expression of proliferation-associated molecules in individual micrometastatic carcinoma cells. J Natl Cancer Inst 1993; 85: 1419–23.
11. Fujimaki T, Ellis LM, Bucana CD et al. Simultaneous radiolabel, genetic tagging and proliferation assays to study the organ distribution and fate of metastatic cells. Int J Oncol 1993; 2: 895–901.
12. Al Mehdi AB, Tozawa K, Fisher AB et al. Intravascular origin of metastasis from the proliferation of endothelium-attached tumor cells: a new model for metastasis. Nature Med 2000; 6: 100–2.
13. Orr WF, Wang HH, Lafrenie RM et al. Interactions between cancer cells and the endothelium in metastasis. J Pathol 2000; 190: 310–29.
14. Chambers AF, Naumov GN, Varghese HJ et al. Critical steps in haematogenous metastasis: an overview. Surg Oncol N Am 2001; 10: 243–55.
15. Schoppmann SF, Horvat R, Birner P. Lymphatic vessels and lymphangiogenesis in female cancer: mechanisms, clinical impact and possible implications for anti-lymphangiogenic therapies. Oncol Rep 2002; 9: 455–60.
16. Eccles SA. Cell biology of lymphatic metastasis: the potential role of c-erbB signalling. Recent Results Cancer Res 2000; 157: 41–54.
17. Brodt P. Adhesion mechanisms in lymphatic metastasis. Cancer Metast Rev 1991; 10: 23–32.
18. Kainz C et al. Immunohistochemical detection of adhesion molecule CD44 splice variants in lymph node metastases of cervical cancer. Int J Cancer 1996; 69: 170–3.
19. Holmgren L, O'Reilly MS, Folkman J. Dormancy of micrometastases: balanced proliferation and apoptosis in the presence of angiogenesis suppression. Nature Med 1995; 1: 149–53.
20. Eccles SA. Dormancy in experimental solid tumour systems. In Stewart T, Wheelock F. (eds), Cellular Immune Mechanisms and Tumor Dormancy. CRC Press: Boca Raton, FL, 1992: 27–51.
21. Welch DR, Steeg PS, Rinker-Schaeffer CW. Molecular biology of breast cancer metastasis: genetic regulation of human breast carcinoma metastasis. Breast Cancer Res 2000; 2: 408–16.
22. Arap W, Kolonin MG, Trepel M et al. Steps towards mapping the human vasculature by phage display. Nature Med 2002; 8: 121–7.

23. Kolonin M, Pasqualini R, Arap W. Molecular addresses in blood vessels as targets for therapy. Curr Opin Chem Biol 2001; 5: 308–13.

24. Cooper CR, McLean L, Walsh M et al. Preferential adhesion of prostate cancer cells to bone marrow endothelial cells as compared to extracellular matrix components in vitro. Clin Cancer Res 2000; 6: 4839–47.

25. Iguchi H, Tanaka S, Ozawa Y et al. An experimental model of bone metastasis by human lung cancer cells: the role of parathyroid hormone-related protein in bone metastasis. Cancer Res 1996; 56: 4040–3.

26. Radinsky R. Paracrine growth regulation of human colon carcinoma organ-specific metastasis. Cancer Metast Rev 1993; 8: 3037–42.

27. Kallioniemi OP, Holli K, Visakorpi T et al. Association of c-erbB-2 protein overexpression with high rate of cell proliferation, increased risk of visceral metastasis and poor long-term survival in breast cancer. Int J Cancer 1991; 49: 650–5.

28. Muller A, Homey B, Soto H et al. Involvement of chemokine receptors in breast cancer metastasis. Nature 2001; 410: 50–6.

29. Bar-Yehuda S, Barer F, Volfsson L, Fishman P. Resistance of muscle to tumor metastases: a role for a3 adenosine receptor antagonists. Neoplasia 2001; 3: 125–31.

30. Yoshida B, Solokoff MM, Welch DR, Rinker-Schaeffer CW. Metastasis-suppressor genes: a review and perspective on an emerging field. J Natl Cancer Inst 2000; 92: 1717–30.

31. Simone NL, Paweletz CP, Charboneau L et al. Laser capture microdissection: beyond functional genomics to proteomics. Mol Diagn 2000; 5: 301–7.

32. Fidler IJ, Radinsky R. Search for genes that suppress metastasis. J Natl Cancer Inst 1996; 88: 1700–3.

33. Welch DR, Rinker-Schaeffer CW. What defines a useful marker of metastasis in human cancer? J Natl Cancer Inst 1999; 91: 1351–3.

34. O-charoenrat P, Rhys-Evans PH, Archer DJ, Eccles SA. c-erbB receptors in squamous cell carcinomas of the head and neck: clinical significance and correlation with matrix metalloproteinases and vascular endothelial growth factors. Oral Oncol 2002; 38: 73–80.

35. Eccles SA. The role of c-erbB2/HER2/neu in breast cancer progression and metastasis. J Mamm Gland Biol Neoplasia 2001; 6: 393–406.

36. Yi B, Williams PJ, Niewolna M et al. Tumor-derived platelet-derived growth factor BB plays a critical role in osteosclerotic bone metastasis in an animal model of human breast cancer. Cancer Res 2002, 62: 917–23.

37. Eccles S. c-erbB-2 as a target for immunotherapy. Exp Opin Invest Drugs 1998; 7: 1879–96.

38. Izumi Y, Xu L, di Tomasso E et al. Tumour biology: herceptin acts as an antiangiogenic agent. Nature 2002; 416: 279–80.

39. Shawver L, Slamon D, Ulrich A. Smart drugs: tyrosine kinase inhibitors in cancer therapy. Cancer Cell 2002; 1: 117–23.

40. Fidler IJ. Angiogenesis and cancer metastasis. Cancer J Sci Am 2000; 6: S134–41.

41. Maniotis AJ, Folberg R, Hess A et al. Vascular channel formation by human melanoma cells in vivo and in vitro: vasculogenic mimicry. Am J Pathol 1999; 155: 739–52.

42. Sood AK, Fletcher MS, Hendrix MJ. The embryonic-like properties of aggressive tumour cells (1). J Soc Gynaecol Invest 2002; 9: 2–9.

43. Bissell MJ. Tumor plasticity allows vasculogenic mimicry, a novel form of angiogenic switch. A rose by any other name? Am J Pathol 1999; 155: 675–9.

44. Lyden D, Hattori K, Dias S et al. Impaired recruitment of bone-marrow-derived endothelial and haematopoietic precursor cells blocks tumour angiogenesis and growth. Nature Med 2001; 7: 1194–201.

45. Falardeau P, Champagne P, Poyet P et al. Neovastat, a naturally occurring multifunctional antiangiogenic drug, in Phase III clinical trials. Semin Oncol 2001; 28: 620–5.

46. Bergers G, Brekken R, McMahon G et al. Matrix metalloproteinase-9 triggers the angiogenic switch during carcinogenesis. Nature Med Biol 2000; 2: 737–44.

47. Mirjami MT, Ruohola JK, Karpanen T et al. VEGF-C induced lymphangiogenesis is associated with lymph node metastasis in orthotopic MCF-7 tumours. Int J Cancer 2002; 98: 946–51.

48. Stacker S, Caesar C, Baldwin ME et al. VEGF-D promotes the metastatic spread of tumor cells via lymphatics. Nature Med 2001; 7: 186–91.

49. Semenza GL. HIF-1 and tumor progression: pathophysiology and therapeutics. Trends Molec Med 2002; 8(suppl): S62–7.

50. O-charoenrat P, Rhys-Evans P, Modjtahedi H, Eccles SA. Vascular endothelial growth factor family members are differentially regulated by c-erbB signaling in head and neck squamous carcinoma cells. Clin Exp Metast 2000; 18: 155–61.

51. Christofori G. The role of fibroblast growth factors in tumour progression and angiogenesis. In Bicknell R et al. (eds), Tumour Angiogenesis. Oxford University Press: Oxford, 1997; 201–37.

52. Fidler IJ. Critical determinants of cancer metastasis: rationale for therapy. Cancer Chemother Pharmacol 1999; 43(suppl): S3–10.

53. Yancopoulos GD, Davis S, Gale NW et al. Vascular specific growth factors and blood vessel formation. Nature 2000; 407: 242–8.

54. Jiang W. E-cadherin and its associated protein catenins, cancer invasion and metastasis. Br J Surg 1996; 83: 437–46.

55. Christofori G, Semb H. The role of the cell adhesion molecule E-cadherin as a tumour-suppressor gene. Trends Biochem Sci 1999; 24: 73–6.

56. Van Roy F, Mareel M. Tumour invasion: effects of cell adhesion and motility.Trends Cell Biol 1992; 2: 263–9.

57. Biswas C et al. The human tumour cell-derived collagenase stimulating factor (renamed EMMPRIN) is a member of the immunoglobulin superfamily. Cancer Res 1995; 55: 434–9.

58. Pignatelli M. Integrins, cadherins, and catenins: molecular cross-talk in cancer cells. J Pathol 1998; 186: 1–2.

59. Janda E, Lehman K, Killisch I et al. Ras and TGFβ cooperatively regulate epithelial cell plasticity and metastasis: dissection of Ras signalling pathways. J Cell Biol 2002; 156: 299–313.

60. Savagner P. Leaving the neighbourhood: molecular mechanisms involved during epithelial–mesenchymal transition. Bioessays 2001; 23: 912–23.

61. Khoury H, Dankort DL, Sadekova S et al. Distinct tyrosine autophosphorylation sites mediate induction of

epithelial–mesenchymal like transition by an activated ErbB-2/Neu receptor. Oncogene 2001; 20: 788–99.

62. Pece S, Gutkind JS. E-cadherin and Hakai: signalling, remodelling or destruction? Nature Cell Biol 2002; 4: E72–4.

63. Petersen OW, Lind Neilsen H, Gudjonnnson T et al. The plasticity of human breast carcinomas is more than epithelial to mesenchymal conversion. Breast Cancer Res 2001; 3: 213–17.

64. Radisky D, Muschler J, Bissell MJ. Order and disorder: the role of the extracellular matrix in epithelial cancer. Cancer Invest 2002; 20: 139–53.

65. Berman AE, Kozlova NI. Integrins: structure and function. Membr Cell Biol 2000; 13: 207–44.

66. Schwartz MA, Ginsberg MH. Networks and crosstalk: integrin signalling spreads. Nature Cell Biol 2002; 4: E65–8.

67. Sung V, Stubbs JT III, Fisher I et al. Bone sialoprotein supports breast cancer cell adhesion proliferation and migration through differential usage of the α(v), β3 and α(v) β5 integrins. J Cell Physiol 1998; 176: 482–94.

68. Tawil NJ et al. Integrin α3β1 can promote adhesion and spreading of metastatic breast carcinoma cells on the lymph node stroma. Int J Cancer 1996; 66: 703–10.

69. Mercurio AM, Bachelder RE, Chung J et al. Integrin laminin receptors and breast carcinoma progression. J Mamm Gland Biol Neoplasia 2001; 6: 299–309.

70. Yamada KM, Even-Ram S. Integrin regulation of growth factor receptors. Nature Cell Biol 2002; 4: E75–6.

71. Brooks B et al. Localization of matrix metalloproteinase MMP-2 to the surface of invasive cells by interaction with integrin αvβ3. Cell 1996; 85: 683–93.

72. Krause T, Turner GA. Are selectins involved in metastasis? Clin Exp Metast 1999; 17: 183–92.

73. Bourguignon LYW. CD44-mediated oncogenic signalling and cytoskeleton activation during mammary tumor progression. J Mamm Gland Biol Neoplasia 2001; 6: 287–97.

74. Stracke ML, Liotta LA. Multi-step cascade of tumor cell metastasis. In Vivo 1992; 6: 309–16.

75. Murrey MJ, Lessey BA. Embryo implantation and tumor metastasis: common pathways of invasion and angiogenesis. Semin Reprod Endocrinol 1999; 17: 275–90.

76. Yoshida BA et al. Prostate cancer metastasis-suppressor genes: a current perspective. In Vivo 1998; 12: 49–58.

77. Paweletz CP, Charboneau L, Bichsel VE et al. Reverse phase protein microarrays which capture disease progression show activation of pro-survival pathways at the cancer invasion front. Oncogene 2001; 20: 1981–9.

78. Nam SW, Clair T, Kim Y-S et al. Autotaxin (NPP-2) a metastasis-enhancing motogen, is an angiogenic factor. Cancer Res 2001; 61: 6938–7044.

79. Webb DJ, Parsons JT, Horwitz AF. Adhesion assembly, disassembly and turnover in migrating cells—over and over and over again. Nature Cell Biol 2002, 4: E97–100.

80. Ridley A. Molecular switches in metastasis. Nature 2000; 406: 466–7.

81. Frame MC, Fincham VJ, Carragher NO, Wyke JA. V-src's hold over actin and cell adhesions. Nature Rev Mol Cell Biol 2002; 3: 233–46.

82. O-Charoenrat P, Modjtahedi H, Rhys-Evans P et al. Epidermal growth factor-like ligands differentially upregulate matrix metalloproteinase-9 in head and neck squamous carcinoma cells. Cancer Res 2000; 60: 1121–8.

83. Lochter A, Bissell MJ. An odyssey from breast to bone: multistep control of mammary metastases and osteolysis by matrix metalloproteinases. APMIS 1999; 107: 128–36.

84. Nemeth JA, Yousif R, Herzog M et al. Matrix metalloproteinase activity, bone matrix turnover and tumor cell proliferation in prostate cancer bone metastasis. J Natl Cancer Inst 2002; 94: 17–25.

85. McCawley LJ, Matrisian LM. Matrix metalloproteinases: multifunctional contributors to tumor progression. Mol Med Today 2000; 6: 149–56.

86. Chang C, Werb Z. The many faces of metalloproteases: cell growth, invasion, angiogenesis and metastasis. Trends Cell Biol 2001; 11: S37–43.

87. Sounni NE, Devy L, Hajitou A et al. MT1-MMP expression promotes tumor growth and angiogenesis through an upregulation of vascular endothelial growth factor expression. FASEB J 2002; 16: 555–64.

88. Egeblad M, Werb Z. New functions for the matrix metalloproteinases in cancer progression. Nature Rev Cancer 2002; 2: 161–74.

89. O-charoenrat P, Rhys-Evans P, Eccles SA. A synthetic matrix-metalloproteinase inhibitor prevents squamous carcinoma cell proliferation by interfering with epidermal growth factor receptor autocrine loops. Int J Cancer 2002; 100: 527–33.

90. Noel A, Albert V, Bajou K et al. New functions of stromal proteases and their inhibitors in tumor progression. Surg Oncol N Am 2001; 10: 417–32.

91. Rabbani SA, Mazar AP. The role of the plasminogen activation system in angiogenesis and metastasis. Surg Oncol Clin N Am 2001; 10: 393–415.

92. Duffy MJ, Maguire TM, McDermott EW, O'Higgins N. Urokinase plasminogen activator: a prognostic marker in multiple types of cancer. J Surg Oncol 1999; 71: 130–5.

93. Pedersen H, Brunner N, Francis D et al. Prognostic impact of urokinase, urokinase receptor and type 1 plasminogen activator inhibitor in squamous and large cell lung cancer tissue. Cancer Res 1994; 54: 4671–5.

94. Devy L, Blacher S, Grignet-Debrus C et al. The pro- or antiangiogenic effect of plasminogen activator inhibitor is dose-dependent. FASEB J 2002; 16: 147–54.

95. Mignatti P, Rifkin D. Plasminogen activators and matrix metalloproteinases in angiogenesis. Enzyme Protein 1886; 49: 117–37.

96. Frosch BA, Berquin I, Emmert-Buck MR et al. Molecular regulation, membrane association and secretion of tumor cathepsin B. APMIS 1999; 107: 28–37.

97. McKerrow JH, Bhargava V, Hansell E et al. A functional proteomics screen of proteases in colorectal carcinoma. Mol Med 2000; 6: 450–60.

98. Rochefort H, Garcia M, Glondu M, Laurent V. Cathepsin D in breast cancer: mechanisms and clinical applications, a 1999 overview. Clin Chim Acta 2000; 291: 157–70.

99. Kos J, Werle B, Lah T, Brunner N. Cysteine proteinases and their inhibitors in extracellular fluids: markers for diagnosis and prognosis in cancer. Int J Biol Markers 2000; 15: 84–9.

100. Van Noorden CJ, Jonges TG, Meade-Tollin LC, Smith RE, Koehler A. In vivo inhibition of cysteine proteinases delays the onset of growth of human pancreatic cancer explants. Br J Cancer 2000; 82: 931–6.

101. Kostoulas G, Lang A, Nagase H, Baici A. Stimulation of angiogenesis through cathepsin B inactivation of the tissue inhibitors of matrix metalloproteinases. FEBS Lett 1999; 455: 286–90.

102. Keppler D, Sameni M, Moin K et al. Tumor progression and angiogenesis: cathepsin B and Co. Biochem Cell Biol 1996; 74: 799–810.

103. Mai J, Waisman DM, Sloane BF. Cell surface complex of cathepsin B/annexin II tetramer in malignant progression. Biochim Biophys Acta 2000; 1477: 215–30.

104. Aziz S, Pervez S, Khan S et al. Immunohistochemical cathepsin D expression in breast cancer: correlation with established pathological parameters and survival. Pathol Res Pract 2001; 197: 551–7.

105. Arkona C, Wiederanders B. Expression, subcellular distribution and plasma membrane binding of cathepsin B and gelatinases in bone metastatic tissue. Biol Chem 1996; 377: 695–702.

106. Kawamata H, Nakashiro K, Uchida D et al. Possible contribution of active MMP-2 to lymph node metastasis and secreted cathepsin L to bone invasion of newly established human oral squamous cancer cell lines. Int J Cancer 1997; 70: 120–7.

107. Park IC, Lee SY, Jeon DG et al. Enhanced expression of cathepsin L in metastatic bone tumors. J Korean Med Sci 1996; 11: 144–8.

108. Ishakawa T, Kamiyama M, Tani-Ishii N et al. Inhibition of osteoclast differentiation and bone resorption by cathepsin K antisense oligonucleotides. Mol Carcinogen 2001; 32: 84–91.

109. Katunuma N, Tsuge H, Nukatsuka M et al. Structure based design of specific cathepsin inhibitors and their application to protection of bone metastasis of cancer cells. Arch Biochem Biophys 2002; 397: 305–11.

110. Liu D, Shriver Z, Venkataraman G et al. Tumor cell surface heparan sulfate as cryptic promoters or inhibitors of tumor growth and metastasis. Proc Natl Acad Sci USA 2002; 99: 568–73.

111. Vlodavsky I, Miao H-Q, Benezra M et al. Involvement of the extracellular matrix, heparan sulfate proteoglycans and heparan sulfate degrading enzymes in angiogenesis and metastasis. In Lewis CE, Bicknell R, Ferrara N (eds), Tumour Angiogenesis. Oxford University Press, Oxford, 2001; 125–40.

112. Smorenburg SM, Van Noorden CJ. The complex effects of heparins on cancer progression and metastasis in experimental studies. Pharmacol Rev 2001; 53: 93–105.

113. Eccles SA. Heparanase: breaking down barriers in tumors. Nature Med 1999; 5: 735–6.

114. Liotta LA, Kohn EC. The microenvironment at the tumour–host interface. Nature 2001; 411: 375–9.

115. Giordano FJ, Johnson RS. Angiogenesis: the role of the microenvironment in flipping the switch. Curr Opin Genet Dev 2001; 11: 35–40.

116. Fidler IJ. Seed and soil revisited: contribution of the organ microenvironment to cancer metastasis. Surg Oncol Clin N Am 2001; 10: 257–69.

117. Freije JMP, Lawrence J, Hollingshead MG et al. Identification of compound with preferential inhibitory activity against low-Nm-23 expressing breast carcinoma and melanoma cell lines. Nature Med 1997; 3: 395–400.

118. Petricoin EF, Ardekani AM, Hitt BA et al. Use of proteomic patterns in serum to identify ovarian cancer. Lancet 2002; 359: 572–7.

119. Dimitroff CJ, Sharma A, Bernacki RJ. Cancer metastasis: a search for therapeutic inhibition. Cancer Invest 1998; 16: 279–90.

120. Chambers AF et al. Clinical targets for anti-metastasis therapy. Adv Cancer Res 2000; 79: 91–121.

121. Cherrington JM, Strawn LM, Shawver LK. New paradigms for the treatment of cancer: the role of anti-angiogenesis agents. Adv Cancer Res 2000; 79: 1–38.

Parathyroid Hormone-related Protein and Bone Metastases

T. J. Martin[1], Janine A. Danks[1] and Michael A. Henderson[2]

[1]*St Vincent's Institute for Medical Research, Melbourne, Australia*
[2]*University of Melbourne, Melbourne, Australia*

BONE METASTASES IN CANCER

It has long been recognised that human cancers have preferential sites of distant spread, suggesting that metastasis is a highly specific and regulated process rather than a random event. Indeed, for cancers to grow in distant organs they need special properties that allow them to flourish in these sites. Over 100 years ago the predilection for breast cancer to spread to bone was recognised by the surgeon Steven Paget [1] on the basis of an extensive autopsy study of women who had died of breast cancer. He proposed the "seed and soil" hypothesis to explain site-specific metastasis, and that bone provides a favourable and specific "soil", or microenvironment, for the growth of specific "seed", such as breast cancer cells. Breast cancer is the most common malignancy in women and a leading cause of cancer-related death, with a mortality rate that is exceeded only by lung cancer in Europe and the USA. It is thus a major public health problem. As is the case with other solid cancers, death in breast cancer usually results after a debilitating illness from metastatic disease, with bone metastases playing a major role in this illness.

Breast cancer is one of several tumours, including prostate, thyroid and kidney, that display a remarkable and specific predilection for metastasis to bone. Bone is the commonest site of metastasis from breast cancer and at least 80% of patients who develop metastatic breast cancer will at some time during the course of their disease develop bone metastases [2,3]. Although most patients also have metastases at other sites, about 15–17% have no evidence of metastatic disease other than in bone [4,5]. Bone represents the first site of metastasis in over 50% of patients who fail systemically [5]. Survival after the diagnosis of bone metastases is primarily related to the presence of other non-bone metastases, with a wide variation in survival after diagnosis of bone metastases, most series reporting a median survival in the order of 20–30 months [6]. In contrast, the median survival of patients with visceral metastases is in the order of 6 months. Apart from the absence of metastatic disease in other organs, a number of factors are known to influence survival after diagnosis of bone metastases. The length of disease-free survival prior to bone involvement is an important predictor of outcome, as is premenopausal rather than postmenopausal status [7]. The presence of osteosclerosis as seen on X-ray as the predominant form of metastasis is associated with improved survival, a finding which has been interpreted as indicating a slower rate of growth [8]. Unfortunately, over 80% of bone metastases from breast cancer noted on plain X-rays are osteolytic in appearance. It is generally accepted that the development of radiological sclerosis in a previously osteolytic lesion indicates tumour regression with healing [4]. Yamashita et al. [9] have demonstrated prolonged survival in patients developing an osteosclerotic response compared to those patients who have failed to exhibit such a

Textbook of Bone Metastases. Edited by C. Jasmin, R. E. Coleman, L. R. Coia, R. Capanna and G. Saillant
© 2005 John Wiley & Sons Ltd: ISBN 0 471 87742 5

response. Oestrogen receptor status of the primary tumour is associated with improved survival, but whether this represents an intrinsic property of the tumour or increased likelihood of a favourable response to therapy is unknown. Other properties of the primary tumour that favour development of bone metastases include lower histological grade, the extent of angiogenesis and increased plasminogen activator activity [7,10].

Although in some cases bone lesions may be asymptomatic, they are nevertheless a major cause of morbidity, with bone pain that can be severe and resistant to analgesic control, together with susceptibility to fractures that require surgery. The complication of spinal cord compression following vertebral fracture is an especially difficult problem.

PATHOGENESIS OF METASTASIS TO BONE

For tumour cells to metastasise successfully, a series of highly specific and ordered events must occur. Tumour cell growth at the primary tumour site is associated with new vessel formation and alterations in the relationship between extracellular matrix and tumour cells, providing tumour cells with the opportunity to escape the primary site and enter the circulation. The tumour cells then need to attach and adhere to the extracellular matrix in the target organ before further tumour cell growth and induction of new vessel formation can occur. Bone represents a particularly harsh microenvironment for successful tumour cell establishment and growth.

Cells in the circulation need to attach and adhere to extracellular matrix components and to other cells. Important to this process are integrins, which are heterodimeric molecules that bind to the extracellular matrix through RGD sequences present in matrix proteins. For example, the $\alpha_v\beta_3$ integrin, which is important in osteoclast attachment to bone, is expressed at high levels in breast cancer cells in bone [11]. It may help breast cancer cells to lodge in bone by its ability to bind bone proteins vitronectin, bone sialoprotein and collagen type-1. This integrin is also expressed in endothelial cells, and neutralising antibodies have been shown to inhibit breast tumour growth and angiogenesis [12]. Recent studies of primary breast tumours indicate that $\alpha_v\beta_3$ integrin expression is elevated in tumours of patients with metastatic disease, and may have prognostic value in predicting metastatic progression [13]. Certain bone matrix proteins are expressed in breast cancer cells and may contribute to the affinity these cells appear to have

for bone. In the invasion process the cancer cells must broach the basement membrane and extend through the extracellular matrix. This requires that the normal balance between proteases and their inhibitors is disturbed. The matrix metalloproteinase family of enzymes is central to the invasion process, and the balance between activation and inactivation is controlled by endogenous inhibitors (TIMPs) [14]. Indeed, transfection of metastatic breast tumour cells with TIMP-2 has been shown to reduce bone metastases in an animal model of growth of breast cancer in bone [15].

There is little doubt that the most important specific property required of cancer cells to grow as metastases in bone is the ability to promote bone resorption, thereby providing a pathway of entry of tumour cells and their expansion in this otherwise hostile environment (Figure 2.1). Older ideas of pathogenesis suggested that tumour cells may themselves also directly cause bone breakdown (e.g. [16,17]). Milch and Changus [8] noted a relative paucity of osteoclasts in the region of bone resorption, and concluded that the process of malignant bone destruction was most likely due to direct tumour pressure or a physicochemical process due to the presence of tumour cells. Furthermore, when human breast cancer cells were grown on mouse calvaria *in vitro*, calcium release occurred [18], suggesting that direct resorption of bone by tumour cells might take place. However, such results are probably explained by release of tissue degrading enzymes rather than true resorption with the classical Howship's lacunae in bone resulting from osteoclast activity.

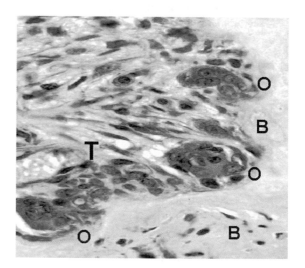

Figure 2.1. Human breast cancer metastases in bone (B), showing active multinucleated osteoclasts (O) on bone surface and adjacent to tumour cells (T) ($\times 100$)

Ample histological evidence has now accumulated that human breast tumour deposits in bone are surrounded by active osteoclasts [19,20] and there is similar evidence from animal models of tumour osteolysis [20–22] and of metastasis to bone [23]. Furthermore, clinical [24,25] and experimental studies [15,26] have shown that inhibition of osteoclast-mediated bone resorption is effective in reducing the metastatic burden in bone. The appearance of active osteoclasts at the site of tumour growth and further bone resorption results from the generation of new osteoclasts derived from haematopoietic precursors. This process can be driven by a number of cytokines and hormones, a complex process that has only recently become understood. Certain properties of breast cancer cells and of the microenvironment of bone are important in the process, and these will be discussed.

Osteoclast Formation

Since osteoclasts are so important in bone metastasis formation and growth, several recent discoveries in osteoclast biology provide new points of interest and possibly of therapeutic development. The development of active osteoclasts requires intimate contact between osteoblastic stromal cells and osteoclast precursors of the monocyte/macrophage lineage. This process is influenced by a variety of osteotrophic factors, including 1,25-dihydroxyvitamin D_3, parathyroid hormone (PTH), prostaglandin E_2 (PGE_2), interleukin-6 (IL-6) and IL-11, all of which enhance osteoclast formation, whilst other cytokines such as IL-4, IL-10, IL-13 and IL-18 are inhibitory [27]. These factors are unable to mediate osteoclast differentiation in the absence of osteoblastic stromal cells and have been defined as acting directly on the osteoblast population, rather than on the osteoclast precursors. This observation led to the proposal of an osteoclast differentiation factor of osteoblastic origin [28], the nature of which has been discovered in the last few years. Receptor activator of nuclear factor κB (RANKL) is a member of the tumour necrosis factor (TNF) ligand family, produced by osteoblastic stromal cells as well as T cells, and acts upon its receptor, RANK, in mononuclear cells to programme osteoclast differentiation and maintain their activity [29,30]. Together with the soluble TNF receptor molecule, osteoprotegerin (OPG), a decoy receptor which is a powerful inhibitor of RANKL/RANK interaction [31], they comprise an exquisitely regulated system that ensures controlled osteoclast formation from haematopoietic precursors,

as well as the maintenance of active osteoclasts. Treatment with OPG is effective in preventing the increased bone resorption associated with ovariectomy in the rat, as well as in experimental models of cancer hypercalcaemia, bone metastasis, arthritis and periodontal disease [32–34].

These molecules are intimately involved in the increased osteoclast formation around breast cancer metastases in bone. Their disturbed control by tumour products and, by factors in the bone microenvironment, all contribute to the ability of breast cancers to erode bone and progress as metastases. These mechanisms will be dealt with in subsequent sections.

Parathyroid Hormone-related Protein, an Osteolytic Cancer Product

The discovery of parathyroid hormone-related protein (PTHrP) as an important cause of hypercalcaemia of malignancy has provided new insights into the pathogenesis of skeletal complications in cancer. It reveals PTHrP as a previously unrecognised hormone, which is important in foetal development and exerts paracrine actions in a number of foetal and adult tissues. When produced in excess in certain cancers, it is also involved in the pathogenesis of hypercalcaemia. The term "humoral hypercalcaemia of malignancy" (HHM) was used to describe patients with certain cancers in whom the blood calcium is elevated in the absence of skeletal metastases [35]. The most common cause of this is squamous cell carcinoma of the lung, as well as squamous cell cancers at other sites, including skin, oesophagus, head and neck, and also renal cortical carcinoma, primary liver cancer, pancreatic cancer, bladder carcinoma and melanoma. HHM is unusual in breast cancer and rare in prostate cancer. In the absence of secondary lesions, removal of the primary tumour leads to resolution of the hypercalcaemia [36,37]. The syndrome of HHM was explained by the purification and cloning of PTHrP [38] and the realisation that it actively promotes bone resorption. It does so in a manner identical to that of PTH, by acting upon the receptor it shares with PTH (PTH1R), which is located on cells of the osteoblast lineage and programmes the formation and activation of osteoclasts [39]. Both PTHrP and PTH promote cyclic AMP and phosphorus excretion and reduce calcium excretion. Other actions of PTHrP that reflect those of PTH include the ability to relax vascular and other smooth muscle. This response may reflect more a physiological function of PTHrP rather than of PTH and is consistent with PTHrP production and local action on smooth muscles at various sites [40].

In addition to the PTH-like actions of PTHrP, there is increasing evidence for other biological activities within the PTHrP molecule, not shared with PTH, and giving rise to the concept that PTHrP is a polypeptide precursor of a number of biological activities, analogous with pro-opiomelanocortin. Of great interest is the discovery that PTHrP is localised in either the nucleus or the cytoplasm of cells, and that its location is cell cycle-dependent [41,42]. In quiescent cells, nuclear/nucleolar location is evident, but with predominant cytoplasmic location and increased production and secretion as cells move towards mitosis [42]. The nuclear transport of PTHrP is carried out by specific binding to importin β and phosphorylation of Thre[85] of PTHrP by the cyclin-dependent protein kinases, CDK2 and CDC2, favouring extrusion of PTHrP from the nucleus [43]. The nuclear/nucleolar locations, its phosphorylation control, cell cycle-dependence and specific nuclear import mechanism, all suggest that the protein exerts important function(s) in the nucleus, the nature of which remain to be determined.

PTHrP AND OTHER BONE-RELATED MOLECULES IN THE DEVELOPING AND ACTIVATED BREAST

There is much evidence to indicate a role for PTHrP in the normal processes of breast development and lactation. Thiede and Rodan [44] demonstrated prolactin-responsive production of PTHrP by the lactating rat breast. This finding led to the detection of large concentrations of immunoreactive PTHrP in the milk from several species [45,46], suckling-induced rises in urinary phosphate and cyclic AMP in the rat [47], a venous arterial concentration gradient of plasma PTHrP in the goat [48] and elevated levels of PTHrP in lactating women [46]. All of these studies identify PTHrP as a major product of the activated breast. Both the duct epithelial cells and myoepithelial cells produce large amounts of PTHrP during lactation. No plasma assay convincingly detects PTHrP in normal adult subjects, but circulating levels of PTHrP can be readily measured in the majority of lactating women [46] although the proportion decreases with the length of lactation. Although some of the expected features of raised levels of PTHrP can be found in many lactating women (increased urinary cAMP, reduced calcium excretion), the significance of PTHrP in human lactation is yet to be fully explained.

Whether it does indeed function as a hormone in that circumstance, or simply reflects 'spillover' into the circulation from the lactation process, is not known.

Production of PTHrP by the activated breast may be relevant to the place of PTHrP in breast cancer, but its involvement in breast development is likely to be at least as significant. Mice in which the PTHrP gene is ablated die very soon after birth with predominantly skeletal deformities. Rescue of these mice, by directing PTHrP production to cartilage with use of the collagen II promoter, has allowed study of the effect of the PTHrP null phenotype on several other organs. In the case of the breast, the 'rescued' PTHrP null mice show failure of early breast ductal development, providing clear evidence of a role for PTHrP in promoting branching morphogenesis [49,50]. In the developing mouse mammary gland, PTHrP is expressed by both lumenal and myoepithelial cells, while myoepithelial cells and other stromal cells alone express PTHrP receptors. Communication between epithelial cells and mesenchymal cells appears to be necessary for normal breast development, and studies in PTH/PTHrP receptor (PTH1R) null mice indicate that the developmental effects of PTHrP appear to be mediated through the PTH1R. With such dramatic expressions of PTHrP involvement both in early breast development and in activation of the mature breast, it is perhaps not surprising that PTHrP emerges as a factor important in breast cancer biology.

A further, and most intriguing, link between breast and bone has been provided by the discovery that mice rendered null for the genes encoding RANKL, or its receptor, RANK, fail to lactate because of lack of development of lobulo-alveolar structures during pregnancy. All the earlier stages of mammary development are normal in these mice, including the mammary buds and rudimentary ductal tree in the embryo and the branching morphogenesis taking place at puberty. Implantation of RANKL into the mammary tissue of pregnant RANKL $-/-$ mice restored lobulo-alveolar differentiation and milk production [51], although of course it did not rescue the RANK $-/-$ phenotype. The RANKL $-/-$ and RANK $-/-$ mice are severely osteopetrotic because they are unable to develop osteoclasts. Involvement of these molecules at a crucial stage of breast development makes a fascinating link between breast development and bone. It might be noted also that the breast phenotypes in the RANKL $-/-$ and RANK $-/-$ mice resemble closely those in cyclin D_1 $-/-$ mice [52], and in mice in which a dominant negative form of Erb B2 is expressed [53]. Both cyclin D_1 and Erb B2 have significant roles in breast cancer.

Finally, the studies of RANKL effects on lobulo-alveolar development of Fata et al. [51] showed that both prolactin and PTHrP induce expression of RANKL by mammary epithelial cells. Such an effect might require epithelial–mesynchymal–epithelial signalling to take place, since the PTHrP is produced by mammary epithelium, whereas its receptor (PTH1R) is located on stromal cells [54].

The possible significance for breast cancer of these findings in breast development will be discussed in relation to mechanisms of bone metastasis formation.

PTHrP AND SKELETAL COMPLICATIONS OF MALIGNANCY

Expression of PTHrP mRNA and protein had been demonstrated in a large number of tumour types and tumour-derived cell lines. The experiments of Kukreja et al. [55], in which hypercalcaemia was treated and prevented by anti-PTHrP antisera in a nude mouse model of HHM, provided strong support for the importance of PTHrP in contributing to the mechanism of hypercalcaemia. Subsequent studies detected PTHrP in > 90% of squamous cell carcinomas by either immunohistochemical or *in situ* hybridisation techniques, and close to 100% of tumours are positive when the two techniques are combined. Tumour production of PTHrP has also been demonstrated in haematological malignancies, particularly in adult T cell leukaemia/lymphoma [56], but also in cases of multiple myeloma and in lymphomas of B cell lineage. The regulation of PTHrP gene expression has been extensively studied in adult T cell leukaemia/lymphoma, a malignancy associated with human T cell leukaemia virus type 1 (HTLV-1) infection. This malignancy is frequently associated with hypercalcaemia.

Further confirmation of the aetiological link between elevated levels of PTHrP and hypercalcaemia associated with malignancy came from measurements of circulating levels by radioimmunoassay and immunoradiometric assays, which documented circulating levels of PTHrP in subjects with malignancy-associated hypercalcaemia [36,37]. Elevated PTHrP levels were found also in 65% of patients with hypercalcaemia and breast carcinoma metastatic to bone [37]. Patients with solid tumours other than breast carcinoma who had hypercalcaemia and bone metastases also had elevated PTHrP levels, particularly those with squamous cell carcinoma, where 100% had detectable PTHrP immunoreactivity. In normal subjects, no PTHrP assay has convincingly measured PTHrP in the circulation. This is consistent with the view that in normal physiology PTHrP acts as a cytokine, or local regulator, in the many tissues in which it is produced. This includes skin, bone, uterus, brain and breast. Apart from its role in the foetus, and its appearance in the circulation during lactation, PTHrP only functions as a hormone postnatally when it is produced in sufficient excess by cancers. In the case of breast cancer it seems that PTHrP can exert both paracrine and endocrine roles. In extensive studies over several years (e.g. [57,58]) we have found no detectable levels of PTHrP in the plasma of patients with breast cancer that had not yet metastasised.

Breast Cancer

In studying breast cancers removed at surgery, Southby et al. [57] found immunohistochemically detectable PTHrP in 60% of primary tumours but not in the accompanying normal breast tissue, a finding that has been amply confirmed [59–62]. Positive staining was related to progesterone (PR) status of the tumour ($p=0.04$) but not to ER receptor status, patient age, tumour size, histological grade or nodal status. Although there was very limited follow-up in this group of patients, the development of hypercalcaemia and bone metastases appeared to occur more frequently in patients with PTHrP-positive tumours. To overcome the problem of limited follow-up, PTHrP status was related to a prognostic index. This indicated, apparently paradoxically, that the presence of PTHrP in the primary tumour appeared to be related to improved survival.

When our restrospective analysis of primary breast cancers and metastases in bone and soft tissue revealed that 92% of metastasis in bone were positive for PTHrP, compared with 17% of those in non-bone tissues [63], we proposed that production of PTHrP as a bone-resorbing factor might be a property of breast cancers that would favour their growth in bone. Subsequent to this, compelling evidence for a role for PTHrP in bone metastasis formation has been obtained from experimental approaches.

Prostate Cancer

The focus of this discussion on breast cancer reflects its seriousness as a clinical problem, but bone metastases are a frequent and serious complication also in prostate cancer, and there are likely to be a number of mechanisms common to the two diseases. Although the bone metastases in prostate cancer are predominantly sclerotic, and research efforts have concentrated on identifying the 'bone-forming' factors, it is increasingly recognised that osteoclast formation contributes to bone invasion in a manner similar to that in breast cancer. A number of human prostate cancer cell lines have been found to produce PTHrP [64]. In a rat model, intracardiac injection of human prostate cancer cells overexpressing PTHrP led to osteosclerotic lumbar vertebral metastases [65].

Clinical studies also reveal an intriguing link with PTHrP. In a small series of primary prostate tumours and bone metastases, 95% of the primary tumours were positive for the PTHrP protein, while only 50% of bone secondaries were positive [66]. This study also found that 100% of bone metastases from other primary tumours were positive for PTHrP. Clearly, the PTHrP antigen status of the bony metastases from prostate primary tumours is different from the metastases to bone from other types of primary tumours. In another series of 20 bony metastases, 58% were found to be positive for the PTHrP protein but only 58% of the 97 primary prostatic tumours were also positive (M. Richardson, J. A. Danks, unpublished). This is in line with the percentage of positive primary breast tumours (57%) but differs from the study of Iddon et al. [66] as well as the 100% positivity seen in another series of 33 primary prostatic tumours [67]. All three studies utilised either monoclonal or polyclonal antisera made to different portions of the PTHrP molecule, which may account for the differing results. There is a need for more extensive clinical studies to provide a clearer picture of the proportion of primary prostatic tumours that contain PTHrP as well as the significance of PTHrP-positive bone metastases.

Experimental Models: Role of the Bone Microenvironment

Guise et al. [68] used the human breast cancer cell line, MDA-MB-231, in a model of tumour-mediated osteolysis in which the cells were injected into the left ventricle of nude mice, and radiology and histology were used to examine and quantitate the lytic bone deposits. These typically developed after 3 weeks, with the tumour-bearing mice not exhibiting a rise in PTHrP or calcium levels in peripheral blood, but showing elevated PTHrP levels in marrow plasma. Importantly, treatment of tumour-injected animals with a neutralising monoclonal antibody against PTHrP largely prevented tumour growth and histological evidence of bone invasion. In these studies, tumours growing in bone were characterised by prolific osteoclast appearance at the tumour–bone interface, an appearance that was lost with anti-PTHrP treatment. The success of anti-PTHrP treatment mirrored that seen earlier in models of humoral hypercalcaemia of malignancy [55], in which hypercalcaemia was prevented and treated by neutralising anti-PTHrP antibody.

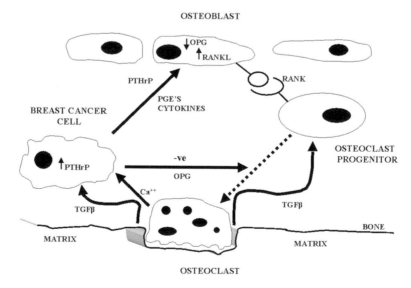

Figure 2.2. Bone microenvironment and bone metastasis process. PTHrP produced by cancer cells promotes osteoclast development. TGFβ released during invasion can promote further PTHrP production, a process enhanced by Ca^{2+} released in resorption. Discontinuous line indicates formation and activation of osteoclasts

In a model of spontaneous metastasis of a mouse breast cancer to bone, intramammary inoculation also results in osteolytic metastases and elevated circulating PTHrP and calcium [23]. This model is unique in that it represents the entire metastasis pathway from the primary site to bone. Subcloning of the original mouse tumour has given rise to cell lines which either do not metastasise or which metastasise to different sites, including lymph nodes, lung and bone. Although all the clones secrete low levels of PTHrP, secretion is greatest in the clone that spreads to bone. This model promises to be useful in defining the roles of PTHrP in the early invasive processes as well as in the establishment of bone secondaries.

The importance of bone as the favourable 'soil' for the growth of breast cancer cells as 'seed' [1], is illustrated beautifully by experiments indicating that TGFβ, released from bone matrix during resorption, can enhance further tumour invasion in bone by promoting PTHrP production by the cancer cells (Figure 2.2). This evidence was obtained by expressing a dominant negative TGFβ receptor in the MDA-MB-231 cells, and finding a substantial reduction in tumour establishment and growth in bone [69]. Thus, the copious store of TGFβ in the bone matrix is a source of active TGFβ released during bone resorption, and available to act upon the tumour cells to enhance further the production of PTHrP [70]. The potential of TGFβ to amplify this pathological process may indeed be even greater than previously thought, with some recent insights into the growth factor's secretion and action. First, TGFβ significantly enhances osteoclast formation from precursor haematopoietic cells prepared *in vitro* in the absence of osteoblastic stromal cells with RANKL and M-CSF [71]. Second, elevating the ambient calcium concentration significantly enhances PTHrP production by the human breast cancer cells, MCF-7, in culture, as well as amplifying the TGFβ-induced elevation of PTHrP [72]. Each of these processes could contribute significantly to the bone resorption and invasion process in the disturbed anatomy accompanying metastatic establishment in bone, and each might provide new pathways to drug development in intervention.

These processes illustrate the prime importance of the microenvironment in determining the establishment and progress of metastases in bone. The microenvironment is also an important consideration in the final specific steps of osteoclast formation, in that RANKL action upon haematopoietic precursors is essential. When the human breast cancer cell line, MCF-7, was engineered to overexpress PTHrP, these cells yielded large lytic tumours when given by intracardiac injection to nude

mice [73]. The cells produced mRNA for OPG and RANK, but RANKL mRNA could not be detected by RT-PCR. When they were co-cultivated with mouse calvarial osteoblasts together with haematopoietic cells, osteoclasts were generated without the need for treatment with bone-resorbing agents. Furthermore, expression of RANKL mRNA was enhanced in the co-cultures and OPG mRNA was decreased. This is taken to indicate that the tumour cells, nearby to host bone cells, could promote the formation of osteoclasts by inducing appropriate changes in the production of those molecules that are crucial in the process (Figure 2.2).

These experiments have helped in proving the concept that tumour production of a bone-resorbing cytokine, in this case PTHrP, could facilitate cancer establishment in bone. They do not exclude contributions from other cytokines, e.g. IL-1, IL-6, TNFα, or of cyclooxygenase products, which could be produced by tumour or by host cells in response to the tumour, and these possibilities are conceded in the schema proposed in Figure 2.2. Many of these cytokines act upon bone in a manner similar to PTHrP, and could potentially contribute in this way or by additive or synergistic effects with PTHrP. However, the accumulating data showing the frequency with which PTHrP is produced in primary and metastatic breast cancer focuses attention on its role. The other important feature of these experiments was the prominent part played by osteoclasts in the tumour invasion process.

Bone Proteins and Matrix Metalloproteinases

Although much attention in the study of bone metastases is directed at promotion of bone resorption, there are other likely specific properties that enhance the ability of breast cancers to grow in bone. First is the need to be able to attach to and interact with bone extracellular matrix. It is increasingly recognised that breast cancers produce certain proteins that are typical of the osteoblast, and this may be a relevant property. Second, the matrix metalloproteinases (MMPs) comprise a large family (at least 20 members) of endopeptidases with substrate specificities for several collagens and non-collagenous proteins of the extracellular matrix [74]. They are involved in the tissue remodelling that occurs in bone remodelling, normal breast development and wound healing, as well as in tumour invasion and metastasis [75].

The production by breast cancer of proteins of bone is quite a striking property of tumour cells. Bone sialoprotein (BSP) is commonly expressed in breast cancers [76,77], and the suggestion has been made that this property relates to bone metastasis development [78] and poor patient survival [79], although it would be reassuring to see prospective studies. This protein possesses an integrin-binding RGF domain which could promote interactions between breast cancer cells and bone matrix. Evidence in favour of this was obtained in studies of human breast cancer cell adhesion and migration, in which promotion by BSP appeared to be through $\alpha\beta3$ and $\alpha\beta5$ integrin receptors [80].

Osteopontin is another bone protein related to BSP, also possessing an RGD sequence and able to bind to bone mineral as well. It was expressed in 100% of a small series of primary breast cancers [77]. It too could contribute to breast cancer attachment to bone via the vitronectin receptor. Osteonectin is associated with morphogenesis and tissue remodelling, influencing several cell functions including spreading and adhesion. Also, it is produced in breast cancers [81] and has been shown to induce MMP-2 activation in human breast cancer cell lines [82]. When these various proteins are produced by breast cancer cells, they could combine to confer upon the cells special properties that, when combined with their ability to promote bone resorption, equip them to establish as metastatic growths in bone.

The fact that MMPs are involved in tissue invasion by cancers, including those of breast, is accepted. In the case of invasion and metastasis in bone, ECM tissue remodelling is necessary as well as the specific osteoclast-mediated bone invasion. In that sense, MMP involvement is likely but there is little direct information at present.

PTHrP AND METASTASIS: CLINICAL STUDIES

In our initial clinical studies a role for PTHrP in the bone metastasis process was suggested, and the prognostic index data in the study by Southby et al. [57] indicated that presence of PTHrP in the primary tumour was related to improved survival. These were studies of relatively few patients, however, and of short duration.

In a later retrospective study of patients with widely varying prognosis, a relationship between positive PTHrP status, the development of bone metastases and hypercalcaemia was noted [83]. Three groups of patients were evaluated: first, a favourable prognosis group who had not experienced any evidence of metastatic disease during a minimum of 3 years of

follow-up; second, a group of patients who developed distant metastases within 3 years of diagnosis; and a final group consisting of patients who presented with distant disease. No differences in the PTHrP status of the primary tumours were found amongst the three patient groups (66%, 65% and 61%, respectively). A further study of patients who developed hypercalcaemia demonstrated a slightly higher rate of primary tumours containing PTHrP (76%). Again, a relationship between positive PR status and the presence of PTHrP in the primary breast tumours was found, but no association with ER status, nodal status, tumour size or age was noted. In this group of 33 patients, all but two developed bone metastases. Subsequently these results were confirmed by Bundred et al. [84], who found that 65% of primary tumours contained PTHrP, but that amongst patients who developed bone metastases, PTHrP staining was much more common (88%) compared with patients who did not develop bone metastases (53%). This was a small prospective study with limited follow-up (128 cases followed for a median of 48 months). Liapis et al. [60] also found approximately two-thirds of breast carcinomas contained immunohistochemically detectable PTHrP and that its presence was inversely correlated with tumour stage and nodal status. There was no significant correlation with tumour grade, patient age or ER or PR status. A small study by Bouizar et al. [61] noted a much higher frequency of PTHrP gene expression in the primary tumours of patients developing bone metastases compared to patients who did not develop bone metastases.

These preliminary studies were characterised by small numbers, case selection, limited follow-up and/ or retrospective accrual, but in summary indicated that PTHrP could be found in approximately two-thirds of primary breast tumours and appeared to be associated with the development of skeletal complications, i.e. bone metastases and hypercalcaemia. With the exception of the study by Southby et al. [57], they suggested that PTHrP status was associated with worse survival. The shortcomings of these various studies were evident enough and it was becoming clear that long-term, prospective studies of unselected patients were needed.

Long-term Prospective Study of the Role of PTHrP in Breast Cancer

This clinical investigation was established to study the significance of PTHrP in primary breast cancer for the subsequent development of skeletal complications. It was based on our findings that two-thirds of breast cancers were PTHrP-positive by immunohistology [57], that bone metastases appeared to be enriched for PTHrP production [63] and that elevated plasma levels of PTHrP occurred commonly in breast cancer [37].

The long-term prospective follow-up study of a consecutive series of patients was commenced in 1989, and over the following 5 years a total of 367 eligible patients were accrued, with analysis carried out in 1999 [58]. The median follow-up was 67 months. The median age at diagnosis was 60 years and the majority were post-menopausal (70%); the median tumour size was 26 mm and most patients were axillary lymph node-negative (60%). PTHrP was detected in 265 (72% of primary breast tumours) patients by immuno-histology, and positive PTHrP status was associated with ER status, PR status, presence of tumour calcification but not with menopausal status, tumour size, nodal status, tumour grade or the presence of lymphatic/vascular invasion by tumour. Crude 5 year cancer-specific survival for all patients was 82%. Patients who had primary tumours containing PTHrP had a crude 5 year cancer-specific survival of 87% (95% CI = 82–91%), compared to patients with PTHrP-negative tumours with a crude 5 year cancer survival of 73% (95% CI = 63–81%). Other factors associated with improved survival included stage, tumour size, nodal status, ER status, PR status, tumour calcification, the absence of tumour lympha-tic/vascular invasion and tumour grade, but not menopausal status [58].

Multivariate analysis of these prognostic factors using Cox proportional hazards modelling indicated that positive PTHrP status was independently asso-ciated with improved survival ($p=0.003$), as were the

absence of axillary lymph node involvement ($p < 0.00001$), small tumour size ($p < 0.00001$) and low tumour grade ($p=0.007$). The hazard rate for death from breast cancer in women with PTHrP-positive tumour was 45% of that in women with a PTHrP-negative tumour [58].

The study also demonstrated that patients with PTHrP-positive primary tumours were less likely to develop metastases at any site, including bone, at any time after surgery (Figure 2.3). Bone metastases developed in 12% of patients with PTHrP-positive tumours but in 27% of patients with PTHrP-negative tumours. Patients with PTHrP-negative tumours were also more likely to have metastases to lung, liver and other soft tissue sites compared to PTHrP-positive tumours (Figure 2.3). On univariate analysis, factors found to be predictive for the development of bone metastases were negative PTHrP status, negative ER and negative PR status, positive nodal status, large tumour size, high tumour grade, lymphatic and vascular invasion, and the absence of calcification in the primary tumour. The crude cumulative 5 year risk for the development of bone metastases was 26% for patients with PTHrP-negative primary tumours, com-pared to 13% for patients with PTHrP-positive tumours.

Multivariate analysis of the factors associated with development of bone metastases, using a Cox propor-tional hazards model, demonstrated that negative PTHrP status ($p=0.002$), as well as the number of axillary lymph nodes involved with tumour ($p=0.00001$), the presence of lymphatic or vascular invasion ($p=0.002$) and the absence of PR staining ($p=0.04$), were associated with the development of bone metastases. The hazard rate for development of bone metastases in women with PTHrP-positive tumours was 39% that of women with PTHrP-negative tumours.

The study found a relationship between PTHrP status and ER and PR status, but not with other recognised prognostic factors. In contrast to previous reports, this long-term study assessed ER status by the more sensitive and specific immunohistochemical assay (compared to the older competitive radioligand bind-ing assay). Although there is *in vitro* evidence that oestrogen can promote PTHrP production in human breast cancer cell lines, any clinical significance remains to be established. Although ER and PR status were individually associated with improved survival, they were eliminated from the final multivariate Cox model, indicating that with PTHrP in the model they were not independently predictive of outcome.

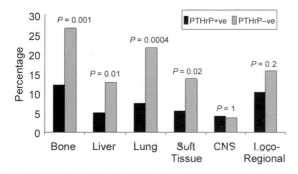

Figure 2.3. For each tissue site, the percentage of patients who developed metastases at any time for 265 patients with primary breast cancers containing PTHrP (black columns), and for 102 patients with PTHrP-negative primary tumours (open columns). *p* Values (Fisher exact test) are indicated in each case. Data from Henderson et al. [58]

A large number of factors were individually predictive of the development of bone metastases, including positive nodal status, larger tumours, high grade and negative PTHrP, ER and PR status. A relationship between positive ER status and the development of bone metastases has been consistently reported previously, but not by all studies. A recent large study with prolonged follow-up (median of 11 years) demonstrated that nodal status (> 3 nodes), young age, larger tumours and positive ER were independently predictive for the development of bone metastases [85]. The effect of positive ER status on the development of bone metastases did not become obvious until after prolonged follow-up, indicating that patients with ER-positive tumours took longer to develop bone metastases. It should also be noted that patients who died of breast cancer without bone metastases were more likely to be ER-negative, and presumably, if they had survived longer, may have developed bone metastases. The data from our long-term study [58] was analysed to explore the possibility that PTHrP was a time-dependent variable, as ER appears to be, but no effect due to time delay was found. As noted above, hormone receptor status in the long-term study was estimated by immunohistochemistry, rather than the old competitive ligand-binding assays. To the present time, no comparable large long-term studies evaluating immunohistochemical analysis of ER and PR are available.

The implication of these findings is that production of PTHrP by the breast cancer cells confers upon them a less malignant phenotype, one that is less invasive and less likely to result in metastasis formation. The finding is apparently at odds with the starting hypothesis, which was that expression of PTHrP in primary breast cancers would correlate with subsequent development of bone metastases, but it is by no means inconsistent with a role for PTHrP in bone metastasis development. This clinical study suggests that PTHrP-negative breast cancers may be relatively enriched in general invasive properties that are needed for metastasis establishment. Upon reaching the bone marrow and exerting these functions, the resulting microenvironment would provide the special properties necessary for invading bone, i.e. enhanced production of PTHrP by cancer cells through the actions of local factors, especially TGFβ, calcium and perhaps other growth factors, leading to increased osteoclast formation and bone resorption (Figure 2.4).

Implications for the Treatment and Prevention

The importance of osteoclast formation and activity in the development of skeletal complications of breast cancer has led to bone resorption inhibitors having a central place in treatment. The most widely used are the bisphosphonates, analogues of pyrophosphate which concentrate in bone and are, to date, the most effective inhibitors of resorption. Treatment with parenteral bisphosphonates, e.g. pamidronate, given intravenously every 3–4 weeks, is associated with reduction in skeletal complications of breast cancer, including hypercalcaemia, pathological fractures and their sequelae, and reduced treatment requirements (surgery, irradiation) (reviewed in [24,25,86–88]). However, there is no evidence that such reduction in morbidity leads to prolonged patient survival, and there have been only a few small prospective clinical studies that ask whether bisphosphonates can provide benefit when used in an adjuvant setting in women with breast cancer which has not yet metastasised to bone. Appropriate large adjuvant studies are needed, whether carried out with bisphosphonates, with newer inhibitors of bone resorption as they are developed [89], or in combination with drugs targeting other aspects of the bone metastasis process, such as the matrix metalloproteinases.

As understanding of the bone metastasis process increases, and as new prospects for therapeutic intervention present themselves, it should be possible to develop approaches to preventing bone metastasis formation. Rather than facing the prospect of designing trials involving unselected patients from the time of breast cancer, selected groups at high risk of bone metastasis could provide the basis for such prevention studies. A recent example is provided by the outcome

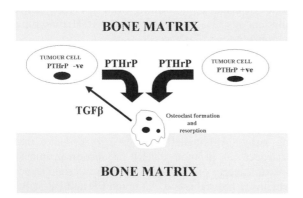

Figure 2.4. Bone microenvironment interaction with tumour cells. It is proposed that the more invasive PTHrP-negative tumour cells respond to local influences, especially TGFβ, to enhance PTHrP production and promote osteoclast formation

of the International Breast Cancer Study Group trial, which identifies two patient populations who were subject to a high incidence of bone metastases. These were patients with four or more involved axillary lymph nodes and patients who had a first recurrence in local, regional or distal soft tissue sites. The former group had a cumulative incidence of 14.9% and the latter group an incidence of 18.2% after 2 years [85].

CONCLUSIONS

Metastasis to bone requires that tumour cells are able to promote bone resorption, in addition to their general invasive properties. The promotion of osteoclast formation is the single most important requirement, a function that metastatic tumour cells fulfil by producing bone-resorbing cytokines. The most intensely studied of these is PTHrP, which may be an important local mediator of breast cancer invasion of bone, although contributions by other factors (e.g. IL-6, IL-11, PGE_2) are not excluded. The bone microenvironment plays a crucial role in determining the successful growth of tumour in bone, with locally generated TGFβ and calcium-enhancing production of PTHrP by tumour cells. The finding from a prospective clinical study in breast cancer, that primary production of PTHrP is associated with fewer metastases (including bone) and improved survival, raises the interesting possibility that PTHrP production confers upon the tumour cells a less invasive phenotype. This is nevertheless not inconsistent with a role for PTHrP in bone, contributing in a specific way to bone metastases formation.

REFERENCES

1. Paget S. The distribution of secondary growths in cancer of the breast. Lancet 1889; 1: 571–3.
2. Tubiana-Hulin M. Incidence, prevalence and distribution of bone metastases. Bone 1991;12 (suppl 1): S9–10.
3. Galasko CS. Mechanisms of lytic and blastic metastatic disease of bone. Clin Orthop 1982; 169: 20–7.
4. Hortobagyi GN, Libshitz HI, Seabold JE. Osseous metastases of breast cancer. Clinical, biochemical, radiographic, and scintigraphic evaluation of response to therapy. Cancer 1984; 53: 577–82.
5. Coleman RE, Rubens RD. The clinical course of bone metastases from breast cancer. Br J Cancer 1987; 55: 61–6.
6. Theriault RL. Medical treatment of bone metastases. In Harris JR, Lippman ME, Morrow M, Hillman S (eds), Diseases of the Breast. Lippincott-Raven: Philadelphia, PA, 1996: 819–27.
7. Scher HI, Yagoda A. Bone metastases: pathogenesis, treatment, and rationale for use of resorption inhibitors. Am J Med 1987; 82: 6–28.
8. Milch RA, Changus GW. Response of bone for tumour invasion. Cancer 1956; 9: 340–51.
9. Yamashita S, Koyama H, Inayi H. Prognostic significance of bone metastasis from breast cancer. Clin Orthop 1995; 312: 89–94.
10. Sherry MM, Greco FA, Johnson DH, Hainsworth JD. Metastatic breast cancer confined to the skeletal system. An indolent disease. Am J Med 1986; 81: 381–6.
11. Liapis H, Flath A, Kitazawa S. Integrin αvβ3 expression by bone-residing breast cancer metastases. Diagn Mol Pathol 1996; 5: 127–35.
12. Brooks PC, Stromblad S, Klemke R et al. Anti integrin αvβ3 blocks human breast cancer grown and angiogenesis. J Clin Invest 1995; 96: 1815–22.
13. Gasparini G, Brooks PC, Biganzoli E et al. Vascular integrin α(v)β3: a new prognostic indicator in breast cancer. Clin Cancer Res 1998; 4: 2625–34.
14. McCawley LJ, Matrisian LM. Matrix metalloproteinases: multifunctional contributors to tumour progression. Mol Med Today 2000; 4: 149–56.
15. Yoneda T, Sasahi A, Dunstan C et al. Inhibition of osteolytic bone metastasis of breast cancer by combined treatment with the bisphosphonate ibandronate and tissue inhibitor of the matrix metalloproteinase-2. J Clin Invest 1997; 99: 2509–17.
16. Gutman AB, Tyson TL, Gutman EB. Serum calcium, inorganic phosphorus and phosphatase activity in hyperparathyroidism, Paget's disease, multiple myeloma and neoplastic diseases of bone. Arch Intern Med 1936; 57: 379–413.
17. Farrow JH, Woodard HQ. Influence of androgenic and estrogenic substances on serum calcium in cases of skeletal metastases from mammary cancer. J Am Med Assoc 1942; 118: 339–43.
18. Eilon G, Mundy GR. Direct resorption of bone by human breast cancer cells in vitro. Nature 1978; 276: 726–8.
19. Mundy GR, Martin TJ. The hypercalcemia of malignancy: pathogenesis and management. Metabolism 1982; 31: 1247–77.
20. Clohisy DR, Ranmaraine ML. Osteoclasts are required for bone tumours to grow and destroy bone. J Orthop Res 1998; 16: 660–6.
21. Clohisy DR, Palkert D, Ranmaraine ML et al. Human breast cancer induces osteoclast activation and increases the number of osteoclasts at sites of tumour osteolysis. J Orthop Res 1996; 14: 396–402.
22. Clohisy DR, Perkins SL, Ranmaraine ML. Review of cellular mechanisms of tumour osteolysis. Clin Orthop 2000; 373: 104–14.
23. Lelekakis M, Moseley JM, Martin TJ et al. A novel orthotopic model of breast cancer metastasis to bone. Clin Exp Metast 1999; 17: 163–70.
24. Hillner BE, Ingle JN, Berenson JR et al. American Society of Clinical Oncology guideline on the role of bisphosphonates in breast cancer. American Society of Clinical Oncology Bisphosphonates Expert Panel. J Clin Oncol 2000; 18: 1378–91.
25. Lipton A, Theriault RL, Hortobagyi GN et al. Pamidronate prevents skeletal complications and is effective palliative treatment in women with breast carcinoma and osteolytic bone metastases: long-term follow-up of two randomized, placebo-controlled trials. Cancer 2000; 88: 1082–90.

26. Yoneda T, Michigami T, Yi B et al. Actions of bisphosphonates on bone metastasis in animal models of breast carcinoma. Cancer 2000; 88: 2979–88.

27. Suda T, Takahashi N, Udagawa N et al. Modulation of osteoclast differentiation and function by the new members of the tumor necrosis factor receptor and ligand families. Endocr Rev 1999; 20: 345–57.

28. Suda T, Takahashi N, Martin TJ. Modulation of osteoclast differentiation. Endocr Rev 1992; 13: 66–80.

29. Yasuda H, Shima N, Nakagawa N et al. Osteoclast differentiation factor is a ligand for osteoprotegerin/osteoclastogenesis-inhibitory and is identical to TRANCE/RANKL. Proc Natl Acad Sci USA 1998; 95: 3597–602.

30. Lacey DL, Timms E, Tan TL et al. Osteoprotegerin ligand is a cytokine that regulated osteoclast differentiation and activation. Cell 1998; 93: 165–76.

31. Simonet WS, Lacey DL, Dunstan CR et al. Osteoprotegerin: a novel secreted protein involved in the regulation of bone density. Cell 1997; 89: 309–19.

32. Kong Y-Y, Feige U, Sarosi I et al. Activated T cells regulate bone loss and joint destruction in adjuvant arthritis through osteoprotegerin ligand. Nature 1999; 402: 304–9.

33. Capparelli C, Kostenuik PJ, Morony S et al. Osteoprotegerin prevents and reverses hypercalcemia in a murine model of humoral hypercalcemia of malignancy. Cancer Res 2000; 60: 783–7.

34. Teng YT, Nguyen H, Kong YY et al. Functional human T-cell immunity and osteoprotegerin ligand control alveolar bone destruction in peridontal infection. J Clin Invest 2000; 106: R59–67.

35. Martin TJ, Atkins D. Biochemical regulators of bone resorption and their significance in cancer. Essays Biochem 1979; 4: 49–82.

36. Burtis WJ, Brady TG, Orloff JJ et al. Immunochemical characterization of circulating parathyroid hormone-related protein in patients with humoral hypercalcemia of cancer. N Engl J Med 1990; 322: 1106–12.

37. Grill V, Ho P, Body JJ et al. Parathyroid hormone-related protein: elevated levels in both humoral hypercalcemia of malignancy and hypercalcemia complicating metastatic breast cancer. J Clin Endocrinol Metab 1991; 73: 1309–15.

38. Moseley JM, Kubota M, Diefenbach-Jagger H et al. Parathyroid hormone-related protein purified from a human lung cancer cell line. Proc Natl Acad Sci USA 1987; 84: 5048–52.

39. Evely RS, Bonomo A, Schneider HG et al. Structural requirements for the action of parathyroid hormone-related protein (PTHrP) on bone resorption by isolated osteoclasts. J Bone Min Res 1991; 6: 85–93.

40. Martin TJ, Moseley JM, Williams ED. Parathyroid hormone-related protein: hormone and cytokine. J Endocrinol 1997; 154: S23–37.

41. Lam MH, Olsen SL, Rankin WA et al. PTHrP and cell division: expression and localization of PTHrP in a keratinocyte cell line (HaCaT) during the cell cycle. J Cell Physiol 1997; 173: 433–46.

42. Lam MH, Briggs LJ, Hu W et al. Importin β recognizes parathyroid hormone-related protein with high affinity and mediates its nuclear import in the absence of importin α. J Biol Chem 1999a; 274: 7391–8.

43. Lam MH, House CM, Tiganis T et al. Phosphorylation at the cyclin-dependent kinases site (Thr85) of parathyroid hormone-related protein negatively regulates its nuclear localization. J Biol Chem 1996b; 274: 18559–66.

44. Thiede MA, Rodan GA. Expression of a calcium-mobilizing parathyroid hormone-like peptide in lactating mammary tissue. Science 1988; 242: 278–80.

45. Budayr AA, Halloran BP, King JC et al. High levels of parathyroid hormone-like protein in milk. Proc Natl Acad Sci USA 1989; 86: 7183–5.

46. Grill V, Hillary J, Ho PM et al. Parathyroid hormone-related protein: a possible endocrine function in lactation. Clin Endocrinol 1992; 37: 405–10.

47. Yamamoto M, Fisher JE, Thiede MA et al. Concentrations of parathyroid hormone-related protein in rat milk change with duration of lactation and interval from previous suckling, but not with milk calcium. Endocrinology 1992; 130: 741–7.

48. Ratcliffe WA, Thompson GE, Care AD, Peaker M. Production of parathyroid hormone-related protein by the mammary gland of the goat. J Endocrinol 1992; 133: 87–93.

49. Wysolmerski JJ, McCaughern-Carucci JF, Daifotis AG et al. Overexpression of parathyroid hormone-related protein or parathyroid hormone in transgenic mice impairs branching morphogenesis during mammary gland development. Development 1995; 121: 3539–47.

50. Wysolmerski JJ, Philbrick WM, Dunbar ME et al. Rescue of the parathyroid hormone-related protein knockout mouse demonstrates that parathyroid hormone-related protein is essential for mammary gland development. Development 1998; 125: 1285–94.

51. Fata JE, Kong YY, Li J et al. The osteoclast differentiation factor osteoprotegerin-ligand is essential for mammary gland development. Cell 2000; 103: 41–50.

52. Brisken C, Kaur S, Chavarrie TE et al. Prolactin controls mammary gland development via direct and indirect mechanisms. Dev Biol 1999; 210: 96–106.

53. Jones FE, Stern DF. Expression of dominant-negative ErbB2 in the mammary gland of transgenic mice reveals a role in lobuloalveolar development and lactation. Oncogene 1999; 18: 3481–90.

54. Martin TJ, Gillespie MT. Receptor activator of nuclear factor κB (RANKL): another link between breast and bone. Trends Endocrinol Metabol 2001; 12: 4–6.

55. Kukreja SC, Rosol TJ, Wimbiscus SA et al. Tumour resection and antibodies to parathyroid hormone-related protein cause similar changes on bone histomorphometry in hypercalcemia of cancer. Endocrinology 1990; 127: 305–10.

56. Moseley JM, Danks JA, Grill V et al. Immunocytochemical demonstration of PTHrP protein in neoplastic tissue of HTLV-1 positive human adult T cell leukaemia/lymphoma: implications for the mechanism of hypercalcaemia. Br J Cancer 1991; 64: 745–8.

57. Southby J, Kissin MW, Danks JA et al. Immunohistochemical localization of parathyroid hormone-related protein in human breast cancer. Cancer Res 1990; 50: 7710–16.

58. Henderson MA, Danks JA, Moseley JM et al. Parathyroid hormone-related protein production by breast cancers associated with improved survival and reduction in bone metastases. J Natl Cancer Inst 2001; 93: 234–7.

59. Bundred NJ, Walker RA, Ratcliffe WA et al. Parathyroid hormone related protein and skeletal morbidity in breast cancer. Eur J Cancer 1992; 28: 690–2.

60. Liapis H, Crouch EC, Grosso LE et al. Expression of parathyroid-like protein in normal, proliferating and neoplastic breast tissue. Am J Pathol 1993; 143: 1169–78.

61. Bouizar Z, Spyratos F, Deytieux S et al. Polymerase chain reaction analysis of parathyroid hormone-related protein gene expression in breast cancer patients and occurrence of bone metastases. Cancer Res 1993; 53: 5076–8.

62. Vargas SJ, Gillespie MT, Powell GJ et al. Localization of parathyroid hormone-related protein mRNA expression in breast cancer and metastatic lesions by in situ hybridization. J Bone Min Res 1992; 8: 971–9.

63. Powell GJ, Southby J, Danks JA et al. Localization of parathyroid hormone-related protein in breast cancer metastases: increased incidence in bone compared with other sites. Cancer Res 1991; 51: 3059–61.

64. Iwamura M, Abrahamsson PA, Foss KA et al. PTHRP: a potential autocrine growth factor in human prostate cancer cell lines. Urology 1994; 43: 675–9.

65. Rabbani SA, Gladu J, Harakidas P, Jamison B, Goltzman D. Overproduction of parathyroid hormone-related peptide results in increased osteolytic skeletal metastasis by prostate cancer cells in vivo. Int J Cancer 1999; 80: 257–64.

66. Iddon J, Bundred NJ, Hoyland J et al. J Pathol 2000; 191: 170–4.

67. Iwamura M, Wu G, diSant'Agnese PA et al. Immunohistochemical localization of parathyroid hormone-related protein in human prostate cancer. Cancer Res 1993; 53: 1724–6.

68. Guise TA, Yin JJ, Taylor SD et al. Evidence for a causal role of parathyroid hormone-related protein in the pathogenesis of human breast cancer-mediated osteolysis. J Clin Invest 1996; 98: 1544–9.

69. Yin JJ, Selander K, Chirgwin JM et al. TGF-β signaling blockade inhibits PTHrP secretion by breast cancer cells and bone metastases development. J Clin Invest 1999; 103: 197–206.

70. Kiriyama T, Gillespie MT, Glatz JA et al. TGFβ stimulation of parathyroid hormone-related protein (PTHrP): a paracrine regulator? Mol Cell Endocrinol 1993; 92: 55–62.

71. Sells Galvin RJ, Gatlin CL, Horn JW, Fuson TR. TGF-β enhances osteoclast differentiation in hematopoietic cell cultures stimulated with RANKL and M-CSF. Biochem Biophys Res Commun 1999; 265: 233–9.

72. Sanders JL, Chattopadhyay N, Kifor O et al. Extracellular calcium-sensing receptor expression and its potential role in regulating parathyroid hormone-related peptide secretion in human breast cancer cell lines. Endocrinology 2000; 141: 4357–64.

73. Thomas RJ, Guise TA, Yin JJ et al. Breast cancer cells interact with osteoblasts to support osteoclast formation. Endocrinology 1999; 40: 4451–8.

74. Benaud C, Dickson RB, Thompson EW. Roles of the matrix metalloproteinases in mammary gland development and cancer. Breast Cancer Res Treat 1998; 50: 97–116.

75. Rudolph-Owen LA, Matrisian LM. Matrix metalloproteinase in remodelling of the normal and neoplastic mammary gland. J Mamm Gland Biol Neoplasia 1998; 3: 177–89.

76. Bellahcene A, Merville MP, Castronovo V. Expression of bone sialoprotein, a bone matrix protein, in human breast cancer. Cancer Res 1994; 54: 2823–6.

77. Gillespie MT, Thomas RJ, Pu ZY et al. Calcitonin receptors, bone sialoprotein and osteopontin are expressed in primary breast cancers. Int J Cancer 1997; 73: 812–15.

78. Bellahcene A, Kroll M, Liebens F, Castronovo V. Bone sialoprotein expression in primary human breast cancer is associated with bone metastases development. J Bone Min Res 1996; 11: 665–70.

79. Bellahcene A, Menard S, Bufalino R et al. Expression of bone sialoprotein in primary human breast cancer is associated with poor survival. Int J Cancer 1996; 69: 350–3.

80. Sung V, Stubbs JT III, Fisher L et al. Bone sialoprotein supports breast cancer cell adhesion proliferation and migration through differential usage of the α(v)β3 and α(v)β5 integrins. J Cell Physiol 1998; 176: 482–94.

81. Graham JD, Balleine RL, Milliken JS et al. Expression of osteonectin mRNA in human breast tumours is inversely correlated with oestrogen receptor content. Eur J Cancer 1997; 33: 1654–60.

82. Gilles C, Bassuk JA, Pulyaeva H et al. SPARC/ osteonectin induces matrix metalloproteinase 2 activation in human breast cancer cell lines. Cancer Res 1998; 58: 5529–36.

83. Kissin MW, Henderson MA, Danks JA et al. Parathyroid hormone-related protein in breast cancers of widely varying prognosis. Eur J Surg Oncol 1993; 19: 134–42.

84. Bundred NJ, Walls J, Radcliffe WA. Parathyroid hormone-related protein, bone metastases and hypercalcaemia of malignancy. Ann R Coll Surg Engl 1996; 78: 354–8.

85. Colleoni M, O'Neill A, Goldhirsch A et al. Identifying breast cancer patients at high risk for bone metastases. Clin Oncol 2000; 18: 3925–35.

86. Hortobagyi GN, Theriault RL, Porter L et al. Efficacy of pamidronate in reducing skeletal complications in patients with breast cancer and lytic bone metastases. Protocol 19, Aredia Breast Cancer Study Group. N Engl J Med 1996; 335: 1785–91.

87. Hortobagyi GN, Theriault RL, Lipton A et al. Long-term prevention of skeletal complications of metastatic breast carcinoma with pamidronate. J Clin Oncol 1998; 16: 2038–44.

88. Berenson JR, Lipton A. Bisphosphonates in the treatment of malignant bone disease. Ann Rev Med 1999; 50: 237–48.

89. Rodan GA, Martin TJ. Therapeutic approaches to bone diseases. Science 2000; 289: 1508–14.

3

Osteoblastic Metastases

Peter I. Croucher

University of Sheffield Medical School, Sheffield, UK

INTRODUCTION

A number of tumours commonly metastasise to bone, the best examples of which are breast cancer and prostate cancer. The presence of tumour cells in bone can result in the development of either osteolytic bone lesions, an osteoblastic disease or a mixed osteolytic/ osteoblastic disease. Osteoblastic metastases occur most commonly in prostate cancer. However, other tumours that metastasise to bone or grow in bone, e.g. breast cancer, can also give rise to an osteoblastic disease. Prostatic carcinoma is one of the most prevalent cancers in men, accounting for 29% of new diagnoses [1]. A major clinical feature of prostate cancer is the development of bone metastases, which are a major cause of morbidity. It has been estimated that 80–100% of men who die from prostate carcinoma have bone metastases [2]. The majority of such metastastes are osteoblastic in nature.

Our understanding of the mechanisms that lead to the development of osteoblastic metastases are poor; however, recent studies have begun to shed new light on this complex area. The purpose of this chapter is to discuss our current understanding and some of these new developments. Since prostatic carcinoma is the tumour most commonly associated with osteoblastic metastases, the chapter will focus on data drawn from this area. However, lessons have also been learnt from other tumour types.

TUMOUR CELL METASTASIS TO BONE

With the exception of those tumours that grow in bone, tumour cells that metastasise to bone require a unique set of characteristics that enable them to find their way from the primary tumour site to bone, where they are able to grow and survive. These features include the ability of tumour cells to detach from the primary tumour. This is likely to require a change in tumour cell phenotype, with modulation of expression of adhesion molecules, proteinases and growth factors. Metastatic tumour cells utilise these features to enter the circulation and migrate to a distant site. Tumour cells that arrest in a capillary bed in bone leave the circulation by a process known as extravasation. On entry into the bone marrow microenvironment, tumour cells encounter an entirely different environment, to which they respond by growth and survival. A consequence of these cells within the marrow microenvironment is the development of local changes in bone. The events that lead to the changes in phenotype, and whether these changes continue throughout the metastatic process, are unclear. However, they are also likely to involve the regulated expression of adhesion molecules, growth factors and proteinases, with expression influenced by the properties of adjacent stromal and bone cells.

The reason why some tumours, but not others, metastasise to bone and give rise to osteoblastic metastases is unclear. It has been suggested that this results from a number of characteristics, including anatomical features, tumour cell-specific features and the suitability of the bone marrow microenvironment [3]. The importance of this latter feature was originally recognised by Paget in the "seed and soil" hypothesis [4]. Paget proposed that tumour cells, the "seed", could be disseminated widely, but only grow when they localise in an appropriate environment, the "soil".

Textbook of Bone Metastases. Edited by C. Jasmin, R. E. Coleman, L. R. Coia, R. Capanna and G. Saillant

Whether the metastatic processes that give rise to osteoblastic disease differ from those that give rise to osteolytic disease is unclear. However, it appears likely that tumours that metastasise to bone will have many features in common. Subtle differences in cellular phenotype, and interactions with the local bone microenvironment, may be more important in determining whether there is a predominantly osteoblastic or osteolytic response in bone.

BONE REMODELLING AND TUMOUR METASTASES

Under normal circumstances, bone is constantly being turned over by a process known as bone remodelling. A quantum of bone is resorbed by osteoclasts and this is replaced with new, structurally competent bone by osteoblasts. These events take place in discrete sites throughout the skeleton and are known as basic multicellular units. The processes of bone resorption and formation are coupled in both time and space, with the amount of bone resorbed being approximately equal to that formed. Under these circumstances there is no net loss of bone. However, as we age the amount of bone resorbed is marginally greater than that formed; we enter a period of negative remodelling balance and, as a result, we gradually lose bone. If tumour cells metastasise to bone, or grow in bone, they are ideally placed to influence this remodelling cycle. Clearly, tumour cells can influence the cells of bone in a number of ways and in doing so they can have very different consequences, e.g. tumour cells can stimulate an increase in osteoclast activity, which can result in an increase in bone loss and the development of an osteolytic disease. Alternatively, tumour cells can stimulate bone formation, which can give rise to an osteosclerotic disease. In addition, by increasing the frequency of these remodelling units the magnitude of any response can be increased significantly (Figure 3.1).

MECHANISMS OF OSTEOBLASTIC METASTASES DEVELOPMENT

Once tumour cells find their way to the local bone marrow microenvironment they can modulate bone remodelling. Those tumours that give rise to predominantly osteoblastic metastases can do so in several

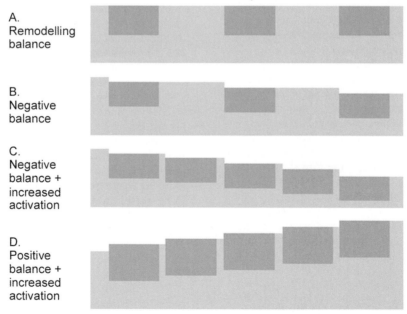

A. Remodelling balance

B. Negative balance

C. Negative balance + increased activation

D. Positive balance + increased activation

Figure 3.1. Diagrammatic representation of the possible consequences of altering remodelling activity within individual bone remodelling units; (A–D) represent the cumulative effect of remodelling activity over time. The dark boxes represent the remodelling activity of an individual remodelling unit. (A) Remodelling balance—the amount of bone resorbed is equal to that formed. (B) Negative remodelling balance—the amount of bone resorbed exceeds that formed. (C) Negative remodelling balance and increased activation of new remodelling units. (D) Positive remodelling balance and increased activation frequency—the amount of bone resorbed is less than that formed, coupled with an increase in the frequency of activation of remodelling units, leading to a rapid increase in bone deposition

ways (Figure 3.2). Tumour cells can promote an increase in bone remodelling, with the remodelling balance favouring bone formation rather than bone resorption. In this situation the increased osteoblastic activity would be preceded by bone resorption. Alternatively, bone formation could occur in the absence of prior resorption (Figure 3.2). However, of these two possibilities there is now increasing evidence to suggest that osteoblastic metastasis is associated with prior bone resorption.

Histomorphometric studies have reported an increase in bone resorption in bone biopsies taken from both metastatic sites and from unaffected areas of patients with prostate cancer [5,6]. A number of studies have also demonstrated that biochemical markers of bone resorption are elevated in men with prostate cancer and evidence of osteoblastic metastases. For example, Nemoto et al. [7] have reported that pyridinoline concentrations may be increased in some patients with metastatic prostate cancer when compared to subjects with locally confined disease. In addition, Maeda et al. [8] and Noguchi and Noda [9] have demonstrated that serum concentrations of pyridinoline cross-linked carboxyterminal telopeptide of type I collagen (ICTP) are also increased in patients with prostate cancer with bone metastases when compared to those without metastases. Indeed, the magnitude of serum ICTP increase was associated with the extent of metastasis [9]. Urinary markers of type I collagen telopeptides are also increased in patients with prostate cancer with evidence of metastases, when compared to those without metastases or patients with benign prostatic hyperplasia. Interestingly, treatment

of patients with bone metastases with the bisphophonate pamidronate resulted in a significant decrease in markers of bone resorption but had no effect on indices of bone formation [10]. However, as yet it is not clear whether these increases in biochemical indices reflect a true increase in bone resorption preceding new bone formation. It remains possible that the increases in resorption markers are a response to the increase in bone formation seen within the metastatic site [11].

A number of in vivo models of osteoblastic metastases have also been described. These models are likely to play an important role in establishing the mechanisms involved in the development of osteoblastic metastases. These studies are already beginning to provide important evidence to support the suggestion that increased osteoclastic activity may be critical in the development of an osteoblastic disease. Yi et al. [12] have demonstrated that MCF-7 breast cells transfected with platelet-derived growth factor give rise to osteoblastic metastases after injection into nude mice. Importantly, this study also demonstrated that there was an initial phase of osteoclastic bone resorption prior to the development of the osteoblastic disease. More recently, Zhang et al. [13] have reported that C4-2B cells, which are derived from the LNCaP human prostate cancer cell line, when injected into the tibia of SCID mice resulted in the development of both osteolytic and osteoblastic lesions. Histological examination revealed the presence of increased numbers of osteoclasts at the tumour interface.

Should bone resorption play a role in the development of osteoblastic metastases, then inhibitors of

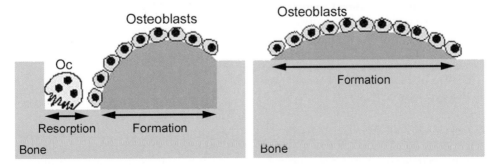

Figure 3.2. Diagrammatic representation of two of the possible mechanisms responsible for the development of osteoblastic metastases. (A) Positive remodelling balance. Osteoclastic bone resorption precedes osteoblastic activity, with the amount of bone formed by osteoblasts being greater than that resorbed by osteoclasts (Oc). (B) Formation without resorption. Bone formation by osteoblasts occurs on quiescent bone surfaces without prior resorption

bone resorption would be predicted to be an effective treatment strategy [14]. Although bisphosphonates have been utilised in patients with osteolytic metastases, there are few studies investigating their effect in osteoblastic metastases (reviewed by Adami [14] and Papapoulos et al. [15]). However, studies have shown that bisphosphonates are effective at reducing biochemical markers of bone resorption in patients with bone metastases, including those with prostate cancer [10,16,17]. In addition, these responses are also associated with a reduction in the bone pain associated with the development of osteoblastic metastases [17,18].

Taken together, these data support the suggestion that increased osteoclastic activity and bone resorption may play an important role in the development of osteoblastic metastases.

FACTORS INVOLVED IN THE DEVELOPMENT OF OSTEOBLASTIC METASTASES

Although there is evidence to suggest that the development of osteoblastic bone metastases is more complex than first thought, with bone resorption preceding bone formation, our understanding of the cellular and molecular mechanisms responsible for the induction of these events is poor. It is therefore likely that tumour cells have the capacity to influence both bone resorption and bone formation. The mechanism by which this is achieved remains unclear. However, tumour cells may be able to produce factors themselves to modulate bone remodelling or to influence the production of factors by the local bone microenvironment. Furthermore, these events could be mediated by the release of soluble factors, or occur via direct cell-to-cell communication.

Factors Implicated in Stimulating Osteoclast Formation in Osteoblastic Metastases

Few studies have examined the ability of tumours that give rise to osteoblastic metastasis to promote osteoclastic activity. However, two factors have been implicated in this activity.

Parathyroid Hormone-related Protein (PTHrP)

Parathyroid hormone-related protein was originally identified as a product of tumour cells that could induce hypercalcaemia [19,20]. Subsequently, studies have demonstrated that PTHrP may play an important role in the development of bone metastases (see

Chapter 5), including mediating breast cancer-induced osteolysis [21]. However, the role of PTHrP in the development of osteoblastic metastases is less clear. Iwamura et al. [22] have reported that samples taken from patients with localised prostate cancer expressed PTHrP, with the staining intensity correlating with increasing tumour grade. Similar observations have been reported by other groups [23,24]. PTHrP has also been shown to be expressed in bone metastases from patients with prostate cancer, although only 50% of specimens were reported to be positive [24]. Studies have demonstrated that overexpression of PTHrP in rat prostate cancer cells results in increased osteoclastic activity when injected *in vivo* [25], although this was not necessarily associated with an increase in the number or size of metastatic lesions [26]. However, the role of PTHrP in the development of osteoblastic metastases remains unclear, as prostate-specific antigen (PSA) has been shown to cleave PTHrP [27]. Furthermore, cleavage has been shown to reduce the ability of PTHrP to stimulate cAMP production in murine osteoblast-like cells, suggesting that PSA may be able to regulate its biological activity [27].

Receptor Activator of NF-κB (RANKL)

The receptor activator of NF-κB ligand (RANKL [28], also known as osteoprotegerin (OPG) ligand [29], osteoclast differentiation factor [30], or TRANCE [31]) has recently been shown to play a critical role in normal osteoclast development (see Chapter 8). RANKL is expressed by stromal cells and osteoblasts in the local bone marrow microenvironment, where it can bind to its receptor RANK [28] on the surface of osteoclast precursors. The binding of RANKL to RANK plays an important role in promoting osteoclast differentiation and bone resorption. A soluble decoy receptor, known as osteoprotegerin (OPG), has also been identified [32]. OPG binds RANKL, inhibiting its interaction with RANK and preventing osteoclast formation. The importance of this system in normal osteoclast formation has resulted in considerable interest in its role in pathological conditions, including breast cancer-induced bone disease and multiple myeloma. Recent studies have also begun to investigate the role of this system in prostate cancer. Brown et al. [33] have examined expression of RANKL and OPG in tissue from patients with prostate cancer. RANKL was expressed by the majority of prostate cancer samples, whereas OPG could only be detected in 2/10 specimens. The proportion of tumour cells expressing RANKL was reported to be increased in bone metastases when compared to the primary tumour [33]. Zhang et al. [13] have also reported that C4-2B cells directly stimulated the formation of murine tartrate-resistant, acid phosphatase-positive, multinucleate, osteoclast-like cells *in vitro*. This activity was reported to be mediated by the release of a soluble form of RANKL. In addition, treatment of animals bearing C4-2B cells with osteoprotegerin prevented the establishment of both osteolytic and osteoblastic metastases induced by the C4-2B cells [13]. In contrast, OPG has no effect on subcutaneously implanted tumours.

Factors Stimulating Bone Formation in Osteoblastic Metastases

The factors responsible for stimulating osteoblastic activity are also unclear. Simpson et al. [34] demonstrated that conditioned media from *Xenopus* oocytes injected with the mRNA from a human prostate cancer cell line stimulated the growth of rat osteosarcoma and production of alkaline phosphatase activity. Perkel et al. [35] demonstrated that PC-3-conditioned media stimulated the proliferation of human osteoblasts but not fibroblasts. Similarly, Martinez et al. [36] reported that PC-3 cell-conditioned media could stimulate proliferation of foetal rat calvarial cells; however, in this model conditioned media inhibited alkaline phosphatase activity. In contrast, extracts from prostatic adenocarcinoma tissue were reported to stimulate both the proliferation of osteoblast-like cells and alkaline phosphatase activity [37]. More recently, studies have shown that a bone-derived prostate cancer cell line, MDA Pca 2b, induced the proliferation of murine osteoblasts and promoted their differentiation [38]. This osteoblastic response was confirmed *in vivo* by intrafemoral injection of MDA PCa 2b cells into SCID mice. The increase in osteoblastic differentiation was associated with an upregulation of Cbfa1, an osteoblast-specific transcription factor [38]. Although these studies suggest that prostate cancer cells are able to produce factor(s) that can stimulate an osteoblastic response, the specific identity of this activity remains unknown and may represent more than one activity. A number of growth factors have now been implicated in mediating the increased osteoblastic response, although in the majority of cases there is no direct evidence to support a causal role.

Transforming Growth Factor Beta (TGFβ)

TGFβ plays an important role in promoting osteoblast differentiation. It is synthesised by osteoblasts in a latent form, which can be activated by proteolytic activity or by acid pH to release active TGFβ. TGFβ stimulates expression of a range of molecules important for osteoblast function, including type I collagen, alkaline phosphatase, osteonectin and osteocalcin. Local injection of TGFβ results in an increase in new bone formation. These observations make TGFβ a strong candidate for the activity responsible for inducing the osteoblastic response in prostate cancer. Indeed, prostate cancer cells have been reported to produce TGFβ, expression of which may be greater than that seen in normal prostate tissue. Steiner et al. have shown that prostate cancer cells produce TGFβ in the latent form, although, much of this can be activated by the tumour cells [39]. In contrast, Eklov et al. [40] have demonstrated that malignant, but not benign, prostate tissue produces TGFβ but not the latent transforming growth factor binding protein. However, other than by association there are currently no data directly linking expression of TGFβ with induction of new bone formation in prostate tumour metastases.

Bone Morphogenetic Proteins (BMPs)

BMPs are members of the larger TGFβ superfamily. BMPs were originally identified as molecules that can stimulate bone formation *in vivo*; however, they have now been shown to exhibit other biological activities. The BMPs appear to initiate a complex cascade of events that lead to new bone formation, including the recruitment of mesenchymal cells, their differentiation to chondrocytes, angiogenesis and osteoblast differentiation [41]. BMPs also have effects on committed osteoblast precursors, promoting upregulation of alkaline phosphatase, type I collagen and expression of osteocalcin [42,43]. Given this ability, a number of early studies explored the possibility that these molecules may play a role in the development of osteoblastic metastases. Bentley et al. [44] and Harris et al. [45] showed that members of the BMP family, including BMPs-2, -3, -4 and -6, were expressed by both benign and malignant prostate tissue and by a number of prostate cancer cell lines. However, levels of expression varied between normal and metastatic tissue. The study by Bentley et al. [44] reported that BMP-6 expression was present in more than 50% of patients with metastatic prostate cancer but not in patients with non-metastatic or benign disease. This observation prompted more extensive investigations into the expression of BMP-6. Hamdy et al. [46] reported that BMP-6 mRNA was expressed in prostatic epithelial cells from 95% of patients with metastatic disease but only 18% of patients with localised disease. The BMP-6 protein was also found in all patients with metastatic disease. Furthermore, BMP-6 mRNA was detected in 11/13 bone metastases from patients with prostatic cancer, and in three paired samples of prostate carcinoma and osteoblastic metastases [47]. However, immunohistochemistry analysis also demonstrated expression of BMP-6 in benign prostatic hyperplasia [46]. Although BMP-6 has been shown to be over-expressed, there is no direct evidence to suggest a functional link between expression and the ability to promote osteoblastic metastases.

Thomas et al. [48] have recently reported that a new member of the BMP family, placental bone morpho-genetic protein, is expressed at high levels in normal prostate. Interestingly, this member of the family is downregulated in the prostate as the tumour progresses. However, this molecule was shown to be expressed at sites of osteoblastic metastases, raising the possibility that this member of the family may also be involved in the development of the osteoblastic disease.

Insulin-like Growth Factors (IGF)

The insulin-like growth factor system is a complex system that includes IGF1 and IGF2, two receptors and at least six IGF binding proteins (IGFBPs), which regulate the activity of the IGFs. IGF1 and IGF2 are synthesised by osteoblasts and present in bone matrix. The IGFs are released from bone during the process of bone resorption and are made available to regulate osteoblastic activity. Studies have shown that these molecules are able to stimulate the proliferation of osteoblast-like cells and upregulate type I collagen synthesis *in vitro*. IGFs stimulate bone formation *in vivo* and mice with a mutation in the IGF receptor have abnormalities in skeletal development [49].

When cultured *in vitro*, prostatic epithelial cells express IGFs and IGFBPs [50]. Furthermore, IGFBP2 and IGFBP3 are expressed by malignant cells in prostate tissue, with IGFBP2 expression being increased and IGFBP3 decreased [51]. Studies have also shown that the serum IGFBP2 concentrations are increased in prostate cancer and that this is positively correlated with prostate-specific antigen concentrations [52,53]. Cohen et al. reported that serum IGFBP3 levels were not significantly different in patients with prostate cancer when compared to controls [52]. However, serum IGFBP3 concentrations have been shown to be lower in patients with prostate cancer and bone metastases when compared to controls [53].

Therefore, based upon the observations that prostate cancer cells express components of the IGF system, and that IGFs regulate the activity of osteoblasts, it has been suggested that local production of IGFs in bone may contribute to the development of new bone formation in prostate cancer metastases [3].

Fibroblast Growth Factors (FGF)

FGFs are a family of heparin-binding growth factors that are potent regulators of cell proliferation and differentiation. There are at least nine members of the family, with the prototypes acidic FGF and basic FGF being FGF1 and FGF2, respectively. The FGF/FGF receptor (FGFR) system is believed to play an important role in skeletal biology. FGFs are stored in bone matrix and released during the process of resorption. These molecules stimulate the proliferation of osteoblasts and regulate synthesis of other growth factors that are important in bone formation. The importance of these molecules in skeletal biology has been further demonstrated by the identification of genetic mutations that lead to skeletal abnormalities. Mutations in FGFR1 and FGFR2 are found in the craniosynostosis syndromes [54], whereas mutations in FGFR3 are associated with the development of achondroplasia [55].

Several studies have demonstrated that prostate cancer cell lines and primary tissues are able to express the genes for, or produce, FGFs [56,57]. Expression has also been observed in tissues from patients with benign prostatic hyperplasia and at a higher level than in normal prostate [58]. In addition to prostate cancer cells, other tumour cells that can give rise to an osteoblastic disease have also been reported to produce FGFs. For example, Izbicka et al. isolated an extended form of FGF2 from an amniotic tumour that has been shown to stimulate new bone formation *in vivo* [59]. These observations therefore raise the possibility that the FGFs, produced by tumour cells, could also contribute to the development of an osteoblastic response in cells that metastasise to bone.

Endothelin-1 (ET1)

ET1 is most commonly known as a potent vasocon-strictor; however, this molecule can also stimulate osteoblastic activity. Nelson et al. [60] have reported that prostate cancer cell lines express the ET1 mRNA and secrete the protein. Plasma ET1 concentrations are significantly elevated in men with metastatic prostate cancer when compared to those with organ-confined disease [60]. ET1 has also been shown to be a potent mitogen for osteoblast-like cells and modulates alkaline phosphatase levels *in vitro* [61]. It has therefore been suggested that ET1 may play a critical role in the development of osteoblastic metastases in prostate cancer [60]. Studies have also shown that co-culturing human prostate cancer cells with bone increases expression of ET1 [62].

The role of ET1 in the development of osteoblastic metastases has also been investigated in a number of murine models of osteoblastic metastases. Studies have demonstrated that the WISH tumour cell line, which is derived from amnion, produces ET1 and can stimulate new bone formation *in vivo* [63]. Nelson et al. [63] demonstrated that overexpression of ET1 in these cells results in a significant increase in new bone formation *in vivo* when compared to WISH cells expressing normal levels of ET1. New bone formation was significantly decreased in animals treated with an endothelin A receptor antagonist [63]. Yin et al. [64] have also reported that the human breast cancer cell line, ZR-75-1, also gives rise to osteoblastic metastases when injected into the cardiac ventricle of nude mice. ZR-75-1 cells promoted a significant increase in cancellous bone volume in the long bones when compared to control animals or those injected with the MDA-231 cell line, a line that gives rise to osteolytic disease in this model. A comparison of factors produced by these two lines revealed that the ZR-75-1 cell line produced significantly more ET1 than MDA-231 cells. A number of other growth factors that have been reported to stimulate bone formation were produced at similar levels.

Prostate cancer cells have also been reported to decrease osteoclastic bone resorption *in vitro* [62]. This effect was inhibited with antibodies to ET1 [62]. This raises the possibility that ET1 could play a role in both the suppression of osteoclastic acitivity and stimulation of new bone formation. This uncoupling of the normal process of bone remodelling could contribute significantly to the development of osteoblastic metastases.

Other Factors

Although the factors described above have been implicated in the development of osteoblastic metastases, there is often little direct evidence for a causal role. This raises the possibility that, in the future, other factors that are demonstrated to promote bone formation may also be shown to be produced by tumour cells and able to promote osteoblastic metastases. These factors need not be confined to soluble growth factors and cytokines, but may include direct cell-to-cell communication, via adhesion molecules or other molecules such as proteinases. Although there are little data investigating the role of adhesion molecules in this process, studies have begun to investigate the role of proteinases.

Prostate-specific antigen (PSA) is a serine proteinase produced by prostatic epithelial cells. PSA has been reported to cleave IGFBP3 [65] and to promote the proliferation of osteoblasts, possibly by activating TGFβ [66]. Furthermore, as discussed previously, PSA is also able to cleave PTHrP and modulate its biological activity. Prostate cancer cells also produce urokinase-type plasminogen activator (uPA) [67] and levels may be increased in bone metastases when compared to the primary tumour [68]. uPA is a serine proteinase and can cleave extracellular matrix proteins, including fibronectin and laminin, and may therefore play a role in tumour cell migration. However, Rabbani et al. [69] have reported that a fragment of uPA can stimulate the proliferation of osteoblasts *in vitro*. Overexpression of uPA in the Mat LyLu rat prostate cell line has been shown to result in a shorter time to hind limb paralysis [70]. This was also associated with tumour metastases occurring sooner. Osteoblastic metastases were a significant feature in animals bearing the uPA-overexpressing cells. Whether this reflects an increase in the ability of tumour cells to metastasise to bone or an effect on the osteoblasts themselves is not clear. However, Koutsilieris et al. [71] have shown that uPA may be able to cleave IGFBPs, raising the possibility that uPA may be able to mediate a direct effect on bone formation via the IGF system.

CONCLUSIONS

The development of osteoblastic bone metastases is a complex process requiring a coordinated sequence of events. These include the ability of metastatic cells to detach from the primary tumour, their capacity to migrate to bone and their ability to stimulate new bone formation. It is likely that a series of local growth factors, adhesion molecules and proteinases contribute to this activity, although their identity remains unclear. Studies over recent years have also suggested that the osteoblastic response may be preceded by osteoclastic bone resorption. These observations have resulted in a search for factors that are produced by tumour cells, and that may be responsible for inducing both bone resorption and new bone formation (Figure 3.3).

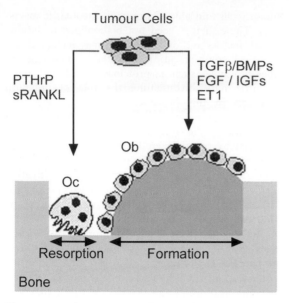

Figure 3.3. Diagram illustrating the role that different growth factors and cytokines may play in the development of osteoblastic metastases. Tumour cells arising in bone may produce factors that can stimulate osteoclast formation and bone resorption. In addition to promoting bone resorption, tumour cells also produce factors that stimulate osteoblast recruitment and differentiation and the synthesis of new bone

Studies have implicated PTHrP and, more recently, RANKL in promoting bone resorption in prostate cancer. Furthermore, a number of candidates have been implicated in stimulating new bone formation in osteoblastic metastases, including TGFβ, the BMPS, FGFs, IGFs and ET1. However, in the majority of cases no direct functional link has been identified. This will continue to remain an important challenge over coming years. The suggestion that osteoclastic bone resorption may contribute to the development of osteoblastic metastases may provide new therapeutic opportunities. The bisphosphonates remain the most promising of such candidates; however, new approaches to inhibiting bone resorption, e.g. with osteoprotegerin, may also prove to be important. Similarly, the identification of the factors that stimulate new bone formation will continue to provide new targets, e.g. by blocking the activity of ET1 with receptor antagonists. It is therefore likely that continued improvements in our understanding of the mechanisms that lead to the development of osteoblastic metastases, and the identification of the factors involved, will lead to new therapeutic opportunities in the future.

REFERENCES

1. Carlin BI, Andriole GL. The natural history, skeletal complications, and managment of bone metastases in patients with prostate carcinoma. Cancer 2000; 88: 2989–94.
2. Whitmore WJ. Natural history and staging of prostate cancer. Urol Clin N Am 1984; 11: 209–20.
3. Guise TA, Mundy GR. Cancer Bone Endocr Rev 1998; 19: 18–54.
4. Paget S. The distribution of secondary growths in cancer of the breast. Lancet 1889; 1: 571–3.
5. Urwin GH et al. Generalised increase in bone resorption in carcinoma of the prostate. Eur J Urol 1985; 57: 721–3.
6. Clarke NW, McClure J, George NJR. Morphometric evidence for bone resorption and replacement in prostate cancer. Br J Urol 1991; 68: 74–80.
7. Nemoto R et al. Serum pyridinoline cross-links as markers of tumour-induced bone resorption. Br J Urol 1997; 80: 274–80.
8. Maeda H et al. Correlation between bone metabolic markers and bone scan in prostate cancer. J Urol 1997; 157: 539–43.
9. Noguchi M, Noda S. Pyridinoline cross-linked carboxy-terminal telopeptide of type I collagen as a useful marker for monitoring metastatic bone activity in men with prostate cancer. J Urol 2001; 166: 1106–10.
10. Garnero P et al. Markers of bone turnover for the management of patients with bone metastases from prostate cancer. Br J Cancer 2000; 82: 858–64.
11. Roodman GD. Biology of osteoclast activation in cancer. J Clin Oncol 2001; 19: 3562–71.
12. Yi B et al. Evidence that osteolysis precedes osteoblastic lesions in a model of human osteoblastic metastases. J Bone Miner Res 2000; 15: S177.
13. Zhang J et al. Osteoprotegerin inhibits prostate cancer-induced osteoclastogenesis and prevents prostate tumor growth in bone. J Clin Invest 2001; 107: 1235–44.
14. Adami S. Bisphosphonates and prostate carcinoma. Cancer 1997; 80: 1674–9.
15. Papapoulos SE, Hamdy NAT, van der Pluijm G. Bisphosphonates in the management of prostate carcinoma metastatic to the skeleton. Cancer 2000; 88: 3047–53.
16. Vinholes J et al. Metabolic effects of pamidronate in patients with metastatic bone disease. Br J Cancer 1996; 73: 1089–95.
17. Pelger RC et al. Effects of the bisphosphonate olpadronate in patients with carcinoma of the prostate metastatic to the skeleton. Bone 1998; 22: 403–8.
18. Adami S et al. Dichlormethylene-diphosphonate in patients with prostate carcinoma metastatic to the skeleton. J Urol 1985; 134: 1152–4.
19. Moseley JM et al. Parathyroid hormone-related protein purified from a human lung cancer-cell line. Proc Natl Acad Sci USA 1987; 84: 5048–52.
20. Strewler GJ et al. Parathyroid hormone like protein from renal carcinoma cells. Structural and functional homology with parathyroid hormone. J Clin Invest 1987; 80: 1803–7.
21. Guise TA et al. Evidence for a causal role of parathyroid hormone-related protein in the pathogenesis of human breast cancer-mediated osteolysis. J Clin Invest 1996; 98: 1544–9.

22. Iwamura M et al. Immunohistochemical localization of parathyroid hormone-related protein in prostate cancer. Cancer Res 1993; 53: 1724–6.

23. Asadi F et al. Enhanced expression of parathyroid hormone-related protein in prostate cancer as compared to benign prostatic hyperplasia. Hum Pathol 1996; 27: 1319–23.

24. Iddon J et al. Expression of parathyroid hormone-related protein and its receptor in bone metastases from prostate cancer. J Pathol 2000; 191: 170–4.

25. Rabbani SA et al. Overproduction of parathyroid hormone-related peptide results in increased osteolytic skeletal metastasis by prostate cancer cells in vivo. Int J Cancer 1999; 80: 257–64.

26. Blomme EA et al. Skeletal metastasis of prostate adenocarcinoma in rats: morphometric analysis and role of parathyroid hormone-related protein. Prostate 1999; 39: 187–97.

27. Cramer SD, Chen Z, Peehl DM. Prostate specific antigen cleaves parathyroid hormone-related protein in the PTH-like domain: inactivation of PTHrP-stimulated cAMP accumulation in mouse osteoblasts. J Urol 1996; 156: 526–31.

28. Anderson DM et al. A homologue of the TNF receptor and its ligand enhance T-cell growth and dendritic cell function. Nature 1997; 390: 175–9.

29. Lacey DL et al. Osteoprotegerin ligand is a cytokine that regulates osteoclast differentiation and activation. Cell 1998; 93: 165–76.

30. Suda T, Takahashi N, Martin TJ. Modulation of osteoclast differentiation. Endocr Rev 1992; 13: 66–80.

31. Wong BR et al. TRANCE is a novel ligand of the tumor necrosis factor receptor family that activates c-Jun N-terminal kinase in T cells. J Biol Chem 1997; 272: 25190–4.

32. Simonet WS et al. Osteoprotegerin: a novel secreted protein involved in the regulation of bone density. Cell 1997; 89: 309–19.

33. Brown JM et al. Osteoprotegerin and rank ligand expression in prostate cancer. Urology 2001; 57: 611–16.

34. Simpson E et al. Identification of a messenger ribonucleic acid fraction in human prostatic cancer cells coding for a novel osteoblast-stimulating factor. Endocrinology 1985; 117: 1615–20.

35. Perkel VS et al. Human prostatic cancer cells, PC3, elaborate mitogenic activity which selectively stimulates human bone cells. Cancer Res 1990; 50: 6902–7.

36. Martinez J, Silva S, Santibanez JF. Prostate-derived soluble factors block osteoblast differentiation in culture. J Cell Biochem 1996; 61: 18–25.

37. Koutsilieris M et al. Characteristics of prostate-derived growth factors for cells of the osteoblast phenotype. J Clin Invest 1987; 80: 941–6.

38. Yang J et al. Prostate cancer cells induce osteoblast differentiation through a Cbfa1-dependent pathway. Cancer Res 2001; 61: 5652–9.

39. Steiner MS et al. Expression of transforming growth factor-β1 in prostate cancer. Endocrinology 1994; 135: 2240–7.

40. Eklov S et al. Lack of the latent transforming growth factor β binding protein in malignant, but not benign prostatic tissue. Cancer Res 1993; 53: 3193–7.

41. Reddi AH. Bone morphogenetic proteins: an unconventional approach to isolation of first mammalian morphogens. Cytokine Growth Factor Rev 1997; 8: 11–20.

42. Chen TL et al. Bone morphogenetic protein-2b stimulation of growth and osteogenic phenotype in rat osteoblast-like cells: comparison with TGF-β1. J Bone Min Res 1991; 6: 1387–93.

43. Takuwa Y et al. Bone morphogenetic protein-2 stimulates alkaline phosphatase activity and collagen synthesis in cultured osteoblastic cells, MC3T3-E1. Biochem Biophys Res Commun 1991; 174: 96–101.

44. Bentley H et al. Expression of bone morphogenetic proteins in human prostatic adenocarcinoma and benign prostatic hyperplasia. Br J Cancer 1992; 66: 1159–63.

45. Harris SE et al. Expression of bone morphogenetic protein messenger RNAs by normal rat and human prostate and prostate cancer cells. Prostate 1994; 24: 204–11.

46. Hamdy FC et al. Immunolocalization and messenger RNA expression of bone morphogenetic protein-6 in human benign and malignant prostatic tissue. Cancer Res 1997; 57: 4427–31.

47. Autzen P et al. Bone morphogenetic protein 6 in skeletal metastases from prostate cancer and other common human malignancies. Br J Cancer 1998; 78: 1219–23.

48. Thomas R et al. Placental bone morphogenetic protein (PLAB) gene expression in normal, pre-malignant and malignant human prostate: relation to tumor development and progression. Int J Cancer 2001; 93: 47–52.

49. Liu JP et al. Mice carrying a null mutation of the genes encoding insulin-like growth factor I and type I IGF receptor. Cell 1993; 75: 59–72.

50. Cohen P et al. Insulin-like growth factors (IGFs), IGF receptors and IGF binding proteins in primary cultures of prostate epithelial cells. J Clin Endocrinol Metab 1991; 73: 401–7.

51. Tennant MK et al. Insulin-like growth factor-binding protein-2 and -3 expression in benign human prostate epithelium, prostate intraepithelial neoplasia, and adenocarcinoma of the prostate. J Clin Endocrinol Metab 1996; 81: 411–20.

52. Cohen P et al. Elevated levels of insulin-like growth factor-binding protein-2 in the serum of prostate cancer patients. J Clin Endocrinol Metab 1993; 76: 1031–5.

53. Kanety H et al. Serum insulin-like growth factor binding protein-2 (IGFBP-2) is increased and IGFBP-3 is decreased in patients with prostate cancer: correlation with serum prostate specific antigen. J Clin Endocrinol Metab 1993; 77: 229–33.

54. Muenke M, Schell U. Fibroblast-growth factor receptor mutations in human skeletal disorders. Trends Genet 1995; 11: 308–13.

55. Rousseau F et al. Mutations in the gene encoding fibroblast growth factor receptor-3 ub achondroplasia. Nature 1994; 371: 252–4.

56. Mansson PE et al. Heparin-binding growth factor gene expression and receptor characteristics in normal rat prostate and two transplantable rat prostate tumors. Cancer Res 1989; 49: 2485–94.

57. Nakamoto T et al. Basic fibroblast growth factor in human prostate cancer cells. Cancer Res 1992; 52: 571–7.

58. Mori H et al. Increased expression of genes for basic fibroblast growth factor and transforming growth factor type β2 in human benign prostatic hyperplasia. Prostate 1990; 16: 71–80.

59. Izbicka E et al. Human amniotic tumor that induces new bone formation *in vivo* produces growth-regulatory activity *in vitro* for osteoblasts identified as an extended form of basic fibroblast growth factor. Cancer Res 1996; 56: 633–6.

60. Nelson JB et al. Identification of endothelin-1 in the pathophysiology of metastatic adenocarcinoma of the prostate. Nature Med 1995; 1: 944–9.

61. Takuwa Y, Masaki T, Yamashita K. The effects of endothelin family peptides on cultured osteoblastic cells from rat calvariae. Biochem Biophys Res Commun 1990; 170: 998–1005.

62. Chiao JW et al. Endothelin-1 from prostate cancer cells is enhanced by bone contact which blocks osteoclastic bone resorption. Br J Cancer 2000; 83: 360–5.

63. Nelson JB et al. New bone formation in an osteoblastic tumor model is increased by endothelin-1 overexpression and decreased by endothelin A receptor blockade. Urology 1999; 53: 1063–9.

64. Yin JJ et al. Role of endothelin-1 in osteoblastic metastases to bone. Bone 1998; 23: S377.

65. Fielder PJ et al. Biochemical analysis of prostate specific antigen-proteolysed insulin-like growth factor binding protein-3. Growth Regul 1994; 4: 164–72.

66. Killian CS et al. Mitogenic response of osteoblast cells to prostate-specific antigen suggests an activation of latent TGF-β and proteolytic modulation of cell adhesion receptors. Biochem Biophys Res Commun 1993; 192: 940–7.

67. Hollas W et al. Expression of urokinase and its receptor in invasive and non-invasive prostate cancer cell lines. Thromb Haemostas 1992; 68: 662–6.

68. Kirchheimer JC et al. Plasminogen activator activity in bone metastases of prostatic carcinomas as compared to primary tumors. Invasion Metast 1985; 6: 344–5.

69. Rabbani SA et al. An amino-terminal fragment of urokinase isolated from a prostate cancer cell line (PC-3) is mitogenic for osteoblast-like cells. Biochem Biophys Res Commun 1990; 173: 1058–64.

70. Achbarou A et al. Urokinase overproduction results in increased skeletal metastasis by prostate cancer cells *in vivo*. Cancer Res 1994; 54: 2372–7.

71. Koutsilieris M et al. Urokinase-type plasminogen activator: a paracrine factor regulating bioavailability of IGFs in PA-III cell-induced osteoblastic metastases. Anticancer Res 1993; 13: 481–6.

4

The Role of RANK, RANK Ligand and Osteoprotegerin in the Lytic Effects and Growth of Bone Metastases

Colin R. Dunstan

ANZAC Research Institute, Sydney, NSW, Australia

BONE RESORPTION IS REGULATED BY CELLS OF THE OSTEOBLAST LINEAGE

In 1981, Rodan and Martin [1] proposed that osteoblasts mediate the regulation of bone resorption by calciotropic hormones and other resorptive factors, such as parathyroid hormone-related protein (PTHrP). The basis of their hypothesis was that osteoclasts did not appear to have receptors for parathyroid hormone (PTH), PTHrP and other calciotropic hormones, whereas osteoblasts did have the relevant receptors. In addition, it was noted that osteoblasts or marrow stromal cells had to be present to mediate the resorptive effects of calciotropic hormones and cytokines in *in vitro* cultures of osteoclasts [2]. However, determining the nature of this mediating signal, necessary for the local regulation of bone resorption, proved to be elusive.

DISCOVERY OF THE ROLE OF RANKL, RANK AND OPG IN BONE RESORPTION

The discovery that resolved the mechanism of local regulation of bone resorption was unexpected. Workers at Amgen in California [3] and at Snow Brand Milk Company in Japan [4] independently identified a novel protein, which they named osteoprotegerin (OPG) or osteoclastogenesis inhibitory factor (OCIF), respectively, that *inhibited* the differentiation of osteoclasts *in vitro* and *in vivo*. OPG was found to be a large (120 kDa) dimeric secreted protein with an N-terminal region with homology to the ligand-binding domains of the tumour necrosis factor receptor (TNFR) family. However, the protein had no transmembrane domain or apparent signal transduction sequences. Instead it had a large C-terminal domain, which served to covalently dimerise the molecule and provide heparin-binding capability, and which had weak homology with the death domains of some intracellular proteins [5]. It was found that only the putative ligand-binding domain was required for inhibition of osteoclast differentiation [3].

Yasuda et al. [6] and Lacey et al. [7], again working independently, were able to use OPG as a probe to identify a TNF family member with high affinity for OPG. This molecule was found to have a transmembrane domain, in common with other members of this family, and both the membrane-bound form and a soluble extracellular domain were able to promote osteoclast formation *in vitro*. This molecule had been previously identified as a molecule with potential activity in the immune system, regulating interactions of T cells and dendritic cells, initially as TRANCE [8] and then as a ligand and ligand receptor pair, receptor activator of NF-κB (RANK) and RANK ligand (RANKL) [9]. RANK has been definitively demonstrated to be the relevant receptor for RANKL effects

Textbook of Bone Metastases. Edited by C. Jasmin, R. E. Coleman, L. R. Coia, R. Capanna and G. Saillant

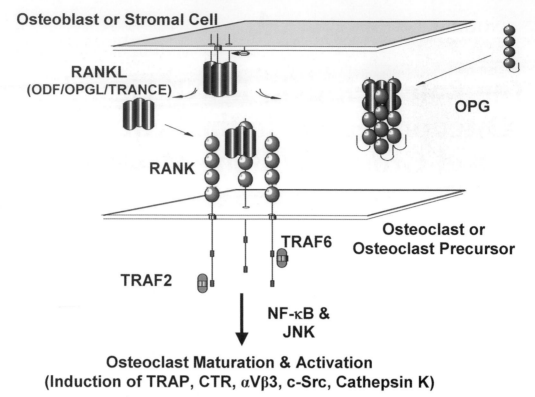

Figure 4.1. Signalling pathway for RANKL. RANKL is expressed initially as a membrane-bound ligand by cells of the osteoblast lineage. In either the membrane-bound form, or when the extracellular domain is released as a soluble form, RANKL binds its receptor RANK on osteoclasts and their precursors to initiate signal transduction. OPG opposes this action by binding and inactivating both soluble and membrane-bound forms of RANKL

on osteoclasts [10,11]. Figure 4.1 illustrates the interactions or RANKL, OPG and RANK molecules to produce and modulate RANK signalling.

RANKL can, with mCSF, replace the requirement for stromal cells for osteoclast generation *in vitro*. RANKL is able to activate freshly isolated mature rat osteoclasts to increase bone resorption [12,13], as indicated by increased pit formation and ultra-structural reorganisation, culminating in the formation of actin ring structures [13]. *In vitro*, RANKL appears to be exposed initially on the cell membrane, with gradual protease-mediated release of a soluble form into the surrounding media [14]. Both RANKL and mCSF appear to be survival factors for osteoclasts and osteoclast precursors [15,16]. In addition, RANKL, when injected into mice, produces profound hypercalcaemia and osteoclast-mediated bone destruction [7]. Thus, RANKL appears to be a potent osteoclast differentiation [7], activation [13] and survival [17] factor which, when administered systemi-cally, is a potent stimulator of bone resorption.

Consistent with an important regulatory role, the expression of both OPG and RANKL are influenced by most of the bone-active hormones and cytokines. Factors like PTHrP that increase bone resorption, increase RANKL expression and, with some exceptions, decrease OPG expression. Thus, the balance of RANKL and OPG expression is changed by these factors. It is likely that the balance of OPG and RANKL levels, rather than the absolute levels, is important [18].

PHYSIOLOGICAL IMPORTANCE OF OPG, RANK, AND RANKL HAVE BEEN DEMONSTRATED BY GENE KNOCKOUT AND OVEREXPRESSION

Targeted disruption of the OPG gene in mice produces animals which develop a severe osteoporotic pheno-type [19,20] (Figure 4.2). These animals are characterised by skeletal deformities, pathological fractures, high bone turnover and increased cortical

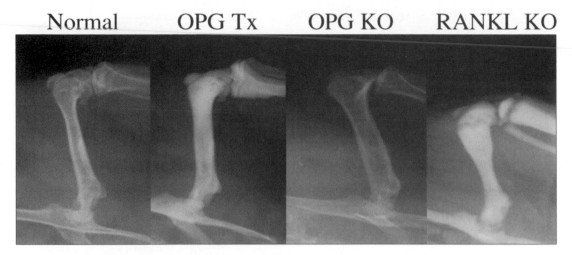

Figure 4.2. Radiographs illustrating the effects on bone of genetic manipulations increasing or abrogating OPG expression, or abrogating RANKL expression. OPG transgenic mice have bones that are increased in density; however, size and shape of the bones are normal. OPG-deficient mice develop osteoporosis, as indicated by the increased radiolucency of the bone. Mice deficient in RANKL have dense bones characteristic of osteopetrosis and in addition the bones are shortened and club-shaped, indicating inhibition of both the growth and modelling of the bones

porosity, and thus share many features with human osteoporosis. In contrast, OPG overexpression results in osteopetrosis [3]. Mice lacking a functional RANKL or RANK gene have been produced and were found to have profoundly severe osteopetrosis, with characteristic small body size, dense bones, failed tooth eruption and club-shaped long bones (Figure 4.2). Histological evaluation of these mice, including long bone metaphyses, vertebra, jaw and calvaria, demonstrated a complete absence of osteoclasts. This study confirms that in mice there is an absolute requirement for RANKL signalling for normal osteoclast formation [21].

and their precursors. Expression of RANKL and OPG is differentially regulated by calciotropic hormones. When PTHrP and pro-resorptive cytokines bind to their respective receptor osteoblasts or their precursors (marrow stromal cells) within the bone marrow, they increase the level of RANKL expression relative to that of OPG [22,23]. RANKL is then available to interact with its receptor RANK on osteoclast precursors to promote differentiation, and on mature osteoclasts to activate bone resorption. Other factors, such as oestrogen, may act to increase expression of OPG relative to RANKL and thus downregulate bone resorption [24].

MECHANISM OF RANKL/OPG/RANK OSTEOBLAST MEDIATION OF THE REGULATION OF BONE RESORPTION

Figure 4.1 illustrates the molecular mechanism of action of OPG, RANK and RANKL in directly regulating the differentiation [7], activation [13] and survival [17] of osteoclasts. Multiple systemic and local signals that modulate bone resorption, including those generated by tumour cells, converge on the RANK signalling pathway to regulate osteoclast differentiation and activity [18] (Figure 4.3). Together, RANKL and OPG form a ligand–ligand inhibitor pair which modulates RANK signalling in osteoclasts

RECOMBINANT OPG IS ABLE TO INHIBIT THE HYPERCALCAEMIC AND PRO-RESORPTIVE EFFECTS OF THE MAJOR PRO-RESORPTIVE HORMONES AND CYTOKINES IN MICE

The ability of OPG to oppose the *in vivo* effects of exogenous cytokines and hormones has been evaluated [24,25,26]. The role of RANKL signalling in mediating a wide range of hormonal and cytokine signalling is supported by the ability of OPG treatment to oppose the hypercalcaemic effects of administered PTH, PTHrP, $1,25(OH)_2D_3$, IL-1β and TNFα. In each case this was associated with inhibition of the increase in osteoclast number produced by these treatments [24].

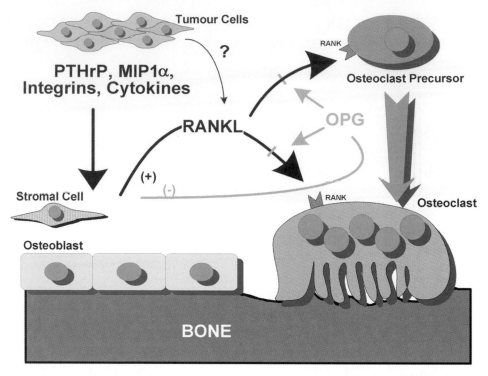

Figure 4.3. Pathway for OPG and RANKL regulation of bone resorption in cancer. Cancer cells produce factors that act in the local microenvironment to increase osteoclastic bone resorption. PTHrP, MIP1α or other factors interact with their respective receptors on osteoblasts and/or stromal cells, which modulates the expression of OPG and RANKL to produce excess production of RANKL relative to OPG, thus increasing the differentiation, activation and survival of osteoclasts

Mice maintained on a low-calcium (0.02%) diet were able to maintain normal blood calcium levels; however, when treated concurrently with recombinant OPG, these mice developed hypocalcaemia, indicating that OPG is also able to inhibit mobilisation of skeletal calcium by endogenous hormones [24].

OPG treatment was also demonstrated to provide almost complete inhibition of bone resorption in an acute inflammatory model of rheumatoid arthritis, despite having no discernible antiinflammatory activity. This model is associated with very high expression levels of the inflammatory cytokines TNFβ and IL-1β [27]. Together these data support the concept that RANKL is at least an essential permissive factor for bone resorption induced by the major pro-resorptive factors, and is likely to be the major mediator of their activity.

ROLE OF REGULATION OF RANKL AND OPG IN NORMAL HUMAN BONE PHYSIOLOGY

Most of the studies of OPG and RANKL have been completed in rodent models. However, there is growing evidence that the same pathways are important in humans. Osteoclast precursors in the human peripheral circulation express RANK and respond *in vitro* to RANKL and m-CSF to form functional osteoclasts [28,29]. In addition, RANK [30], RANKL(7) and OPG(3) are expressed in human tissues and detectable levels of OPG are present in the circulation of healthy adult humans [31,32]. A recent report indicates that bone resorption is inhibited in humans by systemic administration of recombinant OPG. Subcutaneous injection of a single dose of OPG in healthy post-menopausal women dose-dependently suppressed the surrogate marker of bone resorption, urinary N-telopeptide of collagen (N-Tx). Suppression of N-Tx was rapid, with significant effects seen 12 h after dosing, with maximal suppression of approximately 80% occurring 3–4 days after treatment (Figure 4.4) [33]. The congenital condition familial expansile osteolysis, a disease marked by high bone remodelling, has been found to be the result of an activating mutation of RANK [34]. Together these results demonstrate the relevance of this pathway in normal human bone metabolism.

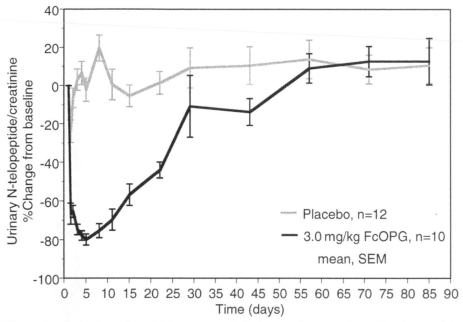

Figure 4.4. Effects of a single dose of an OPG construct (FcOPG) on urinary N-telopeptide of collagen levels in healthy postmenopausal women. Following a single subcutaneous dose of FcOPG, biological activity was determined in healthy postmenopausal women with the surrogate marker of bone resorption, urinary N-telopeptide of collagen. This marker is a cross-linked product of bone collagen breakdown that is secreted in the urine. OPG rapidly and profoundly suppressed bone resorption as assessed by this marker, confirming the importance of RANKL in normal human physiological bone resorption

ROLE OF RANKL/OPG/RANK IN OTHER SYSTEMS

While OPG and RANK are widely expressed, the expression of RANKL is restricted to areas of bone resorption, mammary glands, and to organs of the immune system. RANK- and RANKL-deficient mice lack lymph nodes and are unable to suckle their young, indicating roles in lymph node organogenesis [21,30] and in mammary gland development [35]. In mammary gland, RANKL is required for the differentiation of epithelial cells to form the lobular alveolar structure in pregnant mice. This defect can be prevented by the local delivery of RANKL to the mammary gland [35]. Whether the role of RANKL in normal mammary gland plays any role in the development of mammary tumours or their propensity to metastasise to bone has not been studied in detail.

RANKL may have additional roles in the modulation of immune function. Indeed RANKL has been described as a protein produced by activated T cells [8,9]. In each of these cases it was proposed that RANKL functioned in the interaction of T cells and dendritic cells. RANKL has been proposed to be a survival factor for dendritic cells [8]. OPG has been reported to also bind and inactivate soluble forms of TRAIL (with lower affinity than with RANKL), another TNF family member with potential cytotoxic activity [36]. However, OPG was previously reported to have little or no affinity to membrane-expressed TRAIL [3], and the original observation of binding may have been partly explained by an *in vitro* artefact. However, in adult animals the role of RANKL and OPG in the immune system remains unclear. In OPG-transgenic animals with high circulating levels of OPG throughout life, organs of the immune system were normal and mice had a normal life expectancy, implying a functional immune system [3].

CIRCULATING OPG AND RANKL LEVELS IN NORMAL HUMAN POPULATIONS AND IN DISEASE

It is likely that in human bone disease, dysregulation of calciotropic hormones, inflammatory cytokines or other factors also increase the expression of RANKL relative to that of OPG, producing increased bone resorption. Our understanding of how specific diseases impact on the regulation of OPG and RANKL is in its

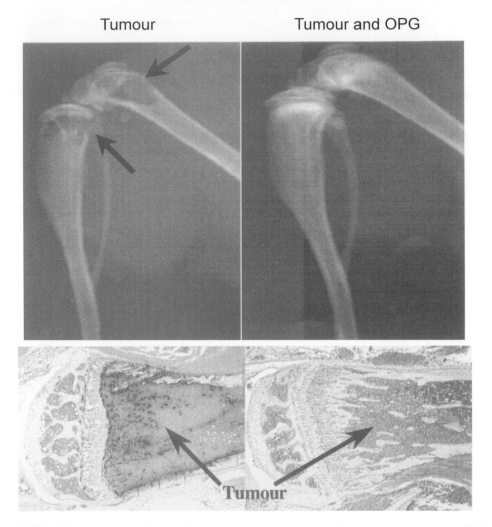

Figure 4.5. OPG inhibits osteolysis and increased osteoclast number in models of metastatic breast cancer. Nude mice were inoculated via the left venticle with human breast cancer cells (MDA-231). After 4 weeks, lytic lesions were apparent in radiographs of the proximal tibia and distal femur (arrows, upper left panel). Histologically, these tumour foci in the bone were associated with increased numbers of osteoclasts (dark TRAP-stained cells) and marked bone destruction (lower left panel). Treatment with OPG completely prevented the appearance of lytic lesions on radiographs (upper right panel), profoundly inhibited the appearance of osteoclasts, and preserved bone structure (lower right panel) (see [56] for complete data)

infancy. RANKL is initially expressed in membrane-bound form but can be released in an active soluble form by protease activity [14]; however, measurement of circulating levels has not been reported, perhaps due to the lack of appropriate antibodies. OPG, while a soluble protein, has an affinity for heparin and, when injected systemically in rats, has a very short half-life of 20–30 minutes in the circulation [37]. Clearance mechanisms for OPG have not been determined. Detectable levels of OPG are present in the peripheral circulation and measurement of these in various disease states may help elucidate the underlying pathology. There have been reported marked elevations of OPG with ageing, with greater increases in osteoporotic patients, suggesting a compensatory increase of OPG in osteoporosis [31]. However, this was not found with another assay, in which only marginal increases were observed with ageing [32]. OPG is expressed in many tissues where it is likely that it predominantly acts locally, and it is likely that what is measured in the serum is either at levels below that required for systemic activity, or in inactive monomeric fragments.

OPG levels have been reported to be elevated in endstage prostate cancer, perhaps related to OPG expression by osteoblasts associated with extensive bone metastases [38]. In contrast, OPG levels have been reported to be reduced in the blood of multiple myeloma patients (39). Possible reasons for this could be direct or indirect inhibition by myeloma cells of OPG expression, or increased OPG clearance resulting from increased RANKL expression [40]. An alternative mechanism for myeloma cell-mediated direct clearance of OPG could be through binding and internalisation of OPG following binding to sulphated proteoglycans on the myeloma cell surface. Syndecan-1 is expressed on the myeloma cell surfaces, and can bind to heparin binding site on OPG [41]. If multiple myeloma cells suppress OPG levels in the bone microenvironment, that would be one explanation for the increased bone resorption in this disease. OPG deficiency in mice is associated with high bone resorption and bone loss [19].

ROLE OF RANKL, RANK AND OPG IN BONE RESORPTION IN HYPERCALCAEMIA AND CANCER METASTASIS

Lytic bone metastases are associated with pain and with other serious morbidities, such as fracture and paralysis, and are frequently evident when there is cancer metastasis to bone. It is likely that the mechanism of bone destruction in cancer is predominantly osteoclastic bone resorption. Bone samples from resected lytic tumours show scalloped surfaces characteristic of osteoclast action [42,43]. Bisphosphonate inhibitors of bone resorption inhibit progression of lytic lesions and are highly effective in protecting the skeleton in animal models of metastatic bone disease [44].

Although cancer cells can produce some of the enzymes associated with the osteoclastic bone resorption, such as matrix metalloproteinases [45] and cathepsin K (46), it is likely that the contribution of these to bone dissolution is small, due to the requirement for bone demineralisation to occur before these enzymes can access the bone matrix.

It is likely that increased bone resorption around cancer foci in bone results from increased RANKL expression. RANKL expression is increased around tumours [38] and is induced in stromal cells by coculture with tumour cells [47]. Cancer cells interact with osteoblasts or stromal cells to induce osteoclast formation from osteoclast precursors *in vitro* [48]. Cancer cells could increase RANKL expression in several ways. Tumour cells could themselves express RANKL, as has been reported for prostate cancer cells [38] and a squamous carcinoma-derived cell line [49]. Many tumour cells produce PTHrP, which has been clearly shown able to increase RANKL and decrease OPG expression in stromal cells [50]. Other factors, such as inflammatory cytokines and, in myeloma, MIP1α [51], may also be expressed either by the tumour cells or by host cells in response to tumour and indirectly increase RANKL and/or decrease OPG expression [52]. Binding of cancer cell-expressed integrins with their receptors on stromal cells can induce increased osteoclastogenic activity that is possibly related to increased RANKL expression [53].

EFFECTIVENESS OF INHIBITION OF RANK SIGNALLING IN ANIMAL MODELS OF CANCER-RELATED BONE DISEASES

Further evidence of the role of RANKL in cancer-mediated bone destruction is found in the effectiveness of OPG treatment for inhibiting cancer-related bone destruction. In mice, OPG is protective against bone humoral hypercalcaemia of malignancy, due to high PTHrP expression [54,55]. OPG [56] and soluble RANK [57] are each protective against bone resorption in animal models of lytic bone metastasis (Figure 4.5). In addition, OPG [58] is able to reduce bone destruction in a mouse model of multiple myeloma.

Cancer growth in bone is associated with bone pain. There is evidence in animal models that osteoclast-mediated bone resorption produces significant bone pain, as specific inhibition of osteoclastic bone resorption by OPG can diminish bone pain [59].

Thus, OPG is able to inhibit the resorptive effects of the osteotropic factors involved in metabolic, inflammatory and cancer-related diseases associated with pathological levels of bone resorption. The effectiveness of OPG in rodent models of bone disease provides strong support for the central role of RANKL upregulation in bone resorption in disease, as well as for physiological regulation of bone resorption. However, these results could also be explained if RANKL were an essential permissive factor for bone osteoclast differentiation and other factors were involved in mediating the effects of these hormones and cytokines. *In vivo* studies of the local regulation of RANKL and OPG expression in bone by these factors, and in disease states, are required to confirm the importance of their regulation in normal pathology and disease.

It is also likely that other factors may function to modify the responsiveness of the OPG–RANKL–RANK axis, as has been suggested for PGE$_2$ [60]. However, the ability of OPG to block the resorptive effects of all these factors indicates a wide potential application in cancer for therapeutics directed at this pathway.

OPG SUPPRESSES BONE RESORPTION IN PATIENTS WITH METASTATIC BONE RESORPTION AND MULTIPLE MYELOMA

In preliminary reports, treatment with OPG was found in human studies to profoundly suppress surrogate markers of bone resorption in patients with metastatic breast cancer [61] and multiple myeloma [62]. Thus, cancer-related bone resorption is likely to be osteoclast-mediated, and RANK signalling either mediates this increase or is at least permissive for the stimulation of bone resorption.

BONE RESORPTION MAY INDUCE CANCER CELLS TO TARGET TO BONE

In growing mice, intracardiac delivery of MDA-231 cancer cells results in the appearance of lytic bone lesions associated with tumour foci. Tumour cells appear to target the region of the growth plates of the long bones most commonly. These are the regions of bone with the highest levels of bone resorption and vascularisation. It is possible that the presence of bone resorption itself is either chemotactic to cancer cells or provides a fertile environment for cancer cells to lodge and grow [63]. TGFβ, which is released from bone matrix in active form by osteoclastic bone resorption, would be a candidate for enabling invasion of cancer cells into bone from the vasculature [64]. Human breast cancer cells can be induced to target calvarial bone if bone resorption is increased there by the local injection of IL-1 [65], although this targeting could also be related to the increased inflammation and inflammatory cell infiltration associated with IL-1 treatment. Thus, profound inhibition of bone resorption, as can be achieved by inhibition of RANK signalling, could provide a way to decrease metastasis to bone in subjects who are at high risk of metastatic disease.

ROLE OF BONE RESORPTION IN PROMOTING THE GROWTH OF CANCER CELLS IN BONE

The propensity of some tumour types, such as breast and prostate cancer, to metastasise to bone has given rise to theories about the basis for this targeting. One theory gaining credence is that some tumour cell types can induce the release of growth and survival factors from bone matrix through the induction of bone resorption, and thus make the bone marrow environment fertile for tumour growth [63]. Continued growth of the tumour sets up a vicious cycle (Figure 4.6), whereby tumours release factors that increase osteoclastic bone resorption, which in turn releases growth factors from bone matrix which promote tumour growth. If this is true, effectively blocking bone resorption should accomplish the dual purposes of preserving bone strength and diminishing cancer progression in the bone environment.

It is likely that the major factor released by solid tumours to increase bone resorption is PTHrP. Expression of tumour-derived PTHrP can be increased by TGFβ released through bone resorption, providing additional magnification of the vicious cycle [66]. As PTHrP appears to act through upregulation of RANKL and downregulation of OPG [50] (Figure 4.6), therapeutic use of OPG could provide an effective inhibitor of this destructive cycle. Support for this concept is provided by the reduction of tumour growth in bone achieved through inhibition of PTHrP activity directly [63] or through inhibition of bone resorption by bisphosphonate or OPG treatment.

There is as yet no clear demonstration of anti-tumour effects of inhibiting bone resorption in human disease, as data with bisphosphonates are contradictory [67,68]. However, this is clearly an area requiring further study.

There are intriguing data in animal models indicating that inhibition of RANKL signalling inhibits cancer growth in the bone, in addition to blocking bone resorption. OPG treatment has not been shown to have any effects on tumour growth in soft tissues; however, treatment with OPG or soluble RANK has reduced tumour growth within the bone in models of breast cancer metastasis [56,69], multiple myeloma [58] and prostate cancer [70]. Due to the lack of effects in non-bone tissues, it is unlikely that RANKL blockade directly blocks cancer growth. It is more likely that this effect is mediated through the inhibition of bone resorption and the release of factors from bone and/or osteoclasts that stimulate tumour growth.

POTENTIAL THERAPEUTIC ROLE FOR RANK SIGNALLING BLOCKADE IN CANCER

It is likely that the OPG–RANKL–RANK axis is as important in humans as it is in rodents, given the profound suppression of surrogate markers of bone

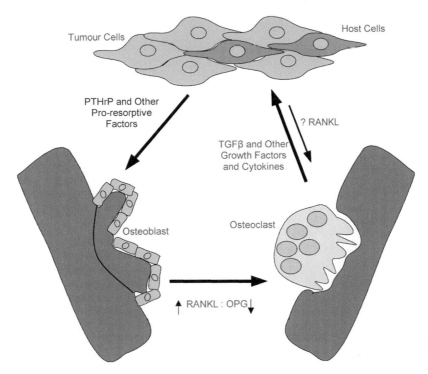

Figure 4.6. Cancer cells may interact with bone cells to increase RANKL expression to produce a vicious cycle that destroys bone while promoting tumour growth. Tumour cells produce factors which increase RANKL expression by cells of the osteoblast lineage. An increase in RANKL levels mediates the increase in bone resorption which releases and activates growth factors sequestered in bone matrix. These factors potentially then support additional tumour growth

resorption following single dose of OPG constructs in healthy postmenopausal women [33] (Figure 4.4), and patients with breast cancer [61] or multiple myeloma [62]. In this case, it is apparent that therapeutic interventions directed at this regulatory pathway have great clinical potential for inhibiting pathological bone resorption associated with cancer. At the simplest level this could involve treatment with recombinant OPG or soluble RANK. Inhibition of the signalling pathway for RANKL or modulation of expression of OPG or RANKL are alternative strategies. The signal transduction pathway for RANKL is beginning to be delineated with the identification of RANK as the receptor, with its several binding sites for proteins of the TRAF family, including TRAF 6 [11,71]. The recent discovery that TRAF 6-deficient mice have non-functional osteoclasts and osteopetrosis [72] implicates this molecule at least in the activation of osteoclasts. NF-κB-deficient mice have osteopetrosis with a similar absence of osteoclasts to RANKL-deficient mice [73]. NF-κB transcription factors are important in the signalling of many TNF family members, and activation

of these factors may be an endpoint of the RANKL/RANK signalling pathway in osteoclasts.

Blockade of RANK signalling is very likely to be an effective strategy for the inhibition of osteolytic effects of bone metastases. There may be a therapeutic advantage for inhibition of RANK signalling, as RANK blockade inhibits osteoclast formation as opposed to the inhibitory and apoptotic effects of bisphosphonates on mature osteoclasts. An additional effect of blockade of RANK signalling may be retarding of tumour growth in bone, which could in some cases have benefit for patient morbidity and possibly even survival. If osteoclastic bone resorption is important for cancer to lodge and grow in bone from micrometastasis, RANK blockade may have benefit in preventing the appearance of bone metastasis in patients at high risk of relapse.

Whether OPG treatment or some other form of RANK signalling blockade will be superior to, or synergistic with, bisphosphonate treatment, remains to be determined. However, the ability of OPG to prevent osteoclast formation, rather than, as do bisphosphonates, inactivate and kill existing osteoclasts, at least is encouragement that this therapeutic strategy be evaluated.

CONCLUSION

Osteoblasts and marrow stromal cells mediate the bone resorptive effects of osteotropic hormones and cytokines. Recent discoveries have elucidated a signalling pathway that provides the basis for this mediation. RANK, RANKL and OPG form a receptor, ligand (agonist), and decoy receptor (antagonist) triad essential for osteoclast formation and the maintenance of normal bone mass. RANKL is a potent stimulator of osteoclast differentiation, activation and survival. OPG is a soluble secreted inhibitor of osteoclastogenesis that acts by binding and inactivating RANKL. RANK is the membrane-bound receptor that mediates the effects of RANKL on bone resorption. Gene deletion studies in mice have shown that OPG is essential to maintain normal bone mass in mice and that RANKL is essential for osteoclast formation. Cancer cells can induce bone resorption by expressing or upregulating expression of factors such as PTHrP, which regulate OPG and RANKL expression in osteoblasts and marrow stromal cells to increase the signal for bone resorption. Cancer-induced bone resorption can be inhibited by blocking RANKL signalling by treatment with OPG or a soluble RANK construct, protecting against bone destruction and possibly inhibiting tumour growth in bone. The potential of this target invites further clinical studies of RANK signalling inhibition to evaluate the bone-protective effects, the effects on bone pain, and potential effects on metastasis and growth of tumour in bone.

Although RANKL/RANK signalling is central in the local regulation of bone resorption in normal physiology and in many disease states, clearly many other factors may directly or indirectly interact with osteoclasts to modulate their activity and differentiation. The identification of other factors that result in increased bone destruction in cancer is required to produce therapies that are more targeted to the disease process.

The use of circulating levels of OPG, RANK and RANKL as diagnostic indicators of disease is also an area requiring further investigation. OPG levels are reduced in multiple myeloma and increased in endstage prostate cancer, highlighting the potential utility of this measurement. Circulating levels for the extracellular domains of RANK or RANKL have not been reported but could be of great interest.

REFERENCES

1. Rodan GA, Martin TJ. Role of osteoblasts in hormonal control of bone resorption—a hypothesis. Calcified Tissue Int 1981; 33: 349–51.
2. Chambers TJ. The regulation of osteoclastic development and function. CIBA Foundation Symposium 1988; 136: 92–107.
3. Simonet WS, Lacey DL, Dunstan CR et al. Osteoprotegerin: a novel secreted protein involved in the regulation of bone density. Cell 1997; 89: 309–19.
4. Tsuda E, Goto M, Mochizuki S-I et al. Isolation of a novel cytokine from human fibroblasts that specifically inhibits bone osteoclastogenesis. Biochem Biophys Res Commun 1997; 234: 137–42.
5. Yamaguchi K, Kinosaki M, Goto M et al. Characterization of the structural domains of human osteoclastogenesis inhibitory factor. J Biol Chem 1998; 273: 5117–23.
6. Yasuda H, Shima N, Nakagawa N et al. Osteoclast differentiation factor is a ligand for osteoprotegerin/osteoclastogenesis-inhibitory factor and is identical to TRANCE/RANKL. Proc Natl Acad Sci USA 1998; 95: 3597–602.
7. Lacey DL, Timms E, Tan H-L et al. Osteoprotegerin ligand is a cytokine that regulates osteoclast differentiation and activation. Cell 1998; 93: 165–76.
8. Wong BR, Josien R, Lee SY et al. TRANCE (tumor necrosis factor (TNF)-related activation-induced cytokine), a new TNF family member predominantly expressed in T cells, is a dendritic cell-specific survival factor. J Exp Med 1997; 186: 2075–80.
9. Anderson DM, Maraskovsky E, Billingsley WL et al. A homologue of the TNF receptor and its ligand enhance T cell growth and dendritic cell function. Nature 1997; 390: 175–9.
10. Nakagawa N, Kinosaki M, Yamaguchi K et al. RANK is the essential signaling receptor for osteoclast differentiation factor in osteoclastogenesis. Biochem Biophys Res Commun 1998; 253: 395–400.
11. Hsu H, Lacey DL, Dunstan CR et al. The TNFR-related protein RANK is the osteoclast differentiation and activation receptor for osteoprotegerin ligand. Proc Natl Acad Sci USA 1999; 96: 3540–5.
12. Hakeda H, Kobayashi Y, Yamaguchi K et al. Osteoclastogenesis inhibitory factor (OCIF) directly inhibits bone-resorbing activity of isolated mature osteoclasts. Biochem Biophys Res Commun 1998; 251: 796–801.
13. Burgess TL, Qian Y-X, Kaufman S et al. The ligand for osteoprotegerin (RANKL) directly activates mature osteoclasts. J Cell Biol 1999; 145: 527–38.
14. Lum L, Wong BR, Josien R et al. Evidence for a role of a tumor necrosis factor-α (TNF-α)-converting enzyme-like protease in shedding of TRANCE a TNF family member involved in osteoclastogenesis and dendritic cell survival. J Biol Chem 1999; 274: 18613–18.
15. Fuller K, Wong B, Fox S et al. TRANCE is necessary and sufficient for osteoblast-mediated activation of bone resorption in osteoclasts. J Exp Med 1998; 188: 997–1001.
16. Jimi E, Akiyama S, Tsurukai T et al. Osteoclast differentiation factor acts as a multifunctional regulator in murine osteoclast differentiation and function. J Immunology 1999; 163: 434–42.

17. Lacey DL, Tan HL, Lu J et al. Osteoprotegerin ligand modulates murine osteoclast survival *in vitro* and *in vivo*. Am J Pathol 2000; 157: 435–48.

18. Horwood NJ, Elliott J, Martin TJ, Gillespie MT. Osteotropic agents regulate the expression of osteoclast differentiation factor and osteoprotegerin in osteoblastic stromal cells. Endocrinology 1998; 139: 4743–6.

19. Bucay N, Sarosi I, Dunstan CR et al. Osteoprotegerin-deficient mice develop early onset osteoporosis and arterial calcification. Genes Dev 1998; 12: 1260–8.

20. Mizuno A, Amizuka N, Irie K et al. Severe osteoporosis in mice lacking osteoclastogenesis inhibitory factor/osteoprotegerin. Biochem Biophys Res Commun 1998; 247: 610–15.

21. Kong Y-Y, Yoshida H, Sarosi I et al. OPGL is a key regulator or osteoclastogenesis, lymphocyte development and lymph-node organogenesis. Nature 1999; 397: 315–23.

22. Dunstan CR. Osteoprotegerin and osteoprotegerin ligand mediate the local regulation of bone resorption. Endocrinologist 2000; 10: 18–21.

23. Hofbauer LC, Khosla S, Dunstan CR et al. The roles of osteoprotegerin and osteoprotegerin ligand in the paracrine regulation of bone resorption. J Bone Mineral Res 2000; 15: 2–12.

24. Hofbauer LC, Khosla S, Dunstan CR et al. Estrogen stimulates gene expression and protein production of osteoprotegerin in human osteoblastic cells. Endocrinology 1999; 140: 4367–70.

25. Morony S, Capparelli C, Lee R et al. A chimeric form of osteoprotegerin inhibits hypercalcemia and bone resorption induced by IL-1β, TNFα, PTH, PTHrp, and 1,25-dihydroxyvitamin D₃. J Bone Min Res 1999; 14: 1478–85.

26. Yamamoto M, Murakami T, Nishikawa M et al. Hypocalcemic effect of osteoclastogenesis inhibitory factor/osteoprotegerin in the thyroparathyroidectomized rat. Endocrinology 1998; 139: 4012–15.

27. Kong YY, Feige U, Sarosi I et al. Activated T cells regulate bone loss and joint destruction in adjuvant arthritis through osteoprotegerin ligand. Nature 1999; 402: 304–9.

28. Matsuzaki K, Udagawa N, Takahashi N et al. Osteoclast differentiation factor (ODF) induces osteoclast-like cell formation in human peripheral blood mononuclear cell cultures. Biochem Biophys Res Commun 1998; 246: 199–204.

29. Shalhoub V, Faust J, Boyle WJ et al. Osteoprotegerin and osteoprotegerin ligand effects on osteoclast formation from human peripheral blood mononuclear cell precursors. J Cell Biochem 1999; 72: 251–61.

30. Li J, Sarosi I, Yan XQ et al. RANK is the intrinsic hematopoietic cell surface receptor that controls osteoclastogenesis and regulation of bone mass and calcium metabolism. Proc Natl Acad Sci USA 2000; 97: 1566–71.

31. Yano K, Tsuda E, Washida N et al. Immunological characterization of circulating osteoprotegerin/osteoclastogenesis inhibitory factor: increased serum concentrations in postmenopausal women with osteoporosis. J Bone Min Res 1999; 14: 518–27.

32. Arrighi HM, Hsieh A, Wong V et al. Osteoprotegerin serum levels in healthy volunteers. Bone 1998; 23: S298.

33. Bekker PJ, Holloway D, Nakanishi A et al. The effect of a single dose of osteoprotegerin in postmenopausal women. J Bone Min Res 2001; 16: 348–60.

34. Hughes AE, Ralston SH, Marken J et al. Mutations in TNFRSF11A, affecting the signal peptide of RANK, cause familial expansile osteolysis. Nature Genet 2000; 24: 45–8.

35. Fata JE, Kong Y-Y, Li J et al. The osteoclast differentiation factor osteoprotegerin-ligand is essential for mammary gland development. Cell 2000; 103: 41–50.

36. Emery JG, McDonnell P, Burke MB et al. Osteoprotegerin is a receptor for the cytotoxic ligand TRAIL. J Biol Chem 1998; 273: 14363–7.

37. Tomoyasu A, Goto M, Fujise N et al. Characterization of monomeric and homodimeric forms of osteoclastogenesis inhibitory factor. Biochem Biophys Res Commun 1998; 245: 382–7.

38. Brown JM, Corey E, Lee ZD et al. Osteoprotegerin and RANK ligand expression in prostate cancer. Urology 2001; 57: 611–16.

39. Seidel C, Hjertner O, Abilgaard N et al. Serum osteoprotegerin levels are reduced in patients with multiple myeloma with lytic bone disease. Blood 2001; 998: 2269–71.

40. Giuliani N, Bataille R, Mancini C et al. Myeloma cells induce imbalance in the osteoprotegerin/osteoprotegerin ligand system in the human bone marrow environment. Blood 2001; 98: 3527–33.

41. Borset M, Standal T, Hjertner O et al. Binding, internalization and degradation of osteoprotegerin in human myeloma cells (abstr). Blood 2001; 98: 636a.

42. Boyde A, Maconnachie E, Reid SA et al. Scanning electron microscopy in bone pathology: review of methods. Potential and applications. Scanning Electron Microsc 1986; IV: 1537–44.

43. Taube T, Elomaa I, Blomqvist C et al. Histomorphometric evidence for osteoclast-mediated bone resorption in metastatic breast cancer. Bone 1994; 15: 161–6.

44. Sasaki A, Boyce BF, Story B et al. Bisphosphonate risedronate reduces metastatic human breast cancer burden in bone in nude mice. Cancer Res 1995; 55: 3551–7.

45. Sanchez-Sweatman OH, Lee J, Orr FW, Singh G. Direct osteolysis induced by metastatic murine melanoma cells: role of matrix metalloproteinases. Eur J Cancer 1997; 33: 918–25.

46. Littlewood-Evans AJ, Bilbe G, Bowler WB et al. The osteoclast-associated protease cathepsin K is expressed in human breast carcinoma. Cancer Res 1997; 57: 5386–90.

47. Mancino AT, Klimberg VS, Yamamoto M et al. Breast cancer increases osteoclastogenesis by secreting M-CSF and upregulating RANKL in stromal cells. J Surg Res 2001; 100: 18–24.

48. Chikatsu N, Takeuchi Y, Tamura Y et al. Interactions between cancer and bone marrow cells induce osteoclast differentiation factor expression and osteoclast-like cell formation *in vitro*. Biochem Biophys Res Commun 2000; 267: 632–7.

49. Nagai M, Kyakumoto S, Sata N. Cancer cells responsible of humoral hypercalcemia express mRNA encoding a secreted form of ODF/TRANCE that induces osteoclast formation. Biochem Biophys Res Commun 2000; 269: 532–6.

50. Nakchbandi IA, Weir EE, Insogna KL et al. Parathyroid hormone-related protein induces spontaneous osteoclasts formation via a paracrine cascade. Proc Natl Acad Sci USA 2000; 97: 7296–300.

51. Han J-J, Choi SJ, Kurihara N et al. Macrophage inflammatory protein-1 is an osteoclastogenic factor in myeloma that is independent of receptor activator of nuclear factor B ligand. Blood 2001; 97: 3349–53.

52. Pearse RN, Sordillo EM, Yaccoby S et al. Multiple myeloma disrupts the TRANCE/osteoprotegerin cytokine axis to trigger bone destruction and promote tumor progression. Proc Natl Acad Sci USA 2001; 98: 11581–6.

53. Michigami T, Shimizu N, Williams PJ et al. Cell–cell contact between marrow stromal cells and myeloma cells via VCAM-1 and α(4)β(1)-integrin enhances production of osteoclast stimulating activity. Blood 1998; 96: 1953–60.

54. Akatsu T, Murakami T, Onon K et al. Osteoclastogenesis inhibitory factor exhibits hypocalcemic effects in normal mice and in hypercalcemic nude mice carrying tumors associated with humoral hypercalcemia of malignancy. Bone 1998; 23: 495–8.

55. Capparelli C, Kostenuik PJ, Morony S et al. Osteoprotegerin prevents and reverses hypercalcemia in a murine model of humoral hypercalcemia of malignancy. Cancer Res 2000; 60: 783–7.

56. Morony S, Capparelli C, Sarosi I, Lacey DL, Dunstan CR, Kostenuik PJ. Osteoprotegerin (OPG) inhibits osteolysis and decreases skeletal tumor burden in syngeneic and nude mouse models of experimental bone metastasis. Cancer Res 2001; 61: 4432–6.

57. Oyajobi BO, Anderson DM, Traianedes K et al. Therapeutic efficacy of a soluble receptor activator of nuclear factor B-IgG Fc fusion protein in suppressing bone resorption and hypercalcemia in a model of humoral hypercalcemia of malignancy. Cancer Res 2001; 61: 2572–8.

58. Croucher PI, Shipman CM, Lippitt J et al. Osteoprotegerin inhibits the development of osteolytic bone disease in multiple myeloma. Blood 2001; 98: 3534–40.

59. Honore P, Luger NM, Sabino MAC et al. Osteoprotegerin blocks bone cancer-induced skeletal destruction, skeletal pain and pain-related neurochemical reorganization of the spinal cord. Nature Med 2000; 6: 521–8.

60. Wani MR, Fuller K, Kim NS et al. Prostaglandin E_2 cooperates with TRANCE in osteoclast induction. J Biol Chem 1997; 272: 25190–4.

61. Body J-J, Lipton A, Coleman RE et al. An OPG construct decreases bone resorption profoundly in breast cancer bone metastasis. J Bone Min Metab 2001; 19(suppl): 51.

62. Greipp P, Facon T, Williams CD et al. A single subcutaneous dose of an osteoprotegerin (OPG) construct (AMGN-0007) causes a profound and sustained decrease of bone resorption comparable to standard intravenous bisphosphonate in patients with multiple myeloma. Blood 2001; 98(11): 775a.

63. Guise TA. Molecular mechanisms of osteolytic bone metastases. Cancer 2000; 88 (suppl): 2892–8.

64. Welch DR, Fabra A, Nakajima M. Transforming growth factor stimulates mammary adenocarcinoma cell invasion and metastasis. Proc Natl Acad Sci USA 1990; 87: 7678–82.

65. Myoui A, Sasaki P, Williams P et al. Bone-derived growth factors enhance breast cancer metastasis to bone. J Bone Min Res 1996; 11(suppl 1): S481 (abstr).

66. Yin JJ, Selander K, Rankin W et al. The effects of transforming growth factor-β on breast cancer-mediated osteolysis are mediated by parathyroid hormone-related protein via the Smad signaling pathway. J Bone Min Res 1999; 14(suppl 1).

67. Diel IJ, Solomayer EF, Costa SD et al. Reduction in new metastases in breast cancer with adjuvant clodronate treatment. N Engl J Med 1998; 339: 356–63.

68. Saarto T, Blomqvist C, Virkkunen P, Elomaa I. Adjuvant clodronate treatment does not reduce the frequency of skeletal metastases in node-positive breast cancer patients: 5-year results of a randomized controlled study. J Clin Oncol 2001; 19: 10–17.

69. Clohisy DR, Ramnaraine ML, Scully S et al. Osteoprotegerin inhibits tumor-induced osteoclastogenesis and bone tumor growth in osteopetrotic mice. J Orthop Res 2000; 18: 967–76.

70. Zhang J, Dai J, Qi Y et al. Osteoprotegerin inhibits prostate cancer-induced osteoclastogenesis and prevents prostate tumor growth in the bone. J Clin Invest 2001; 107: 1235–44.

71. Wong BR, Josien R, Lee SY et al. The TRAF family of signal transducers mediates NF-κB activation by the TRANCE receptor. J Biol Chem 1998; 273: 28335–59.

72. Lomaga MA, Yeh WC, Sarosi I et al. TRAF6-deficient mice are osteopetrotic and defective in interleukin-1, interleukin-18, CD40 and LPS signaling. Genes Dev 1999; 13: 1015–24.

73. Iotsova V, Caamano J, Loy J et al. Osteopetrosis in mice lacking NF-κB1 and NF-κB2. Nature Med 1997; 3: 1285–9.

2

Clinical Features and Assessment

Section Editor: Robert E. Coleman

5

Clinical Features and Prognosis of Bone Metastases

T. A. Plunkett and R. D. Rubens

Guy's Hospital, London, UK

INCIDENCE AND DISTRIBUTION OF BONE METASTASES

The skeleton is commonly affected by metastatic cancer. Tumours of the breast and prostate are particularly likely to disseminate to bone; at post mortem examination approximately 70% of patients dying from these cancers have evidence of skeletal metastatic disease (Table 5.1) [1]. Carcinomas of the thyroid, kidney and bronchus also commonly give rise to bone metastases, with an incidence at post mortem of 30–40%, although tumours of the gastrointestinal tract rarely produce bone metastases. It is likely that these figures are underestimates of the true incidence, as they depended upon macroscopic rather than microscopic identification of metastatic deposits in bone.

Bone metastases most commonly affect the axial skeleton, which contains the red marrow in the adult, and this suggests that properties of the circulation, cells and extracellular matrix within this region could assist in the formation of bone metastases. There is evidence that blood from some anatomical sites may drain directly into the axial skeleton. In post mortem studies of animals and humans, Batson [2] demonstrated that venous blood from the breasts and pelvis flowed not only into the venae cavae, but also into a vertebral venous plexus of vessels extending from the pelvis throughout the epidural and perivertebral veins. The drainage of blood to the skeleton via the vertebral venous plexus may, at least in part, explain the tendency of breast and prostate cancers, as well as those arising in kidney, thyroid and lung, to produce metastases in the axial skeleton and limb girdles.

The vertebral venous plexus does not provide the entire explanation for these cancers to metastasise to the skeleton. Molecular and cellular biological characteristics of the tumour cells and the tissues to which they metastasise influence the pattern of metastatic spread. In breast cancer, the development of metastatic bone disease has been associated with primary tumours that express PTHrP [3] and that are well-differentiated [4] or steroid hormone (oestrogen and/or progesterone) receptor-positive [5]. In prostate cancer, the development of bone metastases is associated with poorly differentiated tumours [6]. It is likely that many other factors are also important in the metastatic spread of cancer to the skeleton.

DIAGNOSIS OF BONE METASTASES

Bone metastases typically affect multiple sites and cause pain, tenderness and increasing disability. The diagnosis is usually straightforward, but can occasionally be confused with benign skeletal pathology. In particular, bone metastases can be confused with osteoporosis or Paget's disease. Osteoporosis is common in the elderly, and can be accelerated by certain anticancer treatments, e.g. premature menopause secondary to ovarian ablation or cytotoxic chemotherapy in patients with breast cancer [7,8], tamoxifen use in pre-menopausal patients with breast cancer [9] and androgen blockade in patients with prostate cancer

Textbook of Bone Metastases. Edited by C. Jasmin, R. E. Coleman, L. R. Coia, R. Capanna and G. Saillant
© 2005 John Wiley & Sons Ltd: ISBN 0 471 87742 5

Table 5.1. Incidence of bone metastases at post mortem examination in different cancers

Primary tumour	Incidence of bone metastases (%)
Breast	73
Prostate	68
Thyroid	42
Kidney	35
Lung	36
Gastrointestinal tract	5

From [1].

[10]. In all cases, appropriate imaging tests are required and should be interpreted in conjunction with the clinical context, serum markers of bone turnover and, if relevant, serum tumour markers.

Plain Radiographs

Plain radiographs of the skeleton demonstrate the net result of bone destruction and repair. The predominance of lysis or sclerosis gives rise to the characteristic appearance of bone metastases. Lytic metastases form when bone resorption predominates (e.g. breast, lung, thyroid, renal, melanoma and gastrointestinal cancers). For a destructive lesion in trabecular bone to be identified on such images, it must be greater than 1 cm in diameter, with loss of approximately 50% of the bone mineral content [11]. In sclerotic metastases, excessive new bone formation results in thickened, coarse trabeculae that appear radiographically as nodular, rounded lesions (e.g. prostate, breast, lung, carcinoid and medulloblastoma tumours). However, both osteolysis and new bone formation are accelerated in affected bone. Although this is probably a general phenomenon, it is most apparent in "mixed lesions", seen most commonly in breast cancer, in which both sclerotic and lytic lesions are visible.

Radionuclide Bone Scans

Radionuclide bone scans identify areas of active bone formation. The bone scan therefore reflects the metabolic activity of osteoblasts, irrespective of the disease process, e.g. infection, trauma, primary tumour, metastatic disease. Scintigraphic and radiographic appearances therefore do not necessarily correlate, although most comparative analyses demonstrate the bone scan to be the more sensitive [12].

Although not specific, the pattern of bone scan abnormalities may suggest a specific diagnosis. Metastases are usually multiple, irregularly distributed and generally affect the axial skeleton. As the radionuclide uptake depends upon new bone formation, a false negative scan may result in cases of pure lytic disease. This is typical of myeloma, which is best investigated by plain radiographs, but may occur in other tumour types. Rarely, so-called "cold spots" (photon-deficient areas) may develop at sites of significant bone destruction. In extensive disease, the focal lesions may coalesce to produce a "super-scan", with increased contrast between bone and background soft tissue.

Computed Tomography and Magnetic Resonance Imaging

Computed tomography (CT) produces excellent soft tissue and contrast resolution and both lytic and sclerotic deposits can be demonstrated. It is usually reserved for assessment of patients with a positive bone scan but negative plain radiographs. In one such series of patients with breast cancer, 50% had metastases on CT, 25% a benign pathology, and in 25% no abnormality was observed. None of this latter group subsequently developed metastases [13].

Magnetic resonance imaging (MRI) is also useful in the evaluation of patients with suspected metastases. MRI involves no radiation, and provides multi-planar images. It is now the method of choice for the investigation of spinal cord compression. MRI has been suggested as a method to screen for bone metastases in patients with prostate cancer [14]. The authors used a 30 min examination of the axial skeleton, sternum and proximal femora, and predicted that the method would detect more than 90% of bone metastases. Although MRI differentiates between osteoporotic and metastatic vertebral collapse, this method did not identify 9% of metastatic lesions, most often in the peripheral skeleton. However, as the methods are refined MRI may become a useful staging tool.

Biochemical Measurements

Numerous biochemical tests of bone resorption and formation are available. Although these may be helpful in predicting and assessing the response to treatment, there are no convincing data that demonstrate their usefulness in the detection of bone metastases.

PATHOPHYSIOLOGY OF MORBIDITY FROM BONE METASTASES

The symptoms from bone metastases predominantly result from osteoclastic bone resorption. Normal bone is in a dynamic state, being continually resorbed and reformed throughout life by the coordinated action of osteoclasts and osteoblasts, acting both on trabecular surfaces and in Haversian systems as discrete bone remodelling units. The balance between bone resorption and formation is upset in metastatic bone disease. Bone metastases are typically referred to as "lytic", "sclerotic" or "mixed", depending on the radiographic appearances. In lytic bone lesions, osteolysis predominates over new bone formation (e.g. multiple myeloma, breast cancer, lung cancer, thyroid, renal and gastrointestinal malignancies) and in sclerotic lesions the converse is true (e.g. prostate cancer in particular, but also breast, lung, carcinoid and medulloblastoma tumours). However, both processes are typically accelerated in affected bone. Evidence for this includes "mixed" radiographic appearances (i.e. both lytic and sclerotic lesions in the same patient), increased osteoclastic activity and resorption cavities within sclerotic bone lesions [15] and from biochemical evaluation of bone turnover [16].

These data suggest that, despite the differing radiographic appearances, the pathological processes are similar in bone metastases from different primary cancers. The morbidity from bone metastases differs between cancers; this is largely a result of differences in survival from the diagnosis of skeletal metastatic disease.

PROGNOSIS

Although bone metastases are common in many cancers, the survival from diagnosis varies between different tumour types (Table 5.2). The median survival from diagnosis of bone metastases from prostate cancer or breast cancer is approximately 20 months. In contrast, the median survival from the diagnosis of advanced lung cancer is approximately 3

Table 5.2. Survival from diagnosis of bone metastases

Cancer type	Median survival (months)
Breast	20
Prostate	20
Lung	3

months. As a result of the high prevalence of breast and prostate cancers and their relatively long clinical courses, these two cancers account for the majority of patients with metastatic bone disease.

Breast Cancer

Coexisting non-osseous metastatic disease is important in determining prognostic differences between patients with bone metastases from the same type of tumour. In advanced breast cancer, metastatic disease confined to the skeleton is associated with a relatively good prognosis. For example, in a study from the Guy's Hospital Breast Unit, the median survival was 24 months in those patients with metastatic disease apparently confined to the skeleton, compared to 3 months after first relapse in the liver (Figure 5.1; $p < 0.00001$) [4].

In a study of 718 patients with metastatic breast cancer at a single institution, more than 50% of women developed skeletal complications (hypercalcaemia, spinal cord compression, surgery to bone, radiotherapy to bone or pathological fracture) [17]. The patients were classified according to the sites of disease at first relapse: 37% had metastatic disease confined to the skeleton; 21% had disease in the skeleton and at other sites; and 42% had no skeletal involvement. Of the women with bone-only disease at first relapse, 81% developed skeletal complications,

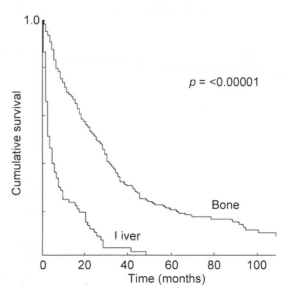

Figure 5.1. Survival of patients with breast cancer after first relapse. From [4]

compared to 60% of women with bone plus extra-osseous metastatic disease and 21% of women with no bone metastases at first relapse.

In women with disease confined to the skeleton at first relapse, the median time to first skeletal complication was 11 months. This compared with 20 months in women with bone and extra-osseous disease and 56 months in women without bone metastases at diagnosis of first relapse (there were no significant differences between the groups in the type of first skeletal complication). There may be a lead time bias in this analysis. Patients without extra-osseous disease are likely to have been investigated specifically for symptoms suggestive of bone metastases, whereas in patients with extra-osseous disease, the bone metastases may have been asymptomatic and instead were detected as part of the staging procedure.

In a multivariate analysis, the most significant predictor of subsequent skeletal complications was the presence of bone metastases at diagnosis of metastatic breast cancer, regardless of other sites of metastatic disease. However, in this analysis patients were classified as "bone only", "bone plus other sites" or "no bone disease" at first relapse. The group of patients termed "bone plus other sites" is necessarily heterogeneous, and there is evidence that prognosis differs between such patients depending on the sites of additional extra-osseous disease.

A retrospective analysis of 859 patients who developed bone metastases from breast cancer at Guy's Hospital between 1975 and 1991 was performed to identify factors that predict for complications from skeletal disease [18]. The patients were divided into four groups according to the sites of disease at diagnosis of bone metastases: bone disease only ($n=243$); bone and soft tissue disease ($n=268$); bone and pleuro-pulmonary disease ($n=237$); and bone and liver disease ($n=111$). Survival from diagnosis of bone metastases was longest for patients with metastatic disease confined to the skeleton (median survival 24 months; Figure 5.2, $p < 0.001$) and was least for patients with concomitant bone and liver metastases (median survival 5.5 months).

The case notes of all patients were reviewed and the following factors related to skeletal complications were recorded: number of fields of radiotherapy at diagnosis of bone metastases and subsequently; date and site of pathological fractures; date of spinal cord compression; date of first episode of hypercalcaemia (Table 5.3). There were no differences between the groups of patients in time to pathological long bone fracture. However, since patients with bone disease confined to the skeleton at diagnosis lived longest,

most long bone fractures occurred in this group (Table 5.3). Forty-two long bone fractures occurred in patients with bone disease only (i.e. one pathological long bone fracture in every 5.8 patients) compared to five such fractures in patients with bone and liver disease (i.e. one fracture in every 22.2 patients).

Patients with disease confined to the skeleton at diagnosis of bone metastases were more likely to have received radiotherapy to bone than patients with additional extra-osseous disease. Of patients with bone-only disease, 83% required radiotherapy for painful skeletal deposits and 60% of these patients required more than one treatment. In contrast, 47% of patients with bone and liver metastases required radiotherapy to bone for pain relief, and only 21% of these required more than one treatment. There were no significant differences between the groups in response to first systemic treatment following the diagnosis of bone metastases. Therefore, the increased need for radiotherapy and the greater number of pathological long bone fractures in patients with bone-only disease at diagnosis of skeletal metastases may reflect their prolonged survival compared with other groups of patients.

For patients with advanced breast cancer and metastatic disease confined to the skeleton at first relapse, the probability of survival is influenced by the subsequent development of metastases at extra-osseous sites. In a study of 367 patients with bone metastases from breast cancer, those that later developed extra-osseous disease had a median survival of 1.6 years, compared to 2.1 years for those with disease that remained clinically confined to the skeleton (Figure 5.3; $p < 0.001$) [19]. A number of factors in the primary

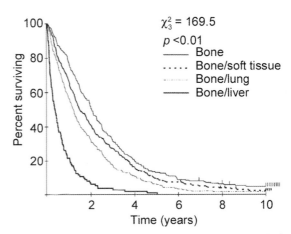

Figure 5.2. Survival from diagnosis of bone metastasis in patients with breast cancer. From [18], with permission from Elsevier © 2000

Table 5.3. Skeletal-related events for patients with advanced breast cancer—all groups of patients shown

Event	All patients (*n*=859)	Bone only (*n*=243)	Bone and soft tissue (*n*=268)	Bone and pleuro-pulmonary (*n*=237)	Bone and liver (*n*=111)
Any pathological fracture*	299 (34%)	128 (53%)	91 (34%)	55 (23%)	22 (20%)
Vertebral fractures*	176 (20%)	79 (33%)	47 (18%)	31 (13%)	16 (14%)
Long bone fractures*	102 (12%)	42 (17%)	37 (14%)	18 (8%)	5 (5%)
Fractures at other sites*	108 (13%)	37 (15%)	40 (15%)	24 (10%)	7 (6%)
Hypercalcaemia*	162 (19%)	62 (25%)	44 (16%)	30 (13%)	26 (23%)
Spinal cord compression*	67 (8%)	36 (15%)	15 (6%)	11 (5%)	2 (2%)

*Total number of patients that developed complications.
From [18].

tumour have been identified that predict for disease remaining confined to the skeleton (Table 5.4). These patients are more likely to be older, have lobular or low-grade ductal tumours and had little or no axillary lymph node involvement at initial diagnosis/surgery.

Prostate Cancer

Prostate cancer is the most prevalent non-dermatological cancer in males. At presentation, approximately 10% of patients have bone metastases, and almost all patients who die of prostate cancer have bone metastases [20]. The clinical course of patients with metastatic prostate cancer can be relatively long, and several prognostic factors have been identified; these include performance status, tumour grade, haemoglobin, serum lactate dehydrogenase, PSA and alkaline phosphatase [21–23]. For example, in patients with good performance status and disease confined to the

axial skeleton, median survival is 53 months. For patients with additional visceral disease median survival was 30 months, and for patients with poor performance status with bone and visceral disease the median survival was 12 months [21].

Several studies have attempted to correlate the extent of skeletal metastatic involvement with survival in patients with advanced prostate cancer. A staging system based upon distribution of bone metastases according to bone scintigraphy (axial vs. appendicular) demonstrated a significant association with survival [24]. A different system, based upon the number of lesions identified by bone scintigraphy, was also predictive for survival [25]. However, although both systems were able to discriminate between patients at

Table 5.4. Characteristics of patients with breast cancer with first relapse in bone in relation to the concomitant or subsequent development of bone metastases

	Metastases		
	Bone only	Bone plus other sites	*p*-Value
Mean age	59 years	54 years	<0.001
Pre-menopausal	24%	37%	
Post-menopausal	63%	43%	<0.009
Nodal status			
0	29%	18%	
1–3	24%	19%	
>3	16%	30%	<0.02
Histology			
IDC grade I	2%	1%	
IDC grade II	39%	38%	
IDC grade III	19%	32%	<0.0001
Lobular	21%	12%	<0.04

IDC, infiltrating ductal carcinoma.
From [19].

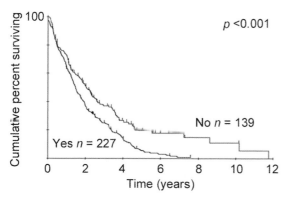

Figure 5.3. Survival after bone metastases by subsequent development of non-osseous metastases or disease confined to the skeleton. From [4]

the extremes of their respective scales, neither was particularly effective at discriminating between patients towards the centre of the range.

A bone scan index (BSI) has been developed to quantify the extent of skeletal involvement by tumour [26]. It is based on the known proportional weights of each of the 158 bones derived from the so-called "reference man", a standardised skeleton in which post mortem-based individual bone weights were reported for the average adult [27]. The bones were considered individually and assigned a numerical score representing the percentage involvement with tumour multiplied by the weight of the bone (derived from the reference man). The BSI represented the sum of the numerical scores from each bone in the skeleton. Despite the seemingly complex method, there was little inter- or intra-observer error in calculating the BSI [26].

In a study of 191 patients with androgen-independent prostate cancer, patients with low, intermediate or extensive skeletal involvement according to the BSI had median survivals of 18.3, 15.8 and 8.1 months, respectively [26]. In a multiple-variable proportional analysis, BSI was associated with survival, as were age, haemoglobin, LDH and therapy received. It is not known whether changes in BSI correlate with response to therapy, or whether this method can be applied to patients with other cancers. There are no data comparing BSI to morbidity from bone metastases. However, the BSI may represent a useful tool in prognostic stratification of patients with bone metastases.

Studies have also been reported on the correlation of serum markers of bone turnover and prognosis in prostate cancer. In a study of 48 patients, the serum levels of carboxy-terminal telopeptide of type I procollagen (PICP) and carboxy-terminal telopeptide of type collagen, alkaline phosphatase (ALP) and PSA were evaluated as prognostic markers [28]. Patients with low PICP or ALP had significantly longer survival times compared to those with high values. However, these markers were not significant in a multivariate analysis and they need to be studied in larger numbers of patients before any definite conclusions can be drawn.

Multiple Myeloma

In patients with multiple myeloma, the median survival is 2–3 years. There are several established prognostic factors [29]. For example, the median survival of patients with high levels of both C-reactive protein and β2-microglobulin was 6 months compared to 54

months for patients with low serum levels of these markers [30]. Other candidate markers for prognosis include neopterin, IL-6, plasma cell labelling index and LDH.

A recent study investigated the relationship between serum markers of bone turnover with prognosis and morbidity from bone metastases in patients with myeloma [31]. The study of 313 patients demonstrated a correlation between serum carboxy-terminal telopeptide of type I collagen (ICTP), and also the bone isoform of alkaline phosphatase with bone pain, number of skeletal lesions and pathological fractures. In univariate analysis, serum ICTP correlated with survival; the median survival time for patients with low ICTP was 4.1 years compared to 3.5 years for those with high levels. These findings require confirmation in larger prospective studies, but suggest that markers of bone turnover may be helpful in assessing prognosis and in identifying patients most at risk of skeletal complications from myeloma bone disease.

CLINICAL FEATURES

Skeletal metastatic disease is the cause of considerable morbidity in patients with advanced cancer (Table 5.5). In a recent study of 243 patients with first relapse in bone from breast cancer, 17% developed pathological long bone fractures, 26% hypercalcaemia and 15% spinal cord compression [18]. In multiple myeloma, the prevalence of skeletal complications was assessed in 254 patients with myeloma [32]. Bone pain was reported in 75% of patients, 54% had radiographic evidence of vertebral fracture and 33% had hypercalcaemia at diagnosis.

Pain

Bone metastases are the most common cause of cancer-related pain [33]. The pathophysiological mechanisms of pain in patients with bone metastases are poorly understood. Although approximately 80% of patients with advanced breast cancer develop

Table 5.5. Complications of bone metastases

Pain
Pathological fracture
Spinal cord compression
Cranial nerve palsies
Hypercalcaemia
Bone marrow suppression

osteolytic bone metastases, about two-thirds of such sites are painless [34].

Many nerves are found in the periosteum and others enter the bone alongside blood vessels. Rapidly growing tumours in bone cause invasion and distension of the periosteum and an increase in intra-osseous pressure, which activates pressure-sensitive nerves and results in pain. Bone metastases may be associated with inflammation. The release of prostaglandins, bradykinin and other mediators of inflammation produced by osteoclasts and macrophages may stimulate local nociceptors. Pain can also result from mechanical stresses in weakened, tumour-infiltrated bones. The spread of tumour from bone to surrounding neurological structures, such as the spinal cord, nerve roots, and brachial and lumbosacral plexuses are also significant causes of pain.

Different sites of bone metastases are associated with distinct clinical pain syndromes. Common sites of metastatic involvement associated with pain are the base of skull (in association with cranial nerve palsies, neuralgias and headache), vertebral metastases (producing neck and back pain, with or without neurological complications secondary to epidural extension), and pelvic and femoral lesions, producing pain in the back and lower limbs (often associated with mechanical instability and incident pain).

The spine is the most commonly affected site of metastatic spread from breast and prostate cancers. Pain at the site of involvement is common and may be associated with radicular pain if the tumour involves adjacent nerve roots. Extension of the tumour may lead to spinal cord compression. Several pain patterns have been described. Damage to the lower cervical and upper thoracic spine may be referred to the interscapular region; involvement of the lower thoracic and upper lumbar spine may cause unilateral or bilateral pain in the region of the iliac crest or sacro-iliac joints.

Bone pain may be poorly localised and is difficult to evaluate. Various methods have been devised to assess pain, including linear analogue scales and categorical systems. These systems and the management of patients with pain from bone metastases are discussed elsewhere.

Hypercalcaemia

Hypercalcaemia most often occurs in those patients with squamous cell lung cancer, breast and kidney cancers, and certain haematological malignancies (in particular myeloma and lymphoma). In most cases hypercalcaemia is a result of bone destruction, and osteolytic metastases are present in 80% of cases [35].

In breast cancer, there is an association between hypercalcaemia and the presence of liver metastases. In a series of 498 patients with first relapse in bone, hypercalcaemia was more common in patients who later developed liver metastases than in patients with disease that remained confined to the skeleton (31% vs. 15%; $p < 0.001$) [36]. In a prospective study of 35 patients with hypercalcaemia, the 18 patients with liver metastases had higher levels of renal tubular calcium reabsorption and higher levels of cyclic AMP excretion than patients without liver metastases. These differences could be due to the production of some humoral factor in patients with liver metastases, or the decreased clearance of humoral factors in such patients.

Secretion of humoral and paracrine factors by tumour cells stimulates osteoclast activity and proliferation, and there is a marked increase in markers of bone turnover [37]. Several studies have established the role of PHTrP in the majority of cases of malignant hypercalcaemia [38]. The levels of circulating PTHrP are elevated in two-thirds of patients with bone metastases and hypercalcaemia and in almost all patients with humoral hypercalcaemia (hypercalcaemia in cancer patients without bone metastases) [38]. The kidney also has a role in malignant hypercalcaemia; as a result of volume depletion and the action of PTHrP, renal tubular resorption of calcium is increased, further increasing serum calcium levels.

The signs and symptoms of hypercalcaemia are nonspecific, and the clinician should have a high index of suspicion. Common symptoms include fatigue, anorexia and constipation (Table 5.6). If untreated, a progressive rise in serum calcium results in deterioration of renal function and mental status. Death ultimately results from renal failure and cardiac arrhythmias.

It is unusual for the aetiology of hypercalcaemia to be in doubt, but non-malignant causes should be considered. In the community, hyperparathyroidism is the most common cause; measurement of serum PTH is useful in cases where doubt exists over the cause of hypercalcaemia.

The treatment of hypercalcaemia is described in detail elsewhere. Treatment depends on the calcium level, symptoms and life expectancy of the patient.

Table 5.6. Clinical features of hypercalcaemia

Neurological	Weakness, lethargy, confusion, delirium
Renal	Polyuria, thirst, dehydration
Gastrointestinal	Anorexia, gastroparesis, abdominal pain, nausea, constipation

Pathological Fractures

The destruction of bone by metastatic disease reduces its load-bearing capabilities and results initially in micro-fractures, which cause pain. Subsequently, fractures occur, most commonly in the ribs and vertebrae. The fracture of a long bone or the epidural extension of tumour into the spine causes most disability. As the development of a long bone fracture has such detri-mental effects on quality of life in patients with advanced cancer, efforts have been made to predict sites of fracture and to use prophylactic surgery.

In a retrospective analysis, patients with evidence on radionuclide bone scan of deposits in the femora or humeri at diagnosis of bone metastases from breast cancer were significantly more likely than other patients to fracture these bones subsequently ($p < 0.0001$) [18]. Patients with bone scan evidence of metastases in the femur or humerus were divided according to the presence of osteolytic disease in these bones on plain radiographs. Patients with both scintigraphic and radiographic abnormalities in the same bone at diagnosis of skeletal metastatic disease were not at greater risk of subsequent fracture than patients with scintigraphic evidence alone. It is possible that the use of alternative imaging modalities may have better predicted those at later risk of fracture, but these data emphasise the long natural history of skeletal metastatic disease and the need for continued radio-graphic monitoring of known sites of disease.

Fractures are common through lytic lesions in weight-bearing bones. Damage to both cortical and trabecular bone are structurally important. Several radiological features have been identified that may predict imminent fracture; fracture is likely if lesions are large, predominantly lytic and erode the cortex. A scoring system has been proposed based upon the site, nature, size and symptoms from a metastatic deposit (Table 5.7) [39]. Using this system, lesions that scored greater than seven generally require

Table 5.7. Scoring system for assessment of metastatic deposits

	Score		
	1	2	3
Site	Upper limb	Lower limb	Peri-trochanteric
Pain	Mild	Moderate	Severe
Lesion	Blastic	Mixed	Lytic
Size	<1/3	1/3–2/3	>2/3

From [37].

surgical intervention; deposits that scored 10 or more had an estimated risk of fracture of greater than 50%.

Prophylactic internal fixation is the treatment of choice for such lesions, followed by radiation therapy to inhibit further tumour growth and avoid further bone destruction. Before surgery, a radionuclide bone scan and radiographs of the affected bone should be obtained. This ensures stabilisation of all potential sites of pathological fracture and that these sites are included in the radiation therapy field.

Pathological fractures are not necessarily a manifes-tation of terminal disease, and primary internal stabilisation followed by radiotherapy is usually the treatment of choice and certainly the modality most likely to restore function and relieve pain [40]. Untreated pathological fractures rarely heal and although local radiation therapy may provide local tumour control, bony union remains unlikely. Patho-logical femoral neck fractures rarely unite despite internal fixation, and in such cases replacement arthroplasty is required. Careful pre-operative assess-ment of the pelvis and femur is needed. If the acetabulum is affected by metastatic disease, then total replacement arthroplasty may be required, or even pelvic reconstruction.

The surgical approaches to prophylaxis and to treatment of pathological fractures are discussed in detail elsewhere.

Compression of the Spinal Cord or Cauda Equina

Spinal cord compression is a medical emergency and suspected cases require urgent evaluation and treat-ment. The prompt and appropriate use of corticosteroids, radiation therapy and/or surgery can reduce permanent neurological damage. There may be few specific warning signs or symptoms of spinal cord compression and clinicians need to maintain a high index of suspicion. In a retrospective analysis of 70 patients with spinal cord compression secondary to breast cancer, 96% of those ambulant prior to therapy maintained the ability to walk [41]. In those unable to walk, 45% regained ambulation, with radiotherapy and surgery equally effective. Median survival was 4 months. The most important predictor of survival was the ability to walk after treatment (Figure 5.4). These results suggest that earlier diagnosis and intervention may improve both outcome and survival.

Pain occurs in the majority of patients, is localised to the area overlying the tumour and often worsens with activities that increase intradural pressure, e.g. coughing, sneezing or straining. The pain is usually

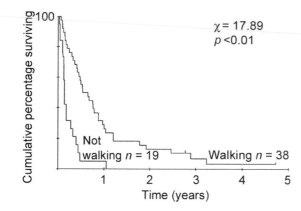

Figure 5.4. Survival from time of diagnosis of spinal cord compression

worse at night, which is the opposite pattern to pain from degenerative disease. There may also be radicular pain radiating down a limb or around the chest or upper abdomen. Local pain usually precedes radicular pain and may pre-date the appearance of other neurological signs by weeks or months.

The majority of patients with spinal cord compression will have weakness or paralysis. Late sensory changes include numbness and anaesthesia distal to the level of involvement. Urinary retention, incontinence and impotence are usually late manifestations of cord compression. However, lesions at the level of the conus medullaris can present with early autonomic dysfunction of the bladder, rectum and genitalia.

In the retrospective analysis of 70 patients with spinal cord compression secondary to breast cancer, mentioned earlier, the most frequent symptom was motor weakness (96%), followed by pain (94%), sensory disturbance (79%) and sphincter disturbance (61%) [41]; 91% of patients had at least one symptom for more than 1 week.

Definitive diagnosis of spinal cord compression is usually made by MRI scanning. MRI is the study of choice because of its high sensitivity for metastatic disease and its ability to detect lesions throughout the spine and to detail tumour present in the spinal canal and the degree of cord compression. CT scan, with or without myelography, may be used if MRI is either contraindicated or unavailable. Extradural compression accounts for more than 95% of cases of spinal cord compression. In more than one-third of cases there are multiple non-contiguous levels.

Corticosteroids should be administered to those patients in whom spinal cord compression is suspected. In a randomised, controlled trial, high-dose dexamethasone (dexamethasone 96 mg i.v. bolus, then 24 mg p.o. q.d.s. for 3 days, then tapered for 10 days) was compared to no steroids in patients with spinal cord compression treated with radiotherapy [42]. There was a statistically and clinically significant benefit for patients treated with steroids (81% ambulatory post-treatment vs. 63% controls). Significant side-effects were reported in 11% of those who received high-dose steroids.

In a historical case-control series, high-dose dexamethasone was compared to moderate-dose dexamethasone (10 mg i.v. bolus, then 4 mg i.v. q.d.s., tapered over 2 weeks) in patients receiving radiotherapy [43]. Significantly fewer side-effects were seen in patients receiving the lower dose of steroids. There was no difference in the post-treatment ambulatory rate between the groups, although these data were not formally reported.

The optimal treatment of epidural spinal cord compression remains controversial. As a result of the lack of well-designed, prospective clinical trials, the decision to choose a specific therapy is primarily based on judgement and experience. Patients can be divided into three categories: ambulatory, non-ambulatory and paraplegic. These patients either have stable, intact vertebral bodies or unstable, collapsed vertebral bodies. Patients with stable spines are treated with corticosteroids, radiotherapy, surgery or a combination of these, whereas patients with unstable spines are usually treated by surgery.

Ambulatory patients with stable spines are usually treated non-operatively. After corticosteroids and radiotherapy, the majority of these patients retain the ability to walk [44]. Radiation therapy is started soon after the administration of corticosteroids.

The optimal treatment for non-ambulatory patients with a stable spine is unclear. Post-treatment ambulatory rates following radiotherapy and corticosteroids are variable and there are no well-controlled studies comparing these treatments with surgery. Paraplegic patients with stable spines have the lowest post-treatment ambulatory rates [44]. The addition of a laminectomy does not increase the ambulatory rate [45].

Spinal instability or vertebral body collapse associated with spinal cord compression is ideally treated with vertebral body resection and spinal stabilisation [46]. Stabilising the spine also promotes mobilisation. Many surgeons would also consider surgery in the following cases: progressive neurological deterioration during radiotherapy; bone extending into the thecal canal, causing thecal compression; radiculopathy with uncontrolled or progressive symptoms; direct tumour extension from primary tumours; and cord compression in a previously irradiated area. Surgery has the potential for considerable morbidity and mortality and the patient's general condition and life expectancy should be taken into account when making these decisions.

Spinal Instability

Back pain is a frequent symptom in patients with advanced cancer, and in 10% of cases is due to spinal instability. The pain, which can be severe, is mechanical in origin and frequently the patient is only comfortable when lying still. Surgical stabilisation is often required to relieve the pain; such major surgery is associated with considerable morbidity and mortality. However, with appropriate patient selection, excellent results can be obtained.

Cranial Nerve Palsies

Cranial nerve palsies are a common consequence of metastases to the base of skull. They are frequently associated with head, neck or facial pain and may be aggravated by neck movements. Frontal, periorbital or retro-orbital pain may be caused by orbital or parasellar lesions and may be accompanied by proptosis and/or diplopia. Involvement of the sphenoid or ethmoid sinuses may cause bifrontal, bitemporal or retro-orbital pain, sometimes associated with feelings of fullness in the head, nasal stuffiness or diplopia. Neurological symptoms and signs may enable the precise anatomical site of a metastasis to be determined. For example, tumours near the jugular foramen often produce occipital pain, radiating to the vertex or ipsilateral side of the neck or shoulder, and are accompanied by dysfunction of the ninth, tenth and eleventh cranial nerves, producing hoarseness, dysarthria and dysphagia.

Bone Marrow Suppression

Infiltration of the bone marrow by metastatic cells results in impaired haematopoiesis and the development of a leukoerythroblastic anaemia characterised by the appearance of immature red cells and granulocytes in the peripheral blood. The associated thrombocytopenia and leukopenia predispose to haemorrhage and infection, respectively. These effects on bone marrow function can limit the doses of both radiotherapy and chemotherapy that can be safely administered.

SUMMARY

Bone metastases are the cause of considerable morbidity in patients with advanced cancer. Patients with metastatic breast or prostate cancers are particularly likely to develop complications from bone metastases. The principal problems that arise are pain, pathological fractures, spinal cord compression, hypercalcaemia and bone marrow suppression. Together, these problems are responsible for a high proportion of days spent in hospital as a result of cancer, and therefore are costly to both the patient and the healthcare provider. Preliminary studies have suggested certain clinical or biochemical features that might predict which patients with bone metastases are at particular risk of developing the most serious complications, and this can assist in the selection of patients for optimal treatment and towards the prevention of serious morbidity.

Although the recent introduction of the bisphosphonates is reducing the complication rate from bone metastases, much more progress still needs to be made to lessen this problem as a major cause of disability and suffering in patients with cancer. In the meantime, the management of patients with skeletal metastases requires close cooperation between medical oncologists, radiation oncologists, nuclear medicine physicians, symptom control teams and orthopaedic surgeons to palliate symptoms and to prevent complications.

REFERENCES

1. Galasko C. The anatomy and pathways of skeletal metastases. In Weiss L, Gilbert A (eds), Bone Metastases. GK Hall: Boston, 1981: 49–63.
2. Batson O. The role of vertebral veins in metastatic processes. Ann Intern Med 1942; 16: 38–45.
3. Bundred N et al. Parathyroid hormone related protein and skeletal morbidity in breast cancer. Eur J Cancer 1992; 28: 690–2.
4. Coleman R, Rubens R. The clinical course of bone metastases in breast cancer. Br J Cancer 1987; 77: 336–40.
5. Koenders P et al. Steroid hormone receptor activity of primary human breast cancer and pattern of first metastasis. Breast Cancer Res Treat 1991; 18: 27–32.
6. Fang K, Peng C. Predicting the probability of bone metastasis through histological grading of prostate carcinoma: a retrospective correlative analysis of 81 autopsy cases with ante-mortem transurethral resection specimens. J Urol 1983; 57: 715–20.

7. Rivkees A, Crawford J. The relationship of gonadal activity and chemotherapy-induced gonadal damage. J Am Med Assoc 1988; 259: 2123–5.

8. Saarto T et al. Chemical castration induced by adjuvant cyclophosphamide, methotrexate and fluorouracil chemotherapy causes rapid bone loss that is reduced by clodronate: a randomised study in premenopausal breast cancer patients. J Clin Oncol 1997; 15: 1341–7.

9. Powles T et al. The effect of tamoxifen on lumbar bone mineral density in pre- and post-menopausal women. J Clin Oncol 1996; 14: 78–84.

10. Daniell H. Osteoporosis after orchiectomy for prostate cancer. J Urol 1997; 157: 439–44.

11. Edelstyn G, Gillespie P, Grebbel F. The radiological demonstration of osseous metastases: experimental observations. Clin Radiol 1967; 18: 158–61.

12. Fogelman I, Coleman R. The bone scan and breast cancer. In Freeman L, Weisman H (eds), Nuclear Medicine Annual. Raven: New York, 1988: 1–14.

13. Muindi J et al. The role of computed tomography in the detection of bone metastases in breast cancer patients. Br J Cancer 1983; 56: 233–6.

14. Traill Z et al. Magnetic resonance imaging versus radionuclide scintigraphy in screening for bone metastases. Clin Radiol 1999; 54: 448–51.

15. Urwin G et al. Generalised increase in bone resorption in carcinoma of the prostate. Br J Urol 1985; 57: 721–3.

16. Garnero P et al. Markers of bone turnover for the management of patients with bone metastases from prostate cancer. Br J Cancer 2000; 82: 858–64.

17. Domchek S et al. Predictors of skeletal complications in patients with metastatic breast carcinoma. Cancer 2000; 89: 363–8.

18. Plunkett T, Smith P, Rubens R. Risk of complications from bone metastases in breast cancer: implications for management. Eur J Cancer 2000; 36: 476–82.

19. Coleman R, Smith P, Rubens R. Clinical course and prognostic factors following bone recurrence from breast cancer. Br J Cancer 1998; 77: 336–40.

20. Landis S et al. Cancer statistics. CA Cancer J Clin 1999; 49: 8–29.

21. Robson M, Dawson N. How is androgen-dependent metastatic prostate cancer best treated? Hematol Oncol Clin North Am 1996; 10: 727–47.

22. Eisenberger M, Crawford E, Wolf M. Prognostic factors in stage D2 prostate cancer: important implications for future trials. Semin Oncol 1994; 21: 613–19.

23. Matzkin H, Perito P, Soloway M. Prognostic factors in metastatic prostate cancer. Cancer 1993; 72(suppl 12): 3788–92.

24. Crawford E, Eisenberger M, McLeod K. A controlled trial of leuprolide with and without flutamide in prostatic carcinoma. N Engl J Med 1989; 321: 419–24.

25. Soloway M, Hardeman S, Hickey D. Stratification of patients with metastatic prostate cancer based on extent of disease on initial bone scan. Cancer 1988; 61: 195–202.

26. Sabbatini P et al. Prognostic significance of extent of disease in bone in patients with androgen-independent prostate cancer. J Clin Oncol 1999; 17: 948–57.

27. International Commission on Radiological Protection. Report of the Task Force Group on the Reference Man. Pergamon Press: New York, 1975.

28. Akimoto S et al. Inability of bone turnover marker as a strong prognostic indicator in prostate cancer patients with bone metastasis: comparison with the extent of disease (EOD) grade. Prostate 1999; 38: 28–34.

29. Smith M, Newland A. Treatment of myeloma. Qu J Med 1999; 92: 11–14.

30. Bataille R, Boccadoro M, Klein B. C-reactive protein and β-2 microglobulin produce a simple and powerful myeloma staging system. Blood 1992; 80: 733–9.

31. Fonseca R et al. Prognostic value of serum markers of bone metabolism in untreated multiple myeloma patients. Br J Haematol 2000; 109: 24–9.

32. McCloskey E et al. Natural history of skeletal disease in multiple myelomatosis and treatment with clodronate. Bone Min 1992; 28(suppl 1): S27–31.

33. Mercadante S. Malignant bone pain: pathophysiology and treatment. Pain 1997; 69: 1–18.

34. Front D et al. Bone metastases and bone pain in breast cancer. J Am Med Assoc 1979; 242: 1747–8.

35. Muggia F. Overview of cancer-related hypercalcaemia: epidemiology and etiology. Semin Oncol 1990; 17(suppl 5): 3–9.

36. Coleman R, Fogelman I, Rubens R. Hypercalcaemia and breast cancer: an increased humoral component in patients with liver metastases. Eur J Surg Oncol 1988; 14: 423–8.

37. Body J, Delmas P. Urinary pyridinium crosslinks as markers of bone resorption in tumor-associated hypercalcaemia. J Clin Endocrinol Metab 1992; 74: 471–5.

38. Grill V et al. Parathyroid hormone-related protein: elevated levels in both humoral hypercalcaemia of malignancy and hypercalcaemia complicating metastatic breast cancer. J Clin Endocrinol Metab 1991; 73: 1309–15.

39. Mirels H. Metastatic disease in long bones: a proposed scoring system for diagnosing impending pathological fractures. Clin Orthoped Clin Res 1989; 249: 256–64.

40. Douglass H, Shukla S, Mindell E. Treatment of pathological fractures of long bones excluding those due to breast cancer. J Bone Joint Surg Am 1976; 58: 1055–61.

41. Hill M et al. Spinal cord compression in breast cancer: a review of 70 cases. Br J Cancer 1993; 68: 969–73.

42. Sorensen S et al. Effect of high-dose dexamethasone in carcinomatous metastatic spinal cord compression treated with radiotherapy. Eur J Cancer 1994; 1: 22–7.

43. Heimdal K et al. High incidence of serious side effects of high-dose dexamethasone treatment in patients with epidural spinal cord compression. J Neurooncol 1992; 12: 141–4.

44. Maranzano E, Latini P. Effectiveness of radiation therapy without surgery in metastatic spinal cord compression: final results from a prospective trial. Int J Radiat Oncol Biol Phys 1995; 32: 959–67.

45. Young R, Post E, King G. Treatment of spinal epidural metastases. Randomised prospective comparison of laminectomy and radiotherapy. J Neurosurg 1980; 53: 741–8.

46. Loblaw D, Laperriere N. Emergency treatment of malignant extradural spinal cord compression: an evidence-based guideline. J Clin Oncol 1998; 16: 1613–24.

6

Radioisotope and PET Imaging of Bone Metastases

Gary J. R. Cook[1] and Ignac Fogelman[2]

[1]*Royal Marsden Hospital, Sutton, and* [2]*Guy's Hospital, London, UK*

INTRODUCTION

Bone scintigraphy remains one of the most widely used methods for the diagnosis and surveillance of metastatic skeletal disease and was first described by Fleming and colleagues in 1961 using strontium-85 (^{85}Sr) [1]. Since then there have been many developments in both radiopharmaceuticals and scanning techniques to aid evaluation of metastatic bone disease. In recent years, technetium-99m (^{99m}Tc)-labelled diphosphonates have become the most widely used radiopharmaceuticals, particularly ^{99m}Tc methylene diphosphonate (MDP). Improvements in gamma camera design, including the increased availability of tomographic scintigraphy (single photon emission computed tomography, SPECT), have also helped nuclear medicine techniques maintain their clinical utility, in spite of the major advances in cross-sectional anatomical imaging techniques such as computed tomography (CT) and magnetic resonance imaging (MRI).

In addition to non-specific skeletal tracers, there are a number of radiopharmaceuticals which exist for specific types or groups of tumours and which, in addition to evaluating soft tissue metastases, can be helpful in assessing the skeleton. Examples include iodine-131 (^{131}I) for differentiated thyroid cancer metastases, ^{123}I or ^{131}I meta-iodobenzylguanidine (mIBG) and Indium-111 (^{111}In) octreotide for neuroendocrine tumours, including neuroblastoma and carcinoid. Some non-specific tumour-avid radiopharmaceuticals have also been assessed in the evaluation

of skeletal metastases, including thallium-201 (^{201}Tl), ^{99m}Tc sestamibi and ^{99m}Tc pentavalent dimercaptosuccinic acid (V-DMSA). However, compared to the diphosphonates and tumour-specific tracers, they are rarely used in clinical practice to specifically evaluate the skeleton.

Positron emission tomography (PET) was previously regarded as a research tool but there has been an enormous increase in clinical applications in recent years, particularly in the field of oncology. Imaging can be performed on dedicated PET scanners or, more recently, on the lower cost option of hybrid gamma cameras.

Although the bone-specific tracer ^{18}F-fluoride was first described for skeletal imaging in the 1960s [2], with the increased availability in clinical PET there has been renewed interest in this tracer. The most commonly used tracer in clinical PET is ^{18}F-fluorodeoxyglucose (^{18}FDG), a non-specific tumour agent in which there has been some interest for the evaluation of skeletal metastases.

RADIOPHARMACEUTICALS AND MECHANISMS OF UPTAKE

The uptake of bone agents such as the diphosphonates depends on both local blood flow and, more importantly, local osteoblastic activity. The exact mechanism of uptake is still not fully understood but it is thought that the diphosphonate groups are chemisorbed on to the surface of bone and are incorporated into the

Textbook of Bone Metastases. Edited by C. Jasmin, R. E. Coleman, L. R. Coia, R. Capanna and G. Saillant
© 2005 John Wiley & Sons Ltd: ISBN 0 471 87742 5

hydroxyapatite crystal, especially at sites of new or reactive bone formation. Therefore, sclerotic metastases, as commonly seen in prostatic cancer for example, in which newly formed bone is laid down without prior resorption, are associated with markedly increased uptake of bone tracers. Although osteolytic metastases, caused by osteoclastic bone resorption stimulated by tumour derived cytokines, are more commonly seen in most cancers, this type of metastasis also is nearly always accompanied by reactive bone formation, leading to uptake of bone radiopharmaceuticals. In tumours where osteolysis predominates, such as myeloma, there may be little in the way of an osteoblastic response and hence there may be little or no abnormality visible on bone scintigraphy. It is rare for a bone scan to be completely normal in myeloma patients but a radiographic skeletal survey may be a better method to assess the extent of skeletal disease [3]. With improved spatial resolution on modern gamma cameras it may be possible to detect purely cold lesions. This is a fact that is worth considering when interpreting a bone scan of a patient with a malignancy that is known to produce predominantly lytic lesions, such as myeloma or renal cell carcinoma, as these may not be obvious on initial inspection. Predominantly cold lesions may also be seen in very aggressive metastases where surrounding bone is unable to mount an osteoblastic response (Figure 6.1).

It is the functional nature of bone scintigraphy and the fact that most skeletal metastases are accompanied by an osteoblastic response, whether they are predominantly sclerotic or lytic in nature, which makes it such a sensitive technique. It has been estimated that at least 50% of bone must be destroyed before a lesion is evident radiographically [4]. Galasko reported a lead-time of 12–18 months for bone scintigraphy over radiography [5], and in a serial study of 6 monthly bone scans a median lead-time of 4 months (range 0–18 months) was found [6].

When using bone-specific tracers to assess response to treatment, it must be noted that an increase in activity of lesions, or even an increase in the number of lesions, does not always correspond to disease progression. The well-recognised flare response on the bone scan, whereby an increase in uptake in responding metastases due to a local bone osteoblastic reaction in the early months following instigation of systemic therapy, has been described as a result of chemotherapy and hormone therapy in both breast and prostate cancer [7,8]. This may be indistinguishable from truly progressive disease. The appearance of new uptake in hitherto undetected lesions has also been described as part of this phenomenon [9]. The

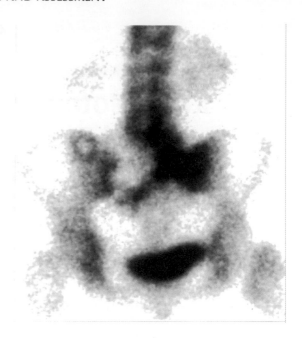

Figure 6.1. ^{99m}Tc MDP bone scan of the posterior pelvis in a woman with known myeloma, demonstrating a large photopoenic abnormality with a rim of increased activity in the left of the sacrum, consistent with a predominantly lytic lesion

increased uptake as a result of the flare response may last for as long as 6 months after therapy before a subsequent decrease in uptake in individual lesions is noted, but has been reported to be associated with a more favourable prognosis [10]. An early reduction in uptake after treatment virtually always indicates a response, except in the instances where very aggressive lytic disease may continue to progress without an osteoblastic response, an observation that is, however, rare.

If a bone scan is performed at a time beyond which the flare response can occur, then an increase in the number of skeletal lesions is usually taken as incontrovertible evidence of disease progression. Similarly, allowing for technical acquisition and display factors, an increase in intensity in known skeletal metastases is also generally regarded as evidence of disease progression [11], although it is not as reliable a sign [12].

Other single-photon radiopharmaceuticals have been used in the assessment of both primary and metastatic bone tumours and are most commonly non-specific tumour agents rather than acting as bone tracers. Thallium-201 (^{201}Tl), an analogue of potassium, enters tumour cells via the Na^+/K^+ ATPase pump but, as well as reflecting the metabolic status of the cell, uptake also depends on blood flow. ^{99m}Tc-labelled sestamibi shows a similar distribution to ^{201}Tl but has a different mechanism of accumulation and is thought to reflect cell viability, and is mainly associated in cells with the mitochondria. Interestingly, this agent is a substrate for the membrane glycoprotein P-glycoprotein, which is associated with tumour multi-drug resistance and, when present, leads to the transport of sestamibi back out of the cell. ^{99m}Tc V-DMSA uptake has also been described in bone metastases, the exact mechanism of uptake being uncertain (Figure 6.2) [13].

The majority of bone metastases initially seed in bone marrow and there is therefore the potential to use bone marrow scintigraphy as a method to detect bone metastases at an early stage, by demonstrating focal areas of marrow replacement [14]. There are a number of limitations to this technique, including difficulty in visualising the spine because of overlying hepatic and splenic activity, and the inability to assess areas of the skeleton where red marrow is scarce. Because of this, the technique is unlikely to be used to routinely detect and determine the extent of skeletal metastases but may nevertheless be useful in certain cases in conjunction with ^{99m}Tc MDP scintigraphy, where the specificity for individual lesions may be improved.

A number of nuclear medicine tracers exist which are specific to a type or group of tumours. These localise in both skeletal and soft tissue metastases and are often valuable in assessing the total extent of disease. Examples include ^{131}I for differentiated thyroid cancers; ^{131}I- and ^{123}I-labelled meta-iodobenzoylguanidine (mIBG), which behaves as a noradrenaline analogue localising in a number of neuroendocrine tumours, including neuroblastoma, medullary thyroid cancer and carcinoid tumours; and indium-111 (^{111}In)-labelled octreotide, which localises in tumours bearing somatostatin receptors, including a number of neuroendocrine tumours.

Currently available PET tracers with a potential role for assessing skeletal metastases include ^{18}F-fluoride ion and ^{18}FDG. The mechanism of uptake of ^{18}F-fluoride is similar to other bone tracers used in nuclear medicine and depends on both regional blood flow and osteoblastic activity. It is preferentially deposited at sites of high bone turnover and remodelling by chemisorption onto bone surfaces, exchanging with hydroxyl groups in hydroxyapatite crystal of bone to form fluoroapatite [15].

As tumour uptake of ^{18}FDG depends on glycolysis and membrane glucose transporters, both of which are known to be increased in malignant tissue [16,17], the mechanism of uptake, and hence the information

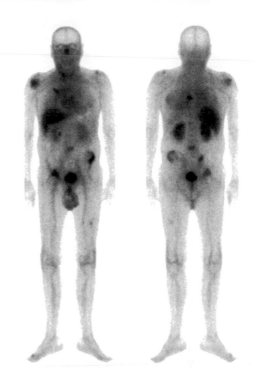

Figure 6.2. Anterior (left) and posterior (right) ^{99m}Tc pentavalent DMSA scan of a patient with medullary thyroid cancer, demonstrating metastases in the right humerus, a right anterior rib, the spine and the pelvis

available from this tracer in the skeleton, are significantly different to ^{18}F-fluoride. The uptake of ^{18}FDG is obviously not restricted to tumour involving the skeleton and has the advantage of demonstrating all metastatic sites in a cancer patient, whether they are in soft tissue or bone.

SCANNING TECHNIQUES

Although many ^{99m}Tc MDP bone scans have been acquired as multiple overlapping spot views of the skeleton in the past, modern dual-headed gamma cameras allow high resolution, whole-body images of the entire skeleton in a short acquisition time, including both anterior and posterior images. Most modern gamma camera systems also have the ability to acquire additional tomographic images (SPECT), allowing an increased sensitivity for lesion detection because of the resultant improvement in contrast compared to planar imaging, and a better three-dimensional localisation of abnormalities, which aids specificity. It has been suggested that SPECT imaging not only increases sensitivity in the detection of vertebral metastases in cancer patients but, by being able to examine the pattern and position of lesions tomographically, it may be possible to improve differentiation between metastases and coincidental benign lesions. For example, lesions that extend from the vertebral body into the posterior vertebral elements, or involve the pedicle, are more likely to represent metastases than lesions confined to the facet joints, anterior vertebral body or either side of a disc (Figure 6.3) [18,19].

PET is a branch of nuclear medicine which, although not yet widely available, has a growing list of clinical applications in oncology. It depends on the detection of two coincident 511 keV γ-rays, which are emitted at 180° from one another following the annihilation of a positron (a positively charged, antimatter equivalent of an electron from an unstable nucleus). The synchronous detection of the two photons allows accurate placement of the point of emission and, with standard image reconstruction algorithms, tomographic images can be acquired and displayed. There are a number of advantages over conventional nuclear medicine techniques. PET shows higher spatial resolution and accurate, absolute quantitation, the latter because of the ability to accurately correct for the effects of attenuation of photons within the body. In addition, PET radionuclides include isotopes of oxygen, carbon and nitrogen, biologically important elements that allow the labelling of naturally occurring compounds rather than analogues. At present clinical PET centres are not widespread but there is a growing interest and increasing evidence of cost-effectiveness, especially in oncology, and PET is likely to play a more significant role in patient management in the future.

PATTERNS IN THE SCINTIGRAPHIC EVALUATION OF BONE METASTASES

The typical pattern of widespread focal areas of increased uptake of ^{99m}Tc diphosphonates, predominantly in the axial skeleton in the distribution of red marrow, is easily recognised (Figure 6.4). However, peripheral skeletal metastases may occur and are most commonly seen in clinical practice in lung, prostate

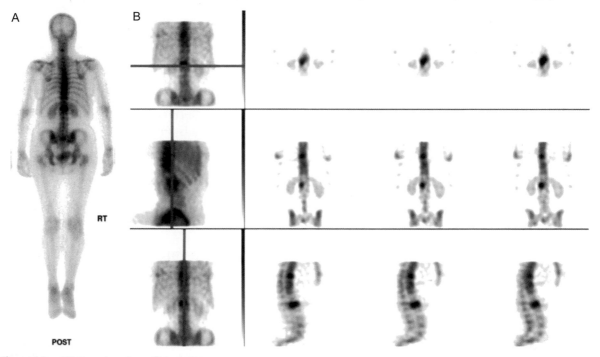

Figure 6.3. (A) Posterior planar ^{99m}Tc MDP bone scan in a patient with breast cancer. (B) Transaxial, coronal and sagittal (top to bottom) tomographic (SPECT) images of the lumbar spine from the same study. Focal abnormalities are seen in the mid-cervical, mid-thoracic and upper lumbar spine. On transaxial SPECT images, the upper lumbar spine abnormality can be seen to extend posteriorly from the vertebral body into the posterior elements, a pattern that is likely to represent a metastatic deposit rather than coincidental degenerative disease

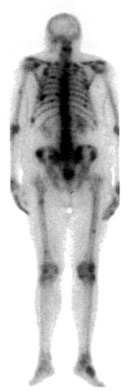

Figure 6.4. Posterior ^{99m}Tc MDP bone scan of a patient with prostate cancer, demonstrating multiple irregularly scattered lesions, predominantly in the axial skeleton, a pattern typical of bone metastases

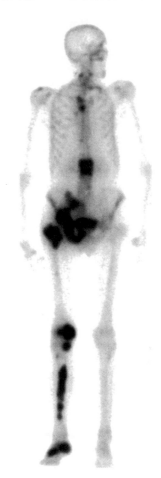

Figure 6.5. Anterior ^{99m}Tc MDP bone scan in a man with prostate cancer. In addition to some spinal and pelvic abnormalities, a number of lesions show an unusual peripheral distribution in the right leg

and breast cancer (Figure 6.5) [20]. It has previously been somewhat controversial as to whether to include the peripheries in all patients having a bone scan. With most modern gamma cameras it is much easier to obtain whole-body scans in a single acquisition with greater time efficiency than the multiple overlapping spot view technique of old. In addition to detecting peripheral metastases, a potential bonus of including the peripheries is the detection of hypertrophic pulmonary osteoarthropathy (HPOA) associated with malignancy. The typical scintigraphic appearance of HPOA is of increased uptake in the cortex of the ends of long bones, giving rise to the "tram-line sign", and is often noted at the wrists, distal tibiae or distal femora.

Of course, increased uptake of tracer on a bone scan is not specific for malignancy. Although there is usually little doubt as to the metastatic nature of irregularly distributed lesions in the axial skeleton of cancer patients, solitary lesions may be more problematic and are not uncommon. In a retrospective analysis

of 301 patients with a variety of cancers, 11% had malignancy confirmed in solitary new lesions [11]. In a further study of patients with breast cancer, 21% relapsed with a solitary new bone metastasis in the spine [21]. A single focal rib lesion is usually regarded as having a low probability of being metastatic (~10%) in patients with known cancer [22,23], although a more recent study found that more than 40% of such lesions subsequently proved to be metastatic in nature [24].

It is not uncommon to see a solitary upper rib lesion in patients with breast cancer due to osteonecrotic fracture following radiotherapy. Focal rib lesions are otherwise commonly a result of trauma that may not even be recalled by the patient, but lesions that appear to extend along the length of a rib are more suspicious of malignant infiltration. However, a line of foci in adjacent ribs is almost certainly indicative of a traumatic aetiology.

The interpretation of lesions in the spine may be especially problematic, as there is a high incidence of benign disease, such as osteoarthritis, in this region that may mimic metastases. Because of the large amount of haematopoietic marrow in vertebrae, the spine is also a common site for metastases. Solitary spinal lesions have been reported to have a benign aetiology in 57% of patients in one series [25]. A feature that has been described as being more commonly associated with benign disease is that of peripheral vertebral lesions that extend outside the vertebral margin, in contrast to complex irregular lesions, which are more commonly associated with metastases. These observations were made on planar bone imaging and, as mentioned above, it is possible that the addition of tomographic scintigraphic images may improve specificity further.

Linear increased uptake within a vertebral body is a typical feature of vertebral body fracture but it is not possible to differentiate vertebral collapse due to osteoporosis from that due to tumour infiltration on a bone scan alone. The presence of multiple other irregularly distributed lesions would point towards a malignant aetiology, whereas fading activity over a period of a few months would suggest a benign cause for fracture, but otherwise it may be difficult to characterise these lesions on bone scintigraphy alone. Spinal radiographs do not commonly add further information, other than confirming that the bone scan findings are due to vertebral collapse, but correlative MRI or CT may show specific findings to suggest malignancy.

Interval bone scans may be helpful in characterising otherwise non-specific bone scan findings. For example, in a small series of patients with a variety of known cancers, 19/21 metastases became more intense, whilst benign lesions either remained unchanged (47%) or resolved (41%) [11]. Benign rib, pelvic and peripheral lesions tended to resolve within 12–24 months, whilst benign vertebral and skull lesions persisted, probably reflecting the different nature of benign lesions tending to occur at different skeletal sites. Even using all the available information from a bone scan, there are a number of abnormalities that require further investigation to be accurately characterised. It is common practice to acquire radiographs in the first instance and, if there is a benign abnormality to explain a bone scan lesion, then there is less than a 1% chance that a coincident metastasis will be missed [26]. Because radiographs are much less sensitive than bone scinti-

graphy, the converse is not true and a negative radiograph does not exclude metastatic disease. In this situation, with currently available imaging technology, cross-sectional imaging with CT or MRI may be the most appropriate next investigation in evaluating indeterminate bone scan lesions. The role of ^{18}FDG PET is still being assessed in this situation but would appear to be a promising alternative method for differentiating benign from malignant tissue.

In common with any imaging technique, it is important that potential pitfalls, including normal variations, benign causes of uptake and artefacts, are recognised to aid accurate interpretation. A number of variants that may mimic metastases have been described. These include focal activity at the confluence of the sutures at the pterion in the skull, the deltoid muscle insertion on the humerus, and symmetrical paraspinal muscle insertions in the ribs, resulting in a stippled appearance.

Abnormalities seen at joints are generally benign, with increased uptake seen on either side of a joint being a reassuring feature. This pattern may be more difficult to discern in the spine but the addition of SPECT and correlative radiographs may again be helpful in this situation.

In some areas of the world, Paget's disease may be present in up to 5% of the population over the age of 40 [27]. This disease is multifocal in the majority and is often asymptomatic but may be difficult to differentiate from metastases. Factors that may aid correct interpretation include the presence of diffuse uptake throughout a bone, abnormal activity extending from a joint into the diaphysis of a long bone, with a flame-shaped leading edge, or the appearance of expansion or bowing. Even if there are characteristic scintigraphic features, it is often advisable to confirm the diagnosis with radiographs. Even so, radiographic appearances may be difficult to differentiate from confluent osteoblastic metastases such as those commonly seen in prostate cancer.

On occasion, when bone metastases are very extensive and become confluent, the diffuse nature of uptake may make the bone scan appear normal on first inspection. However, the "superscan", so-called because of the apparent exceptional quality of the scan, has a number of characteristic features that should alert the interpreter. In addition to the apparent high quality of the scan, soft tissue activity, including the kidneys, becomes inconspicuous due to the increased uptake of tracer by the skeleton and resultant increase in bone:soft tissue ratio (Figure 6.6). On close inspection there are often some areas of inhomogeneity of tracer uptake, particularly

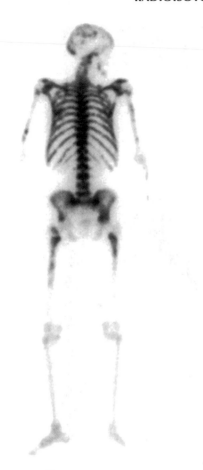

Figure 6.6. Posterior ^{99m}Tc MDP bone scan in a man with prostate cancer. Note the increased contrast between bone and soft tissue, with no visualisation of renal tissue. The irregularity of uptake in the long bones, ribs and skull indicate that this is a superscan due to extensive metastatic disease

in the ribs and long bones, indicating the metastatic nature and differentiating it from metabolic causes of superscans, such as hyperparathyroidism.

BONE SCINTIGRAPHY IN SPECIFIC CANCERS

The clinical use of bone scans is governed to a large extent by the frequency of skeletal metastases in individual cancers. Breast and prostate cancer are the most frequent indications for bone scintigraphy in many institutions, although specific roles exist in many other types of cancer.

Although controversy still exists as to the requirement of skeletal scintigraphy at different disease stages,

a number of general situations arise where it is potentially valuable. Examples include initial evaluation as a baseline staging procedure, in the surveillance of asymptomatic patients, evaluating treatment response and investigating individuals with clinical or biochemical features suggesting possible skeletal metastases.

Breast Cancer

Breast cancer is common and the skeleton is the most frequent site to which breast cancer spreads. Skeletal metastases are the reason for much of the morbidity and disability caused by this disease. The clinical course may be prolonged, with the median survival for those in whom the disease remains confined to the skeleton being 24 months and with 20% remaining alive at 5 years [28]. The costs of treating bone metastases and complications make a major demand on health care resources [29]. In skeletal metastases from breast cancer there is usually a predominance of osteoclastic activity, leading to lytic lesions that are generally associated with greater morbidity, but mixed or purely osteoblastic lesions may also occur.

Controversy exists as to the best time to use the bone scan in patients with breast cancer, in part due to conflicting results from early studies in the 1970s and 1980s. Small numbers of subjects within studies, different radiopharmaceuticals, varied criteria for diagnosis of metastases and inconsistent use of correlative radiography are factors that are likely to be responsible for discrepancies between early studies. More recent reports, using similar modern radiopharmaceuticals and imaging equipment, have shown more uniform results.

In the initial staging of breast cancer early studies showed detection rates of 0–18% for stage I [30–34] and 0–41% for stage II [30–35]. These figures compared to 0–6% and 0.2–10%, respectively [36–39], in later studies when radiopharmaceuticals, equipment and reporting criteria were more standardised. The apparently high incidence of metastases resulting from some of the early studies led to the belief that all women with breast cancer should have a staging bone scan. This is no longer universally held but many clinicians find a baseline scan may be useful for subsequent comparison. Stage III disease is associated with a detection rate of 6–62% in these studies and, as such, many believe that this would justify routine bone scans in this group. Surprisingly, the gain from bone scans in this group may be less than expected, as many with locally advanced disease may be inoperable and require local radiotherapy and chemotherapy, even with a positive scan. However, the bone scan may still be valuable in detecting metastases at risk of pathological fracture or spinal cord compression, thereby aiding in directing palliative radiotherapy.

In one of the largest studies (1267 patients) in which clinical staging, scintigraphic technique and scan interpretation were well standardised, where correlative radiographs were used and there was at least 1 year of follow-up data on each patient, the fraction of patients with bone metastases was 0% for stage I, 3% for stage II, 7% for stage III and 47% for stage IV [36]. When staging by tumour size alone, it was found that T1 tumours (0–2 cm) were only rarely associated with bone metastases (0.3%), but T2 (2–5 cm), T3 (> 5 cm) and T4 (> 5 cm + infiltration/ulceration) cases had scan-positive rates of 3%, 8% and 13%, respectively. It was therefore felt that bone scans are appropriate in those with stage II or above, or in those with tumours greater than 2 cm. As expected, a positive baseline scan also has prognostic significance [39,40].

In the screening of asymptomatic patients, most authors conclude that serial scans are not required and probably not cost-effective. The majority of patients may seek medical attention between scans and have relapses that are clinically evident [41]. Even if routine serial scans lead to the detection of more metastases than clinical follow-up alone, it is unlikely that survival would be changed [42]. Rather than serially scanning all patients, it has been suggested that identifying those with adverse prognostic features (T4 tumours, more than four involved axillary lymph nodes, inoperable tumour) is worthwhile [6].

In symptomatic patients, few would argue that a bone scan is justified and may be helpful in decisions on subsequent local or systemic palliative therapy, as well as providing prognostic information. The bone scan is particularly valuable in those with new symptoms, or in those in whom there are clinical, laboratory or radiological features that are worrying and may play an important role in identifying metastases at risk of complications such as fracture. Metastases identified in the long bones are particularly worth radiological follow-up and may be considered at such risk that prophylactic orthopaedic intervention is required. In hypercalcaemic patients, the bone scan is a convenient method to investigate the cause. Although widespread skeletal metastases are often related, humoral factors may be the cause of hypercalcaemia in 15% [28].

A standardised approach for assessing the response of bone metastases to treatment is to compare serial radiographs. The Union Internationale Contre le Cancer (UICC) defined a number of criteria, including disappearance or reduction in size of lesions and sclerosis of lytic lesions, to indicate various levels of response [43]. This method may be relatively insensitive, as it may take 6–12 months for radiographic evidence of response to be apparent and the assessment of sclerotic disease may be especially problematic. It has also been noted that the response of skeletal disease to systemic therapy is less than apparent overall response, a finding that is felt to reflect the relative insensitivity of the UICC criteria [28]. Although other methods have been proposed to assess skeletal response, including clinical assessment [44], tumour [45] and biochemical markers [46], the bone scan has inherent advantages, as it assesses the whole skeleton whilst localising disease and is very sensitive.

The flare phenomenon may complicate the interpretation of serial bone scans in the first few months after systemic therapy. It has been reported as a consequence of both endocrine and chemotherapy but, if recognised, it is associated with a more favourable prognosis [7,10]. The appearances of the flare phenomenon are maximal at 3 months and it may not be possible to predict response from progression until 6 months following systemic therapy. However, an early reduction in uptake after treatment usually indicates a response, except in the rare instances where very aggressive lytic disease may continue to progress without an osteoblastic response. Similarly, a reduction in the number of visible metastases is associated with disease response. Allowing for these confounding factors, and by only interpreting scans with a detailed knowledge of previous therapy, the bone scan is nevertheless not only a valuable objective measure of response but also gives prognostic information [47]. Even so, the bone scan is limited in its sensitivity to measure treatment effect, with only 52% of responders showing scintigraphic improvement and 62% of non-responders showing scintigraphic deterioration at 6–8 months in one early study [44]. Despite this, approximately one-third of patients in whom radiographs were unhelpful in assessing response showed clear evidence of bone scan changes, but not usually until the 6–8 month follow-up. In an attempt to increase sensitivity of response measurement, some authors have described semiquantitative means of following bone metastases [48,49], but others have found no advantage over visual interpretation [50] and quantitative methods have not gained acceptance into routine practice.

Prostate Cancer

Prostate cancer is one of the commonest to occur in men and frequently metastasises to the skeleton, 85%

of men dying from the disease having evidence of skeletal involvement. Skeletal metastases are most often osteoblastic, leading to sclerotic appearances on radiographs and focal uptake of bone tracers on scintigraphy.

At presentation the fraction of patients with skeletal disease is high and may be 30–50% [51]. The proportion of positive bone scans varies with disease stage. As many as 9% with stage I and 60% with stage IV [52] or 7.1% with T1 and 65% with T2 tumours may be positive [52,53]. These figures would suggest that a bone scan is indicated in every patient presenting with prostate cancer and indeed this is still common practice. However, if using histological staging methods, such as Gleason score, or biochemical measurement of tumour markers, such as prostatic specific antigen (PSA), then it may be possible to define a group who are at very low risk of skeletal disease at presentation. For example, those with a low Gleason score (2–5) or low PSA level (< 10 ng/ml) have a very low probability of bone metastases [54,55]. Of course, most would consider it reasonable to scan all patients who are symptomatic, whatever the initial stage.

PSA measurement may prove helpful in the serial follow-up of patients. Even though a high conversion to bone scan-positive has been reported in the first year (20%) [56], rather than routinely scanning all patients, a rising PSA level might be a better method to select patients for scintigraphy [57].

The flare response may also complicate the measurement of treatment response in prostate cancer and has been described in relation to both hormonal therapy and orchidectomy [8,58]. Whilst some authors have reported only a low incidence of the flare response [59], others have noted this effect much more frequently [60].

It is possible that the measurement of prostate-specific antigen (PSA) may be helpful in deciding which patients warrant bone scintigraphy following treatment. In those with increasing levels, bone scintigraphy may then be helpful in identifying sites of disease recurrence, approximately 50% of such patients being reported to have evidence of skeletal involvement in one study [57]. Those without evidence of skeletal disease usually had recurrence in the prostatic bed, and those with a decreasing PSA level also showed evidence of treatment response on bone scintigraphy.

For those patients in whom bone scan appearances deteriorate despite therapy, prognosis is much worse. Pollen et al. showed that the 1 year survival for those with progression was only 7% compared to 60% in those without [61]. As with carcinoma of the breast, the flare phenomenon may predict a subsequent good clinical response [62].

Miscellaneous Cancers

Reports of the frequency of skeletal metastases in patients presenting with lung cancer vary widely (2–19%) [63]. The variation may indicate different proportions of tumour type in different studies, as small cell carcinoma appears to have a higher incidence of skeletal involvement, approaching 50% [64,65]. A positive bone scan is a poor prognostic sign, as very few patients will subsequently survive 12 months [66]. It remains controversial as to whether all patients should have staging bone scans at presentation but the necessity may diminish as [18]FDG PET becomes more widely available and increasingly utilised as a routine preoperative staging procedure for non-small cell lung cancer [67].

Routine follow-up bone scintigraphy is not frequently practised in asymptomatic lung cancer, as there is no evidence of improvement in survival or morbidity, but it may help in planning appropriate therapy in symptomatic patients and excluding benign causes of symptoms. A relatively common finding in lung cancer on bone scans is hypertrophic pulmonary osteoarthropathy, the appearances of which are described above.

Although renal cell carcinoma is reported to metastasise to bone relatively frequently (7.5–32%) [63], the majority of patients have clinical or biochemical evidence and there would therefore not seem to be a role for routine screening of asymptomatic patients at presentation. Metastases from renal cell carcinoma are frequently predominantly lytic and may not excite much in the way of an osteoblastic response. These types of lesion may therefore be relatively inconspicuous on a bone scan and a careful review for cold lesions should always be made [68].

Neuroblastoma, a solid tumour of childhood, is frequently associated with skeletal involvement. High quality bone scintigraphy is required to avoid false negative interpretations. First, photopoenic lesions may occur that are difficult to resolve in the small paediatric skeleton [69], and second, the only scintigraphic sign may be blurring of epiphyseal activity (Figure 6.7). Accumulation of bone tracers may be seen in the primary tumour and soft tissue metastases [70]. Although [123]I mIBG is a specific tracer for staging and follow-up of neuroblastoma, false negatives have been recorded in relation to the skeleton and a full initial assessment with both bone and mIBG scintigraphy has been recommended [71].

Due to the relatively low incidence of skeletal involvement at presentation in some of the commoner cancers, such as bowel, thyroid, melanoma and head

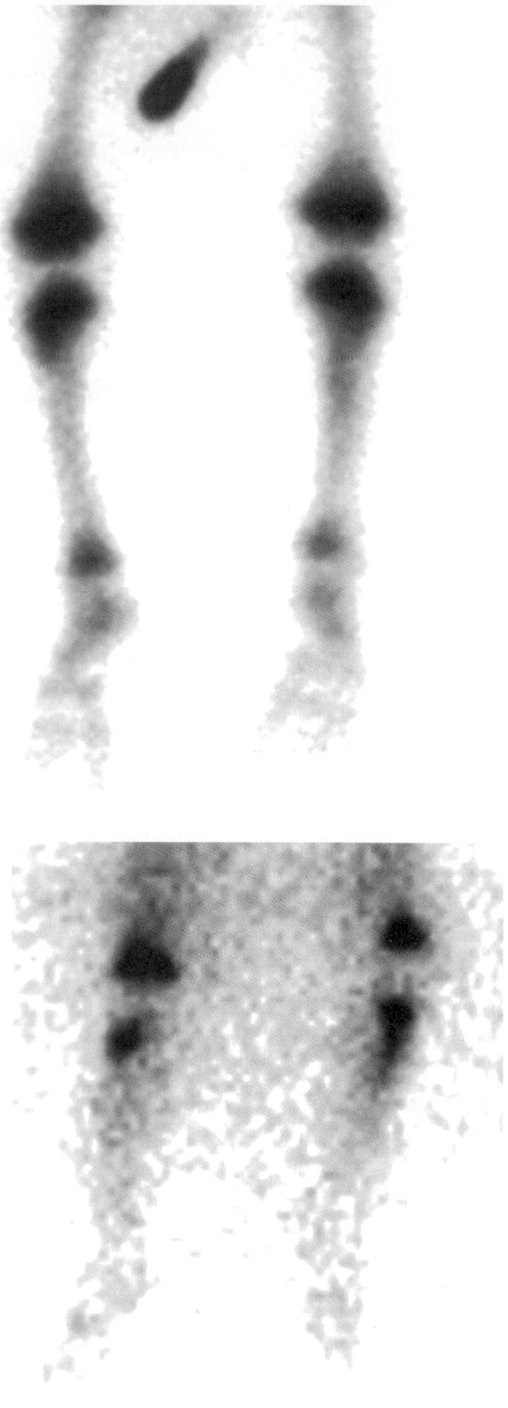

Figure 6.7. (A) Anterior ^{99m}Tc MDP bone scan of the legs. (B) Corresponding ^{123}I mIBG scans in a child with neuroblastoma. The slight blurring of the epiphyses at the knees indicates bone marrow involvement that is confirmed by uptake of ^{123}I mIBG

and neck, bone scintigraphy is usually only performed in patients in whom there is a suspicion of bone metastases and in the assessment of therapy in those with proven skeletal metastases.

POSITRON EMISSION TOMOGRAPHY

PET was previously primarily regarded as a research tool but, with changes in scanner design, allowing imaging of the whole body with relative ease, a number of clinical applications have been realised. This has particularly been in the field of oncology, where in spite of the relatively high capital and running costs compared to other imaging modalities, its use has been shown to be cost-effective in the clinical management of a number of cancers.

Both ^{18}F-fluoride, as a non-specific bone tracer, and ^{18}FDG, as an agent to image altered tumour metabolism, have potential roles in the management of patients with skeletal metastases.

^{18}F-fluoride Ion

Although the increased interest in clinical applications for PET is relatively recent, ^{18}F-fluoride was described as a bone-scanning agent more than 35 years ago [2]. In spite of renewed interest, PET scanners are still not widely accessible and so ^{18}F-fluoride PET is not a routine application. However, the tomographic images of high spatial resolution obtainable with modern PET systems, as well as the high contrast between normal and abnormal bone that is achievable as early as 1 hour post-injection of ^{18}F-fluoride, has led to its use in the evaluation of bone metastases [72–77].

^{18}F-fluoride PET images can be acquired at higher resolution than is possible with conventional bone scintigraphy and tomographic studies of the whole skeleton are routine, unlike ^{99m}Tc MDP SPECT imaging, where an additional tomographic acquisition is made of a relatively localised area following planar views. These factors indicate that there may be potential advantages in both sensitivity and specificity for the detection of bone metastases, a finding that has been supported in studies reported by Schirrmeister and colleagues [74,75]. In a study of 44 subjects with a variety of cancers, including lung, prostate and thyroid, ^{18}F-fluoride and ^{99m}Tc MDP were compared. Results from CT, MRI and ^{131}I-iodine scintigraphy were used as reference. All known skeletal metastases were detected by ^{18}F-fluoride PET and nearly twice as many benign and malignant skeletal abnormalities identified by ^{18}F-fluoride PET compared to ^{99m}Tc MDP. The superior spatial localisation of abnormalities possible with PET enabled lesions to be correctly classified as benign or malignant in a significantly larger number of cases (97% of lesions, compared to 80.5% with ^{99m}Tc MDP), an improvement which was particularly noticeable in the spine. It is possible that the differences between ^{18}F-fluoride and ^{99m}Tc MDP would have not been as large if spinal SPECT scans had been routinely available. Nevertheless, in patients with breast cancer the superior sensitivity of ^{18}F-fluoride PET led to a change in management in 4/34 (12%) patients [76] although the cost-effectiveness of ^{18}F-fluoride PET in cancer patients has not been specifically addressed.

[18]F-fluorodeoxyglucose

The mechanism of uptake of [18]FDG into bone metastases differs greatly from that of ^{18}F-fluoride, and accumulation is assumed to be into viable, metabolically active tumour cells, rather than reactive bone. As uptake of [18]FDG is not restricted to tumour involving the skeleton, it has the advantage of demonstrating both skeletal and soft tissue metastases in patients with cancer (Figure 6.8).

A few early reports exist describing the use of [18]FDG PET specifically in the investigation of bone metastases and in comparison with conventional ^{99m}Tc MDP scintigraphy. In comparing [18]FDG PET with ^{99m}Tc MDP scintigraphy in 110 patients with small cell lung cancer, Bury and colleagues found a similar sensitivity on a patient-by-patient basis (19/21 with bone metastases). Additionally in this study, [18]FDG PET correctly confirmed the absence of skeletal involvement in a much larger proportion of cases (87/89 compared to 54/89) [78]. This is almost undoubtedly due to non-specific uptake of ^{99m}Tc MDP in coincidental benign skeletal lesions, e.g. osteoarthritis, whereas focal skeletal [18]FDG activity is more specific for metastatic involvement.

In a similar study comparing these two agents, PET demonstrated a higher sensitivity and specificity on a lesion-by-lesion basis [79]. The apparent improvement in sensitivity with [18]FDG is partly due to the routine acquisition of tomographic images that were not available for ^{99m}Tc MDP. However, it is also likely that the observed differences are due to the fact that by imaging tumour metabolism directly with [18]FDG, detection may occur at an earlier stage, when only the bone marrow is involved. This may occur before an

A

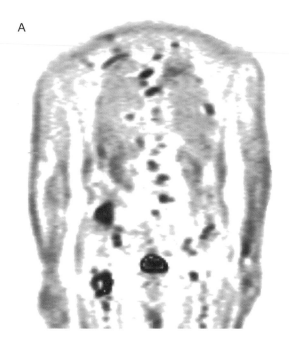

B

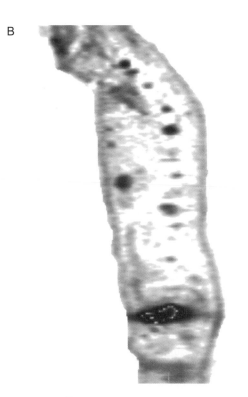

Figure 6.8. [18]FDG scan of a patient with follicular carcinoma of the thyroid, demonstrating multiple skeletal metastases. (A) Coronal and (B) sagittal slices (normal excretion of [18]FDG is seen in the bladder)

identifiable bone reaction, required for abnormal ^{99m}Tc MDP accumulation, has taken place.

In lymphoma, where skeletal metastases are often predominantly marrow-based, it has been found that ^{18}FDG PET is more sensitive than conventional bone scintigraphy [80] and it has been suggested that it might be possible to replace bone marrow biopsy as a staging procedure in these patients [81,82]. There are obvious potential advantages in sensitivity with ^{18}FDG PET in this respect when marrow involvement spares the iliac crest. Following chemotherapy or granulocyte colony-stimulating factors, it is not uncommon for the bone marrow to show a diffuse increase in activity which is reactive, a factor that may limit the use of this method in assessing disease response in bone marrow [83,84].

Although ^{18}FDG PET often detects more skeletal disease than conventional bone scintigraphy, this is not a universal finding. It is interesting to note that there have been a number of reports on the use of ^{18}FDG in prostate cancer, a tumour in which skeletal metastases are usually sclerotic, where a lower sensitivity has been found in the skeleton compared to conventional bone scintigraphy [85,86].

These observations raise the question of whether different tumours or types of skeletal metastasis (e.g. lytic vs. sclerotic) behave differently with regard to uptake of ^{18}FDG. It has been noted that overall a significantly larger number of bone metastases can be identified in breast cancer patients with progressive disease when using ^{18}FDG compared to ^{99m}Tc MDP, but that a subgroup of patients with sclerotic disease have a lower number of lesions identified [87]. In addition, uptake of ^{18}FDG was quantifiably lower in visible sclerotic lesions compared to lytic metastases, and it was found that those with predominantly sclerotic disease had a longer survival than those with lytic disease.

The reason for a greater avidity for ^{18}FDG in lytic metastases is unknown, but may reflect increased glycolyis or expression of glucose membrane transporters. It might also be expected for these more aggressive metastases to become hypoxic, another factor which is known to increase ^{18}FDG accumulation [88]. In contrast, the relative acellularity that may occur in sclerotic metastases [89], with comparatively smaller volumes of tumour tissue in individual lesions, may influence the uptake of ^{18}FDG.

An interesting approach in the use of PET in the investigation of bone metastases is to combine both ^{18}F-fluoride and ^{18}FDG scans. With the simultaneous administration of these tracers, a much better correlation has been found with other imaging methods than when ^{18}FDG PET is used alone. By having bone landmarks available, it has been found that better anatomical localisation of lesions is possible in both the skeleton and soft tissues [90].

REFERENCES

1. Fleming WH, McIraith JD, King ER. Photoscanning of bone lesions utilising strontium-85. Radiology 1961; 77: 635–6.
2. Blau M, Nagler W, Bender MA. A new isotope for bone scanning. J Nucl Med 1962; 3: 332–4.
3. Wolfenden JM, Pitt MJ, Durie BGW, Moon TE. Comparison of bone scintigraphy and radiology in myeloma. Radiology 1980; 134: 723–8.
4. Edelstyn GA, Gillespie PJ, Grebbel FS. The radiological demonstration of osseous metastases. Experimental observations. Clin Radiol 1967; 18: 159–62.
5. Galasko CSB. The significance of occult skeletal metastases detected by scintigraphy in patients with otherwise early breast cancer. Br J Surg 1975; 56: 757–64.
6. Coleman RE, Fogelman I, Habibollahi F et al. Selection of patients with breast cancer for routine follow-up bone scans. Clin Oncol 1990; 2: 328–32.
7. Schneider JA, Divgi CR, Scott AM et al. Flare on bone scintigraphy following Taxol chemotherapy for metastatic breast cancer. J Nucl Med 1994; 35: 1748–52.
8. Johns WD, Garrick MB, Kaplan WD. Leuprolide therapy for prostate cancer. An association with scintigraphic flare on bone scan. Clin Nucl Med 1990; 15: 485–7.
9. Rossleigh MA, Lovegrove FT, Reynolds PM et al. The assessment of response to therapy in bone metastases from breast cancer. Aust NZ J Med 1984; 14: 19–22.
10. Coleman RE, Mashiter G, Whitaker KB et al. Bone scan flare predicts successful systemic therapy for bone metastases. J Nucl Med 1988; 29: 1354–9.
11. Jacobson AF, Cronin EB, Stomper EC et al. Bone scans with one or two new abnormalities in cancer patients with no known metastases: frequency and serial scintigraphic behaviour of benign and malignant lesions. Radiology 1990; 175: 229–32.
12. Condon BR, Buchanan R, Garvie NW et al. Assessment of progression of secondary bone lesions following cancer of the breast or prostate using serial radionuclide imaging. Br J Radiol 1981; 54: 18–23.
13. Lam AS, Kettle AG, O'Doherty MJ et al. Pentavalent 99Tcm-DMSA imaging in patients with bone metastases. Nucl Med Commun 1997; 18: 907–14.
14. Dunker CM, Carrio I, Bernal L et al. Radioimmune imaging of bone marrow in patients with suspected bone metastases from primary breast cancer. J Nucl Med 1990; 31: 1450–5.
15. Blau M, Ganatra R, Bender MA. ^{18}F-fluoride for bone imaging. Semin Nucl Med 1972; 2: 31–7.
16. Warburg O. On the origin of cancer cells. Science 1954; 123: 306–14.
17. Yamamoto T, Seino Y, Fukumoto H et al. Overexpression of facilitative glucose transporter genes in human cancer. Biochem Biophys Res Commun 1990; 170: 223–30.

18. Bushnell DL, Kahn D, Huston B, Bevering CG. Utility of SPECT imaging for determination of vertebral metastases in patients with known primary tumors. Skel Radiol 1995; 24: 13–16.

19. Han LJ, Au-Yong TK, Tong WCM et al. Comparison of bone SPECT and planar imaging in the detection of vertebral metastases in patients with back pain. Eur J Nucl Med 1998; 25: 635–8.

20. Tofe AJ, Francis MD, Harvey WJ. Correlation of neoplasms with incidence and localisation of skeletal metastases. An analysis of 1355 diphosphonate bone scans. J Nucl Med 1975; 16: 986–9.

21. Boxer DI, Todd CE, Coleman RE et al. Bone secondaries in breast cancer: the solitary metastasis. J Nucl Med 1989; 30: 1318–20.

22. Tumeh SS, Beadle G, Kaplan WD. Clinical significance of solitary rib lesions in patients with extraskeletal malignancy. J Nucl Med 1985; 26: 1140–3.

23. Jacobson AF, Stomper PC, Jochelson MS et al. Association between number and sites of new bone scan abnormalities and presence of skeletal metastases in patients with breast cancer. J Nucl Med 1990; 31: 387–92.

24. Baxter AD, Coakley FV, Finlay DB et al. The aetiology of solitary hot spots in the ribs on planar bone scans. Nucl Med Commun 1995; 16: 834–7.

25. Coakley FV, Jones AR, Finlay DB et al. The aetiology and distinguishing features of solitary spinal hot spots on planar bone scans. Clin Radiol 1995; 50: 327–30.

26. Jacobson AF, Stomper MD, Cronin EB et al. Bone scans with one or two new abnormalities in cancer patients with no known metastases: the reliability of interpretation of initial correlative radiographs. Radiology 1990; 174: 503–7.

27. Barker DJP, Clough PWL, Guyer PB et al. Paget's disease of bone in 14 British towns. Br Med J 1977; 1: 1181–3.

28. Coleman RE, Rubens RD. The clinical course of bone metastases from breast cancer. Br J Cancer 1987; 55: 61–6.

29. Richards MA, Braysher S, Gregory WM et al. Advanced breast cancer: use of resources and cost implications. Br J Cancer 1993; 67: 856–60.

30. Nomura Y, Kondo H, Yamagata J et al. Evaluation of liver and bone scanning in patients with early breast cancer based on results obtained from more advanced patients. Eur J Cancer 1978; 14: 1129–36.

31. Davies CJ, Griffiths PA, Preston BJ et al. Staging breast cancer. Role of scanning. Br Med J 1977; 2: 603–5.

32. Gerber FH, Goodreau JJ, Kirchner PT et al. Efficacy or preoperative and postoperative bone scanning in the management of breast carcinoma. N Eng J Med 1977; 297: 300–3.

33. Citrin DL, Furnival CM, Bessent RG et al. Radioactive technetium phosphate bone scanning in preoperative assessment and follow-up study of patients with primary carcinoma of the breast. Surg Gynecol Obstet 1976; 143: 360–4.

34. Campbell DJ, Banks AJ, Davis GD. The value of preliminary bone scanning in staging and assessing the prognosis of breast cancer. Br J Surg 1976; 63: 811–16.

35. Sklaroff RB, Sklaroff DM. Bone metastases from breast cancer at the time of radical mastectomy. Cancer 1976; 38: 107–11.

36. Coleman RE, Rubens RD, Fogelman I. Reappraisal of the baseline bone scan in breast cancer. J Nucl Med 1988; 29: 1045–9.

37. Ciatto S, Pacini P, Bravetti P et al. Staging breast cancer—screening for occult metastases. Tumori 1985; 71: 339–44.

38. Strender LE, Lagergren C, Wallgren A et al. Role of bone scans in the initial assessment of operable patients with breast cancer. Acta Radiol Oncol 1981; 20: 187–91.

39. Kunkler IH, Merrick MV, Rodger A. Bone scintigraphy in breast cancer: a nine year follow-up. Clin Radiol 1985; 36: 279–82.

40. Furnival CM, Blumgart LH, Citrin DL et al. Serial scintiscanning in breast cancer: indications and prognostic value. Clin Oncol 1980; 6: 25–32.

41. Ojeda MB, Alonso MC, Bastus R et al. Follow-up of breast cancer stages I and II. An analysis of some common methods. Eur J Cancer 1987; 23: 419–23.

42. Rosselli Del Turco M, Palli D, Carridi A et al. Intensive diagnostic follow-up after treatment of primary breast cancer. A randomised trial. J Am Med Assoc 1994; 271: 1593–7.

43. Haywood JL, Carbone PP, Heuson JC et al. Assessment of response to therapy in advanced breast cancer. Eur J Cancer 1977; 13: 89–94.

44. Coombes RC, Dady P, Parsons C et al. Assessment of response of bone metastases to systemic treatment in patients with breast cancer. Cancer 1983; 52: 610–14.

45. Palazzo S, Liguori V, Molinari B. Is the carcino-embryonic antigen test a valid predictor of response to medical therapy in disseminated breast cancer? Tumori 1986; 72: 515–18.

46. Hortabagyi GN, Libshitz HI, Seabold JE. Osseous metastases of breast cancer. Clinical, biochemical, radiographic and scintigraphic evaluation of response to therapy. Cancer 1984; 55: 577–82.

47. Bitran JD, Bekerman C, Desser RK. The predictive value of serial bone scans in assessing response to chemotherapy in advanced breast cancer. Cancer 1980; 45: 1562–8.

48. Erdi YE, Humm JL, Imbriaco M et al. Quantitative bone metastases analysis based on image segmentation. J Nucl Med 1977; 38: 1401–6.

49. Pitt WR, Sharp PF. Comparison of quantitative and visual detection of new focal bone lesions. J Nucl Med 1985; 26: 230–6.

50. Condon BR, Buchanan R, Garvie NW et al. Assessment of progression of secondary bone lesions following cancer of the breast or prostate using serial radionuclide imaging. Br J Radiol 1981; 54: 18–23.

51. McKillop JH. Bone scanning in metastatic disease. In Fogelman I (ed.), Bone Scanning in Clinical Practice. Springer-Verlag: Berlin, 1987: 41–60.

52. Paulson DF and the Uro-oncology Research group. The impact of current staging procedures in assessing disease extent in prostatic adenocarcinoma. J Urol 1979; 121: 300–2.

53. Biersack HJ, Wegner G, Distelmaier W, Krause U. Bone metastases of prostate cancer in relation to tumour size and grade of malignancy. Nuklearmedizin 1982; 128: 510–12.

54. Shih WG, Mitchell B, Wierzbinski B et al. Prediction of radionuclide bone imaging findings by Gleason histologic grading of prostate carcinoma. Clin Nucl Med 1991; 16: 763–6.

55. Chybowski FM, Keller JJL, Bergstrahl EJ et al. Predicting radionuclide bone scan findings in patients with newly diagnosed, untreated prostate cancer: PSA is superior to all other clinical parameters. J Urol 1991; 145: 313–18.

56. Huben RP, Schellhammer PF. The role of routine follow-up bone scan after definitive therapy of localised prostate cancer. J Urol 1982; 128: 510–12.

57. Terris MK, Klonecke AS, McDougall IR et al. Utilisation of bone scans in conjunction with PSA levels in the surveillance for recurrent adenocarcinoma after radical prostatectomy. J Nucl Med 1991; 32: 1713–17.

58. Sundkvist GM, Ahlgren L, Lilja B et al. Dynamic quantitative bone scintigraphy in patients with prostatic carcinoma treated by orchiectomy. Eur J Nucl Med 1990; 16: 671–6.

59. Pollen JJ, Witztum KF, Ashburn WL. The flare phenomenon on radionuclide bone scan in metastatic prostate cancer. Am J Roentgenol 1984; 142: 773–6.

60. Levenson RM, Sauerbrunn BJL, Bates HR et al. Comparative value of bone scintigraphy and radiography in monitoring tumour response in systemically treated prostatic cancer. Radiology 1983; 46: 513–18.

61. Pollen JJ, Gerber K, Ashburn WL et al. Nuclear bone imaging in metastatic cancer of the prostate. Cancer 1981; 47: 2585–94.

62. Sundqvist CMG, Ahlgren L, Lilja B et al. Repeated quantitative bone scintigraphy in patients with prostatic carcinoma treated with orchidectomy. Eur J Nucl Med 1988; 14: 203–6.

63. Fogelman I, McKillop JH. The bone scan in metastatic disease. In Rubens RD, Fogelman I (eds), Bone Metastases: Diagnosis and Treatment. Springer-Verlag: London, 1991: 31–5.

64. Bitran JD, Beckerman C, Pinsky S. Sequential scintigraphic staging of small cell carcinoma. Cancer 1981; 47: 1971–5.

65. Levenson RM, Sauerbrunn FJL, Ihde DC et al. Small cell lung cancer: radionuclide bone scans for assessment of tumour extent and response. Am J Roentgenol 1981; 137: 31–5.

66. Gravenstein S, Peltz MA, Poreis W. How ominous is an abnormal bone scan in bronchogenic carcinoma? J Am Med Assoc 1979; 241: 2523–4.

67. Pieterman RM, van Putten JWG, Meuzelaar JJ et al. Preoperative staging of non-small cell lung cancer with positron emission tomography. N Engl J Med 2000; 343: 254–61.

68. Kim EE, Bledin AG, Gutierrez C et al. Comparison of radionuclide images and radiographs for skeletal metastases from renal cell carcinoma. Oncology 1983; 40: 284–6.

69. Fawcett HD, McDougall IR. Bone scan in extraskeletal neuroblastoma with hot primary and cold skeletal metastases. Clin Nucl Med 1980; 5: 49–50.

70. Howman-Giles R, Gilday DL, Ash JM. Radionuclide skeletal survey in neuroblastoma. Radiology 1979; 131: 497–502.

71. Gordon I, Peters AM, Gutman A et al. Skeletal assessment in neuroblastoma: pitfalls of iodine-123-mIBG scans. J Nucl Med 1990; 31: 129–34.

72. Hawkins RA, Choi Y, Huang SC et al. Evaluation of the skeletal kinetics of fluorine-18-fluoride ion with PET. J Nucl Med 1992; 33: 633–42.

73. Hoegerle S, Juengling F, Otte A et al. Combined FDG and [F-18]fluoride whole-body PET: a feasible two-in-one approach to cancer imaging? Radiology 1998; 209: 253–8.

74. Hoh CK, Hawkins RA, Dahlbom M et al. Whole body skeletal imaging with [18F]fluoride ion and PET. J Comput Assist Tomogr 1993; 17: 34–41.

75. Petren-Mallmin M, Andreasson I, Ljunggren et al. Skeletal metastases from breast cancer: uptake of 18F-fluoride measured with positron emission tomography in correlation with CT. Skel Radiol 1998; 27: 72–6.

76. Schirrmeister H, Guhlmann A, Kotzerke J et al. Early detection and accurate description of extent of metastatic bone disease in breast cancer with fluoride ion and positron emission tomography. J Clin Oncol 1999; 17: 2381–9.

77. Schirrmeister H, Guhlmann A, Elsner K et al. Sensitivity in detecting osseous lesions depends on anatomic localization: planar bone scintigraphy versus 18F PET. J Nucl Med 1999; 40: 1623–9.

78. Bury T, Barreto A, Daenen F et al. Fluorine-18 deoxyglucose positron emission tomography for the detection of bone metastases in patients with non-small cell lung cancer. Eur J Nucl Med 1998; 25: 1244–7.

79. Chung JK, Kim YK, Yoon JK et al. Diagnostic usefulness of F-18 FDG whole body PET in detection of bony metastases compared to Tc-99m MDP bone scan. J Nucl Med 1999; 40: 96P.

80. Moog F, Kotzerke J, Reske SN. FDG PET can replace bone scintigraphy in primary staging of malignant lymphoma. J Nucl Med 1999; 40: 1407–13.

81. Carr R, Barrington SF, Madan B et al. Detection of lymphoma in bone marrow by whole-body positron emission tomography. Blood 1998; 91: 3340–6.

82. Moog F, Bangerter M, Kotzerke J et al. 18-F-fluorodeoxyglucose-positron emission tomography as a new approach to detect lymphomatous bone marrow. J Clin Oncol 1998; 16: 603–9.

83. Cook GJ, Fogelman I, Maisey MN. Normal physiological and benign pathological variants of 18-fluoro-2-deoxyglucose positron-emission tomography scanning: potential for error in interpretation. Semin Nucl Med 1996; 26: 308–14.

84. Hollinger EF, Alibazoglu H, Ali A et al. Hematopoietic cytokine-mediated FDG uptake simulates the appearance of diffuse metastatic disease on whole-body PET imaging. Clin Nucl Med 1998; 23: 93–8.

85. Shreve PD, Grossman HB, Gross MD et al. Metastatic prostate cancer: initial findings of PET with 2-deoxy-2-[F-18]fluoro-D-glucose. Radiology 1996; 199: 751–6.

86. Yeh SD, Imbriaco M, Larson SM et al. Detection of bony metastases of androgen-independent prostate cancer by PET-FDG. Nucl Med Biol 1996; 23: 693–7.

87. Cook GJ, Houston S, Rubens R et al. Detection of bone metastases in breast cancer by 18FDG PET: differing metabolic activity in osteoblastic and osteolytic lesions. J Clin Oncol 1998; 16: 3375–9.

88. Clavo AC, Brown RS, Wahl RL. Fluorodeoxyglucose uptake in human cancer cell lines is increased by hypoxia. J Nucl Med 1995; 36: 1625–32.

89. Galasko CSB. Skeletal Metastases. Butterworths: London, 1986.

90. Hoegerle S, Juengling F, Otte A et al. Combined FDG and [F-18]fluoride whole-body PET: a feasible two-in-one approach to cancer imaging? Radiology 1998; 209: 253–8.

7

Imaging of Spinal Bone Metastases

R. Guillevin, J. N. Vallée, N. Martin-Duverneuil, D. Lo,
F. Lafitte, J. C. Maillard and J. Chiras

Hôpital de la Pitié-Salpêtrière, Paris, France

GENERAL CONSIDERATIONS

Bone is a common site of metastasis for many primary malignant tumours, indeed the third location after liver and lung. Metastases are the most frequent bone tumours, and are inaugural in 25% of cases [1,2]. Furthermore, the spine represents the most frequent site of skeletal metastasis. The majority of metastatic lesions in the skeleton are encountered in middle-aged and elderly patients. Carcinomas of breast, prostate, kidney and thyroid, in order of decreasing frequency, account for 80% of skeletal metastases, although these figures are influenced dramatically by the choice of technique used to detect metastatic sites. In men, carcinoma of the prostate (60%), lung and bladder are typical sources of skeleton metastases; in women, carcinomas of the breast (70%) and uterus are common causes. Systematic post mortem anatomical studies have demonstrated that bone metastases are present in 84% of breast and prostate cancers. The frequency is 50% for thyroid cancer, 44% for lung cancer, and 37% for kidney tumours [3,4].

Highly vascularised bone marrow remains present within vertebral bodies until late in life, and thus, fenestration capillaries provide a pathway for myeloid cells to spread into the general circulation. Conversely, metastatic cells can easily traverse the basal membrane, which explains why the posterior aspect of the vertebral body is affected earlier than the posterior arch, the latter rarely being involved alone [5]. Spongeous bone is invaded first, with cortical involvement occurring later, leading to fracture, vertebral instability, and finally the development of an extravertebral, space-occupying mass with compression of the spinal cord. This last-mentioned finding has been observed in 5–10% of persons with metastatic cancer. Spinal metastases predominantly involve the thoracic and lumbar vertebrae. Less frequently lesions are found in the sacrum and rarely in the cervical spine.

In this chapter we review the role of magnetic resonance imaging (MRI), computed tomography (CT), and the more traditional but nonetheless important plain film for the diagnosis and follow-up of bone metastases. Nuclear imaging techniques, e.g. scintigraphy, single photon emission computed tomography (SPECT) and positron emission tomography (PET scan) are discussed in another chapter.

PLAIN FILMS

The performance of radiographs for the detection of spinal metastases depends upon ready absorption of X-rays by bone, providing contrast if their structure is modified. However, X-rays are not always reliable during the early stages of osseous destruction and careful and thorough analysis of radiographs is required to detect lesions. It is generally estimated that around 50% of normal bone tissue must be replaced or destroyed before this can be detected by X-ray [6,7]. Thus, in breast carcinomas, bone metastases are detected 6 months later by radiography than by scintigraphy [8]. The situation of a tumour on the spine and also its location within the vertebra also determine the visibility of the tumour. Because plain films are still widely used in diagnosis and follow-up of skeletal

Textbook of Bone Metastases. Edited by C. Jasmin, R. E. Coleman, L. R. Coia, R. Capanna and G. Saillant
© 2005 John Wiley & Sons Ltd: ISBN 0 471 87742 5

metastases, several issues deserve more detailed discussion.

The most frequent spinal metastases are pure osteolytic lesions. Lodwick [9] has distinguished three different types. *Geographic* osteolysis is a focal destruction of bone tissue, replaced by tumour. "*Moth-eaten*" osteolysis is observed as multiple small holes; complicating the interpretation of this radiological finding is osteoporosis, because of its similar appearance and high frequency. *Pervious* osteolysis, with smaller, millimetric holes, reduces the visibility of the bone frame, and blurred outlines to a vertebral body indicate cortical involvement. Because of the high specificity of this pattern for tumoral involvement, it should be investigated first. The posterior wall of the vertebral body requires specific attention (Figure 7.1). Cortical erasure or posterior convexity of the posterior wall, best seen in precisely positioned lateral radiographs, is highly indicative of malignancy. Conversely, concavity of the posterior wall with backward angulation is highly specific for osteoporotic disease, and cortical lesions are not involved in such cases. The variability of bone involvement is remarkable. Destruction and collapse of the vertebral body by osteolysis is hardly detectable by X-ray plain films prior to major bone destruction. The destruction of one side of the vertebral body is highly specific for malignancy. Common metastatic causes of vertebral body collapse include, in order of decreasing frequency, carcinomas of breast, lung and prostate [10]. More than one vertebral body may collapse sequentially or simultaneously. Angular or irregular distorsion of the vertebral endplates, involvement of the upper thoracic spine, associated soft tissue mass or pedicle destruction are suggestive of metastatic disease. A noteworthy finding, useful for the differentiation of malignant tumours from spondylitis, is preservation of the discal height. Collapse of the vertebral body, which may be the presentation of metastasis, is also evident in osteomalacia, osteoporosis and plasma cell myeloma. Pedicle involvement, a well-known radiographic finding of skeletal metastasis, is best observed in anteroposterior radiographs, revealing the absence of one or both "eyes" in the vertebral body. Cortical involvement may occur in the pedicle earlier than in the vertebral body because of the relative scarcity of spongeous tissue. Thus, metastasis may be visible earlier in the pedicle.

Homogeneous or inhomogeneous sclerotic areas detected on one or more vertebral bodies are further indications of metastatic disease arising from prostate or carcinoid tumours, stomach cancer, plasma cell myeloma and lymphoma [2].

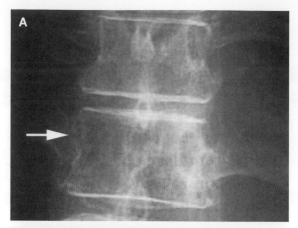

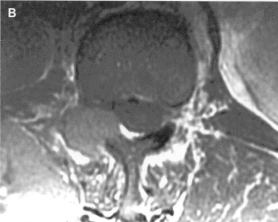

Figure 7.1. Erasing of right pedicle on plain film (A). MRI demonstrates a lytic mass with cortical involvement on right pedicle with soft tissue extension (B)

The site of a metastasis in the spine will strongly influence its visibility. Mainly because of anatomical superimposition, the 7th cervical and 1st to 4th thoracic vertebrae are particularly difficult to study on plain films. After gross survey on plain films, CT and MRI can be used to investigate suspected bone lesions and associated intraspinal or soft tissue masses more reliably.

COMPUTED TOMOGRAPHY

By a combination of X-rays and tomographic rotational slices, CT gives images rebuilt from subduing profiles with a density resolution ten times higher than on plain films, allowing a precise study of trabecular bone. Thus, superimposition is avoided. With contrast

Table 7.1. Osteoporotic vertebral body. Statistical value of CT findings

CT Findings	Sensitivity (%)	Specificity (%)
Cortical fracture on VB side	94	91
Cortical fracture on posterior aspect	56	91
At least one cortical fracture	94	97
Cortical fragment inside medullary canal	35	97
Fracture inside VB	85	72
Circular fracture	26	97
Vacuum sign	15	100
Circular thickness of soft tissues less than 8 mm	41	87

Abbreviations for Tables 7.1–7.5: VB, vertebral body; SE, spin-echo; WI, weighted image; Hypo, hyposignal; Hyper, hypersignal; Iso, isosignal. Data From [11].

intravenous injection, intra- or extracanalicular extensions of tumoral process can be well studied. Helicoidal scan with small rebuilding field, 2–3 mm slice thickness with 1.5 to 2 mm pitch, and frontal and sagittal 2-D reconstructions are good parameters to study images using two filters, soft and bone. In cases of vertebral collapse, porotic or tumoral patterns have been described and are presented in Tables 7.1 and 7.2 [11].

A sclerotic lesion has a heterogeneous, high-density structure (although lower than that of the cortex) with blurred limitation from spongeous bone and also periosteal reaction. Bone trabeculae are no longer visible. Cortical involvement and paravertebral mass are seldom observed. Most often there is a lytic mass, replacing the normal spongeous bone trabeculae by a tissue lesion that may be very small in size and difficult to see. Depending on the stage of the lesion, some trabeculae may remain visible. Sometimes necrosis or,

Table 7.2. Malignant vertebral body collapse. Statistical value of CT findings

CT Findings	Sensitivity (%)	Specificity (%)
VB side cortical destruction	75	97
Posterior VB cortical destruction	69	100
At least one VB cortical destruction	97	97
VB spongeous bone destruction	100	70
At least one pedicle destruction	50	100
Soft tissue mass	56	82
Epidural mass	59	97

For abbreviations, see Table 7.1. Data from [11].

more rarely, calcifications can be seen, as well as cortical or pedicular destruction, epidural encroachment or paravertebral mass. One of the main criteria for tumoral origin of a lesion is cortical involvement (Figure 7.2); almost complete osteolysis of one cortical

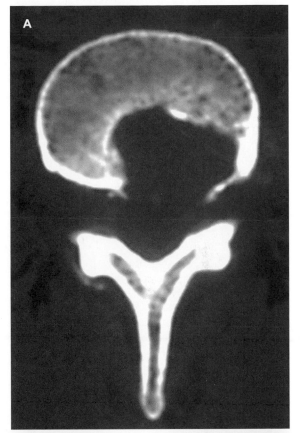

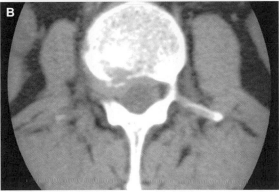

Figure 7.2. Two examples of lytic mass of vertebral bodies replacing normal bone trabeculations and cortical involvement of posterior wall (A), and also right pedicular involvement, epidural and pial extension (B). Bone (A) and soft tissues (B) windowing

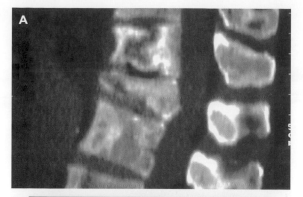

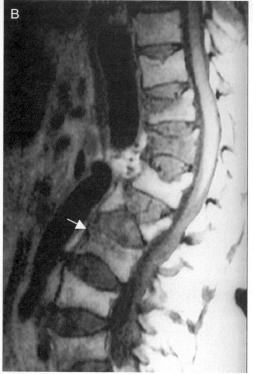

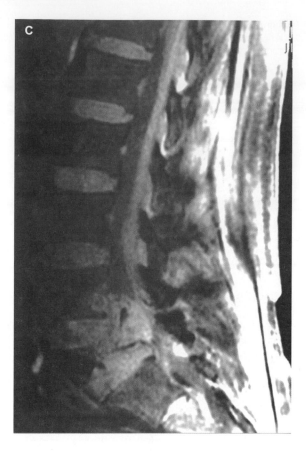

Figure 7.3.   Imaging of vertebral bodies' collapse. Malignant or not? (A) "CT" "Puzzle" aspect, backward angulation of posterior wall of the vertebral body, reduction of height for adjacent discs, vacuum sign of the upper one, all arguments for porotic origin. (B) MRI aspect of porotic collapse. Linear hyposignal of upper part of the vertebral body (small arrow), spongeous herniation (fat arrow). (C) "MRI" Malignancy is well demonstrated by convexity of posterior wall of fifth lumbar vertebra and epidural involvement. Note the entirety of adjacent discs

element, anterolateral or posterior, is quite consistent and specific for diagnosis [11]. Cortical involvement may be visible only by notching of its inner surface. In two-thirds of cases, the posterior wall of vertebral body is also involved. Pedicular involvement is observed in 50% of cases, and foraminal involvement from a pedicular lesion can be well studied on sagittal images. After the injection of intravenous contrast media, CT can be used to demonstrate a soft tissue mass in two-thirds of cases. The "double bag aspect" (see Figure 7.9) may also be noticed in cases of epidural extension. A location above the 7th cervical vertebra and collapse of a single vertebra are very suggestive of malignancy. Conversely, osteoporotic collapse may cause cortical fracture, with bursting and many fragments of different sizes, thus creating puzzle images. Backward angulation is a very specific sign of osteoporotic collapse [11] (Figure 7.3), noticed in one-third of cases. Spongeous bone osteolysis may be present in 30% of cases. In 40% of cases of recent collapse (< 2 months), there is slight thickening of the soft tissues surrounding the vertebral body (< 8 mm).

CT is of great assistance in determining therapeutic orientation, e.g. thorough examination of the pedicles may guide the choice between a transpedicular or posterolateral approach for vertebroplasty.

MRI

Based on the magnetic resonance of protons, the most abundant constituent of water and thus of the human body, MRI has become the elective procedure in soft tissue investigations. Detection of changes in bone marrow constituency is now fundamental to the sensitivity of MR imaging in detection of sites of skeletal metastasis. Identification of such sites using this technique requires the observer to recognise normal age-related marrow changes, particularly in

the spine [12]; (Figure 7.4). These changes relate to the predictable and orderly pattern of cell conversion of red (haematopoietic) to yellow (fatty) marrow that occurs during growth and development [13]. Over the age of 25 years, red marrow, in an adult pattern, is concentrated predominantly in a few sites, among them the vertebrae, with partial occupation of adipocytes, increasing with age [2].

The specific abnormalities seen on MRI related to spinal (and paraspinal) metastatic foci are dependent,

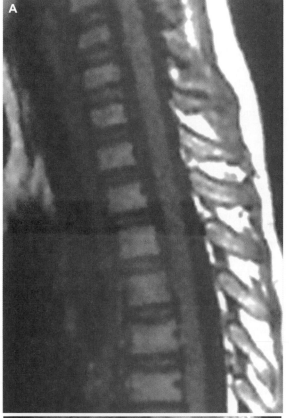

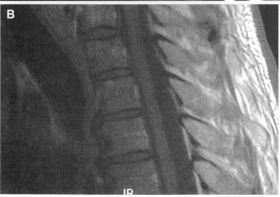

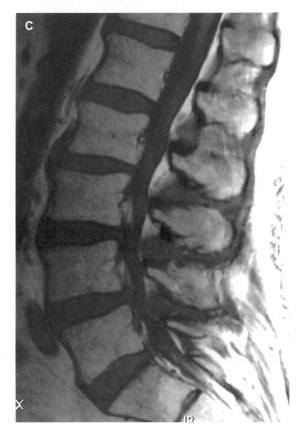

Figure 7.4. Bone marrow signal evolution on MRI (T1-weighted images). Progressive increasing of medullary signal of vertebral bodies with age, due to fatty bone marrow involution

overall, upon the particular imaging parameters employed.

On T1-weighted images, normal bone marrow appears hypointense in children, then progressively iso- and hyperintense in elderly people. The signal for intravertebral lesions is of low intensity and may be very low for sclerotic metastasis (Figure 7.5). Such images can be useful to demonstrate spinal cord compression. Some substances as methaemoglobin-aemia or melanocytes (haemorrhagic metastasis of melanoma), may lead to increase the signal of an involved vertebra.

Intravenous gadolinium administration, by improving the visibility of highly metastatic foci, especially those with extravertebral extension, deserves emphasis. However, the extent of tumour enhancement can be marked, slight or, in the case of sclerotic metastasis, absent. Furthermore, enhancement may be random, initially peripheral with subsequent central spread, or homogeneous. In case of very fat bone marrow, fat suppression or short tau inversion recovery (STIR) must be used. In this case, bearing in mind the risk of equalisation of both signals of metastasis and bone marrow on post-contrast sequences, T1-weighted images without gadolinium should be performed. For the same reason, in a case of fat suppression on T1-weighted images, it will be necessary to make gadolinium administration. The STIR (T2) sequence is more sensitive than T1- and T2-weighted images for detecting metastasis, but conversely is less sensitive for observing extravertebral involvement [14].

On T2-weighted images, the signal characteristics of intravertebral lesions is variable, although an increase in signal intensity is mostly encountered [2]. In some reports (e.g. [15]), T2-weighted images have been considered better than T1-weighted images in appraisal of the subarachnoid space in the absence of cord compression. Because fast or turbo spin-echo sequences show hypersignalling of fat, causing the appearance of metastasis to be isointense in adult bone marrow, fat saturation or STIR are generally used to improve the visibility of lesions (Figure 7.6). One exception is the case of richly haematopoietic bone marrow in the spines of children, where the hyper-intensity of abnormal bone marrow becomes evident on spin-echo sequences as the "flip-flop sign" [16]. On gradient echo sequences the normal appearance of the vertebra is hypointense, because of the magnetic susceptibility effect of the bone bay/marrow interface. However, the appearance of spinal metastases is highly influenced by the choice of imaging parameters (e.g. echo and repetition times, flip angle) [2,5], with the

hypersignal of metastatic foci here due to diminution of the magnetic susceptibility effect caused by trabecular bone destruction by the tumour. Conversely, magnetic susceptibility and metallic artefacts may induce false images of metastatic involvement in patients with cancer (Figure 7.7). For the improvement of T2-weighted images, increased contrast between the normal bone marrow and the tumour may be obtained by using ultrasmall super-paramagnetic particles of iron oxide (USPIO) [5,17,18]. Their specificity for the cells of the reticuloendothelial system induces local high fields in bone marrow (so-called "super-paramagnetic effect"), speeding up phase displacement of water protons and thus shortening the normal bone marrow T2 signal, leading to decreased signal of both yellow and red bone marrow. Bone metastasis, remaining in hypersignal, therefore becomes apparent. Daldrup-Link et al. [18] have shown that the STIR sequence is more sensitive than T1- and T2-weighted TSE images for demonstrating bone marrow signal intensity changes after iron oxide infusion. A strong signal decline is noticed for normal and hypercellular bone marrow 45–60 min after iron oxide administration, whereas no or only a minor signal decline of neoplastic bone marrow lesions is observed. Recent studies [19,20] suggest that histograms provided by quantitative apparent diffusion coefficient (ADC) mapping may provide valuable information in differentiating benign vertebral fractures from metastatic lesions. Zhou et al. [20] have found a mean ADC value of benign lesions 68% higher than that of the metastases. Conversely, qualitative diffusion-weighted imaging, previously described by Baur et al. [21], has shown that benign compression fractures are hypo- to iso-intense relative to adjacent normal vertebral bodies, and that metastatic compression fractures are hyper-intense, without offering advantage over conventional unenhanced MR imaging for detection of vertebral metastases, as shown by Castillo et al. [22,23]. Further, lesions with a high water content and low cellularity may demonstrate hypersignal on T2-weighted images and hypo-intense signal on diffusion-weighted images, owing to the T2 shine-through effect [20].

Both osteolytic and sclerotic lesions can be present on the same patient for the same cancer. Mixed lesions (sclerotic/lytic) are often retrieved, with constant hyposignal on all sequences for sclerotic component, and nodular hypersignal on post-contrast T1-weighted images [2,5]; (Figure 7.5). Association of pure sclerotic metastasis and mixed lesions creates a striped aspect.

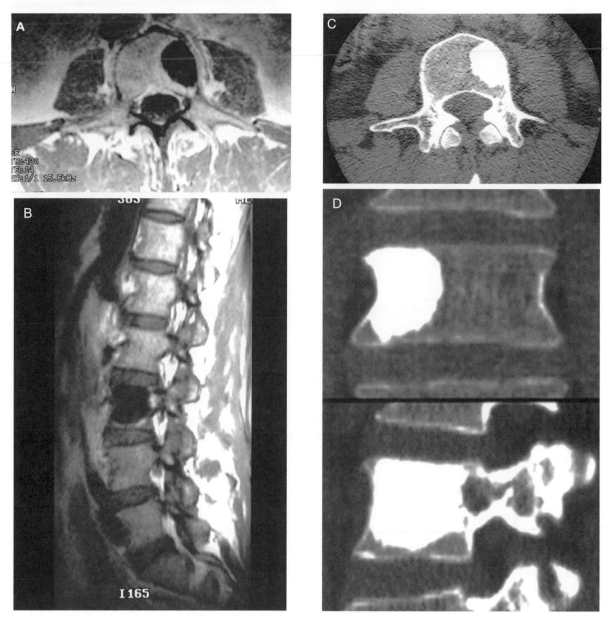

Figure 7.5. Sclerotic metastases. MRI aspects on T1-weighted image (A) and T2-weighted image (B) shows deeply hyposignal, corresponding to hyperdensity on CT images (C,D)

For discriminate vertebral fractures caused by metastasis (or other tumours) and osteoporosis, MRI arguments are presented in Tables 7.3 and 7.4.

The usual appearance on T1-weighted images is low signal intensity, hypersignal on T2-weighted images and heterogeneous hypersignal on T1-weighted images with gadolinium (Figure 7.8). Thus, MRI facilitates study of the entire spinal column, at the same time

searching for other metastatic foci. It also allows an appreciation of the general morphology and the ability to give signals of collapsed vertebrae. In fact, MRI suggests that 65–88% [2,24] of malignant collapses are accompanied by metastatic foci on adjacent vertebrae.

Intradural-extramedullary and intramedullary sites may be involved in metastasis, even without primary bone involvement, as it has been delineated by

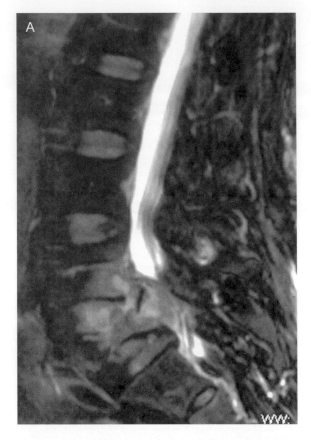

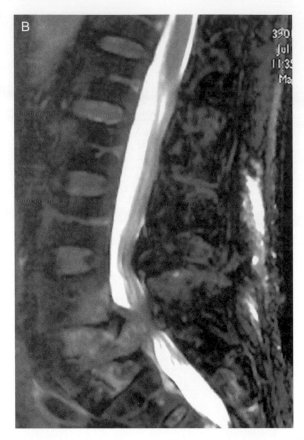

Figure 7.6. MRI. T2-weighted images. STIR (A) and fat sat (B) sequences, by decreasing signal of fatty bone marrow, improve visibility of pathologic bone marrow and epidural extension

Kamholtz and Sze [25]. The great majority of metastases involving the epidural space relate to bone involvement. This pattern is known as the "double bag" type [11], with the same signal as tumour on other sequences (Figure 7.9), and results from the high resistance of the common posterior vertebral ligament to the bulging of tumoral processes. There is considerable interest in gadolinium administration to assess tumour extension into the epidural space. On T1-weighted images, mottling of the fat behind the thecal sac is indicative of epidural metastasis (Figure 7.9). On post-contrast T1-weighted images, a linear streak of enhancement along the dorsal or ventral surface of the spinal cord may represent the site of pial metastasis.

In intradural-extramedullary metastases, MRI provides inconsistent diagnostic results, due to the lack of contrast between the tumour and the surrounding cerebrospinal fluid, the absence of surrounding oedema, and motion artefacts from cerebrospinal fluid pulsations [2,24,26,27]. According to previous considerations, the following pattern of investigations can be proposed:

- Sagittal spin-echo, T1-weighted images on the whole spine.
- Sagittal STIR T2 images, at least on the pathological zone.
- Sagittal post-contrast, spin-echo, fat sat T1-weighted images on the whole spine.
  Axial post-contrast, spin-echo, T1-weighted images on pathological levels.

$Table 7.5 shows the signal of each spinal component on various sequences, previously delineated [5].

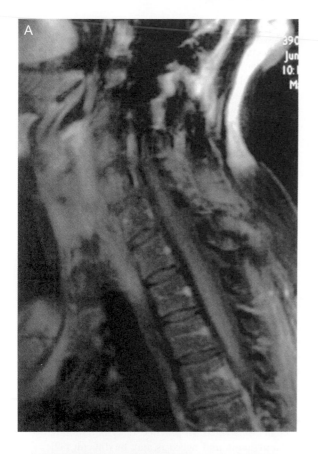

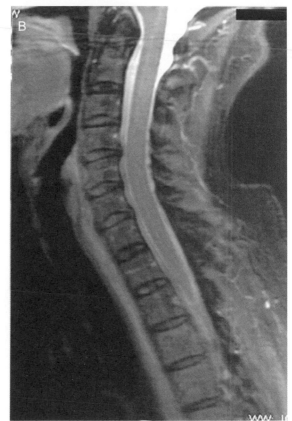

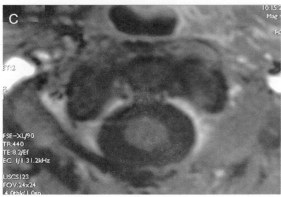

Figure 7.7. MRI and artefacts. Patient with prostate cancer. (A) Typical wrong image with increased signal of C2 on sagittal T1-weighted image after gadolinium due to metallic artefact, no more visible on axial slice (C) neither on sagittal aspect of T2-weighted image (with fat sat) (B)

POST-THERAPEUTIC ASPECTS

After radiation therapy, MRI appears to be a powerful tool for differentiating post-therapeutic changes from tumour recurrence. Post-therapeutic changes include the appearance of areas of increased signal intensity during certain imaging strategies, consistent with either an absolute or a relative increase of fatty tissue; whereas in tumour recurrence a low signal intensity is more characteristic. During the first 2 weeks, marrow oedema and necrosis area are more visible on STIR sequence than on spin-echo. USPIO may also be useful [28]. At 3–6 weeks, fatty bone marrow conversion allows a homogeneous hypersignal on T1-weighted

Table 7.3. Osteoporotic collapse. Statistical value of MRI findings

MRI Findings	Sensitivity (%)	Specificity (%)
VB posterior angle recession into medullary canal	16	100
VB, partly hyposignal on SE T1-WI	68	93
Homogeneous signal of VB on post-contrast T1-WI	84	82
Normal signal of VB or linear hypersignal under fracture on T2-WI	85	90

For abbreviations, see Table 7.1. Data from [23].

Table 7.4. Malignant vertebral body collapse. Statistical value of MRI findings

MRI findings	Sensitivity (%)	Specificity (%)
Backward convexity of VB posterior wall	70	94
Epidural mass	80	100
Pedicle hyposignal on SE T1-WI	80	94
All VB hyposignal on T1-WI	77	81
Heterogeneous hypersignal of VB on T2-WI	85	100
VB heterogeneous or diffuse hypersignal on post-contrast T1-WI	77	100

For abbreviations, see Table 7.1. Data from [23].

images for all vertebrae included in the radiation field [24] (Figure 7.10). Increased visibility of new lesions can be noticed. Medullary conversion arises at the periphery, giving a banded appearance with central hypersignal on T1-weighted images [29]. Marrow recovery depends on the age of patient. A recent study [28] performed on rabbits suggests that late post-contrast images demonstrate a significant positive T1 enhancement of the normal bone marrow, and subsequent increase with irradiation due to increased reticuloendothelial system activity, thus allowing reliable exemplification of irradiation-induced changes in bone marrow physiology. Drug side-effects on osseous tissue can be observed. Osseous remodelling may be altered. Osteopenia, coarsening of trabeculae and secondary neoplasia may be encountered. Vascular lesions may be present, leading to ischaemia and fractures. Thorough examination of MR images allows tumour evaluation and may confirm that extension of the tumour has not occurred. These effects can be observed for up to 5 years [30]. According to some authors [2,31], radiation has a protective effect on the marrow against invasion by tumour cells.

Chemotherapy may produce a similar striped appearance on MR images observed a few weeks after aplasia. Thus, on the STIR sequence, hyposignal will follow hypersignal. After the administration of growth factor, hyperplasia of the marrow can appear as nodes which are difficult to discriminate from metastases because they are both on hypersignal on T1-weighted images.

For the evaluation of vertebral tumours, MRI allows the best imaging of the metastatic process. Necrosis, tumour volume and epidural extension are well demonstrated. In practice, discrimination between haemorrhagia and necrosis may be difficult [32].

Development of a faint sclerotic rim at the periphery of sclerotic lesions is the best sign of a healing response. Progressive bone sclerosis, proceeding from the outside towards the centre, indicating conversion from focal areas of osteolysis to a uniform osteosclerotic zone and sometimes followed by a shrinking appearance prior to disappearance, is a usual pattern of progressive healing. However, in some instances, healing of an osteolytic lesion may be accompanied by progressive ossification at the periphery, leading, even on MR images, to a well-defined and sometimes expanded appearance [33,34]. CT and plain films can

Table 7.5. Signals from spinal components by different imaging techniques

MRI	Fat	Bone	Marrow	CSF	Muscle	Tumour
T2	Hyper	Hypo	Iso	Hyper	Iso	Iso-hyper
STIR	Hypo	Hypo	Iso	Hyper	Iso	Hyper
T1	Hyper	Hypo	Iso	Hypo	Iso	Iso-hypo
T1+G	Hyper	Hypo	Iso	Hypo	Iso	Hyper
T1GFATSAT	Hypo	Hypo	Iso-hyper	Hypo	Iso	Hyper

For abbreviations, see Table 7.1.

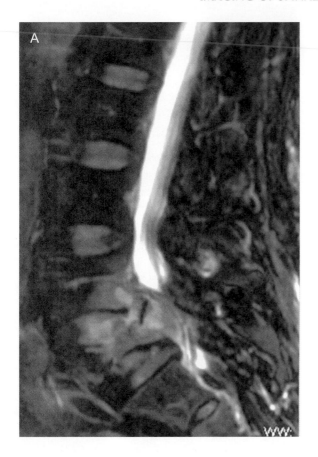

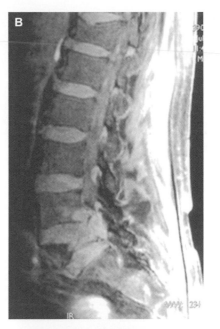

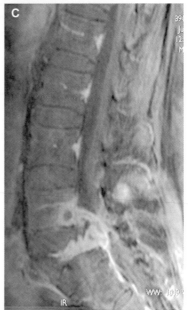

Figure 7.8. Typical sight of malignant vertebral collapse on STIR (T2)- (A), T1-weighted images, before (B) and after (C) gadolinium with fat sat, demonstrating heterogeneous hypersignal of vertebral body on T2-WI, hyposignal on T1-WI, dramatically increased on T1-WI with gadolinium, backward convexity of posterior wall of vertebral body, epidural extension, without evidence of disc destruction

then be useful. A successful response to therapy is demonstrated by sclerotic zones in vertebrae that initially appear normal in appearance, suggesting the existence of non-visible osteolytic lesions. In fact, an osteoblastic reaction suggestive of a successful response to therapy can lead to a dramatic increase in both the size and number of tumoral foci, findings that could easily be interpreted as disease progression [2,35]. Conversely, for sclerotic lesions, a decrease in the size and number of osteoblastic foci could be

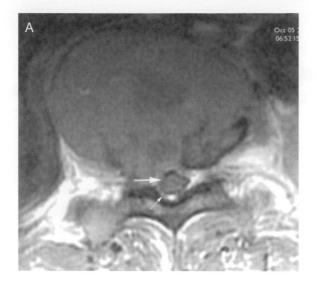

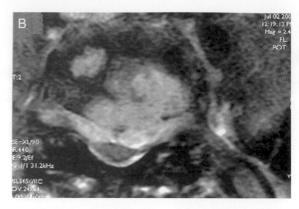

Figure 7.9. Intracanular extension. Axial slices with T1-WI images are mandatory for clear delineation of epidural involvement, here with typical "double bag" aspect (B), arachnoid (small arrow) and pia mater invasion (arrow) (A)

considered as evidence of the healing process. For such tumours as prostate carcinomas, sclerotic areas may remain unchanged, rather than decreasing in size, during tumour remission [2,35]. Thus, correlation of these radiographic changes with clinical and biological data can allow better interpretation of the patient's true condition. In mixed lesions, a successful therapeutic response will be a continuous evolution towards a uniform sclerotic area. Subsequent patterns of the healing process are identical to osteolytic lesions. For reducing artefacts caused by materials introduced after surgery, fast spin-echo sequences are recommended [36].

Since radiographic manifestations of progression or healing of site of skeletal metastasis are fairly constant from one region of the body to another, an abbreviated or shortened examination may suffice when monitoring the tumour's response to therapy.

MANAGEMENT OF IMAGING

The strategy will vary according to clinical manifestations and staging of illness. At the stage of detection and diagnosis of osteophilic neoplastic processes, and even in absence of clinical manifestations, scintigraphy (bone scan) is systematically performed, even with or replaced by SPECT, which greatly improves the predictive value of bone scan in the diagnosis of vertebral metastases [37]. When the scan is positive, MRI is also performed. SPECT is, in fact, considered to produce results comparable to and complementary

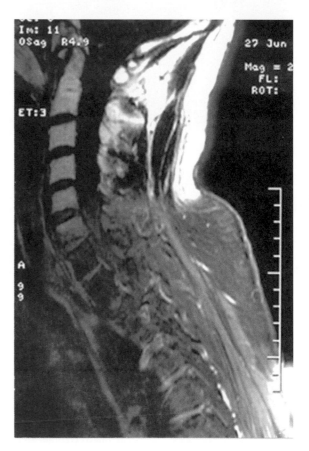

Figure 7.10. Post-therapeutic sight. Striped aspect with hypersignal of bone marrow in the field of previous irradiation of a cervical cancer

with MRI [38]. MRI has equal or greater sensitivity to the detection of osseous metastases as bone scintigraphy, and has greater specificity. Plain films and CT remain a constant part of patient evaluation.

Plain films are useful and easy to perform for metastases monitoring; they allow a good survey of cortical involvement and thus the risk of fracture and neurological complications. Treatment efficiency, by number and size of metastases and staging of rebuilding (or, conversely, progression of destruction) can also be delineated. CT is not used routinely during follow-up, but may be necessary for surveying pure osteoblastic or mixed lesions. MRI is also useful for paravertebral masses and epidural extension. Conversely, MRI has some limitations for appraising tumour necrosis and bone marrow changes but remains mandatory for post-treatment monitoring.

CONCLUSION

Diagnosis and monitoring of spinal metastases has been highly improved with the advent of MRI. Clear knowledge of the performance and limitations of each type of investigation described in this chapter is mandatory for their proper use. The radiologist must remember that X-ray findings can be suggestive of diagnosis without being truly pathognomonic. Searching for bone metastasis should be part of the investigation in any clinical manifestation suggestive of spinal disease, even in patients in whom cancer has not hitherto been suspected.

REFERENCES

1. Bontoux D, Alcalay M. Cancer Secondaire des Os. Expansion Scientifique Française [in French] 1997.
2. Resnik D. Skeletal Metastases. Diagnosis of Bone and Joints Disorders. WB Saunders: Philadelphia, PA, 2002.
3. Bey P, Stines J, Conroy T. Les métastases osseuses inaugurales. Concours Med 1990; 112: 3343–6 [in French].
4. Berretoni BA, Carter JR. Mechanisms of cancer metastasis to bone. J. Bone Joint Surg 1986; 68A: 308–12.
5. Pointillard V, Ravaud A, Palussière J, Dousset V. Imagerie des métastases vertébrales. In Métastases Vertébrales. Springer-Verlag. Paris, 2001 [in French].
6. Edelstyn GA, Gillespie PJ, Grebell FS. The radiological demonstration of osseous metastases. Experimental observations. Clin Radiol 1967; 18: 158–62.
7. Jacobson AF, Stomper PC, Cronin EB, Kaplan WD. Bone scans with one or two new abnormalities in cancer patients with no known metastases: reliability of interpretation of initial correlative radiographs. Radiology 1990; 174: 503–7.
8. Kunkler IH, Merrick MV, Rodger A. Bone scintigraphy in breast cancer: a nine-year follow-up. Clin Radiol 1985; 36: 279–82.
9. Lodwick GS. Reactive response to local injury in bone. Radiol Clin N Am 1964; 2: 209.
10. Fornasier VL, Czsitrom AA. Collapsed vertebrae: a review of 659 autopsies. Clin Orthop 1978; 131: 261.
11. Laredo JD, Lakhdari K, Bellaiche L et al. Acute vertebral collapse: CT findings in benign and malignant non-traumatic cases. Radiology 1995; 194: 41–8.
12. Ricci C, Cova M, Kang YS et al. Normal age-related patterns of cellular and fatty bone marrow distribution in the axial skeleton: MR imaging study. Radiology 1990; 177: 83.
13. Vogler JB III, Murphy WA. Bone-marrow imaging. Radiology 1988; 168: 679.
14. Mehta RC, Marks MP, Hinks RS et al. MR evaluation of vertebral metastases: T1-weighted, short-inversion time recovery, fast spin-echo, and inversion-recovery fast spin-echo sequences. Am J Neuroradiol 1995; 16: 281–8.
15. Smoker WRK, Godersky JC, Knutzon RK et al. The role of MR imaging in evaluating metastatic spinal disease. Am J Roentgenol 1987; 49: 1241.
16. Ruzal-Shapiro C, Berdon WE, Cohen MD et al. MR imaging of diffuse bone marrow replacement in pediatric patients with cancer. Radiology 1991; 181: 587.
17. Seneterre E, Weissleder R, Jaramillo D et al. Bone marrow: ultra-small super-paramagnetic particles iron oxide for MR imaging. Radiology 1991; 179: 529–33.
18. Daldrup-Link HE, Rummeny EJ, Ihssen B et al. Iron oxide-enhanced MR imaging of bone marrow in patients with non-Hodgkin's lymphoma: differentiation between tumor infiltration and hypercellular bone marrow. Eur Radiol 2002; 12(6): 1557–66.
19. Trouard TP, Theilmann RJ, Altbach MI, Gmitro AF. High-resolution diffusion imaging with DIFRAD-FSE (diffusion-weighted radial acquisition of data with fast spin-echo) MRI. Magn Reson Med 1999; 42: 11–18.
20. Zhou XJ, Leeds NE, McKinnon GC, Kumar AJ. Characterization of benign and metastatic vertebral compression fractures with quantitative diffusion MR imaging. Am J Neuroradiol 2002; 23: 165–70.
21. Baur A, Stabler A, Bruning R et al. Diffusion-weighted MR imaging of bone marrow: differentiation of benign versus pathologic compression fracture. Radiology 1998; 199: 349–56.
22. Castillo M, Arbelaez A, Smith JK, Fisher LL. Diffusion-weighted MR imaging offers no advantage over routine non-contrast MR imaging in the detection of vertebral metastases. Am J Neuroradiol 2000; 21: 948–53.
23. Cuenod CA, Laredo JD, Chevret S et al. Acute vertebral collapse due to osteoporosis or malignancy: appearance on unenhanced and gadolinium enhanced MR images. Radiology 1996; 199: 541–9.
24. Yuh WTC, Zagar CK, Barloon TJ et al. Vertebral compression fractures: distinction between benign and malignant causes with MR imaging. Radiology 1989; 172: 215–18.
25. Kamholtz R, Sze G. MRI of spinal metastases. MRI Decisions, 1990; Nov/Dec: 2.
26. Mink JH, Weitz I, Kagen AR et al. Bone scan-positive and radiograph- and CT-negative vertebral lesion in a woman with locally advanced breast cancer. Am J Roentgenol 1987; 148: 341.

27. Barloon TJ, Yuh WTC, Yang CTC et al. Spinal subarachnoid tumor seeding from intracranial metastasis: MR findings. J Comput Assist Tomogr 1987; 11: 242.

28. Daldrup HE, Link TM, Blasius S et al. Monitoring radiation-induced with ultra-small super-paramagnetic iron oxide (USPIO)-enhanced MRI. J Magn Reson Imag 1999; 9: 643–52.

29. Stevens SK, Moore SG, Kaplan ID. Early and late bone-marrow changes after irradiation: MR evaluation. Am J Roentgenol 1990; 154: 745–50.

30. Grignon B, Stines J, Régent D, Gaucher A. Radiolésions osseuses. Encycl Méd Chir Radiodiagn 1990; II: 31185 A10 [in French].

31. Hercbergs A, Werner A, Brenner HJ. Reduced thoracic vertebrae metastasis following post mastectomy para-sternal irradiation. Int J Radiat Oncol Biol Phys 1985; 11: 773–6.

32. Sanchez RB, Quinn SF, Walling A et al. Musculoskeletal neoplasms after intra-arterial chemotherapy: correlation of MR images with pathologic specimen. Radiology 1990; 174: 237–40.

33. Pagani JJ, Libshitz HI. Imaging bone metastases. Radiol Clin N Am 1982; 20: 545.

34. Barry WF Jr, Wells SA Jr, Cox CE et al. Clinical and radiographic correlations in breast cancer patients with osseous metastases. Skel Radiol 1981; 6: 27.

35. Pollen JJ, Shlaer WJ. Osteoblastic response to successful treatment of metastatic cancer of the prostate. Am J Roentgenol 1979; 132: 927.

36. Persilge CA, Lewin JS, Duerk JL et al. Optimizing imaging parameters for MR evaluation of the spine with titanium pedicle screws. Am J Roentgenol 1996; 166: 1213–18.

37. Savelli G, Maffioli L, Maccauro M et al. Bone scintigraphy and the added value of SPECT in detecting skeletal lesions. Qu J Nucl Med 2001; 45(1): 27–37.

38. Kosuda S, Kaji T, Yokoyama H et al. Does bone SPECT actually have lower sensitivity for detecting vertebral metastases than MRI? J Nucl Med 1996; 37(6): 975–8.

8

Monitoring Response to Treatment— the Role of Biochemical Markers

R. E. Coleman and J. E. Brown

Cancer Research Centre, Weston Park Hospital, Sheffield, UK

INTRODUCTION

Advanced cancers frequently metastasise to the bone, and the resulting bone destruction is associated with a variety of skeletal complications, including pathological fractures, bone pain, impaired mobility, spinal cord compression and hypercalcaemia [1]. It is estimated that more than 1.5 million cancer patients worldwide have bone metastases. Current treatment options for patients with bone metastases include radiation therapy, surgery, bisphosphonates and analgesics, in addition to standard anticancer therapy. The primary goal of therapy is to minimise bone pain and morbidity and improve mobility and quality of life. Because of the increasing range of treatment options for metastatic bone disease, there is consequently an increased requirement for practical and accurate methods for assessment of the response to therapy in bone. An ideal approach would be simple and non-invasive to perform, would report changes using a quantitative measure, and would be sufficiently sensitive that an early assessment of response to treatment could be obtained. Although several methods for assessment are available, no single method in current use approaches this ideal.

For metastases in visceral and soft tissues, assessment of treatment response by measurement of tumour dimensions using imaging methods is relatively straightforward. However, in the case of bone metastases, this is much more difficult and controversial because of the length of time before response is detectable by imaging methods, as well as the

difficulties in distinguishing between metastatic progression and bone healing in response to treatment. Although imaging methods are likely to remain central to the management of bone metastases, there is intensive current research into the possible role of bone markers in this context. There is now growing evidence that bone marker measurements may complement imaging methods by allowing more rapid and quantitative evaluation, which can be utilised to influence therapeutic management decisions at an early stage.

BIOCHEMICAL MARKERS OF BONE METABOLISM

Recently, highly specific biochemical markers of bone metabolism have been developed and are increasingly used to predict outcome and monitor therapies for benign bone disease such as osteoporosis [2]. These assays, based on the measurement of bone breakdown and formation products, are now relatively straightforward and convenient to perform (Table 8.1). Data are emerging that suggest that bone markers may be useful in oncology and could be used to augment the imaging techniques currently used for diagnosis and assessment of response. For example, they could be used to identify patients at risk of developing skeletal complications, to aid in diagnosis of skeletal abnormalities, for assessment of response to systemic therapy, and to help define patients who may or may not benefit from bisphosphonate therapy [3]. The clinical utility of

Textbook of Bone Metastases. Edited by C. Jasmin, R. E. Coleman, L. R. Coia, R. Capanna and G. Saillant
© 2005 John Wiley & Sons Ltd: ISBN 0 471 87742 5

Table 8.1. Urine and serum bone markers for assessment of the effects of cancer on bone

Marker (normal range)	Abbreviation	Usual sample source	Type of marker
Calcium 0.28–0.43 mM/mM creatinine		Serum/urine	Resorption
Hydroxyproline 0 1.1 mM/mM creatinine		Urine	Resorption
Pyridinolinium cross-links 19.5–25.1 nM/mM creatinine*	PYD	Urine	Resorption
Deoxypyridinolinium cross-links 4.8–5.5 nM/mM creatinine*	DPD	Urine	Resorption
N-telopeptide 23.2–30.9 nM/mM creatinine*	NTX	Urine/serum	Resorption
C telopeptide 3.9–4.9 nM/mM creatinine*	CTX	Urine/serum	Resorption
Bone alkaline phosphatase 4–20 µg/l	ALP-BI	Serum	Formation
Osteocalcin 3–13 ng/ml		Serum	Formation
Type I procollagen N-terminal propeptide	PINP	Serum	Formation
Type I procollagen C-terminal propeptide	PICP	Serum	Formation
Bone sialoprotein 8.0–9.4 µg/l*	BSP	Serum	Other

* Normal ranges quoted in references 56 and 64.

bone markers in the diagnosis and treatment of malignant bone disease is reviewed in this chapter.

Bone Resorption Markers

The hallmark of metastatic bone disease is increased activity of osteoclasts, associated with variable and typically unmatched amounts of bone collagen synthesis by osteoblasts [4]. This uncoupling of the normal physiology of bone results in abnormal bone remodelling. Osteoclasts produce a number of proteolytic enzymes capable of degrading the organic bone matrix [5,6], thus releasing calcium and a variety of collagen breakdown products into the serum. These by-products of pathological bone resorption are primarily excreted by the kidneys and therefore can also be measured in the urine. The molar ratio of their excretion relative to creatinine excretion provides a reproducible measure of their rate of bone breakdown that is independent of body size or urine dilution.

Urinary calcium and hydroxyproline are traditional biochemical markers that have been widely used for many years to assess bone metabolism in patients with skeletal metastases and other metabolic disorders of the bone. The calcium : creatinine ratio in an early morning urine sample after an overnight fast has been shown to be a reproducible method of quantifying

calcium excretion [7]. Calcium excretion has also been reported to be a useful marker of therapeutic response in patients with osteolytic bone lesions [8,9]. However, subsequent studies have demonstrated that in unselected groups of patients with bone metastases, urinary calcium was not significantly increased compared to controls or subjects without bone metastases [10]. There was also no correlation between urinary calcium and clinical findings or response to bisphosphonate treatment [11]. Moreover, calcium excretion is affected by diet, renal function, uptake of calcium into bone, and circulating levels of parathyroid hormone (PTH) and parathyroid hormone-related protein (PTHrP) [3].

Hydroxyproline is a major amino acid constituent of collagen, and its excretion is typically elevated in the presence of abnormal bone resorption or formation [12]. Although much of the hydroxyproline released from the bone is oxidised in the liver, approximately 15% appears in the urine. Measurements of hydroxyproline can be made on either a 24 h urine collection or on the second voided early morning sample after an overnight fast. Hydroxyproline is not strictly a bone-specific marker, as only approximately 50% of human collagen is derived from bone [13]. Hydroxyproline is also a major constituent of several other human proteins, including acetylcholinesterase, complement factor C1q and elastin. Urinary excretion of hydroxyproline is also strongly influenced by diet [14], age and soft-tissue destruction by tumour. Additionally, there is a circadian rhythm, with a peak between midnight and 8:00 a.m. [15].

Although urinary hydroxyproline is a useful indicator of accelerated collagen breakdown in metastatic bone disease [12], it is not particularly useful or reliable for documenting disease progression or response to therapy. More recently, a number of biochemical markers have been developed that provide more specific and sensitive indications of bone resorption (Table 8.1) [16]. These new markers include several unique breakdown products of type I collagen, including the pyridinium cross-links pyridinoline (PYD) and deoxypyridinoline (DPD), and the peptide-bound cross-links N-telopeptide (NTX) and C-telopeptide (CTX). In comparison with calcium and hydroxyproline, these collagen breakdown products are more specific to bone and are not influenced by diet or extra-osseus metabolism [3].

PYD and DPD cross-links are both specific to bone, and can be quantitated in the urine using reverse-phase high-performance liquid chromatography (HPLC) and/or an enzyme-linked immunosorbent assay (ELISA). Their excretion relative to creatinine is only minimally affected by renal function [17], but does vary substantially throughout the day with a circadian rhythm, and from day to day [3]. Therefore, samples must be taken at the same time each day, and collection of two samples on consecutive days is ideal to establish a reliable baseline value.

In patients with pathological bone resorption, a good correlation has been observed between PYD and DPD excretion and radiological or histomorphometric measures of bone resorption [18]. Moreover, increased excretion of these cross-links correlates well with bone resorption in a variety of pathological conditions, including osteoporosis, Paget's disease and primary hyperparathyroidism.

Immunoassays to measure the N- and C-terminal peptide-bound cross-links of type I collagen in the urine and in serum have also been developed. The CrossLaps™ (Osteometer Biotech A/S, Copenhagen, Denmark) and Osteomark™ (Ostex International, Inc., Seattle, Wash) ELISA, measuring urinary CTX and NTX, respectively, were developed in the early 1990s [19,20]. ELISAs that can be used to measure serum levels of CTX and NTX have become available more recently [16]. These peptide-bound cross-links constitute the major fraction of cross-links from collagen degradation in both the serum and the urine. Therefore, changes in bone metabolism result in greater changes in serum and urine concentrations of NTX and CTX compared with PYD and DPD [20].

This is reflected in larger falls in NTX or CTX compared with PYD or DPD following anti-resorptive therapy. There is an additional C-telopeptide assay in serum called ICTP. This bone collagen product is probably derived from non-osteoclast-mediated bone resorption, utilising matrix metalloproteinases derived from the underlying pathological process, rather than the cathepsin K-mediated pathway associated with physiological bone resorption.

Bone Formation Markers

Type 1 collagen is the major protein of bone and accounts for about 90% of the organic matrix. It is a complex molecule consisting of a heterotrimer of two pro-α1 and one pro-α2 peptide chains. The molecule is tightly coiled due to the presence of regular glycine residues that do not possess a bulky side chain and allow the helical structure to form.

The steps involved in collagen synthesis are multiple and complicated and include a number of post-translational modifications. Essentially, a large precursor protein, Type 1 procollagen, is synthesised by osteoblasts. The three chains are assembled, with intra- and inter-molecular cross-links binding the peptide chains together to make the molecule insoluble. The collagen fibrils are formed by precise spatial alignment of the collagen chains prior to mineralisation of the resulting matrix. The available biochemical markers of bone formation reflect different aspects of this process.

Type 1 procollagen (PICP) is believed to be a marker of early bone formation, appearing principally during the phase of osteoblast proliferation. Assay of the carboxy-terminal propeptide is now possible by radio-immuno-assay [21,22]. Osteoblasts are naturally rich in alkaline phosphatase, and release of the enzyme into the circulation occurs predominantly during the matrix maturation phase of bone formation, and provides a slightly different indication of osteoblast activity. Total alkaline phosphatase is routinely measured in clinical practice, but to exclude the contribution from the liver and other organs, bone isoenzyme estimation (ALP-BI) is required. Raised levels reflect increased new bone formation and in oncology the highest values are found with osteoblastic metastases or in response to healing [22]. Osteocalcin (BGP) is a marker of the late phase of bone formation, appearing during mineralisation [22]. It is also synthesised in osteoblasts, and contains three residues of the vitamin K-dependent amino acid γ-carboxyglutamic acid. Osteocalcin binds strongly to hydroxyapatite, but a small fraction of the newly synthesised protein appears in the circulation, from which it is rapidly cleared by the kidneys. Measurement of serum levels is possible by a variety of radioimmuno-assays.

DIAGNOSIS OF BONE METASTASES

Imaging and Diagnosis

Plain Radiographs

Plain radiograph examination is simple and inexpensive to perform and allows an initial evaluation by the clinician in the outpatient clinic. However, it is of limited sensitivity. For a destructive lesion in trabecular bone to be recognised on a plain radiograph, it must be greater than 1 cm in diameter, with loss of approximately 50% of the bone mineral content [23]. This therefore makes it unreliable as an initial screening test (Figure 8.1). Plain radiographs indicate the net result of bone resorption and repair, and essentially rely on measuring normal tissue reaction to metastatic invasion, rather than measuring lesions themselves [24].

Bone metastases are traditionally classified according to radiological appearance. In breast cancer, lytic, sclerotic and mixed patterns are classically described [25]. When net bone resorption occurs, leading to local bone destruction, radiographs take on a lytic appearance. Sclerotic patterns are seen when osteoblast activity results in net bone formation. However, both histological analysis and bone marker studies have shown that, whether radiographic patterns are lytic or sclerotic, there is an abnormally high level of both bone resorption and bone formation. This is important, as treatments such as bisphosphonates, which are targeted against osteoclasts, can also be effective in patients with apparently sclerotic lesions.

Radionuclide Bone Scanning

Bone scanning or bone scintigraphy utilises the ability of radiopharmaceuticals to accumulate in metabolically active bone and their subsequent detection by a gamma camera. Currently bone scintigraphy with ^{99m}technetium (99mTc)-labelled methylene diphosphonate (MDP) remains the most widely used method for diagnosis and monitoring of bone metastases [26]. Modern equipment allows rapid recording of whole body images of the entire skeleton and also has the ability to focus on specific lesions. The technique is used for initial screening of patients where there is a suspicion of skeletal involvement.

Bone scans have a high sensitivity in detecting lesions, but a rather low specificity. As the technique reflects the rate of bone turnover, "hot spots" can occur in many benign conditions, such as infection and trauma. Indeed, even in those with a previous history of breast cancer, only 50% of solitary "hot spots" are due to metastatic bone disease [26]. The bone scan also lacks anatomical detail. For these reasons it is rarely used alone, but needs to be considered in association with other imaging techniques, such as a plain

Imaging	SENSITIVITY	SPECIFICITY	COST
• Bone scanning	+++	+	+++
• Plain radiographs	+	++	++
• MRI	++++	+++	++++
• CT	+++	+++	+++
Clinical assessment			
• Symptoms	+++	+	+
• Examination	+	+	+
Tumour markers			
• CA 15-3	++	+++	+
• CEA	+	++	+
Bone markers			
• Resorption markers	++	++	+
• Formation markers	+	+	+

Figure 8.1. Sensitivity, specificity and cost of available diagnostic tests for metastatic bone disease

radiograph (X-ray), computed tomography (CT) or magnetic resonance imaging (MRI) to further characterise any abnormalities found. Another potential problem occurs when bone resorption is so dominant in large lytic lesions that there is insufficient new bone formation to trigger radiopharmaceutical detection, with the production of a photon-deficient area, otherwise known as a "cold spot" [27].

Cross-sectional Imaging

CT offers the ability to evaluate the three-dimensional integrity of bone. It is particularly useful to assess early bone destruction as well as extra-osseous soft tissue and intra-osseus medullary spread. CT may also be of benefit in imaging areas such as the sacrum, which present particular technical difficulties with other imaging methods [25,28].

MRI, in contrast to plain radiographs and bone scanning, is able to show changes in the bone marrow itself and hence gives a more direct assessment of bone metastasis [28]. MRI has a higher diagnostic sensitivity than plain radiographs or radioisotope bone scanning [29] and is indicated when these initial investigations appear normal in patients with a strong clinical suspicion of bone metastases. MRI is also usually able to categorise hot spots on bone scans into benign and malignant lesions, although osteoporotic collapse can be difficult to differentiate from metastatic collapse, even with gadolinium enhancement. MRI has now been developed to the point where it offers high spatial resolution, allowing visualisation of fine anatomical detail, and is especially valuable for assessing the spine. This has led to MRI being the investigation of choice for patients presenting with back pain and neurological deficit, particularly when a diagnosis of spinal cord compression is suspected.

Positron Emission Tomography (PET)

PET is a developing technique that is becoming increasingly used in oncology research. Unlike conventional anatomical imaging methods, PET is able to detect dynamic functional and metabolic changes, rather than simply structural features, and is intrinsically more sensitive. For detection of bone metastases in breast cancer patients, most work has been performed with ^{18}F PET (using ^{18}F-fluorodeoxyglucose, FDG). Cook and Fogelman [30] noted that, overall, FDG detected more bone metastases than the conventional ^{99m}Tc MDP bone scan, particularly in those patients with predominantly lytic lesions. PET scans may also show better discrimination between metastatic and benign lesions. There is also evidence that ^{18}F PET may be able to detect small bone lesions at an earlier stage than ^{99m}Tc bone scans [31].

Tumour Markers

In breast cancer there is no single tumour marker identified which is sufficiently specific for diagnostic purposes. However, several markers have been studied which are often elevated in metastatic breast cancer. These include serum carcinoembryonic antigen (CEA), the mucin markers CA 15-3 and CA 549 and tissue plasminogen activator (TPA). A raised level is highly suggestive of metastatic disease [32] but around 35–40% of newly diagnosed patients with bone metastases from breast cancer will have normal CA15-3 or similar mucin marker levels [33].

Prostate-specific antigen (PSA) is a marker of prostatic pathology and may be elevated in any prostate disease—benign prostatic hypertrophy (BPH), prostatitis and cancer. The highest tissue production occurs in prostate cancer and PSA has proved useful in the early diagnosis, staging and follow-up of patients [34]. The level of PSA is dependent on the volume of cancer, the volume of BPH in the prostate and the differentiation of the tumour, with less production of PSA from poorly differentiated tumours.

Use of Bone Markers in the Diagnosis of Metastatic Bone Disease

Bone resorption markers have been shown to be useful in the diagnosis of bone metastases in cancer patients. Many studies have now shown a positive relationship between various bone markers and the presence of metastatic bone disease. Early work was focused on measurements of urinary calcium [8,9] and hydroxyproline [35]. Both may be elevated in patients with metastatic bone disease, but their specificity and sensitivity are too low to be clinically useful. More recently, attention has been focused on the various breakdown products of type I collagen, including PYD, DPD, NTX and CTX (Figure 8.2).

Several studies have shown elevated PYD and DPD in patients with bone metastases [36–39] and it is apparent that these are more reliable indicators of metastatic bone disease. In the majority of patients with bone metastases, excretion of pyridinium

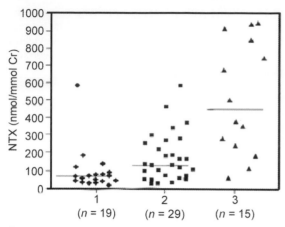

Figure 8.2. N-telopeptide (NTX) values in patients with (1) newly diagnosed bone metastases, (2) progressive bone metastases, or (3) progressive bone metastases and hypercalcaemia. Lines indicate the geometric means. Adapted from [3,64]

cross-links is typically increased by 2.5-fold compared with healthy controls and is also significantly elevated compared with cancer patients without bone metastases [3]. In a study which compared breast cancer patients with bone metastases with healthy premenopausal women, the percentage of elevated values for the cancer group were 47% for urinary calcium, 74% for hydroxyproline, 83% for CTX and 100% for the collagen cross-links PYD and DPD. Alkaline phosphatase but not urinary calcium correlated significantly with the other four bone markers [38]. Patients with breast cancer but without bone metastases may also exhibit slightly increased PYD and DPD excretion [39], possibly due to systemic stimulation of bone resorption by circulating tumour-derived parathyroid hormone-related protein.

Other studies have confirmed these findings, but also highlighted the particular diagnostic value of NTX. On the basis of radiographic and bone scan findings, 127 cancer patients were divided into three groups, including 83 with no bone metastases, 22 with one or two bone metastases and 22 patients with three or more. PYD, NTX and CTX were significantly increased in both groups with bone involvement, indicating the specificity and sensitivity of these markers [39–42]. Lipton et al. [40] have attempted to determine which marker best correlated with skeletal metastases and concluded that NTX was the most predictive for the presence of bone metastases. However, there are data to show that there are some patients who have indolent bone metastases, or only an isolated one or two lesions, that do not break down

sufficient bone matrix to significantly influence serum or urinary concentrations of bone resorption markers. It should also be emphasised that bone markers are not specific for malignant disease and can be elevated in a number of benign bone diseases [43]. Therefore, there is still a need for skeletal imaging to diagnose bone metastases with certainty.

Although bone metastases in prostate cancer are primarily osteosclerotic, increased bone resorption is also evident, and elevated CTX levels correlate with skeletal involvement [44–46]. In a study of 39 prostate cancer patients with bone metastases, urinary serum CTX was increased approximately two-fold compared with 355 healthy, age-matched men [46]. Increases in bone resorption markers were not detected in prostate patients without bone metastases ($n=9$) or in patients with benign prostatic hyperplasia ($n=9$). Levels of bone resorption markers correlate with the extent of bone metastasis in prostate cancer and may be important in predicting clinical outcome [47,48]. Biochemical markers of bone formation, including bone-specific alkaline phosphatase and the amino- and carboxy-terminal propeptides of type I procollagen, have also been shown to correlate with bone metastases in patients with prostate cancer [48,49].

Bone formation markers may also be expected to be raised in metastatic bone disease because of the increased turnover of bone remodelling. Compared with bone resorption markers, there are far fewer data available. Osteocalcin levels [50] and bone-specific alkaline phosphatase levels [51] have both been shown to be significantly raised in patients with metastatic bone disease from breast cancer, compared with normal controls. In such patients, levels of these two formation markers are significantly higher in those with blastic rather than lytic metastases. However, neither of these markers appears to be useful for the early detection of bone metastases. As well as correlating with the presence of bone metastases, it would be useful if markers could give an indication of the extent of bone disease. There is evidence from several studies that a range of markers, including PYD, DPD and alkaline phosphatase, correlated with the number of skeletal areas involved [40,52].

Bone Markers as Predictive/Prognostic Indicators

Since commonly used radiographic methods do not detect bone metastases in the very early stages of development, the question arises whether serial measurements of bone markers may identify the impending development of bone metastases. As yet, data relating to this question are very sparse. Studies carried out on bone sialoprotein (BSP) have proved particularly interesting. BSP is a bone matrix integrin-binding protein synthesised by osteoblasts and osteoclasts, and is expressed ectopically by malignant breast, prostate and other cancer cells [53]. The observations that serum BSP levels were significantly higher in patients with bone metastases than those without [54] ($p < 0.05$), and that levels were 142% greater in postmenopausal women than in premenopausal women [55], suggested that BSP measurement might be useful for monitoring bone resorption. The measurement of serum BSP levels is currently under evaluation as a prognostic factor for bone metastases, disease progression and survival. In an analysis of 388 patients with primary breast cancer without metastasis, Diel et al. [56] showed that a BSP value in excess of 24 ng/ml was highly predictive of subsequent bone metastases. Of the 19 patients who subsequently developed skeletal metastases, only two had normal BSP levels.

In patients diagnosed with bone metastases as the only site of metastatic involvement, the average survival is 2 years. Is the degree of elevation of bone marker related to survival time? There is evidence that this is the case. In a study by Ali et al. [40,57], serum NTX levels were measured in 250 post-menopausal breast cancer patients with bone-only metastases. There was a highly significant correlation between a raised NTX level and poor survival time (Table 8.2). Furthermore, when the data were analysed according to quartiles of NTX level, these differences became even more marked.

ASSESSMENT OF RESPONSE

Imaging Techniques for the Assessment of Response

Plain Radiographs

In spite of the recognised limitations of plain radiography in metastatic bone disease, most of the established criteria for assessing bone response are based on interpretations of plain radiographs. The WHO Response Criteria for skeletal metastases uses changes in radiographic appearance to categorise response [58]. In metastatic bone disease, it is unusual to see a complete response. Partial response in lytic metastasis is said to occur when there is evidence of sclerosis of these lesions with no radiographic evidence of new lesions. However, assignment of apparently

Table 8.2. Median survival according to serum NTX levels in 250 patients with bone-only metastases

	Median survival (years)	
Not elevated	2.6	
Elevated	1.7	($p=0.0001$)
1st (lowest) quartile	3.0	
2nd quartile	2.5	
3rd quartile	2.4	
4th (highest) quartile	1.7	($p=0.0006$)

new areas of sclerosis can be difficult, since these may be due to development of a new metastatic lesion indicating progression or, equally, could be due to the healing of a lesion, previously present, but too small to be detected on previous radiographs.

Response assessment of sclerotic lesions on plain radiographs has proved to be almost impossible, because the radiographic appearance of healing is virtually indistinguishable from the appearance of progressive sclerotic metastases. Such patients are often categorised as "unchanged" following therapy. These difficulties in categorisation may explain, in part, the growing evidence that there is often little correlation between radiographic response and survival outcome [59].

Plain radiographs also have an important role in identifying patients who are at high risk of pathological fractures in weight-bearing bones, and who may benefit from prophylactic surgery. As a general guideline, sequential radiographic examination of selected identified areas of lytic destruction (two or three) should be carried out every 3 months to assess progression and the risk of pathological fracture. There is no value in more frequent routine examination, due to the lack of detectable changes at shorter times. Follow-up radiographs are of little value for sclerotic metastases, for the reasons discussed above.

Isotope Bone Scanning

The use of bone scans to assess response to therapy is of limited value, largely because of the so-called "flare phenomenon" [25]. This occurs following therapy, when the healing of a lesion causes new bone formation. Over a period of up to 6 months, it is impossible to distinguish this healing effect from disease progression. Areas of healing within sites of previous lytic disease can be observed on ^{99m}Tc bone scans [60] and may be confused with disease progression. Therefore, in patients with advanced disease, bone scans should be interpreted with caution within 6 months of a change in therapy. Bone scans are probably most useful for re-staging after relapse to identify sites for radiological assessment and those at risk of pathological fracture.

Cross-sectional Imaging

Although CT offers three-dimensional information and high-quality images, it is impractical to image more than a limited part of the skeleton. Therefore, CT is primarily used as a confirmatory technique and to assess healing of small lytic lesions. CT may have a more important role in the evaluation of response in sclerotic metastases, where plain radiographs and bone scans generally have little to offer. This is because, even in sclerotic metastases, CT is able to identify areas of osteolysis, and if these areas heal, this is a good indication of response to treatment.

MRI may also show a response to treatment with a decrease in tumour bulk and alterations in signal from infiltrating tumours within the bone marrow. However, MRI is not appropriate for routine monitoring of response to treatment, largely because of its expense and limited availability. Clearly, the possibility of using PET scanning to measure local changes in skeletal kinetics offers exciting prospects of using PET to assess more immediate response to systemic treatments than the currently available imaging techniques [30]. Currently PET is an expensive and complex technology, only available in certain tertiary treatment centres and, as yet, it has no established role in routine assessment of response in bone metastases. Nevertheless, there seems little doubt that it will become increasingly considered in patient management.

Tumour Markers

In a study by Kiang et al. [61], the kinetics of CEA and CA 15-3 were assessed in 30 patients with advanced breast cancer, immediately after chemotherapy. Whilst some patients showed the expected increase in markers with progression and decrease in markers with regression, others who responded showed an initial surge in tumour marker, followed later by the expected decline.

Using an index derived from CEA and CA 15-3 in combination with erythrocyte sedimentation rate, an initial study of 65 patients with metastatic breast cancer found a significant correlation with clinical assessment of response, using UICC criteria at 2, 4 and 6 months following systemic endocrine treatment [62]. More recently, this study was widened to include several European centres, using the same index to assess response to therapy in breast cancer patients [63]. The authors concluded that changes in the markers were in line with, and often pre-dated, therapeutic outcome criteria for both remission and progression.

It seems unlikely that any single tumour marker will be adequate for response assessment and the most promising direction will be the establishment of combinations of markers, together with an appropriate quantitative model.

The Role of Bone Markers in Assessment of Response

Objective assessment of response in bone metastases from breast cancer takes up to 6 months using radiological techniques and bone markers have been studied with the aim of providing an earlier indication of response.

Calcium and Hydroxyproline Excretion

Several studies have failed to find a strong correlation between hydroxyproline levels and response to bisphosphonates or radiological response to systemic therapy in breast cancer patients [25,64]. In patients receiving oral or intravenous bisphosphonates, hydroxyproline levels demonstrated poor sensitivity. Indeed, urinary calcium was more sensitive in these studies [65]. In patients receiving only systemic anticancer therapy, hydroxyproline levels increased in 30–40% of patients, despite evidence of stable disease or an objective radiological response of bone lesions [65,66]. Therefore, the hydroxyproline:creatinine ratio is not a sufficiently reliable or sensitive marker of bone resorption. The results from these studies suggest that these traditional markers of bone resorption are suboptimal in terms of selectivity and sensitivity.

Collagen Cross-links

Walls et al. [67] studied the collagen cross-links PYD and DPD as markers in 36 breast cancer patients with bone metastases. In 19 women who developed progressive disease over a median follow-up time of 4 months, both markers increased, with significant changes becoming apparent by 8 weeks. This evidence preceded radiological evidence by a median of 2 months. By contrast, in 17 women who responded to hormone therapy, the markers did not change significantly over a median time of 6 months.

In a study designed to evaluate bone resorption and tumour markers as possible alternatives to plain radiographs for the assessment of response to bisphosphonate therapy, Vinholes et al. [33] studied 37 patients with newly diagnosed bone metastases from breast cancer. NTX levels were significantly lower ($p \leqslant 0.05$) at 1 and 4 months in responding patients compared with those in patients with progressive disease. Similarly, NTX levels at 4 months in patients with either partial or no response were significantly lower in patients with a time to progression of >7 months, compared with patients who progressed in $\leqslant 7$ months. Furthermore, an increase in NTX excretion of $>50\%$ predicted disease progression in 78% of patients. Compared to urinary calcium, hydroxyproline and the tumour markers CA15-3 and cancer-associated serum antigen (CASA), NTX was reported to be the most sensitive marker for assessing response to therapy or progression (Table 8.3).

In a larger, more recent study, 97 evaluable patients with metastatic bone disease from a variety of primary sites were followed during systemic therapy in order to correlate marker changes with response to treatment [68]. Good correlations between urinary NTX, ICTP and bone alkaline phosphatase changes and response were observed, with a rise in NTX of $\geqslant 52\%$ having the highest positive predictive value (71%) for identifying progression.

The Role of Bone Markers in Development and Monitoring of Bisphosphonate Treatments

Whilst it is now well accepted that bone-targeted systemic therapy, particularly the use of the bisphosphonates, can substantially reduce morbidity of skeletal metastases of breast cancer, the optimisation and timing of these therapies remains to be established. Bone markers potentially offer a powerful and relatively simple tool to assist the clinician in developing the most appropriate treatment strategies. Moreover, there is the prospect that it may be possible to use bone markers to tailor treatment to the individual patient. Both NTX and CTX are typically increased two- to seven-fold in 70–80% of patients with bone metastases, compared with healthy controls, and typically decrease by 60–80% in response to bisphosphonate therapy [33,38,69]. Similar dramatic reductions in urinary PYD, DPD, CTX and NTX levels have been reported in patients with post-menopausal osteoporosis treated with 20–30 mg/day risedronate [70].

Several comparative trials have examined bone resorption markers in patients with bone metastases who were treated with bisphosphonates [38,64,69]. These studies have demonstrated significant correlations between baseline and post-treatment levels of PYD, DPD, NTX and CTX. In every study, however, levels of these markers correlated poorly with baseline urinary calcium. In a study of 19 breast cancer patients with extensive bone metastases, mean baseline levels of urinary calcium, hydroxyproline, CTX and collagen cross-links (PYD and DPD) were elevated in 47%, 74%, 83% and 100% of patients, respectively [38]. All of these markers decreased following pamidronate therapy, with the largest decrease observed in CTX (reaching 13% of baseline levels; Figure 8.3). In 29 breast cancer patients with progressing bone metastases, the mean baseline values of NTX, CTX, and DPD were elevated approximately two-fold compared with age-matched controls [69] and, following pamidronate therapy, levels of NTX and CTX decreased significantly ($p=0.001$). In a double-blind study of 32 patients with hypercalcaemia of malignancy, mean baseline levels of NTX were seven-fold above normal, and mean DPD and CTX levels were each five-fold

Table 8.3. Predictive value (PV) of a 50% increase in consecutive markers for the diagnosis of progressive disease

	Positive predictive value (PV$^+$) (%)	Negative predictive value (PV$^-$) (%)	Diagnostic efficiency (DE) (%)
Urine NTX*	81	76	72
Urine Hyp*	69	57	62
Urine calcium*	37	62	51
Serum CA 15-3	75	52	62
Serum CASA	56	52	54

*Corrected for creatinine excretion. Measured on second voided specimen of the morning.
NTX, N-telopeptide; Hyp, hydroxyproline.
Based on data from [33].

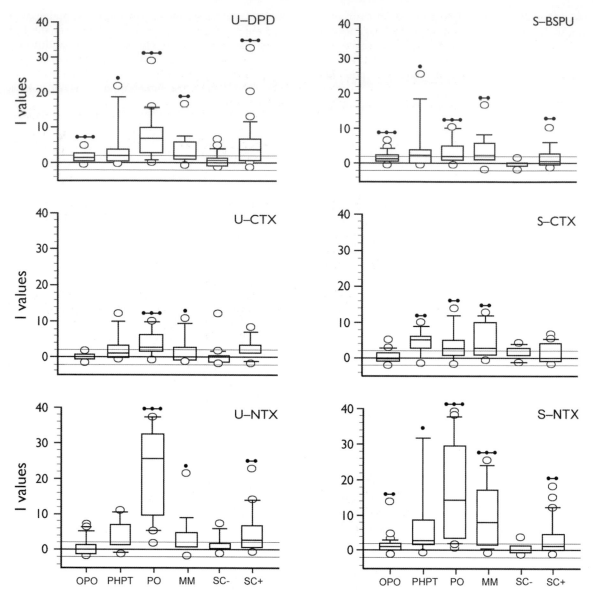

Figure 8.3.   Urinary (U) and serum (S) markers of bone resorption in metabolic and malignant bone disease. Values are expressed as Z scores. The full lines represent the mean and the dotted lines represent ± 2 standard deviations around the mean of healthy controls. $*p < 0.05$; $**p < 0.01$; $***p < 0.001$ vs. healthy controls. DPD, deoxypyridinoline; CTX, C-telopeptide; NTX, N-telopeptide; BSP, bone sialoprotein; OPO, primary vertebral osteoporosis; PHPT, primary hyperparathyroidism; PD, Paget's disease; MM, multiple myeloma; BC⁻, breast cancer without bone metastases; BC⁺, breast cancer with bone metastases. Adapted from [16]

higher than normal [64]. Again, NTX and CTX showed the greatest decrease following pamidronate therapy, reaching 15% and 2% of the baseline values, respectively ($p < 0.01$ vs. any other marker).

Suppression of CTX has also been shown to correlate with response to bisphosphonate treatment

in prostate cancer patients with blastic bone metastases [46,48]. In a study of 39 prostate cancer patients with bone metastases (Figure 8.4), a single injection of pamidronate (120 mg) significantly decreased ($p \leq 0.0015$) urinary α-CTX, urinary β-CTX, and serum CTX [46]. Therefore, CTX may be an important

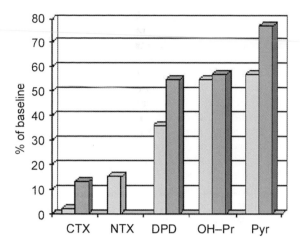

Figure 8.4. The effects of a single infusion of pamidronate on bone resorption markers. Changes are relative to baseline before bisphosphonate therapy. CTX, C-telopeptide; NTX, N-telopeptide; DPD, deoxypyridinoline; OH-Pr, hydroxyproline; Pyr, pyridinoline. Adapted from [38,69]

biochemical marker for monitoring responses to bisphosphonate treatment in prostate cancer patients.

As well as these changes observed in the mean values of resorption marker values following bisphosphonate treatment, there is also evidence that the individual pre-treatment values of a bone marker, particularly NTX, is correlated with response to treatment [11,69]. In one study it was found that almost 50% of patients who received a 2 h infusion of 120 mg pamidronate showed a response in terms of symptomatic pain relief [69]. Baseline values of NTX for non-responding patients were significantly higher ($p < 0.02$) than those of the clinical responders. 0–13% of patients with an initial bone marker value above twice the upper limit of normal responded, compared with 50–70% of those whose initial marker value was normal or below twice the upper level of normal. The precise correlation depended upon the marker chosen and, although baseline values of CTX and DPD were also higher in non-responding patients compared with responders, the NTX value gave the most significant correlation with clinical response ($p < 0.001$) [69]. This study also showed for the first time that, in patients with elevated levels of bone resorption markers, only those who showed a fall in markers subsequent to treatment responded to treatment. Clinical benefit, as indicated by improvement in a pain score, was only seen in those patients (17/32, 60%) whose bone resorption rate normalised after pamidronate, with no responses seen in the 11 patients (35%) with

persistently elevated levels ($p \leqslant 0.01$). This suggested that the aim of bisphosphonate therapy, at least with pamidronate, ought to be to produce a fall in marker levels, preferably into the normal range.

A subsequent study [71] has shown that this principle may be extended to the use of bone markers to distinguish between the benefits of different bisphosphonates; 51 patients, including 24 with metastatic breast cancer, were randomly allocated to treatment with either oral clodronate, intravenous clodronate or intravenous pamidronate. Symptomatic response was more frequent in the pamidronate group than in patients receiving clodronate and this was reflected in a correspondingly greater decrease in the bone resorption markers CTX and NTX. Additionally, biochemical changes correlated with the evolution of a composite pain score after bisphosphonate treatment ($p=0.01$).

The reduction in skeletal events associated with bisphosphonate therapy appears also to be correlated with a reduction in bone resorption markers. Lipton and colleagues [72] investigated the fracture rate in 21 cancer patients with bone metastases who received intravenous pamidronate and whose baseline NTX levels were above the normal range. The bone resorption markers PYD, DPD and NTX were measured at baseline and at 1, 3 and 6 months. In 12/21 patients, NTX levels were normal at 6 months and 9/21 remained abnormally elevated. In the group with NTX returning to normal levels, 42% developed fractures whereas in the group that failed to normalise the corresponding figure was 89% ($p=0.07$). The respective figures for each group of patients who went on to disease progression in bone were 25% and 78% ($p = 0.03$). Although these data represent small numbers of patients, it was suggestive that normalisation of bone resorption should be a goal in reducing the fracture rate in such patients.

With few exceptions [72,73], very little work has been carried out on the possible correlation between bone markers and the occurrence of skeletal events. Despite the obvious clinical benefits of bisphosphonates, it is clear that only a proportion of events are prevented and some patients do not experience a skeletal event despite the presence of metastatic bone disease. It is currently impossible to predict whether an individual patient needs, or will benefit from, a bisphosphonate.

We have recently reported on 121 patients with metastatic bone disease treated at our own institution [74]. These patients had monthly measurements of urinary NTX during treatment with a range of bisphosphonates. All skeletal-related events, plus hospital admissions for control of bone pain and death during the period of observation were recorded. Data were available for 121 and 95 patients over the first (0–3 months) and second (4–6 months) 3 month periods of monitoring, respectively. For 0–3 months the baseline NTX value, and for 4–6 months the NTX value at 3 months were strongly correlated with the number of skeletal-related events and/or death ($r=0.62$, $p < 0.001$ and $r=0.46$, $p < 0.001$, respectively). These data are shown in Table 8.4. Patients with baseline NTX values above 100 nmol/mmol creatinine were many times more likely to experience a skeletal-related event/death than those with NTX below this level ($p < 0.001$). A multivariate logistic regression model was highly predictive of skeletal events and/or death occurring during 0–3 months (baseline NTX correctly predicted 84% of events) and those occurring in 4–6 months (3 month NTX value correctly predicted 52% of events).

Overall, bisphosphonates reduce the frequency of skeletal events by 25–40% [75,76]. However, bisphosphonates are a relatively costly additional intervention in cancer care which is now applicable to a very large proportion of patients with advanced malignancy. The cost-effectiveness has been questioned [77] and prioritisation of bisphosphonate use is needed. It is not known whether the relative benefits of bisphosphonates are the same across the range of possible bone resorption rates. However, on the assumption that they are, with about one-third of

events prevented, our data suggested that the numbers of patients that would need to be treated to prevent one skeletal event would be 31, 17, 3 and 2 for the < 50, 50–100, 100–200, and > 200 nmol/mmol creatinine levels of NTX, respectively [74]. A more cost-effective use of bisphosphonates might be to reserve them until patients have an NTX level above either 50 or 100 nmol/mmol creatinine, and adjust the dose and schedule to maintain a normal rate of bone resorption.

The conclusions of the current study in patients with metastatic bone disease parallel those from studies of bone markers in bone loss due to osteoporosis. In one of the most comprehensive studies, nine bone turnover markers were measured in 375 women aged 50–85 years [78], including NTX and C-telopeptide (CTX). This study concluded that high marker levels were associated with an increased risk of vertebral fracture. There are also many osteoporosis studies that have demonstrated the role of bone markers in assessing response to antiresorptive therapy [79].

Bone marker data are beginning to emerge from clinical studies investigating the latest generation of more potent heterocyclic nitrogen-containing bisphosphonates. Cancer patients with osteolytic metastases have been treated with doses of up to 16 mg zoledronic acid in Phase I trials. In the first study, patients received 0.1–8 mg zoledronic acid monthly for 3 months [80], and sustained dose-dependent decreases in urinary calcium, hydroxyproline, PYD and DPD were observed with doses of zoledronic acid $\geqslant 0.2$ mg.

Table 8.4. Distribution of skeletal events and/or death and adjusted odds ratios according to baseline NTX range for the 0–3 month (top) and 4–6 month (bottom) time periods

Baseline NTX (nmol/mmol creatinine)	Number of patients	Number of patients having any SRE/death	Patients having any SRE/death (%)	Odds ratio*	95% Confidence interval
0–50	31	3	9.7	1	*
> 50–100	34	5	14.7	1.51	0.31, 7.45
> 100–200	26	16	61.5	14.24	3.37, 60.17
> 200	30	25	83.3	42.17	9.01, 197.45
Total	121	49	40.5	*	*

NTX value at 3 months (nmol/mmol creatinine)	Number of patients	Number of patients having any SRE/death	Patients having any SRE/death (%)	Odds ratio*	95% Confidence interval
0–50	35	4	11.4	1	*
> 50–100	24	7	29.2	2.89	0.69, 12.13
> 100–200	11	6	54.5	5.56	1.22, 25.40
> 200	22	14	63.6	13.30	3.35, 52.81
Total	92	31	33.7	*	*

* Adjusted for age, sex and cancer type.

Levels of NTX were suppressed even at the lowest dose, and decreased 70–80% below baseline at doses ≥ 0.8 mg (Figure 8.5). In the second study, doses of zoledronic acid ≥ 2 mg suppressed all urinary bone resorption markers tested, including calcium, hydroxyproline, PYD, DPD and NTX. Importantly, NTX levels were maintained > 50% below baseline for 8 weeks following a single dose of zoledronic acid ≥ 2 mg (Figure 8.5) [81]. These biochemical observations on a relatively small group of patients predicted the subsequent findings of the large Phase II and III development programme of zoledronic acid.

Zoledronic acid and pamidronate have been compared in a randomised, Phase II, multicentre trial for the prevention of skeletal complications (n=280) [82]. Patients with osteolytic lesions due to metastatic breast cancer or multiple myeloma were randomised to double-blind treatment with either zoledronic acid (0.4, 2, or 4 mg) or pamidronate (90 mg) every 4 weeks for up to 10 months. Median NTX values decreased from baseline to end of study by 37%, 59% and 61% in the zoledronic acid groups (0.4, 2, and 4 mg, respectively) and by 58% in the pamidronate group (Table 8.5). Moreover, the 4 mg dose of zoledronic acid resulted in greater decreases in NTX at every time point throughout the duration of the study, compared with 90 mg pamidronate ($p < 0.05$). Consistent with earlier observations, the greater reductions in NTX levels in the groups that received either 2 and 4 mg zoledronic acid or pamidronate correlated with a lower incidence of skeletal-related events, fractures, and the need for radiation to bone, compared with the 0.4 mg zoledronic acid group.

The recently completed Phase III clinical trials of zoledronic acid across the range of tumour types affecting bone have included nearly 3000 patients and prospectively measured bone markers. Patients have been randomly allocated to anticancer treatment plus either zoledronic acid or pamidronate (breast cancer and myeloma patients), or anticancer treatment plus either zoledronic acid or placebo (prostate cancer and other tumours affecting bone). Evaluation of these data should reliably determine whether changes in the bone resorption markers can be used in routine practice to assess response to systemic anticancer treatments and bisphosphonates.

CURRENT STATUS AND FUTURE RESEARCH

Although biochemical markers of bone metabolism are widely used in clinical trials and have provided a wealth of important data, their clinical utility in the management of individual patients remains uncertain.

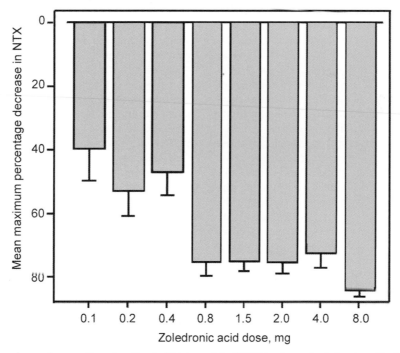

Figure 8.5. Mean maximum decrease from baseline in N-telopeptide (NTX) by dose of zoledronic acid. Adapted from [81]

Table 8.5. Dose-related efficacy (%) of zoledronic acid in breast cancer and multiple myeloma

| | Zoledronic acid | | Pamidronate (%) | |
	0.4 mg	2.0 mg	4 mg	90 mg
Bone alkaline phosphatase	−23	−35	−29	−32
Urine pyridinoline : creatinine ratio	−6	−17	−9	−14
Urine deoxypyridinoline : creatinine ratio	−20	−38	−26	−34
N-telopeptide (NTX)	−37	−59	−61	−58
Serum PTH	+22	+46	+59	+27

Adapted from [82].

New serum assays for NTX and CTX appear promising, but will require extensive validation before they will become routinely used in clinical practice. However, emerging data demonstrating a correlation between the levels of the new-generation, highly sensitive bone markers and clinical outcome may provide the rationale for their widespread acceptance. In clinical practice, markers of bone resorption have a potential role in the diagnosis of bone metastases, in the assessment of disease progression and response to treatment, and in predicting the rate of bone loss and the potential for fracture. In addition, given that bone resorption markers are sensitive indicators of response to bisphosphonate therapy and appear to correlate with clinical outcome, it has been suggested that they could potentially be used to tailor the dose and schedule of bisphosphonates. Reliable definitions of response are required. A > 50% reduction or normalisation of a previously elevated marker would appear to be useful definition for response, while a > 50% increase would be an appropriate definition of progression. Reporting changes in biochemical markers according to these criteria would facilitate comparison of results from different studies.

The treatment of metastatic bone disease in breast cancer patients, particularly with drug therapy, has developed considerably in recent years and this progress looks likely to continue. There is an increasing need for simple and convenient approaches for the quantitative assessment of response. An extensive body of research suggests that markers of bone turnover may play a major role in this assessment. Several studies have shown that the bone resorption markers, especially NTX, are correlated with decreased morbidity, leading to the concept of bone marker directed-therapy. For example, it may be possible to tailor treatment to an individual, with the aim of lowering bone resorption markers into the normal range.

The bone markers will also play an important role in the assessment of new therapeutic approaches, including development of new drugs, such as osteoprotogerin, as well as novel bisphosphonates. The lowering of bone markers towards the normal range will be regarded as a measure of the effectiveness of such therapies. Although bone marker measurements are currently restricted largely to clinical trials and research centres, it is likely that they will become much more routinely used in the near future. The use of bone markers, together with advances in imaging techniques, will enable the clinician to obtain a much more integrated view of the status of the breast cancer patient with metastatic bone disease.

CONCLUSION

The skeletal complications of cancer, including bone pain and fracture, are particularly debilitating to the patient. Imaging techniques, including plain-film radiography, ^{99m}Tc bone scans, MRI and ^{18}F PET, are the current methods for identifying bone lesions and assessing responses to treatment. Unfortunately, these techniques are expensive and some are only available at major medical centres. Because osteolytic lesions are associated with increased bone resorption, patients often have calcium and other bone breakdown products in the serum and urine. Traditional bone resorption markers, including urinary calcium and hydroxyproline, have been used for many years primarily to assess responses to bisphosphonate therapy. However, these traditional markers have been shown to be suboptimal in terms of selectivity and sensitivity.

A number of new biochemical markers involving unique breakdown products of type I collagen have been developed that are more specific and sensitive indicators of bone resorption. These include PYD, DPD, NTX and CTX. These markers are elevated in the majority of patients with bone metastases, suggesting a potential role in the diagnosis of skeletal involvement. In addition, the pre-treatment and post-treatment levels of NTX appear to be useful in predicting clinical outcome. Bisphosphonate therapy results in substantial decreases in the levels of bone resorption markers, and NTX appears to be the most sensitive marker for the assessment of response to treatment. Indeed, the conclusion of several studies has been that the goal of bisphosphonate therapy should be the normalisation of NTX excretion.

Clearly, these new biochemical markers hold much promise for the management of osteolytic disease. In addition, the development of serum assays for NTX and CTX should provide the sensitivity, convenience, and reproducibility lacking in earlier assays. Ongoing clinical trials will provide the rigorous evaluation required for these newly developed biochemical assays to be accepted for routine clinical use.

REFERENCES

1. Coleman RE, Rubens D. The clinical course of bone metastases from breast cancer. Br J Cancer 1987; 55: 61–6.
2. Souberbielle JC, Cormier C, Kindermans C. Bone markers in clinical practice. Curr Opin Rheumatol 1999; 11: 312–19.
3. Vinholes J, Coleman R, Eastell R. Effects of bone metastases on bone metabolism: implications for diagnosis, imaging and assessment of response to cancer treatment. Cancer Treat Rev 1996; 22: 289–331.
4. Bertolini DR, Nedwin GE, Bringman TS et al. Stimulation of bone resorption and inhibition of bone formation in vitro by human tumour necrosis factors. Nature 1986; 319: 516–18.
5. Delaisse JM, Eeckhout Y, Neff L et al. (Pro)collagenase (matrix metalloproteinase-1) is present in rodent osteoclasts and in the underlying bone-resorbing compartment. J Cell Sci 1993; 106: 1071–82.
6. Drake FH, Dodds RA, James IE et al. Cathepsin K, but not cathepsins B, L, or S, is abundantly expressed in human osteoclasts. J Biol Chem 1996; 271: 12511–16.
7. Peacock M, Robertson WG, Nordin BE. Relation between serum and urinary calcium with particular reference to parathyroid activity. Lancet 1969; 1: 384–6.
8. Campbell FC, Blamey RW, Woolfson AM et al. Calcium excretion (CaE) in metastatic breast cancer. Br J Surg 1983; 70: 202–4.
9. Coleman RE, Whitaker KB, Moss DW et al. Biochemical prediction of response of bone metastases to treatment. Br J Cancer 1988; 58: 205–10.
10. Pecherstorfer M, Zimmer-Roth I, Schilling T et al. The diagnostic value of urinary pyridinium cross-links of collagen, serum total alkaline phosphatase, and urinary calcium excretion in neoplastic bone disease. J Clin Endocrinol Metab 1995; 80: 97–103.
11. Vinholes J, Guo CY, Purohit OP et al. Metabolic effects of pamidronate in patients with metastatic bone disease. Br J Cancer 1996; 73: 1089–95.
12. Deacon AC, Hulme P, Hesp R et al. Estimation of whole body bone resorption rate: a comparison of urinary total hydroxyproline excretion with two radioisotopic tracer methods in osteoporosis. Clin Chim Acta 1987; 166: 297–306.
13. Gasser A, Celada A, Courvoisier B et al. The clinical measurement of urinary total hydroxyproline excretion. Clin Chim Acta 1979; 95: 487–91.
14. Mautalen CA. Circadian rhythm of urinary total and free hydroxyproline excretion and its relation to creatinine excretion. J Lab Clin Med 1970; 75: 11–18.
15. Gasser AB, Depierre D, Courvoisier B. Total urinary and free serum hydroxyproline in metastatic bone disease. Br J Cancer 1979; 39: 280–3.
16. Woitge HW, Pecherstorfer M, Li Y et al. Novel serum markers of bone resorption: clinical assessment and comparison with established urinary indices. J Bone Min Res 1999; 14: 792–801.
17. Robins SP, Woitge H, Hesley R et al. Direct, enzyme-linked immunoassay for urinary deoxypyridinoline as a specific marker for measuring bone resorption. J Bone Min Res 1994; 9: 1643–9.
18. Delmas PD, Schlemmer A, Gineyts E et al. Urinary excretion of pyridinoline crosslinks correlates with bone turnover measured on iliac crest biopsy in patients with vertebral osteoporosis. J Bone Min Res 1991; 6: 639–44.
19. Bonde M, Qvist P, Fledelius C et al. Immunoassay for quantifying type I collagen degradation products in urine evaluated. Clin Chem 1994; 40: 2022–5.
20. Hanson DA, Weis MA, Bollen AM et al. A specific immunoassay for monitoring human bone resorption: quantitation of type I collagen cross-linked N-telopeptides in urine. J Bone Min Res 1992; 7: 1251–8.
21. Melkko J, Niemi S, Ristelli J, Risteli L. Radioimmunoassay for human procollagen. Clin Chem 1990; 36: 1328–32.
22. Koizumi M, Maeda H, Yoshimura K et al. Dissociation of bone formation markers in bone metastasis of prostate cancer. Br J Cancer 1997; 75: 1601–4.
23. Edelstyn GA, Gillespie PJ, Grebbel FS. The radiological demonstration of osseus metastases: experimental observations. Clin Radiol 1967; 18: 158–62.
24. Blomqvist C. Assessment of response to systemic therapy focusing on metastatic bone disease. Cancer Treat Rev 2001; 27: 177–80.
25. Coleman RE. Biochemical markers of malignant bone disease. In Rubens RD, Mundy GR (eds), Cancer and the Skeleton. Martin Dunitz: London, 2000: 137–50.
26. Fogelman I, Coleman RE. The bone scan and breast cancer. In Freeman L, Weissman H (eds), Nuclear Medicine Annual. Raven Press: New York, 1988: 1–46.
27. Cook JR, Fogelman I. Diagnostic nuclear medicine. In Rubens RD, Mundy GR (eds), Cancer and the Skeleton. Martin Dunitz: London, 2000: 91–111.
28. MacVicar D. Radiology and magnetic resonance imaging. In Rubens RD, Mundy GR (eds), Cancer and the Skeleton. Martin Dunitz: London, 2000: 113–36.
29. Gold RI, Seeger UL, Bassett LW, Steckel RJ. An integrated approach to the evaluation of metastatic bone disease. Radiol Clin N Am 1990; 28: 471–83.
30. Cook GJR, Fogelman I. The role of positron emission tomography in the management of bone metastases. Cancer 2000; 88(suppl 12): 2927–34.
31. Schirrmeister H, Guhlmann A, Kotzerke J et al. Early detection and accurate description of extent of metastatic bone disease in breast cancer with fluoride ion and

positron emission tomography. J Clin Oncol 1999; 17: 2381–9.

32. Martoni A, Zamagni C, Bellanova B et al. CEA, MCA, CA 15.3 and CA 549 and their combinations in expressing and monitoring metastatic breast cancer: a prospective comparative study. Eur J Cancer 1995; 31A: 1615–21.

33. Vinholes J, Coleman R, Lacombe D et al. Assessment of bone response to systemic therapy in an EORTC trial: preliminary experience with the use of collagen cross-link excretion. European Organization for Research and Treatment of Cancer. Br J Cancer 1999; 80: 221–8.

34. Stamey TA, Yang N, Hay AR et al. PSA as a serum marker of the prostate. N Engl J Med 1987; 317: 909–16.

35. Coombes RC, Dady P, Parsons C et al. Assessment of response of bone metastases to systemic treatment in patients with breast cancer. Cancer 1983; 52: 610–14.

36. Pecherstorfer M, Zimmer-Roth I, Schilling T et al. The diagnostic value of urinary pyridinium crosslinks of collagen, serum, total alkaline phosphatase and urinary calcium excretion in neoplastic bone disease. J Clin Endocrinol Metab 1995; 80: 97–103.

37. Massidda B, Ionta MT, Foddi MR et al. Usefulness of pyridinium crosslinks and CA 15-3 as markers in metastatic bone breast carcinoma. Anticancer Res 1996; 16: 2221–4.

38. Body JJ, Dumon JC, Gineyts E, Delmas PD. Comparative evaluation of markers of bone resorption in patients with breast cancer-induced osteolysis before and after bisphosphonate therapy. Br J Cancer 1997; 75: 408–12.

39. Demers LM, Costa L, Chinchilli VM et al. Biochemical markers of bone turnover in patients with metastatic bone disease. Clin Chem 1995; 41: 1489–94.

40. Lipton A, Costa L, Ali SM, Demers LM. Bone markers in the management of metastatic bone disease. Cancer Treat Rev 2001; 27: 181–5.

41. Miura H, Yamamoto I, Takada M et al. Diagnostic validity of bone metabolic markers for bone metastasis. Endocr J 1997; 44: 751–7.

42. Christianson RH. Biochemical markers of bone metabolism: an overview. Clin Biochem 1997; 30: 573–93.

43. Watts NB. Clinical utility of biochemical markers of bone remodeling. Clin Chem 1999; 45: 1359–68.

44. Tamada T, Sone T, Tomomitsu T et al. Biochemical markers for the detection of bone metastasis in patients with prostate cancer: diagnostic efficacy and the effect of hormonal therapy. J Bone Min Metab 2001; 19: 45–51.

45. Akimoto S, Furuya Y, Akakura K, Ito H. Comparison of markers of bone formation and resorption in prostate cancer patients to predict bone metastasis. Endocr J 1998; 45: 97–104.

46. Garnero P, Buchs N, Zekri J et al. Markers of bone turnover for the management of patients with bone metastases from prostate cancer. Br J Cancer 2000; 82: 858–64.

47. Kylmala T, Tammela TL, Risteli L et al. Type I collagen degradation product (ICTP) gives information about the nature of bone metastases and has prognostic value in prostate cancer. Br J Cancer 1995; 71: 1061–4.

48. Garnero P. Markers of bone turnover in prostate cancer. Cancer Treat Rev 2001; 27: 187–92.

49. Koizumi M, Yonese J, Fukui I, Ogata E. The serum level of the amino-terminal propeptide of type I procollagen is a sensitive marker for prostate cancer metastasis to bone. Br J Urol Int 2001; 87: 348–51.

50. Coleman RE, Mashiter G, Fogelman I, Rubens RD. Osteocalcin: a marker of metastatic bone disease. Eur J Cancer 1988; 24: 1211–17.

51. Berruti A, Pancro A, Angelli A et al. Different mechanisms underlying bone collagen resorption in patients with bone metastases from prostate and breast cancer. Br J Cancer 1996; 73: 1581–7.

52. Berruti A, Torta M, Piovesan A et al. Biochemical picture of bone metabolism in patients with bone metastases. Anticancer Res 1995; 2871–6.

53. Bellahcene A, Merville MP, Castronovo V. Expression of bone sialoprotein, a bone matrix protein, in human breast cancer. Cancer Res 1994; 54: 2823–6.

54. Withold W, Armbruster FP, Karmatschek M, Reinauer H. Bone sialoprotein in serum of patients with malignant bone diseases. Clin Chem 1997; 43: 85–91.

55. Bellahcene A, Kroll M, Liebens F, Castronovo V. Bone sialoprotein expression in primary human breast cancer is associated with bone metastases development. J Bone Min Res 1996; 11: 665–70.

56. Diel IJ, Solomayer EF, Siebel MJ et al. Serum bone sialoprotein in patients with primary breast cancer is a prognostic marker for subsequent bone metastasis. Clin Cancer Res 1999; 5: 3914–19.

57. Ali SM, Demers LM, Leitzel K et al. Elevated serum N-telopeptide predicts poor prognosis in breast cancer patients with bone metastases. Proc Am Soc Clin Oncol 2000; 19(abstr 2549).

58. Hayward JL, Carbone PP, Heuson JC et al. Assessment of response to therapy in advanced breast cancer. Cancer 1977; 3: 1389–94.

59. Howell A, Mackintosh J, Jones M et al. The definition of the "no change" category in patients treated with endocrine therapy and chemotherapy for advanced carcinoma of the breast. Eur J Cancer 1988; 24A: 1567–72.

60. Coleman RE, Mashiter G, Whitaker KB et al. Bone scan flare predicts successful systemic therapy for bone metastases. J Nucl Med 1988; 29: 1354–9.

61. Kiang DT, Greenberg LJ, Kennedy BJ. Tumour marker kinetics in the monitoring of breast cancer. Cancer 1990; 65: 193–9.

62. Robertson JFR, Pearson D, Price MR et al. Objective measurement of therapeutic response in breast cancer using tumour markers. Cancer 1991; 64: 757–63.

63. Robertson JFR, Jaeger W, Syzmendera JJ et al. The objective measurement of remission and progression in metastatic breast cancer by use of serum tumour markers. Eur J Cancer 1999; 35: 47–53.

64. Vinholes J, Guo CY, Purohit O et al. Evaluation of new bone resorption markers in a randomized comparison of pamidronate or clodronate for hypercalcemia of malignancy. J Clin Oncol 1997; 15: 131–8.

65. Blomqvist C, Elomaa I, Virkkunen P et al. The response evaluation of bone metastases in mammary carcinoma. The value of radiology, scintigraphy, and biochemical markers of bone metabolism. Cancer 1987; 60: 2907–12.

66. Coombes RC, Dady P, Parsons C et al. Assessment of response of bone metastases to systemic treatment in patients with breast cancer. Cancer 1983; 52: 610–14.

67. Walls J, Assiri A, Howell A et al. Measurement of urinary collagen cross-links indicate response to therapy

in patients with breast cancer and bone metastases. Br J Cancer 1999; 80: 1265–70.

68. Costa L, Demers LM, Gouveia-Oliveira A et al. Prospective evaluation of the peptide-bound collagen type I cross-links N-telopeptide and C-telopeptide in predicting bone metastases status. J Clin Oncol 2002; 20: 850–6.

69. Vinholes JJF, Purohit OP, Abbey ME et al. Relationships between biochemical and symptomatic response in a double-blind randomised trial of pamidronate for metastatic bone disease. Ann Oncol 1997; 8: 1243–50.

70. Zegels B, Eastell R, Russell RG et al. Effect of high doses of oral risedronate (20 mg/day) on serum parathyroid hormone levels and urinary collagen cross-link excretion in postmenopausal women with spinal osteoporosis. Bone 2001; 28: 108–12.

71. Jagdev SP, Purohit OP, Heatley S et al. Comparison of the effects of intravenous pamidronate and oral clodronate on symptoms and bone resorption in patients with metastatic bone disease. Ann Oncol 2001; 12: 1433–8.

72. Lipton A, Demers L, Curley E et al. Markers of bone resorption in patients treated with pamidronate. Eur J Cancer 1998; 34: 2021–6.

73. Menssen HD, Sakalova A, Fontana A et al. Effects of long term intravenous ibandronate therapy on skeletal-related events, survival, and bone resorption markers in patients with advanced multiple myeloma. J Clin Oncol 2002; 20: 2353–9.

74. Brown JE, Thomson CS, Ellis SP et al. Bone resorption predicts for skeletal complications in metastatic bone disease. Br J Cancer 2003; 89: 2031–2037.

75. Lipton A, Theriault RL, Hortobagyi GN et al. Pamidronate prevents skeletal complications and is effective palliative treatment in women with breast carcinoma and osteolytic bone metastases: long-term follow-up of two randomized, placebo controlled trials. Cancer 2000; 88: 1082–90.

76. Hillner BE, Ingle JN, Berenson JR et al. American Society of Clinical Oncology guideline on the role of bisphosphonates in breast cancer. J Clin Oncol 2000; 18: 1378–91.

77. Hillner BE. Pharmaco-economic issues in bisphosphonate treatment of metastatic bone disease. Semin Oncol 2001; 28:4 (suppl 11), 64–8.

78. Greenfield DM, Hannon RA, Eastell R. The association between bone turnover and fracture risk (Sheffield Osteoporosis study). In Eastell R et al. (eds), Bone Markers—Biochemical and Clinical Perspectives. Martin Dunitz: London, 2000: 225–36.

79. Gonnelli R, Cepollara C, Pondrelli C. The usefulness of bone turnover in predicting the response to transdermal estrogen therapy in postmenopausal osteoporosis. J Bone Min Res 1997; 12: 624–31.

80. Berenson JR, Vescio R, Rosen L et al. A phase I dose-ranging trial of monthly infusions of zoledronic acid for the treatment of osteolytic bone metastases. Clin Cancer Res 2001; 7: 478–85.

81. Berenson JR, Vescio R, Henick K et al. A phase I, open-label, dose-ranging trial of intravenous bolus zoledronic acid, a novel bisphosphonate, in cancer patients with metastatic bone disease. Cancer 2001; 91: 144–54.

82. Berenson JR, Rosen LS, Howell A et al. Zoledronic acid reduces skeletal-related events in patients with osteolytic metastases. Cancer 2001; 91: 1191–200.

9

Surgical Biopsy of Bone Metastases

Moshe Salai[1] and Israel Dudkiewicz[2]

[1]*Orthopedic Department, Rabin Medical Center, Beilinson Campus, Petah Tikva, Israel*
[2]*Chaim Sheba Medical Center, Tel Hashomer, Israel*

INTRODUCTION

During the last 20–30 years, the ability of the medical system to increase the lifespan of patients with malignant disease, and moreover, their quality of life, has improved dramatically. Many patients with malignant diseases live longer, yet with the constant fear of developing metastases, an indication to many of their imminent demise [1]. Any new lesion, especially of the bone, dramatically increases these fears.

The increasing numbers of patients living with malignant diseases also implies that there are more patients with suspected bone metastatic events, in whom biopsy and the results thereof are of utmost importance to their future. Biopsy is not just performed to obtain tissue for diagnosis. Rather, it is the last step in a cascade of events aimed at achieving sufficient tissue for accurate diagnosis, based upon clinical, imaging, and histopathological studies. Although biopsy may seem a simple procedure in patients with known malignancy, this chapter was written with the aim of emphasising the importance of appropriate performance of the biopsy process in patients with even a suspicion of a metastatic event [2–10]. To the best of our knowledge, this is the first occasion in orthopaedic oncology literature that all aspects of surgical biopsy in a suspected metastatic event have been mentioned, and which should serve as guidelines in clinical practice.

PRE-BIOPSY CONSIDERATIONS AND PATIENT EVALUATION

A lesion suspected of being bone metastasis is of major medical, psychological and social insult to patients, their relatives and the treating medical staff. Prior to consideration of the approach towards surgical biopsy in such a patient, several types of medical conditions when a suspected metastatic event presents itself should be identified and treated accordingly:

A. (Case 1, Figure 9.1). A patient with a recent history of known malignancy but no known metastases, who develops a new bony lesion suspected of being bone metastases.
B. (Case 2, Figure 9.2). A patient who has a history of long (occasionally very long) stable malignant disease, such as breast or prostate cancer, or had even been considered cured of the disease, who suddenly develops a new bony lesion.
C. (Case 3, Figure 9.3). A patient with a known history of malignancy who presents with a pathological fracture.
D. (Case 4, Figure 9.4). A patient who had been considered healthy and presents with new multiple bony lesions suspected of being disseminated metastatic disease, yet of unknown origin.
E. A patient who is considered as healthy, but presents with a pathological fracture suspected of being the result of bone metastases of unknown origin [11,12].

Naturally, the most traumatic cases are those presenting with pathological fractures who not only need accurate diagnosis, but also definitive treatment of the fracture [13,14]. Pathological fracture is defined as:

1. A bone fracture with no antecedent trauma.
2. A fracture that has been caused by a trauma that is minor compared to its result.

Textbook of Bone Metastases. Edited by C. Jasmin, R. E. Coleman, L. R. Coia, R. Capanna and G. Saillant
© 2005 John Wiley & Sons Ltd: ISBN 0 471 87742 5

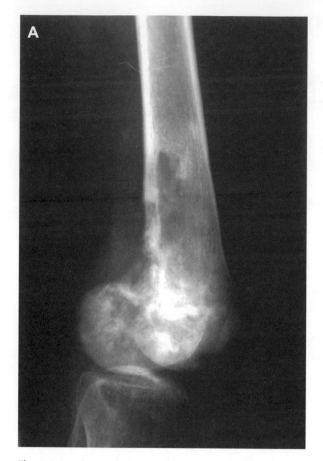 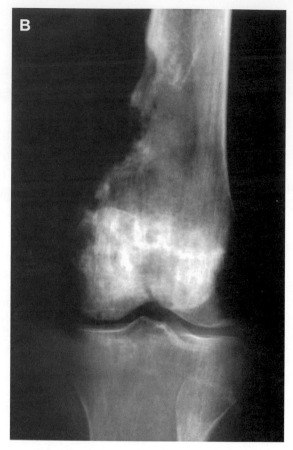

Figure 9.1. Case 1. A 48 year-old male, diagnosed as suffering from lung carcinoma, who presented with obvious lung metastases of the distal femur (A,B)

3. A fracture through a weakening process within the bone.

In any form of presentation, accurate diagnosis of the type of lesion is of utmost importance for management of these patients.

In any form of presentation, rational pre-biopsy strategy, pre-biopsy planning and pre-biopsy evaluation of the patient should be mandatory. These steps should preferably be carried out rapidly, yet without jeopardising management, e.g. performing an open biopsy on a patient with a bony lesion which is a myeloma and could have been identified by blood tests. Moreover, the occurrence of a suspected metastatic event requires rapid teamwork of the entire orthopaedic oncology team adjusted to the kind of event, i.e. the aforementioned types of patients.

In whichever form the suspected metastatic event presents, the patient's status should be carefully evaluated, and the following parameters assessed: type of primary disease (if known) and its clinical behaviour; patient's general medical status; his/her functional performance; and anticipated life expectancy (in certain known tumours with data regarding this delicate issue).

Prior to any surgical intervention aimed at achieving tissue diagnosis throughout rapid staging, studies should be performed in order to achieve maximal information regarding the tumour: its origin, local extent/dimensions, whether it is a single lesion, or whether there are any other lesions amenable to an easier form of biopsy than the one under consideration. Thus, the minimum studies usually necessary are: plain, multidirectional radiographs of the affected lesion (and of others in case of multiple lesions); chest and abdomen computed tomography; and bone scan, which is a sensitive modality for detection of other bone metastases. These studies, as well as

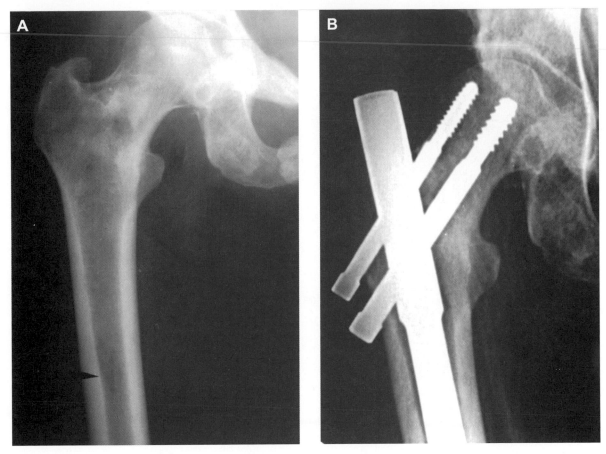

Figure 9.2. Case 2. A 58 year-old lady, presumed cured of breast cancer 10 years previously, who presented with a femoral neck lesion (A). The lesion was diagnosed as breast metastases and surgery proceeded to definitive treatment of a proximal femoral nail (B)

laboratory analysis, can be performed within a few hours in most hospitals, often on an ambulatory basis. The results will provide the treating physician with information regarding other non-tumourous conditions that may emulate bone metastases, such as trauma, metabolic bone diseases, vascular bone disease, haematological diseases such as bone lymphoma, primary, non-metastatic bone tumours and, most importantly, bone infections (Case 5; Figure 9.5).

These studies and considerations of the potential differential diagnosis are mandatory, since unlike the few primary bone tumours which are currently being treated, mostly in assigned major orthopaedic oncology centres, suspected bone metastases events are very common in every hospital, and affect millions of patients throughout the world.

Conversely, our ability to increase the lifespan of patients with metastatic malignant diseases demands such a profound form of evaluation, since prompt

diagnosis of the suspected metastatic event is often a matter of life, or rapidly progressing death, to the patients.

Campanacci [10] reported a small female predominance in the occurrence of bone metastases of 60:40. Over 70% of metastatic events occurred between the 5th and 7th decade of life. The spine was the most common location for bone metastases, followed by the long bones (especially femur and humerus) and the pelvis.

Open surgical biopsy is indicated in all cases where clinico–radiological correlations between bony lesions is unclear. Failing this, either form of closed biopsy usually suffices to establish the final diagnosis.

TYPES OF BONE BIOPSIES

Biopsy is the final step towards evaluation of the suspected metastatic event, and should provide the

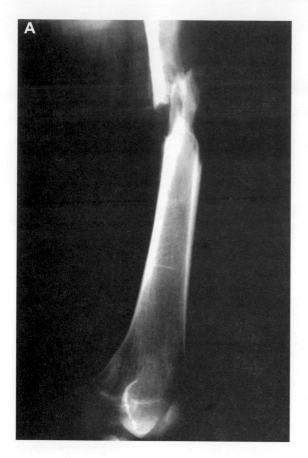
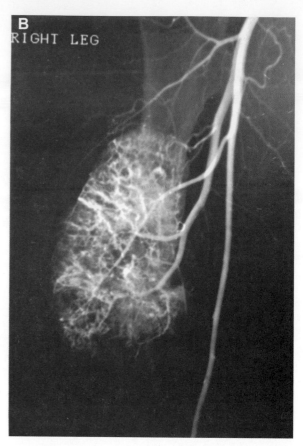

Figure 9.3   *(Caption opposite)*

pathologist with tumoral material for final evaluation. Accuracy of the pathological evaluation depends on the amount and quality of material received for investigation.

Over the last decade, certain centres have developed remarkable skills in the interpretation of specimens of tiny amounts of tissue retrieved through needle, or even fine needle, aspirates. However, the number of such expert centres is small, compared to the large number of patients who need bone biopsy for suspected metastatic events. Thus, for most physicians who face patients with such events, open biopsy is recommended [15–18]. The type of biopsy, whether closed or open, incisional or excisional, should be adjusted to the specific patient, and the specific type of presentation of the suspected metastatic event. This implies needle or core biopsy in known breast cancer patients with multiple bony lesions suspected of being metastatic, as opposed to open biopsy of a single lesion

in patients with a history of so-called "cured" breast cancer 10 years (or more) previously.

The role and different methods of performing closed biopsies are beyond the scope of this chapter; however, it is re-emphasised that where there is any doubt regarding collection of sufficient diagnostic material through closed biopsy, open surgical biopsy is recommended. However, in difficult locations, such as the spine, an attempt at closed biopsy should be considered initially, and only if the material obtained is non-diagnostic should open biopsy be considered [19–21].

Prior to selection of biopsy type, certain definitions should be emphasised: (a) *incisional biopsy*—surgically obtaining tissue from a process for diagnosis. This always involves resection of part of the process, leaving behind most of the tumour; (b) *excisional biopsy*—the surgical process in which the tumour is excised not only for diagnosis, but also for treatment. Several

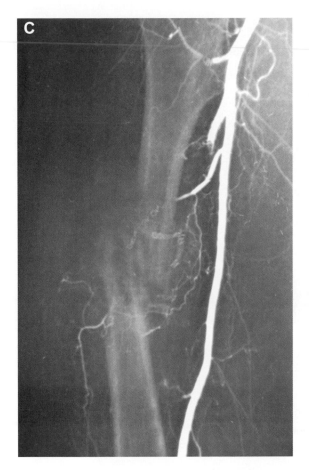

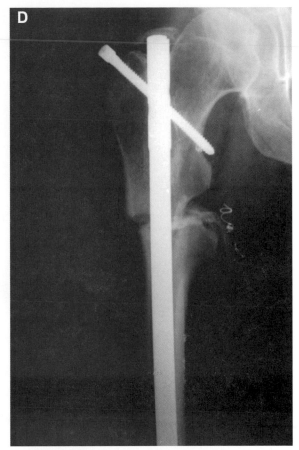

Figure 9.3. Case 3. A 62 year-old man known to suffer from hypernephroma who presented with a pathological femoral fracture (A). Angiography and embolisation preceded the biopsy (B,C) and definitive treatment by resection of the lesion and stabilising the femur with massive bone allograft and interlocking femoral nail (D)

types of excision are used in orthopaedic oncology surgery: (i) *intralesion*—resection of the tumour from within, leaving a shell of tumoural tissue; (ii) *marginal*—resection of a tumour through the reactive zone that encircles the tumour; (iii) *wide*—resection of the tumour through healthy/normal tissue margins; (iv) *radical*—resection of all anatomical compartments involved by the tumour, often implying amputation. These definitions are usually used in the treatment of primary bone or soft-tissue sarcomas. However, with the advancement of treatment for metastases, the definitions are also applicable to metastatic surgery, especially in cases of single metastasis.

Biopsy can be either incisional or excisional, depending on the type of patients at presentation, viz: whether or not there is knowledge of a primary lesion; whether the lesion is single or multiple; the lesion size (whether it is amenable to complete excision during biopsy); and whether or not pathological fracture is present. Accordingly, the surgeon who performs the biopsy should preferably be capable of continuing the biopsy to definitive, reconstructive surgery, and should have appropriate equipment to proceed: prosthesis, plates, rods and bone cement. Failing this, it would be better to transfer the patient to a larger centre capable of completing the procedure.

Excisional biopsy is indicated if the pre-operative diagnosis is fairly obvious and the lesion is small and amenable to resection and reconstruction (if necessary). It is important both clinically and surgically to decide pre-operatively on the type of biopsy. If only incisional biopsy is to be performed, it should be carefully planned so that the biopsy tract is included in

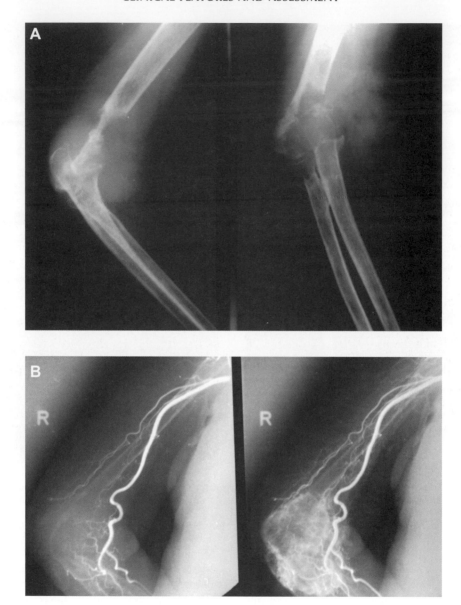

Figure 9.4. Case 4. A 65 year-old woman who presented with highly vascularised destructive lesion of the elbow (A). Angiography and embolisation (B) preceded the biopsy, which revealed metastatic carcinoma of the cervix

the resected specimen of the definitive surgery. As a rule, limb incisions should always be longitudinal, small, yet long enough to obtain sufficient material. Even when planning incisional biopsy, special attention should be paid to tumours such as kidney metastases, which often bleed profusely during surgery, and for which pre-operative angiography and embolisation is mandatory. Today this is a routine procedure during which the supplying vessels to the

tumours are identified and embolised by gel-foam particles, or by metal coils. This procedure reduces blood loss during surgery, and facilitates better surgical resection/management of tumours.

Either of the aforementioned approaches to biopsy should be undertaken with maximal haemostasis, gentle handling of the tissue to prevent local spread and, whenever possible, the direct or shortest approach to the lesion, but with the essential ability to obtain an

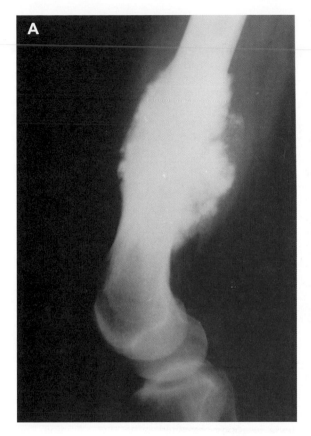
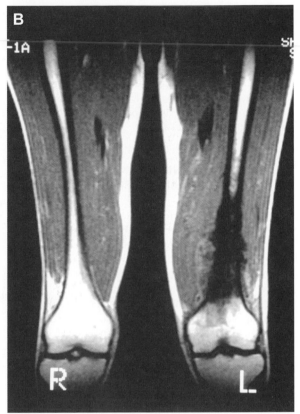

Figure 9.5. Case 5. A 19 year-old male with obvious osteosarcoma of the distal femur (A,B). Core biopsy confirmed the diagnosis

adequate tissue specimen. It should, however, be remembered that often even small holes in the bone may cause a significant decrease in the mechanical properties of the bone, therefore only small, rounded or oblong cuts should be made in the cortical bone in order to prevent pathological fracture [22]. Augmentation by bone cement and/or short bone plate, even in incisional biopsy of cortical bone, is recommended.

The role of a tourniquet in biopsy procedures, and its potential effect on tumour spread, has never been established. However, it is important to release the tourniquet before closure of the surgical wound and to perform meticulous haemostasis, or to use drains along, close and distally to the biopsy tract when necessary. Open biopsy makes it possible to obtain relatively large amounts of tissue, and saves the reported 25–33% of insufficient tissue when closed biopsy techniques are employed. This amount of tissue is also sufficient for frozen sections, even if a definitive surgical procedure is not performed under the same anaesthesia. Open biopsy provides the means to obtain

enough material for examination of the tissue by way of all currently available methods, i.e. simple staining of material embedded in paraffin, electron microscopy, immunohistochemistry, cytology, tissue imprints, tissue cultures, hormone receptors, flow cytometry and, most recently, cytogenetic studies.

Most of these examinations are not possible in closed biopsy techniques due to insufficient tissue for diagnosis (discussed in other chapters). The exceptions to this approach are the clear-cut cases of patients with known malignancy, in whom tiny amounts of tissue are sufficient to confirm the diagnosis. Even with the limitations of bone tissue pathology, and of many inexperienced pathologists, it is recommended that cases and imaging studies be discussed with the pathologist before biopsy, and that a frozen section specimen during biopsy should be obtained. This will provide the surgeon with an option to proceed with definitive surgery if the results of the frozen section confirm metastases. Moreover, it can save the patients and their families days and even weeks of confusion and fearful tension before they receive the result of the biopsy. It also saves the patient from undergoing additional anaesthesia. This approach implies that the surgeon should be prepared to proceed with definitive surgery once the pathology confirms metastasis. This also means that the patient should be prepared, including obtaining informed consent for extension of the surgery from simple open biopsy to definitive reconstruction.

SPECIAL CLINICAL, ANATOMICAL AND SURGICAL CONSIDERATIONS

Prior to performing an open biopsy, the surgeon should be aware of the clinical, immunological and haematological condition of the patients. Often the patients' nutritional status is low, they are immuno-compromised, and suffer from cardiopulmonary compromise due to prior treatments. This makes these patients highly susceptible to infection, bleeding and complications during anaesthesia. Adequate blood replacement should be available, especially in potentially bleeding tumours, such as kidney carcinoma. If possible, malnourished patients should be transfused before surgery. It is almost mandatory that most open surgical biopsies be performed under fluoroscopic guidance to verify and document the proper location of the biopsy.

Prophylactic antibiotics should be given during surgery only after the tissue for frozen sections, other pathological studies, and cultures for bacteriological growth are taken. Duration of antibiotic therapy is determined by the general status of the patient and the extent of the surgical procedure.

The type of anaesthesia for surgery, whether it is regional or general, is usually determined by the anaesthesiologist in collaboration with the surgeon and patient. There are no rules for type of anaesthesia, as long as it makes it possible for the surgeon to perform the biopsy under good anaesthetic conditions and provides the option of proceeding with definitive reconstructive surgery if necessary.

As mentioned previously, limb surgery using a tourniquet is recommended. However, squeezing the limb before closure of the tourniquet is not recommended, since it may cause tumoral cell spread as a result of the pressure bandage. Whether or not biopsy only, or biopsy and reconstruction are planned, the limb should be prepared and draped to allow for a definitive, reconstructive surgical procedure.

Since bleeding disturbances are frequently encountered in these patients, careful closure of the surgical

incision is mandatory. It is recommended that the tourniquet be released before wound closure to prevent haematoma formation. In excessive bleeding, the lesion can be packed with gel foam or polymethylemetacrylate (bone cement). Due to common clotting disturbances in these patients, deep vein thrombosis and thrombo-embolic events may occur, and should be treated by peri-operative thrombophylaxis. Low molecular weight heparin is the treatment of choice for these preventive purposes.

Special surgical anatomical considerations should be taken in regard to the axial skeleton, i.e. spine and pelvis. In the spine, the posterior, trans-pedicular approach is recommended for open biopsy, since it is relatively short and simple. However, it should be remembered that even with the available imaging modalities, surgical events, such as profuse bleeding, adherence of the tumour to neural elements, and even intraoperative vertebral collapse are not rare. Trans-abdominal or trans-thorax approaches for biopsy (either direct, or through modern available scopes), should be avoided due to suspected spillage of tumoral cells in these cavities. In the pelvis, proximity to abdominal and pelvic organs, especially distorted/pushed/retracted by tumoral tissue blood vessels, may impose major surgical hazards. Abdominal and intra-pelvic spillage should be avoided, preferably by using posterior and extra-peritoneal approaches. In both locations, bleeding events are common, yet surgical control is far more difficult than in the limb. Therefore, extra care should be taken to prevent these bleeding events, which can be achieved by using pre-operative angiography and embolisation in any case suspected of having intraoperative bleeding (in certain tumours, such as the kidney, suspected lesions should be embolised even before biopsy).

Finally, surgical biopsy is not complete without the assistance of a psychology expert for the patient and relatives: every step in pre-operative evaluation, surgical procedures, and results of the biopsy should be well explained to the patient and family. These explanations should be simple, precise and clear, to help the patient to continue with the struggle for life.

SUMMARY

Bone biopsy in a patient with a suspected metastatic event is not a simple "off-the-cuff" procedure. It should be carried out following the meticulous guidelines emphasised in this chapter, viz. complete pre-operative staging studies, proper planning of operative strategy, and special specific surgical procedures necessary for treatment of these patients. These guide-lines were not written for only the experienced orthopaedic oncology surgeon, but rather to aid medical students, general practitioners, oncologists and every orthopaedic surgeon who is faced with a suspect bone metastatic event. Adherence to the aforementioned medical/operative guidelines will ensure accurate diagnosis, with a resultant, better clinical result, and preservation of the precious, yet limited, lifespan and quality of life of these patients.

REFERENCES

1. Frassica FJ, Frassica DA, Sim FH. Carcinoma metastatic to bone: pathogenesis and pathophysiology. In Simon MA, Springfield D (eds), Surgery for Bone and Soft-Tissue Tumors. Lippincott-Raven: Philadelphia, PA, 1998; 615–20.
2. Mankin HJ, Lange TA, Spanier SS. The hazards of biopsy in patients with malignant primary bone and soft tissue tumors. J Bone Joint Surg Am 1982; 64A: 1121–7.
3. Mankin HJ, Mankin CJ, Simon MA. The hazards of biopsy, revisited. J Bone Joint Surg Am 1996; 78A: 656–63.
4. Simon MA. Biopsy of musculoskeletal tumors. J Bone Joint Surg Am 1982; 64A: 1253–7.
5. Brostrom L, Harris MA, Simon MA et al. The effect of biopsy on survival of patients with osteosarcoma. J Bone Joint Surg Br 1979; 61B: 209–12.
6. DenHeeten GJ, Oldhoff J, Oosterhuis JW et al. Biopsy of bone tumors. J Surg Oncol 1985; 28: 247–53.
7. Enneking WR. Editorial: the issue of the biopsy. J Bone Joint Surg Am 1982; 64: 1119–20.
8. Simon MA, Biermann JS. Biopsy of bone and soft-tissue lesions. J Bone Joint Surg Am 1982; 75: 1253–60.
9. Bickles J, Jelinek J, Shmookler B et al. Biopsy of musculoskeletal tumors. Clin Orthop 1999; 368: 212–19.
10. Campanacci M. Bone metastases from carcinoma. In Campanacci M (ed.), Bone and Soft Tissue Tumors. Springer-Verlag Aulo Gaggi Editore: Milan, 1990: 677–700.
11. Simon M, Karluk M. Skeletal metastases of unknown origin. Diagnostic strategy for orthopedic surgeons. Clin Orthop 1982; 166: 96–103.
12. Simon M, Bartucci E. The search for the primary tumor in patients with skeletal metastases of unknown origin. Cancer 1986; 58: 1088–95.
13. Haberman ET, Lopez RA. Metastatic disease of bone and treatment of pathological fractures. Orthop Clin North Am 1989; 20: 469–86.
14. Yazawa Y, Frassica FJ, Chao EYS et al. Metastatic bone disease. A study of the surgical treatment of 166 pathological humoral and femoral fractures. Clin Orthop 1990; 251: 213–19.
15. White VA, Fanning CV, Ayala AG et al. Osteosarcoma and the role of the fine-needle aspiration: a study of 51 cases. Cancer 1988; 62: 1238–43.
16. Will'en H. Fine needle aspiration in the diagnosis of bone tumors. Acta Orthop Scand 1997; 273: 47–53.
17. Bommer KK, Ramzy I, Mody D. Fine needle aspiration biopsy in the diagnosis and management of bone lesions: a study of 450 cases. Cancer 1997; 81: 148–56.
18. Ayala AG, Ro JY, Fanning CV et al. Core needle biopsy and fine needle aspiration in the diagnosis of bone and soft-tissue lesions. Hematol Oncol Clin North Am 1995; 9: 633–51.
19. Craig FS. Vertebral-body biopsy. J Bone Joint Surg Am 1956; 38A: 93–105.
20. Ottolenghi CE. Aspiration biopsy of the spine: technique for thoracic spine and results of 28 biopsies in this region and overall results of 1050 biopsies of other spinal segments. J Bone Joint Surg Am 1969; 51A: 1531–40.
21. Harrington KD. Anterior decompression and stabiliza-tion of the spine as a treatment of vertebral collapse and spinal cord decompression for metastatic malignancy. Clin Orthop 1988; 233: 177–97.
22. Clark CR, Morgan C, Sontegard DA et al. The effect of biopsy hole shape and size on bone strength. J Bone Joint Surg Am 1977; 59A: 213–17.

3

Surgical Treatment

Section Editor: Rodolpho Capanna

10

Indications for the Surgical Treatment of Long Bone Metastases

Rodolfo Capanna and Domenico A. Campanacci

Centro Traumatologico Ortopedico, Firenze, Italy

INTRODUCTION

Metastatic carcinoma is the most frequent malignant lesion of bone, and the skeleton represents the third most common site of metastatic spread after lung and liver [1]. Metastatic lesions are most commonly seen in the axial skeleton (spine, pelvis, ribs and skull) and, when the appendicular skeleton is involved, the lesions most frequently occur in the proximal long bones [2].

The treatment of bone metastases has usually a palliative purpose and has to be finalised to achieve adequate pain control and to prevent and cure pathological fractures of long bones. In selected cases, the treatment may have also a curative aim, and the complete resection of an isolated bone metastasis may improve a patient's survival.

The prognosis of patients with bone metastases is extremely variable, depending on the site of the primary cancer, but during the last decades, the life expectancy of patients has considerably improved due to the advances in chemotherapy, immunotherapy, hormonotherapy and radiation therapy [1]. A longer survival of cancer patients leads to an increasing population at risk of developing a bone metastasis and experiencing a pathological fracture. For this reason, the reconstructive procedure requires a longer-term reliability in order to avoid mechanical failures during prolonged survival of the patient.

At present, the patient with bone metastases is followed by different specialists (orthopaedic surgeon, oncologist, radiotherapist) without any rational guideline on the indications for surgical treatment. A protocol of treatment of bone metastases of the appendicular skeleton, describing the guidelines to surgical indications, type of surgery and different kind of reconstructions, was recently introduced. The purpose of this protocol is to offer adequate individual treatment to the patient, avoiding undertreatment and overtreatment, achieving pain control and addressing impending and pathological fractures, so that the longer life expectancy is associated to a better quality of life.

TYPES OF TUMOUR

Prostate

Prostate cancer rarely metastasises to long bones and typical affects the spine and pelvis. The lesions are usually osteoblastic (84%) or mixed (12%) and rarely osteolytic (4%) [3]. Due to the osteoblastic nature, pathological fractures are rarely seen and they have a high potential for union after fixation. The 5 year survival rate for metastatic prostate cancer is 33% [4].

Breast

In metastatic breast cancer, bone lesions are very frequent and as many as 74% of patients will eventually present skeletal involvement [5]. The lesions may be osteolytic, osteoblastic or mixed. At the present time, the 5 year survival rate for metastatic breast cancer is 22% [4].

Textbook of Bone Metastases. Edited by C. Jasmin, R. E. Coleman, L. R. Coia, R. Capanna and G. Saillant
© 2005 John Wiley & Sons Ltd: ISBN 0 471 87742 5

Kidney

Metastatic lesions from kidney cancer are usually located, in order of frequency, in the lung, skeleton and brain. Bone lesions are most often osteolytic with an aggressive aspect: cortex disappearing without periosteal reaction and soft tissue expansion are common. In these lesions, the risk of pathological fracture is high (50%) in both the spine and long bones, with very little potential for spontaneous union [6].

Due to the intense vascularisation of renal cell metastases, pre-operative selective embolisation is recommended to reduce bleeding during operation, expecially for spine, pelvis and shoulder girdle locations. After palliative fixation, repeated embolisations may be used to reduce local progression of the disease.

After resection of a solitary metastasis, the expected 5 year survival rate is 35% and an aggressive approach is justified [6]. In multiple lesions, only palliative surgery is indicated and the median survival is about 12 months. Nevertheless, 25% of patients have a life expectancy of 3–10 years, and therefore long-lasting reconstructive procedures are recommended [6].

Thyroid

Bone metastases are usually osteolytic and hyper-vascularised and a solitary lesion may be observed in 30% of cases [7].

The treatment of choice for solitary and late bone lesions is wide surgical resection followed by radiation therapy. Pre-operative embolisation is recommended before resection or palliative osteosynthesis, because intense bleeding may be expected. In pathological fractures, the union rate after radiation alone is 35% and this rises to 85% if rigid fixation is associated [7].

The overall 5 year survival rate is 44% for metastatic thyroid cancer [4] and the expected survival is less than 1 year for anaplastic tumours, but it is up to 12 years for Hurtle tumours and 3–6 years for other types [7]. In this case also, therefore, the selection of reconstructive techniques must take account of the long-term prognosis.

Lung

The prognosis of patients affected by lung carcinoma have not shown significant improvement in the last decades. The 5 year survival rate was 12% in 1976 and 14% in 1994 [4]. "Small-cell" carcinoma and adeno-carcinoma frequently metastasise to the skeleton, often involving the hands and feet. The bone lesion is usually osteolytic and only 25% of lesions are osteoblastic [8]. Metastatic lung cancer has a very bad prognosis, with a 5 year survival rate of 2% [4]. For this reason, simple osteosynthesis with palliative irradiation (short course/ large fraction) is usually indicated.

SITES OF METASTASES

Hip and Proximal Femur

The proximal femur is the most frequent site of mechanical failure in metastatic patients and surgical treatment is recommended for all impending or pathological fracture in this site, except in bedridden patients with a life expectancy of less than 2 months.

Preoperative MRI of the entire femur and pelvis is indicated in order to: (a) detect any acetabular involvement; (b) define the tumoral extension into the femoral shaft; (c) identify other metastatic foci in the distal medullary canal.

For metastatic lesions limited to the femoral head and neck, a conventional prosthetic replacement is recommended and long-stem prostheses are preferred, in order to reinforce the femoral shaft and to prevent failure in case of disease progression. In some cases, when the calcar area is destroyed, special calcar-replacement prostheses may be required. When the acetabulum is not involved, the use of bipolar cups is indicated because of their intrinsic stability.

For lesions also involving the trochanteric and metaphyseal area, simple osteosynthesis using screw-plate or intramedullary nails often proves inadequate with respect to long-term durability, especially when the medial cortex of the femur is not restored. When the fixation is reinforced with cement to restore the medial bone loss the results are improved, but the high mechanical stresses at this level and the risk of femoral head necrosis due to post-operative irradiation will eventually lead to the failure of the implant. This procedure, which consists of wide exposure, curettage, cement filling and osteosynthesis, has no significant advantages in terms of operative time, amelioration of blood loss, complication rate and recovery time vs. a "more aggressive" wide resection and prosthetic reconstruction. Moreover, intralesional curettage (the technique of choice in benign lesions) has to be considered oncologically inadequate to control a highly malignant tumour such as a metastatic lesion, and local recurrence may be expected in long-term survival and when no other effective adjuvant treatment (cryosurgery, radiation therapy) is utilised.

In metaphyseal lesions, resection of the proximal femur and reconstruction with cemented modular megaprostheses is our preferred method of treatment, and the implant should have the following characteristics: a modular system to be assembled in the operative field according to intraoperative requirements; long-stemmed, in order to reinforce the medullary canal as much as possible; and cemented, because the cement acts as an adjuvant, sterilising any residual tumoral foci in the medullary canal. Cemented implants are not affected by pre- or post-operative radiation therapy, while bone-ingrowth fixation in uncemented implants would be jeopardised by irradiation. Usually, no intramedullary plug for cement restriction is used, allowing the cement to fill the distal metaphysis and reinforce the entire medullary canal, avoiding stress rising at the tip of the stem or along the medullary canal. Drilling of the supracondylar cortex (venting technique) is recommended to prevent possible embolism due to the high-pressure injection of the cement.

All efforts should be made to improve hip stability and avoid post-operative dislocation, a frequent complication due to the lack of muscle control following surgical detachment of major muscles (glutei, quadriceps, ileopsoas) and weak reattachment to the metallic prosthesis. An adequate primary stability is a major goal in metastatic patients in order to allow immediate weight-bearing. The use of intrinsically stable joints, such as bipolar cups, is usually the method of choice. When acetabular replacement is required because of tumoral involvement, associated osteoarthritis or postradiation articular cartilage deterioration, self-retaining (snap-fit) sockets are strongly recommended, together with the use of a large prosthetic femoral head (size 28–32 mm).

The joint capsule should be preserved as much as possible in order to be able to close it around the prosthetic neck. A Marlex mesh tube may be used to reinforce or substitute the joint capsule, wrapping it around the prosthesis and suturing its proximal extremity along the acetabular rim. Muscle reinsertion has to be very accurate, both to the prosthesis and around it. A longitudinal tension band suturing the gluteus medius to the quadriceps is established, and this band provides the anchorage for reattachment of the ileopsoas, gluteus maximus and external rotators. Artificial devices for direct fixation of muscles to the prosthesis (polyethylene plates, artificial ligaments, metallic grips) may improve the fixation temporarily but they are rarely effective alone. To achieve better muscle control some authors suggest, even in metastatic patients, the wider use of a composite prosthesis (allograft with its tendon reinsertions, coupled with a revised long-stemmed conventional prosthesis).

Post-operatively, an external orthosis (articulating pelvic–hip brace) for one month to protect muscle reattachment sutures during weight-bearing is recommended.

Knee and Ankle

The knee and ankle joints undergo loading forces that are mainly compressive and the tensile and torsional forces are lower than in the proximal femur, decreasing the risk of mechanical failure. A metastatic lesion involving less than a half of the epiphyseal or metaphyseal area may be treated successfully by open curettage and plate fixation, filling the defect with PMMA cement. When the lesion involves more than half of the epiphyseal or metaphyseal area, an intra-articular resection is indicated. Distal femur and/or proximal tibia reconstruction may be performed using modular cemented megaprostheses (Figure 10.1). A hinge joint with a posterior axis is recommended to afford passive stability in hyperextension, even in case of large quadriceps excisions [9]. In proximal tibia resection, several techniques have been described to improve patellar tendon reattachment: reinforcement by artificial ligaments or fascia lata grafts; transposition of the proximal gastrocnemius head; multiple osteotomies of the fibula and anteposition of the fibular head; turning down of a patellar–quadriceps osteotendineous graft. However, in metastatic patients, the authors routinely use a flap of the medial gastrocnemius. This technique has been found useful for biological reattachment of the patellar tendon and to achieve better soft tissue coverage, minimising the risk of wound dehiscence and infection (particularly in case of pre- and/or post-operative radiation therapy).

After distal tibia resection, there is no suitable prosthetic device as yet and the only reconstructive option is ankle arthrodesis, using autografts or allografts reinforced by a tibial intramedullary rod, locked proximally into the tibia and distally into the talus and calcaneum. In this case, radiation therapy is not indicated because of its negative effects on graft fusion.

Shoulder and Elbow

The proximal humerus is an area at risk for pathological fractures because of the intense bending

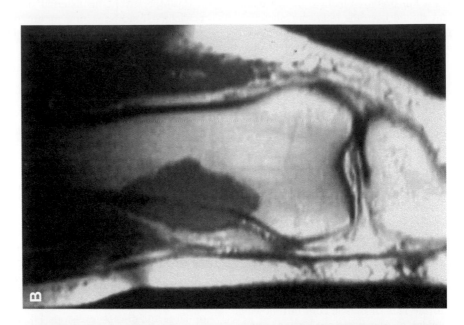

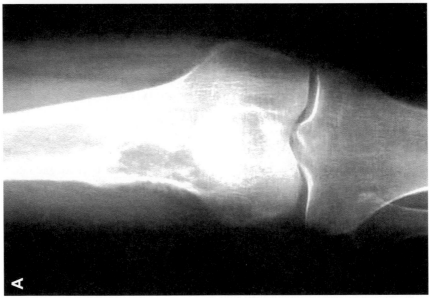

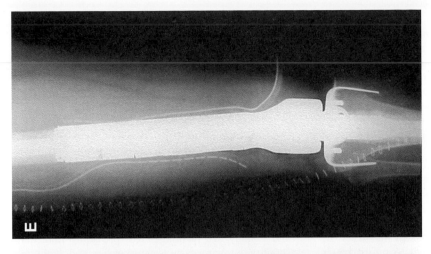

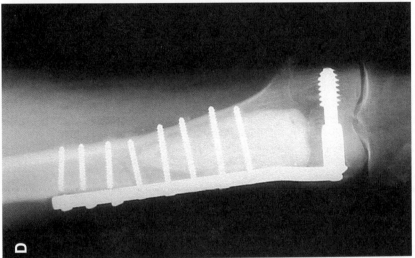

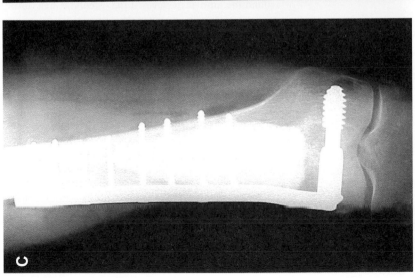

Figure 10.1. (A) Antero-posterior view of an osteolytic metastatic lesion of the distal femur from colon carcinoma. (B) The MRI shows an involvement of less than half of the metaphyseal area. (C) An open curettage was performed and the reconstruction was done with cement filling and screw-plate fixation. (D) Notwithstanding post-operative radiation therapy, disease progression occurred 1 year later, leading to synthesis failure. (E) The patient underwent resection of the distal femur and reconstruction with a modular prosthesis

and rotational forces from the muscle insertions. The humeral metaphysis is largely cancellous and a stable fixation is often difficult to achieve, expecially in older osteoporotic patients. For these reasons, the recommended treatment for proximal humerus metastases is shoulder arthroplasty (Figure 10.2). The epiphyseal lesions may be treated by a conventional cemented long-stem prosthesis, preserving the insertion of the rotator cuff on the greater tuberosity. If the lesion extends to the metaphysis, a modular resection prosthesis must be employed. An accurate reattachment of the rotator cuff, deltoid and pectoralis major to the prosthesis by non-absorbable suture is recommended in order to improve stability and residual function. Recent prostheses have several holes in the metallic body, where strips of artificial ligaments (or fascia lata) may be passed through to afford better muscle reattachment. Shoulder stability may be also improved using suspension bands to the acromion, and wrapping around the prosthetic head an artificial mesh to be sutured to the remaining rotator cuff or to the edges of the glenoid cavity.

The distal humerus and the elbow joint are rarely affected by metastatic lesions, since the meta-epiphyseal region is mainly cortical and less vascularised. When the distal humerus is involved less than half, an open curettage with cement filling and plate fixation may be performed. In a case of joint cavity involvement or extension of the tumour for more than half of the meta-epiphysis, wide resection and modular prosthetic reconstruction is indicated.

Shafts of Major Long Bones

Pathological fracture is a common complication of metastatic lesions of major long bones and the indications for prophylactic fixation depend on the site and size of the defect. The diaphyses more at risk for a pathological fracture are, in descending order, the femur, the humerus and the tibia. There is agreement in accepting the indication to treatment of lesions with a cortical defect in the femur extending for 2.5 cm or more and lesions with interruption of the cortex in either a longitudinal or coronal plane exceeding 50% of the bone diameter [10–13]. A scoring system to define the risk of pathological fracture, taking into consideration the site, pain, radiological appearance and size of the lesion, was introduced by Mirels [12]. The general status of the patient, including life expectancy and the predicted response to adjuvant therapy, must also be considered. In a case of pathological fracture in major long bones, surgical

treatment is always indicated and conservative care is reserved only for patients in a terminal condition [14].

When the general condition and the prognosis of the patient are poor, or in a case of predicted good response to radiation therapy, a simple osteosynthesis without open curettage may be considered. In these cases an intramedullary interlocking nail fixation is preferred, for the following reasons: limited surgical exposure and intraoperative bleeding; surgical access is distant from the lesion and hence there is low risk of wound-healing problems when immediate postoperative irradiation is administered; the rod is closer to the mechanical axis than a plate, and locking screws can be placed in normal bone far away from the lesion. For these reasons, generation nails locked proximally and distally are recommended, providing immediate stability, allowing early weight-bearing and avoiding a telescoping effect in case of massive intercalary resorption. Older generation devices such as Steinmann pins, Rush, Ender or conventional Kuntscher nails are not strong enough and do not prevent telescoping and rotational instability.

For patients in good general condition, with a good prognosis or with a predicted bad response to adjuvants, a more aggressive approach is indicated. A reinforced osteosynthesis may be achieved by accurate curettage of the lesion, polymethylmethacrylate filling and fixation by plate or intramedullary nail. In nail fixation, before rod insertion, the PMMA may be injected under pressure, using a cement gun, into the medullary canal to reinforce the osteosynthesis and prevent failure due to the progression of the disease [15]. The operative working time of the PMMA may be prolonged by cooling the liquid monomer, and a tourniquet inflated around the limb at the level of the osteolytic area during injection may help in preventing cement extrusion into the soft tissues. Some holes drilled (venting technique) in the anterolateral cortex of the femur may decrease the risk of embolic phenomena during cement injection. The cement may also sterilise residual microfoci of the tumour, by either the direct heat of polymerisation or the toxic effect of monomer release.

A higher mechanical strength with the use of two orthogonal plates and cement was observed by Anderson et al. [16], who also reported an increased torsional failure load by × 2.6 and bending failure load by × 4.2 with respect to intramedullary fixation. In our experience, this procedure requires an extensive surgical exposure with excessive blood loss, increasing the risk of local and general complications, and therefore is rarely indicated.

In selected cases of solitary diaphyseal lesions with good prognosis, a wide intercalary resection is

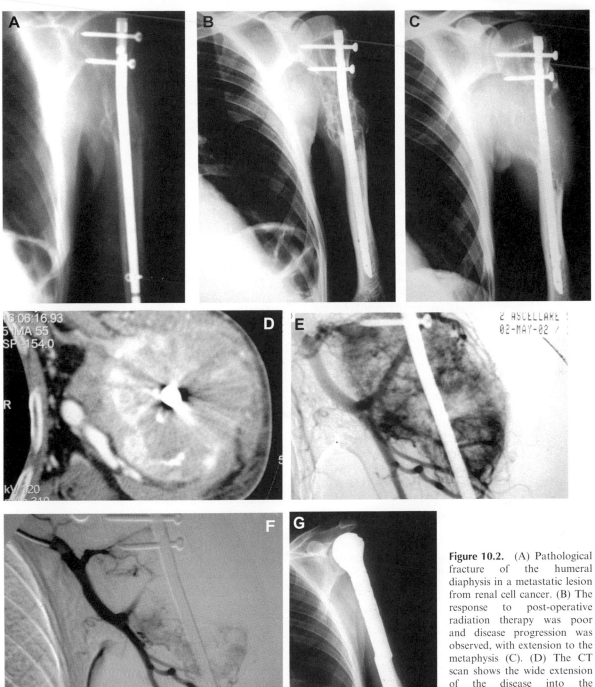

Figure 10.2. (A) Pathological fracture of the humeral diaphysis in a metastatic lesion from renal cell cancer. (B) The response to post-operative radiation therapy was poor and disease progression was observed, with extension to the metaphysis (C). (D) The CT scan shows the wide extension of the disease into the surrounding soft tissues. (E–F) A pre-operative angiography with selective embolisation of the lesion was performed. (G) A resection of the proximal humerus was performed and a modular prosthesis was implanted

indicated and reconstruction may be performed using intercalary prostheses with cemented stems and modular component joined by a morse taper.

Curettage and Local Adjuvants in Bone Metastases

In case of open curettage of the lesion, the cavity walls may be cleaned using curettes, gouges and high-speed burrs, and local adjuvants may be used to improve sterilisation of the margins [17]. Highly concentrated phenol (80%) has proved to be effective in sterilising the surface of the cavity; the technique requires soaking the surface three times, followed by lavage with alcohol and saline solution. The electrocauterisation of the bony walls, expecially if performed with argon, has a haemostatic effect and a sterilising property of 1 mm. PMMA has an adjuvant thermal and toxic effect during polymerisation. The thermal effect is greater in cancellous bone (2–3 mm) and lower in cortical bone (0.5 mm). Cryotherapy represents the most effective local adjuvant, but there are concerns about the bone weakening and possible soft tissue damage [17]. Deep freezing and thawing of the cavity may be performed using liquid nitrogen or by filling the cavity with a sterile gel and inserting a probe connected to a device monitoring temperature and rate of freezing. By repeating the freezing–thawing procedure three times, a ring of necrosis of 1–2 cm is obtained.

GUIDELINES FOR SURGICAL TREATMENT

A multidisciplinary approach is required in the treatment of bone metastases, and interaction between the orthopaedic surgeon, oncologist and radiotherapist is needed, with a clear assessment of their specific roles. In an attempt to address this issue, a prospective protocol has been introduced, containing guidelines on

surgical indications (which patient requires surgery?) and on the type of operation that should be advised (how to perform surgery?). Several different parameters were taken into account: (a) the expected survival; (b) the type and stage of the tumour; (c) the visceral spread; (d) the Karnofsky status [18]; (e) the time interval from primary tumour; (f) the risk of pathological fracture; (g) the predicted sensitivity to chemotherapy, hormone therapy and irradiation.

Indications for Surgical Treatment

Patients are assigned to one of four classes (Table 10.1).

- *Class 1.* Patients with a single metastatic lesion of a primary tumour with good prognosis and a free interval of more than 3 years from primary lesion to the development of bone metastasis. Primary tumours with a favourable prognosis include well-differentiated thyroid, prostate, breast (sensitive to hormone or chemotherapy), clear-cell renal and colorectal carcinomas. Myeloma and lymphoma are included in the protocol, since their biological behaviour and the mechanical implications are similar to metastatic disease.
- *Class 2.* Patients with a pathological fracture in a major long bone.
- *Class 3.* Patients with radiological and/or clinical signs of impending fracture in a major long bone or the periacetabular area.
- *Class 4.* Patients with: (a) osteoblastic lesions at all sites; (b) osteolytic or mixed lesions in non-weight-bearing bones (e.g. fibula, ribs, sternum or clavicle); (c) osteolytic lesions in major bones with no impending fracture; (d) lesions in the iliac wing, anterior pelvis or scapula (excluding patients included in class 1).

Table 10.1. The four different classes of patients of the protocol

Class 1	• Solitary metastatic lesion
	• Primary with good prognosis (well-differentiated tumours of thyroid, prostate, breast sensitive to adjuvants, rectum, clear cell renal, lymphoma, myeloma)
	• Interval after primary over 3 years
Class 2	• Pathological fracture at any site
Class 3	• Impending fracture in a major weight-bearing bone
Class 4	• Osteoblastic lesions at all sites
	• Osteolytic or mixed lesions in non-structural bones (fibula, rib, sternum, clavicle)
	• Osteolytic lesion with no impending fracture in major weight-bearing bone
	• Lesions of the iliac wing, anterior pelvis or scapula, excluding class 1 patients

All patients included in classes 1, 2 and 3 should have a priority referral to an orthopaedic oncologist for surgical treatment. After surgery they should be referred back to the oncologist and/or radiotherapist for adjuvant treatment if indicated. Patients in class 4 should be treated conservatively by chemotherapy, hormone therapy and/or irradiation, according to diagnosis. The response to treatment and the pain control should be carefully evaluated at follow-up. In a case of pathological fracture, or in a case of pain persisting for 2 months after completion of treatment or radiological signs of local progression, these patients should be referred to an orthopaedic surgeon for surgical treatment, having then entered class 2 or 3 (Table 10.2).

Type of Surgery

In Table 10.3, the different osteosynthesis and reconstructive devices are described. Their employment is discussed in relation to the class of the patient and the site of the bone lesion.

Class 1

In these patients, the metastasis is treated as a primary tumour and the operation aims at long-term cure, both oncologically and mechanically. An intra-articular or intercalary resection is performed with wide surgical

Table 10.2. Indications for surgical and conservative treatment by class of patients (see text)

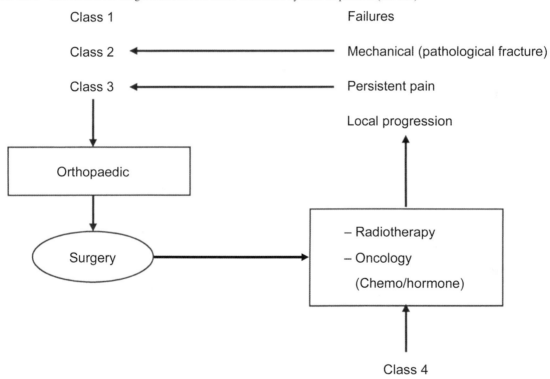

Table 10.3. Different types of surgical reconstruction in long bones

A: Osteosynthesis
A0: Minimal	Single plate; Ender, Rush, Kuntscher nails
A1: Simple	Reconstructive rod locked into solid bone; single plate + cement
A2: Reinforced	Reconstructive rod + cement; double plating + cement

B: Implant
B0	Long-stem prosthesis
B1	Megaprosthesis
B2	Intercalary spacer

Table 10.4. Recommended treatment for meta-epiphyseal lesions in class 2 and class 3 patients

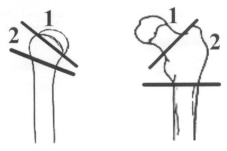

Area 1: B0 (long-stem cemented endoprosthesis)
Area 2 or 1 + 2: B1 (cemented megaprosthesis)

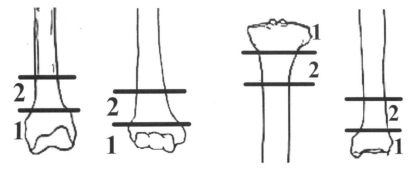

Area 1 or 2 (extension < half): A1 (curettage + plate and cement)
Area 1 or 2 (extension > half): B1 (cemented megaprosthesis or ankle arthrodesis)
Area 1 + 2: B1 (cemented megaprosthesis or ankle arthrodesis)

margins and the defect is reconstructed using a cemented megaprostheses or an intercalary spacer.

Classes 2 and 3

Meta-epiphysis of Long Bones. Table 10.4 shows the recommended treatment for meta-epiphyseal lesions in class 2 and 3 patients. Area 1 (epiphysis) and area 2 (metaphysis) are considered separately.

The risk of pathological fracture is high at the proximal end of the humerus and femur, due to the intense rotational and weight-bearing forces. In these areas, an aggressive approach by resection and prosthetic replacement is recommended in order to allow an early functional recovery and to avoid a subsequent failure due to disease progression. In a case of wide oncological margins post-operative radiation therapy can be avoided, while it is still recommended after marginal or intralesional procedures or in patients presenting with a pathological fracture. In these cases, radiation therapy should be delivered with full doses (3000–5000 cGy) and not for palliative pain control purposes. In epiphyseal involvement, a long-stem cemented conventional prosthesis may be employed, while a metaphyseal resection requires reconstruction by cemented megaprostheses.

The elbow, knee and ankle joint have a lower risk of mechanical failure. For this reason, when less than half of the bone is involved, curettage with cement filling and plate osteosynthesis is considered an adequate treatment. When performing intralesional removal of the lesion, local adjuvants (cryotherapy, phenol, etc.) are strongly recommended and postoperative radiation therapy should be associated for oncological control. When the tumour extends to more than half of the meta-epiphyseal area, an intra-articular resection is recommended and reconstruction is performed by prosthetic replacement of the distal humerus, distal femur and proximal tibia or ankle arthrodesis.

Diaphysis of Long Bones. For diaphyseal metastasis in class 2 and 3 patients, a scoring system has been introduced (Table 10.5) in consideration of expected

Table 10.5. Scoring system and recommended treatment for diaphyseal lesions in class 2 and class 3 patients

Survival	Biomechanics	Size defect	Response to adjuvant therapy
< 1 year=1	Tibia=1	Small (1/3)=1	Yes=0
1–2 years=3	Femur, humerus=2	Large (1/2)=2	No=3
> 2 years=6	Subtrochanteric supracondylar=3	Defective or pathological fracture=3	

<5 points	Minimal or simple osteosynthesis (A0, A1)
5–10 points	Reinforced osteosynthesis (A2)
10–15 points	Megaprosthesis or intercalary spacer (B1, B2)

Table 10.6. Predictive survival and scoring for the protocol

Survival	Sources of metastasis
<1 year (1 point)	Unknown
	Melanoma
	Lung
	Pancreas
	Thyroid (undifferentiated)
	Stomach
1–2 years (3 points)	Colon
	Breast (not responding to adjuvants)
	Liver
	Uterus (responding to adjuvants)
>2 years (6 points)	Thyroid (differentiated)
	Myeloma
	Lymphoma
	Breast (responding to adjuvants)
	Rectum
	Prostate
	Kidney

Table 10.7. Predictive response to adjuvant therapy and scoring for the protocol

Responsive (0 points)	Breast
	Thyroid
	Myeloma
	Lymphoma
	Prostate
Non-responsive (3 points)	Kidney
	Gastrointestinal
	Lung
	Uterus
	Pancreas

survival (Table 10.6), the site and size of the lesion and the response to adjuvants (Table 10.7). The score ranges from 3 to 15 points for each patient. Simple osteosynthesis (A1) is recommended for patients with a low score (< 5 points), reinforced osteosynthesis (A2) for those with a middle score (5–10 points) and resection and prosthetic replacement (B1, B2) is reserved for the higher score (10–15 points). The score is adjusted according to the Karnofsky general status of the patient [18]. A Karnofsky status of under 50 points downgrades from reinforced to simple osteosynthesis, while with a general status of over 50 points the original score is maintained.

REFERENCES

1. Hage WD, Aboulafia AJ, Aboulafia DM. Incidence, location, and diagnostic evaluation of metastatic bone disease. Orthop Clin N Am 2000: 31; 4: 515–28.
2. Silverberg E. Cancer statistics 1986. CA Cancer J Clin 1986; 36: 9–25.
3. Richardson RL, Swee RG, Sim FH et al. Prostate cancer. In Diagnosis and Management of Metastatic Bone Disease: a Multidisciplinary Approach. Raven: New York, 1988: 273–81.
4. Cancer facts and figures. American Cancer Society, Atlanta, GA, 1999: 1–36.
5. Ingle JN, Sim FH, Schray MF et al. Breast cancer. In Diagnosis and Management of Metastatic Bone Disease: a Multidisciplinary Approach Raven: New York, 1988: 251–63.
6. Hahn RG, Sim FH, Scott SM et al. Renal cell cancer. In Diagnosis and Management of Metastatic Bone Disease: a Multidisciplinary Approach. Raven: New York, 1988: 283–90.
7. Hay ID, Rock MG, Sim FH et al. Thyroid cancer. In Diagnosis and Management of Metastatic Bone Disease: a Multidisciplinary Approach. Raven: New York, 1988: 305–17.
8. Frytak S, McLeod RA, Gunderson LL et al. Lung cancer. In Diagnosis and Management of Metastatic Bone Disease: a Multidisciplinary Approach. Raven: New York, 1988: 305–17.
9. Capanna R, Ruggieri P, Biagini R et al. The effects of quadriceps excision on functional results after distal femoral resection and prosthetic replacement of bone tumors. Clin Orthop 1991; 267: 186–96.
10. Bechtol CO. Bone as a structure. In Bechtol CO, Ferguson AB, Laing PG (eds), Metals and Engineering in Bone and Joint Surgery. Willhams & Wilkins: Baltimore, MD, 1959: 127–42.

11. McBroome RY, Hayes WC, Poon P. Strength reduction of endosteal defects in diaphyseal bone. Trans 32nd Ann Meet Orthop Res Soc 1986; 11: 65.

12. Mirels M. Metastatic disease in long bones: a proposed scoring system for diagnosis impending pathologic fractures. Clin Orthop 1989; 249: 256–64.

13. Pugh J, Sherry HS, Futterman B, Frankel VH. Biomechanisms of pathologic fractures. Clin Orthop 1982; 169. 109–14.

14. Yazawa Y, Frassica FJ, Chao EYS et al. Metastatic bone disease: a study of the surgical treatment of 166 pathological humeral and femoral fractures. *Clin Orthop* 1990; 251: 213–19.

15. Sim FM, Daugherty TW, Ivins JC. The adjunctive use of methylmethacrylate in fixation of pathological fractures. J Bone Joint Surg Am 1974; 56-A: 40–8.

16. Anderson JT, Erickson JM, Thompson RC Jr, Chao FY. Pathologic femoral shaft fractures comparing fixation techniques using cement. Clin Orthop 1978; 131: 273–8.

17. Gitelis S, McDonald DJ. Adjuvant agents and filling materials. In Simon MA (ed.), Surgery for Bone and Soft Tissue Tumours. Lippincott-Raven: Springfield, IL, 1998: 133–57.

18. Karnofsky DA, Burchenal JH. The clinical evaluation of chemotherapeutic agents. In McLeod E (ed.), Evaluation of Chemotherapeutic Agents. Columbia University Press: New York, 1949.

11

Prosthetic Replacement in Long Bone Metastases

Bruno Fuchs, Franklin H. Sim and David J. Jacofsky

Department of Orthopedic Surgery, Mayo Clinic, Rochester, MN, USA

INTRODUCTION

Because of technological advances, the treatment of metastases to long bones has improved dramatically. Many reconstructive devices have become available. The selection of the appropriate implant offers unique challenges.

First, it is important to understand the distribution of bone metastasis. Bone metastases predominantly are found in the axial skeleton, particularly the spine, pelvis, sternum, skull and ribs, rather than in the appendicular skeleton [1]. Lesions in the humeri and femora are common, with the proximal long bones most commonly affected. Metastases distal to the elbow and distal to the knee are uncommon [2].

In addition to the location of metastasis, fracture— actual or impending—is another consideration in the treatment decision. The scoring system of Mirels [3] is useful in deciding whether a surgical procedure is indicated in cases of potentially imminent fracture. Others have indicated that a risk of fracture exists when a lesion involves 50% of the cortex, is 2.5 cm in diameter or remains painful on weight-bearing after radiotherapy, or where there is a pathological avulsion fracture of the lesser trochanter [4,5]. Despite such guidelines, it must be remembered that skeletal metastases usually begin in the cancellous marrow and involve the cortex only later in their development [6]. Loss of 30–50% of trabecular mineralisation may be required for radiographic detection.

Three principles should be followed in the decision to treat with prosthetic replacement. First, the patient's estimated survival should exceed the time needed for recovery from the operation. The recovery time needed varies according to the type of procedure. For example, a complex acetabular reconstruction requires a longer recovery period than the insertion of an intramedullary nail. Second, a reconstruction should be stable enough to permit full weight-bearing immediately after the operation and must be durable enough to last the expected lifetime of the patient. Third, any planned reconstruction should address areas of weakened bone that are present at operation, as well as areas that are likely to be weakened subsequently.

As survival rates for patients with tumours improve, surgical reintervention becomes increasingly important. When internal fixation fails, revision is often difficult because now a large skeletal defect may exist from removal of the implant or bone cement (or both) and progression of disease. However, there are devices and prostheses that can be used in several circumstances, such as reconstruction of areas not amenable to internal fixation, including the articular surfaces, the proximal femur, the proximal tibia, and the proximal humerus. These devices can be used in arthroplasty for the hip, knee and shoulder; also available is a modular diaphyseal replacement system for segmental defects in long bones. With the proximal femur, an area of bone loss and high stress, calcar replacements and proximal replacement implants can be used. Improved design has made possible a calcar replacement with a longer neck; this has expanded the options for replacement arthroplasty in patients with peritrochanteric lesions.

Textbook of Bone Metastases. Edited by C. Jasmin, R. E. Coleman, L. R. Coia, R. Capanna and G. Saillant
© 2005 John Wiley & Sons Ltd: ISBN 0 471 87742 5

In general, metastatic involvement, particularly of the long bones, causes serious clinical problems. Advances in techniques and prosthetic designs allow stable and durable fixation and improve the quality of life in patients with bone metastases.

FEMUR

Femoral Head and Neck Fractures

Even for low-demand patients, internal fixation of impending and pathological fractures of the femoral head and neck has an unacceptably high risk of failure due to the high stresses across the proximal femur. Moreover, fractures (including non-displaced fractures) in tumour-destroyed bone in the femoral neck rarely heal before the patient dies. Therefore, these fractures should be managed with replacement arthroplasty. When the involvement does not extend more distally than the level of the femoral neck, a collared prosthesis with bone cement and without calcar replacement may suffice. Implants with long, straight or curved femoral stems are available.

There are two main issues in the use of replacement arthroplasty to treat metastatic involvement of the hip: management of the acetabulum and length of the femoral stem. For patients with a lesion in the proximal femur, management of the acetabulum is under debate. Habermann et al. [7] reported that previously unrecognised acetabular involvement was discovered through biopsy of the acetabulum in 19/23 (83%) of patients with metastatic disease who were having a hip arthroplasty. These authors argue that, in most patients with advanced metastases of the femoral head or neck, the periacetabular bone also is involved and that a single operation to replace the femoral head and acetabulum is preferable to the risk of acetabular fracture later [7,8]. These authors recommended that a total hip arthroplasty be performed routinely whenever a femoral stem is implanted to treat metastatic involvement. However, many authors [8–12] recommend hemiarthroplasty alone under these circumstances, because unrecognised involvement of the acetabular side has not been shown clearly to cause persistent pain or other problems. Hemiarthroplasty is less extensive than total hip arthroplasty and has less risk of hip instability. The use of acetabular prosthetic replacement and local radiation does not ensure that destruction of the periacetabular ilium will not progress, eventually necessitating a more extensive acetabular reconstruction [13]. Furthermore, the additional exposure needed to insert the acetabular

component and the resulting blood loss have discouraged the routine use of total hip arthroplasty in the treatment of metastatic involvement of the femoral head and neck. A major disadvantage of inserting an acetabular component is the added potential of instability, particularly when a megaprosthesis is used. The dislocation rate for patients with megaprostheses is reported to be higher than that in the general population of patients with hip arthroplasty [14]. Therefore, in the absence of clinical acetabular disease, a bipolar endoprosthesis allows greater stability.

Selection of the length of the femoral stem is the second main issue in the use of replacement arthroplasty. The tip of the intramedullary femoral stem should bypass the most distal area of weakness by two bone diameters. Even if imaging studies do not show distal involvement by metastatic disease, an intramedullary prosthesis with a long stem may be inserted prophylactically, particularly if the patient is at substantial risk for multiple lesions, as in multiple myeloma. However, the increased risk of embolisation and cardiac arrest may be a major reason not to use a long-stemmed prosthesis routinely [15]. Venting of the distal femur before reaming may minimise the risk of such complications.

Lane et al. [5] reported on 167 patients treated with endoprosthetic replacement for impending or complete fractures of the hip. The median survival was 5.6 months. No patient had dislocation, loosening or failure of the prosthesis. All patients had dramatic pain relief. In three-quarters of the patients who could walk before the fracture, total long-stemmed hip arthroplasty or the insertion of a long-stemmed femoral endoprosthesis led to improvement of ambulatory status. Patients who benefited little from endoprosthetic replacement were bedridden before the fracture occurred and usually had severe metastatic involvement of the spine.

Other reports also suggest favourable results of prosthetic replacement [14,16]. In their analysis of the treatment of 166 pathological fractures, Yazawa et al. [14] found an overall failure rate of 11% for the treatment of femoral fractures. For proximal femoral fractures fixed with a compression screw or nail plate, the failure rate was 23%. In patients who had arthroplasty, the prosthetic component dislocation rate was 15%. This rate was believed to reflect the extent of femoral resection, prosthetic replacement length, and the poor general health of the patients. Particularly for patients with poor muscle tone, general debilitation or potential prosthetic instability due to excessive bone resection during arthroplasty, the authors recommended that an abduction brace be included as part of the post-operative rehabilitation.

Intertrochanteric Fractures

The operative treatment of pathological intertrochanteric fractures remains controversial. Lesions confined to the intertrochanteric region with minimal medial cortical bone destruction traditionally have been treated with a compression screw and nail plate device. However, this form of treatment has had a high failure rate because of prolonged survival, progression of local disease, poor initial fixation, non-union or delayed union, and lack of load-sharing between the implant device and the residual bone. Many surgeons prefer prosthetic replacement to standard internal fixation supplemented with bone cement. Each technique has advantages and disadvantages.

Classically, a dynamic hip screw combined with curettage and packing of the defect with bone cement is used for internal fixation [6,13]. The main advantages of this technique are the preservation of the hip joint and the surgeon's familiarity with its use. However, because of the mechanics in this region, stable fixation is not always achieved easily. Also, a plate-and-screw device does not prophylactically protect the entire bone from failure due to distal metastatic disease. Given these limitations, fixation may fail because of high stresses placed on the proximal end of the femur, combined with disease progression [14]. Therefore, metastatic involvement of the femoral head and neck with extension into the trochanteric and subtrochanteric regions is rarely managed with these fixation devices.

Prosthetic replacement with calcar or proximal femoral devices is the procedure of choice for managing large tumour-destroyed areas not amenable to internal fixation, and for managing lesions not amenable to radiotherapy alone. Various modular prosthetic designs are available in standard forms or on a custom-made basis. They allow removal of a great portion of the diseased bone, which considerably decreases reliance on that bone for stability and consequently decreases the likelihood of failure due to disease progression. Head and neck replacement devices have been effective for managing most lesions that involve the calcar area (Figure 11.1). They allow preservation of the lateral cortical structures if the bone is intact or reattachment of the greater trochanter to the prosthesis if bone dissolution has occurred. When the prosthesis is augmented with cement,

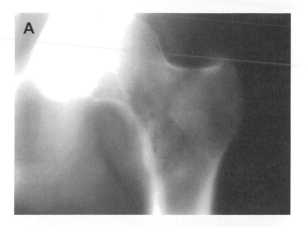

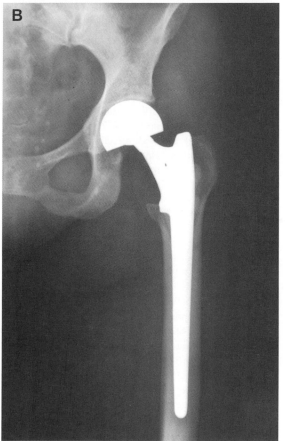

Figure 11.1. For a metastatic lesion in the femoral neck with extension into the intertrochanteric region (A), a short-stemmed hemiprosthesis with a calcar device is used (B)

immediate full weight-bearing can be permitted, and the patient can return to daily activities rapidly.

The main disadvantages of arthroplasty, compared with the use of internal fixation devices, are that it is a more extensive procedure [17] and that its potential complications include instability, fracture of the greater trochanter, loosening of the prosthesis and a reportedly higher risk of infection. However, in one study of arthroplasty for pathological fracture of the hip, the rate of infection was only 1% (2/167 hips) [5]. Another disadvantage of arthroplasty is the potential loss of hip flexor and abductor strength, resulting in a permanent gait disturbance. However, the use of a bipolar femoral component and a modular-design femoral component has helped reduce the incidence of complications due to improper soft tissue tension and dislocation.

Overall, dislocation is the most common complication after proximal femoral and total femoral resection and endoprosthetic reconstruction, with rates of 11–15% [18–23]. Dislocation can be avoided by maintaining proper hip joint compression by using a bipolar cup or a constrained liner, keeping the acetabular component more horizontal with proper anteversion, and providing proper soft tissue reconstruction. Limb length can be equalised, and therefore hip stability improved, with the use of different neck lengths of modular prostheses.

Bickels et al. [24] reported 57 patients who had proximal or total femoral resection with endoprosthetic reconstruction. Bipolar hemiarthroplasty was performed in 49 patients, and fixed unipolar hemiarthroplasty was performed in eight. The acetabulum was spared and not resurfaced in all cases. Soft tissue reconstruction included polyethylene tape capsulorrhaphy over the prosthetic neck, reattachment of the abductor mechanism to the prosthesis, and extracortical bone fixation. After an average follow-up of 6.5 years, there was only one dislocation (1.8%). Aseptic loosening occurred in three patients (5.3%); the limb salvage rate was 98%. Masterson et al. [25] also recommended capsular replacement with synthetic mesh. Thirteen of 88 patients having proximal femoral replacement required capsular replacement, including six patients with pelvic resection. None of the remaining 75 patients had a dislocation. Five of the 13 patients with reconstructed hips had a dislocation after the reconstructive procedure; in one patient the hip remained chronically dislocated.

Another concern is the reconstruction of the abductor mechanism, which is often extremely challenging. The attachment of tendons to prosthetic devices remains crucial, particularly in the reconstruction of the abductor mechanism at the greater trochanter. If the greater trochanter can be preserved, it must be fixed to the prosthesis with wires and cables. Using a sheep model, Gottsauner-Wolf et al. [26] showed that the transplantation of a bone and tendon allograft to an implant resulted in a revitalised, mechanically stable and biologically anchored compound, which could be observed in specimens taken 8 months postoperatively. If the greater trochanter must be resected, the remaining abductor muscles are attached directly to the prosthesis or reefed down to the vastus lateralis [27]. Subsequently, most patients must use a cane to compensate for the loss of the abductor mechanism.

An advantage of using a prosthesis is the availability of long-stemmed prostheses for treating distal disease (Figure 11.2). Clarke et al. [9] reported on 28 patients with pathological lesions in the proximal femur. The patients were treated with implantation of a head and neck prosthesis (23 bipolar hemiarthroplasties, five total hip arthroplasties). In these patients, the greater trochanter and abductor mechanism were intact and the medial cortex was replaced at least as far as the lesser trochanter. At a follow-up of 43 months, 26/28 (93%) of prostheses had survived. Eight patients (29%) had at least one complication (infection in three, instability in only one). Deep infection occurred in three patients, leading to resection in two. Three patients had periprosthetic fractures; one patient with total hip arthroplasty had instability. All patients but one regained ambulatory status.

The results of revision operations after prosthetic replacement have been analysed extensively. The results suggest that revision is feasible and can be done safely without greatly affecting the patient's functional performance. Unwin et al. [28] reported the University of Birmingham's (UK) experience with aseptic loosening of prostheses used for reconstruction of the lower limb. In 1001 custom-made prostheses used with the proximal femur, distal femur and proximal tibia, aseptic loosening was the principal cause of implant failure; 71 patients required revision for aseptic loosening of the cemented intramedullary stem. At 120 months after implantation, implant survival rates were 93.8% for proximal femoral prostheses, 67.4% for distal femoral prostheses, and 58% for proximal tibial prostheses. Age and the percentage of bone removed were significant factors influencing survival in distal femoral but not proximal replacements.

Hsu et al. [29] reviewed the function of 38 patients who needed revision operations for implant failure or other complications (aseptic loosening in 34%) after prosthetic replacement. Fifty-one months after the revision operation, functional results were excellent or good in 72% of the patients. The authors concluded that reoperation for implant failure or other reasons after a limb salvage procedure using custom-designed or modular-segmental bone and joint implants seemed

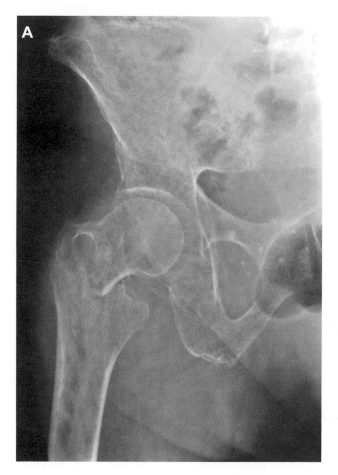
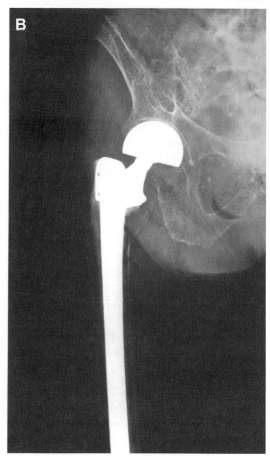

Figure 11.2.   When there is an additional lesion in the distal femur (A), a long-stemmed calcar replacement prosthesis (B) is used

feasible and did not seriously affect subsequent functional performance or patient survival.

Wirganowicz et al. [30] reported on revision operations performed on patients who had received endoprostheses for tumour-weakened bone at the University of California at Los Angeles. Of 278 patients receiving a prosthesis, failure occurred in 64; failure was defined as removal of the prosthesis at revision. The causes for failure were aseptic loosening (44%), fatigue fracture (16%), local recurrence of disease (14%), infection (13%), and failure of the expansion mechanism (6%). In cases of aseptic loosening and mechanical failure, the same type of prosthesis was used again. At 7 years after operation, failure rates for primary and revision reconstructions were 31% and 34%, respectively.

Shin et al. [31] reported on 52 patients who needed revision operations at the Mayo Clinic. The operations included 35 prosthetic revisions, 11 amputations, and four arthrodeses. At 5 and 10 years after operation, prosthetic survival in the group of 35 patients needing revision of the same or another prothesis was 79% and 65%, respectively. The authors concluded that revision is feasible and effective and can be done without jeopardising patient or implant survival and without seriously affecting functional results as compared with pre-operative values.

Subtrochanteric Fractures

The subtrochanteric region, particularly the area extending 5 cm distally from the lesser trochanter, receives great shear and torque stresses. These forces can reach six times body weight [32], which places extreme demands on fixation devices. Treatment of subtrochanteric pathological fractures is more difficult because of the loss of cortical support and the mechanical forces applied on each side of this area. The subtrochanteric area has a less copious blood supply than the intertrochanteric area, and non-union is more common in this area [33,34]. For these reasons, nail plates have an unacceptably high failure rate [14], and have been abandoned widely.

There are two principal options for the fixation of pathological fractures in the subtrochanteric region. Fixation with third-generation intramedullary nails is the preferred method if adequate fixation can be achieved in the remaining proximal bone [6,35–37]. A proximal femoral prosthesis should be considered if there is extensive involvement of the femoral head, femoral neck, and peritrochanteric femur and if fixation is not possible with screws and methyl methacrylate alone. This approach also should be considered if previous fixation of a pathological

fracture has failed. Such fixation is particularly important in the case of lesions resistant to radiotherapy. The use of a proximal femoral megaprosthesis allows replacement of most, if not all, of the weakened proximal femur, providing excellent pain relief and diminishing the risk of local progression and subsequent problems (Figure 11.3). These factors may become more important as the treatment of metastatic cancer improves, resulting in longer survival because the failure rate increases as post-operative survival increases [38].

Care must be taken to bypass the most distal lesion with the intramedullary stem. However, the following two facts should be considered before a proximal femoral megaprosthesis is used. First, these larger implants are far more expensive than standard arthroplasty or internal fixation implants; this much greater cost may be justified in patients with short life expectancies if the use of a less costly implant would

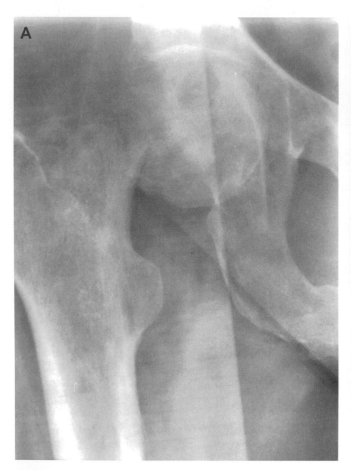 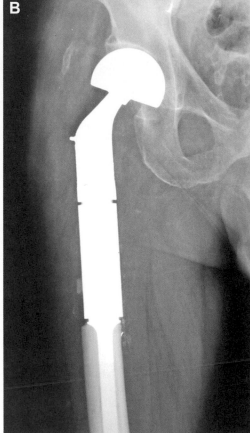

Figure 11.3. When there is extensive involvement of the femoral head, neck and peritrochanteric femur (A), a proximal femoral replacement prosthesis (B) can be considered

likely incur the costs of a second operation after failure. Second, the procedure is more extensive than intramedullary nailing or a standard prosthetic replacement, and the risk of bleeding, neurological injury and infection is higher. The problem of instability, particularly when combined with an acetabular component (inherent with the insertion of a megaprosthesis), has been previously discussed.

Long-term results for cemented large segmental replacement implants of the proximal femur have been favourable and are similar to those for conventional total hip arthroplasty. Sim et al. [27] reported on 140 patients (143 hips) in whom a proximal femoral prosthesis was inserted for various indications. In 77 patients (55%), results were excellent or good. Unsatisfactory results were instability and the need for a cane, both related to weak abductor muscles. In 82 patients, the overall complication rate was 46% (38 patients); this included 22 major complications (27%) and 16 minor complications (20%). Instability was observed in 10 patients (12%). Infection occurred in four patients (5%).

In the replacement of the proximal femur, an allograft–prosthetic composite may be an alternative to a metal device. An allograft–prosthetic composite may allow better restitution of mechanical function in the subtrochanteric area. However, success requires healing of the allograft to the host. An allograft–prosthetic composite is more likely to be considered for patients with primary malignant lesions or selected patients with solitary metastasis who have an overall favorable prognosis and will not require radiotherapy to the allograft–host junction. Jofe et al. [39] found excellent or good results after the reconstruction of the proximal femur with an allograft–prosthetic composite. There were far fewer complications than occurred with use of an allograft reconstruction alone (two failures in 13 patients vs. eight failures in 15 patients). However, others have reported less encouraging results for use of an allograft–prosthetic composite reconstruction. McGoveran et al. [40] suggested that only a few patients benefit from this technique, partly because of the risk of mechanical complications, which can be influenced by careful reconstruction. To identify factors in non-union, Kohles et al. [41] studied types of fixation in reconstructions of the proximal femur using allograft–prosthetic composites. They found that reconstructions with double-plate fixation and a cemented endoprosthesis were structurally stiffer and had greater stiffness at the osteotomy site than other reconstructions. Reconstructions with cement alone or cement and press-fit techniques generally were more compliant than others, structurally and at the osteotomy site.

Diaphyseal Femoral Fractures

One-third of metastatic lesions involving the femur are located in the femoral shaft or supracondylar region. For a pathological fracture of the femoral diaphysis, internal fixation is the procedure of choice. Even though small painful lesions in this region can be treated with radiation alone, the limb must be protected with partial weight-bearing. If the lesion is large and destructive, prophylactic fixation should be considered; if performed, the fracture should not be opened because the intramedullary device may lock statically. If a large amount of the cortex (more than 75% of its diameter) is destroyed, a more extensive procedure must be considered. In such cases the bone will not share any of the load and the nail will be subject to fatigue failure; therefore, the addition of intramedullary curettage and augmentation with methyl methacrylate is beneficial. Prosthetic replacement for lesions in the diaphysis is rarely indicated unless the proximal or distal aspect of the femur is involved.

Abudu et al. [42] reported good clinical and functional results for 18 patients with diaphyseal endoprosthesis reconstruction; 13 of these 18 reconstructions were performed in the femur. After a mean follow-up of 65 months, 77% of the patients achieved 80% or more of their premorbid functional capability. Mechanical loosening, limb shortening and secondary osteoarthritis were the most common complications. Malawer and Chou [43] reported on 82 patients who were treated with a large-segment prosthesis. They found acceptable prosthetic survival rates of 83% at 5 years and 67% at 10 years: 11/12 revisions were successful. The functional results were excellent or good.

Although total femoral replacement is rarely indicated, a total femoral prosthesis may be a realistic alternative to high amputation or hip disarticulation [44]. Ward et al. [45] concluded that total femoral replacement, although not commonly used, provided an option to hip disarticulation. Generally, function was better in younger patients.

Long-term problems with large-segment prostheses are similar to those with conventional total hip arthroplasty: stem loosening, fatigue failure of the metal component, bone resorption due to stress shielding, acetabular loosening, and osteolysis due to wear debris. Femoral stem loosening and cortical bone resorption are persistent problems that have been addressed through the concept of composite fixation, or extracortical bone bridging and ingrowth [46–50]. The concept of extracortical bone bridging was developed to manage the problem of loosening. New bone that forms across the bone–prosthesis junction is believed to improve fixation by controlling the transfer of stresses across the junction and by adding stability to the prosthesis. Shin et al [51] reported on 31 patients who had major reconstruction with devices using this concept. The extracortical bone bridging was maintained for more than 10 years; in one-third of patients more than 75% of the prosthetic circumference was involved.

Distal Femoral Fractures

Comminution and poor bone stock make pathological fractures involving the distal femur challenging problems. Surgical stabilisation is simplified if reconstruction is done before fracture and comminution occur. If their use is possible, condylar nail plate and dynamic screw plate devices, which are available in various lengths, have improved the management of lesions in this area. Augmentation of the device with methyl methacrylate is important because the bone stock in this region is usually poor. In brief, the lesions are curetted and the defects filled with methyl methacrylate. The reconstruction, then, is a composite of the bone remaining, methyl methacrylate and the internal fixation device. Occasionally, when the bone destruction is extensive or the adjacent knee joint is compromised, it is necessary to reconstruct the defect with a proximal femoral replacement or custom-made

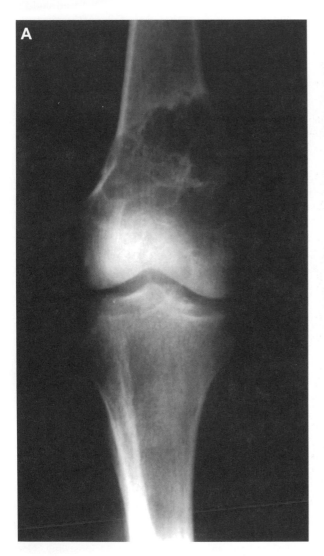
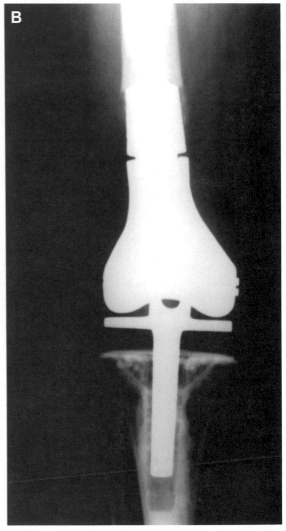

Figure 11.4.   Extensive metastatic lesions in the distal femur (A) can be treated with a prosthetic replacement (B)

total knee implant (Figure 11.4). In these cases, there are three indications for resection and reconstruction: (a) destruction of the articular cartilage such that a painless articulation is not feasible with an internal fixation device; (b) destruction of the metaphyseal bone such that rigid internal fixation is not attainable; and (c) lesion progression after irradiation (especially when progression has occurred after maximum irradiation and further irradiation would exceed normal tissue tolerances). The technique for and results of distal femoral replacement in the management of metastatic disease are similar to those in the management of primary bone tumour. For the prosthetic replacement of the distal femur, various devices provide satisfactory results.

Kawai et al. [52,53] reported the intermediate and long-term results of prosthetic replacement at the distal part of the femur. At a mean follow-up of 8 years, 20 early complications (45% of patients) occurred; aseptic loosening was the most frequent complication. The prosthetic survival rates were 85%, 67% and 48% at 3, 5 and 10 years, respectively. Adverse prognostic factors for prosthetic survival were male gender, resection of at least 40% of the femur, and fixation of the femoral stem with cement. The mean functional Musculoskeletal Tumor Society (MSTS) score was 24.

LEG

Proximal Tibial Fractures

Metastatic deposits in the tibia are not common. When identified early, most proximal lesions can be managed

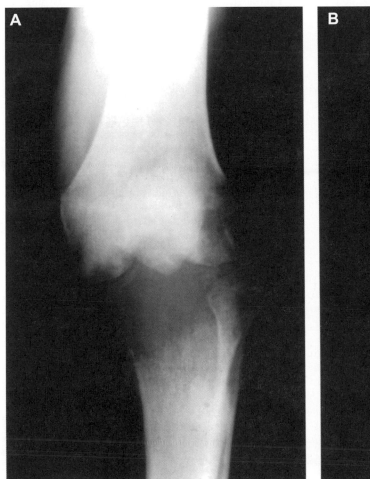
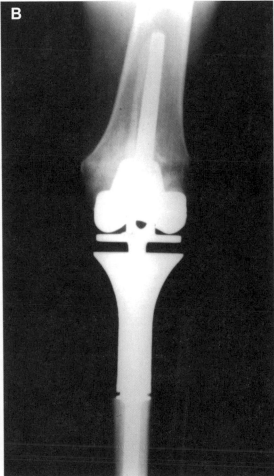

Figure 11.5. Extensive destruction of the proximal tibia, particularly when the weight-bearing articular surface is involved (A), can be treated with a prosthetic replacement (B)

by radiotherapy. Pathological fractures at the proximal tibia are treated in essentially the same way as are those of the distal femur [8]. Indications for prosthetic replacement in fractures of the distal femur apply to proximal tibial fractures as well (Figure 11.5). There is no place for prosthetic replacement in the management of midshaft or distal tibial lesions; these usually are managed with radiotherapy alone, plate and methyl methacrylate fixation, or intramedullary nailing.

Grimer et al. [54] reported on 151 patients with endoprosthetic replacement of the proximal tibia; the study covered a period of 20 years. The authors found that modern techniques of reconstruction at this anatomical site can produce good functional results with an acceptable level of risk. A major issue in prosthetic replacement of the proximal tibia is the type of reconstruction used for the extensor mechanism. Malawer and McHale [55] described a method for reconstructing the extensor mechanism that used a flap of the medial head of the gastrocnemius, which is widely used. Petschnig et al. [56] quantitatively measured the muscle function after reconstruction and found that the best knee extension and flexion strength was achieved with a combination of fibula transposition and gastrocnemius transfer. Prosthetic replacement of the distal leg is extremely rarely indicated but technically feasible. Six cases have been reported with a mean follow-up of 5.3 years [57]. There were two wound infections and one talar collapse. The mean International Symposium on Limb Salvage (ISOLS) score was 24%.

UPPER EXTREMITY

Humeral Fractures

From post mortem examinations of patients who died of metastatic cancer, it is known that the shoulder is involved in approximately 80% of cases. The upper extremity is involved in approximately 20% of cases [58,59]; when the upper extremity is involved, the proximal humerus is by far the most common site, with involvement at this site in approximately 50% of cases. Lesions below the elbow are extremely rare, accounting for less than 1% of osseous metastases. Treatment of upper extremity lesions is prophylactically provided to patients who are experiencing significant pain, who need a stable upper extremity to allow use of external aids, or who are at significant risk for a fracture. Metastatic involvement of the upper extremity interferes markedly with a patient's daily activities and care. Therefore, prophylactic fixation of impending

pathological fractures assumes importance, just as it does in cases of metastasis to the lower extremity. Patients in whom a pathological fracture develops are treated surgically to relieve pain and restore function; a flail upper extremity is usually painful and non-functional, and in many cases conservative management of a pathological fracture does not confer stability or promote healing.

The humerus is the most frequently involved bone in the upper extremity and can be considered as three separate anatomical regions: the humeral head, the humeral shaft and the distal humerus.

Humeral Head

Pathological fractures of the proximal humerus typically occur after extensive destruction of the humeral head and adjacent metaphysis. With rare exceptions, metastatic involvement of the humeral head is best treated with unipolar humeral replacement. Total shoulder replacement usually is not necessary because intra-articular or glenoid metastatic involvement is rare. If involvement includes the upper shaft of the humerus, additional alternatives must be considered. These include proximal humeral replacement with custom components [43,60–65] conventional shoulder replacement using humeral components and intramedullary nails that extend into the uninvolved humerus, use of an allograft–prosthetic composite (Figure 11.6) or use of a free vascularised fibular graft attached through a sling to the acromion to preserve passive scapulohumeral movement [66].

Bos et al. [60] reported on 18 patients who had a proximal humeral reconstruction. The instability rate in this series was high; 10 shoulders had a subluxation and 12 needed a revision. Moeckel et al. [63] reported good to excellent results for reconstruction using a modular hemiarthroplasty. Modular design allows improved soft tissue tensioning and therefore the possibility of a lower instability rate. Osteoarticular allografts for the reconstruction of the upper extremity no longer are used routinely [67] because long-term results have been unsatisfactory; also, recovery time is longer than that required when a prosthesis alone is used. The patient's expected survival time may help determine which device is preferable. An allograft–prosthetic composite allows the attachment of soft tissues to the allograft bone, which may be an advantage. Large custom-made humeral implants have no formal provision for allowing rotator cuff advancement and are therefore less stable.

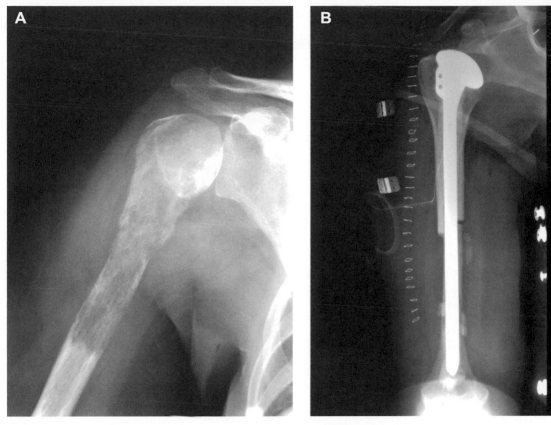

Figure 11.6. For extensive lesions of the proximal humerus (A), one salvage option is the use of an allograft–prosthetic composite (B)

O'Connor et al. [64] analysed various reconstructive procedures at the shoulder girdle for primary bone tumours. Good function was provided by an osteo-articular allograft inserted after intra-articular resection of the proximal aspect of the humerus with preservation of the abductor mechanism. Also, function was superior to that found after reconstruction with a proximal humeral prosthesis. Jensen and Johnston [62] reported on proximal humeral reconstruction with a combination of a long-stemmed cemented Neer prosthesis and allograft or autograft. Function was rated as excellent for 17 patients and good for two patients. There were no failures of fixation, except for two recurrent subluxations and one dislocation.

Harrington [13] reported the use of a large proximal femoral prosthesis or a total hip prosthesis to create inherent stability of the shoulder joint. This approach was used particularly if there was destruction of the rotator cuff and its attachments or there was variable destruction of the glenoid.

Humeral Shaft

Pathological fractures of the humeral shaft are problematic because the humerus is almost entirely cortical at this location and has a very small intramedullary canal. When destruction is sufficient to cause a fracture, bony union fails to occur, even with adequate fixation and in the absence of extensive local post-operative irradiation. The Mirels [3] system for assessing fracture risk in long bones also is applied for assessing risk of fracture caused by metastatic lesions in the upper extremity, particularly at the diaphyseal site. The nature of involvement of the humeral shaft determines whether an open or a closed procedure should be used. Impending pathological fractures of the humeral shaft can be treated effectively with anterograde or retrograde closed intramedullary nailing, performed under fluoroscopic control [68]. Pathological fractures of the humerus often warrant open reduction, removal of the tumour, and augmentation of a selected fixation device with methyl methacrylate. However, unlike the femur, the humerus is subjected to repeated distraction forces that tend to cause separation of the fracture fragments if small intramedullary fixation devices have been used [13]. Another option for the management of humeral shaft fracture is resection combined with shortening if the lesion is less than 4 cm in diameter and if there is no evidence of involvement in the proximal or distal segment. However, shortening of 2 cm or more causes a marked reduction of triceps force [69]. For an isolated diaphyseal metastasis that is larger than 4 cm in diameter, reconstruction by an intercalary prosthesis cemented into the remaining proximal and distal segments is possible [32].

Diaphyseal spacers also may be used in selected cases after internal fixation with other types of devices has failed. There are modular systems that allow the selection of the appropriately sized spacer at the time of operation (Figure 11.7) [70]. Damron et al. [71] reviewed the outcome in 17 cases in which reconstruction with a cemented modular intercalary humeral spacer was used to manage impending fracture, pathological fracture or failure of attempted internal fixation. In these cases an initial prototype was used; radiographic analysis showed that, because of the limited selection of stem lengths, 76% of the distal stems and 47% of the proximal stems were shorter than the ideal length. This has been corrected with the newer designs. Temporary radial nerve injury was the most common complication (three patients). There were three implant failures and two periprosthetic fractures. However, in 88% of the patients, the cemented spacer achieved the goals of immediate and stable humeral fixation, pain relief, and early return of function. Therefore, the use of a diaphyseal spacer is a good option in selected cases.

Distal Humerus

Because of the marked flattening and thinning of bone at the olecranon fossa, supracondylar fractures are particularly difficult to treat. Involvement at or just above the condyles may be best treated with rush rods introduced from the medial and lateral epicondyles. Another option for reconstruction in this area is the use of pelvic reconstruction or periarticular distal humerus plates, reinforced with methyl methacrylate on the medial and lateral columns. In selected cases, a total elbow arthroplasty after tumour resection provides marked pain relief and improvement in function (Figure 11.8) [72]. If the lesion on the distal humerus

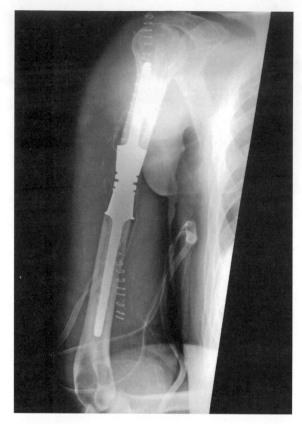

Figure 11.7. An intercalary modular prosthetic design is used for isolated humeral diaphyseal lesions larger than 4 cm, or as a salvage procedure after failed intramedullary nailing with local progression of disease

is so extensive that it cannot be reconstructed with the mentioned approaches, it is preferable to perform reconstruction using a modular prosthesis, a composite allograft–total elbow prosthesis, or an allograft replacement with internal fixation.

Lesions of the Radius and Ulna

Lesions of the radius or ulna may be excised without major reconstructive efforts or managed by radiotherapy alone. There is no indication for prosthetic replacement at this anatomical site.

SUMMARY

In summary, surgical management of long bone metastasis requires considerations pertinent to the

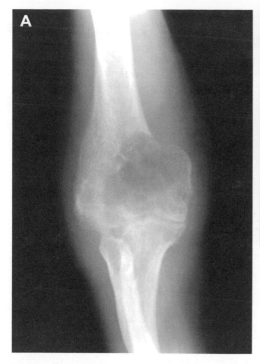

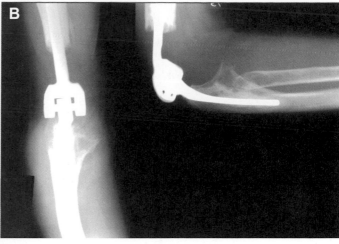

Figure 11.8. For a metastatic lesion that cannot be reconstructed with plates and methyl methacrylate (A), a total elbow replacement (B) is indicated

particular anatomical location and the particular patient. For lesions involving the femoral head and neck, prosthetic replacement is the procedure of choice. Intertrochanteric pathological fractures pose a difficult problem because of neoplastic destruction of the cortex. The surgical repair of peritrochanteric pathological fractures appears controversial. Currently, internal fixation is most commonly advocated if the integrity of the head and neck fragment can allow secure fixation. However, replacement arthroplasty for these lesions is being used more widely. The mechanics of the subtrochanteric region and the associated bone loss have resulted in a high failure rate for internal fixation that uses a dynamic hip screw; however, major advances have been made with the development of third-generation intramedullary nail devices. Prosthetic replacement of the proximal femur may be indicated in patients with extensive destruction and bone stock that cannot provide secure fixation.

The authors cannot overemphasise the importance of a multidisciplinary approach to the treatment of patients with metastatic bone disease. Post-operative radiotherapy to minimise progression of disease and hardware failure, consideration of the use of bisphosphonates and chemotherapy, analgesia, and

management of multiple medical co-morbidities is best carried out in collaboration with experts in these fields.

REFERENCES

1. Harrington KD. Metastatic disease of the spine. J Bone Joint Surg Am 1986; 68: 1110–15.
2. Galasko CSB. The anatomy and pathways of skeletal metastases. In Weiss L, Gilbert HA (eds), Bone Metastasis. GK Hall Medical Publishers: Boston, MA, 1981: 49–63.
3. Mirels H. Metastatic disease in long bones. A proposed scoring system for diagnosing impending pathologic fractures. Clin Orthop 1989; 249: 256–64.
4. Harrington KD. Impending pathologic fractures from metastatic malignancy: evaluation and management. Instr Course Lect 1986; 35: 357–81.
5. Lane JM, Sculco TP, Zolan S. Treatment of pathological fractures of the hip by endoprosthetic replacement. J Bone Joint Surg Am 1980; 62: 954–9.
6. Levy RN, Sherry HS, Siffert RS. Surgical management of metastatic disease of bone at the hip. Clin Orthop 1982; 169: 62–9.
7. Habermann ET, Sachs R, Stern RE et al. The pathology and treatment of metastatic disease of the femur. Clin Orthop 1982; 169: 70–82.
8. Sim FH. Lesions of the pelvis and hip. In Sim FH (ed.), Diagnosis and Management of Metastatic Bone Disease: a Multidisciplinary Approach. Raven: New York, 1988; 183–98.

9. Clarke HD, Damron TA, Sim FH. Head and neck replacement endoprosthesis for pathologic proximal femoral lesions. Clin Orthop 1998; 353: 210–17.

10. Haentjens P, De Neve W, Opdecam P. Prosthetic replacement for pathological fractures of the proximal end of the femur: total prosthesis or bipolar arthroplasty [in French]. Rev Chir Orthop Reparatrice Appar Mot 1994; 80: 493–502.

11. Morris HG, Capanna R, Del Ben M, Campanacci D. Prosthetic reconstruction of the proximal femur after resection for bone tumors. J Arthroplasty 1995; 10: 293–9.

12. Rock MG. The use of Bateman bipolar proximal femoral replacement in the management of proximal femoral metastatic disease. In Enneking WF, Jenett EL (eds), Limb Salvage in Musculoskeletal Oncology. Bristol-Myers/Zimmer Orthopaedic Symposium. Churchill Livingstone: New York, 1987: 437–42.

13. Harrington KD. Orthopaedic management of extremity and pelvic lesions. Clin Orthop 1995; 312: 136–47.

14. Yazawa Y, Frassica FJ, Chao EY et al. Metastatic bone disease. A study of the surgical treatment of 166 pathologic humeral and femoral fractures. Clin Orthop 1990; 251: 213–19.

15. Patterson BM, Healey JH, Cornell CN, Sharrock NE. Cardiac arrest during hip arthroplasty with a cemented long-stem component. A report of seven cases. J Bone Joint Surg Am 1991; 73: 271–7.

16. Algan SM, Horowitz SM. Surgical treatment of pathologic hip lesions in patients with metastatic disease. Clin Orthop 1996; 332: 223–31.

17. Finn HA. Hip and proximal femur. In Simon MA, Springfield D (eds), Surgery for Bone and Soft-tissue Tumors. Lippincott-Raven: Philadelphia, PA, 1998: 683–703.

18. Johnsson R, Carlsson A, Kisch K et al. Function following mega total hip arthroplasty compared with conventional total hip arthroplasty and healthy matched controls. Clin Orthop 1985; 192: 159–67.

19. Kabukcuoglu Y, Grimer RJ, Tillman RM, Carter SR. Endoprosthetic replacement for primary malignant tumors of the proximal femur. Clin Orthop 1999; 358: 8–14.

20. Khong KS, Chao EYS, Sim FH. Long-term performance of custom prosthetic replacement for neoplastic disease of the proximal femur. In Yamamuro T (ed.), New Developments for Limb Salvage in Musculoskeletal Tumors; Kyocera Orthopaedic Symposium. Springer-Verlag: Tokyo, 1989: 403–12.

21. Rechl H, Reinisch M, Plötz W et al. Soft tissue reconstruction about the proximal femur. Oper Techn Orthop 1999; 9: 115–20.

22. Ward WG, Johnston KS, Dorey FJ, Eckardt JJ. Extramedullary porous coating to prevent diaphyseal osteolysis and radiolucent lines around proximal tibial replacements. A preliminary report. J Bone Joint Surg Am 1993; 75: 976–87.

23. Zehr RJ, Enneking WF, Scarborough MT. Allograft–prosthesis composite versus megaprosthesis in proximal femoral reconstruction. Clin Orthop 1996; 322: 207–23.

24. Bickels J, Meller I, Henshaw RM, Malawer MM. Reconstruction of hip stability after proximal and total femur resections. Clin Orthop 2000; 375: 218–30.

25. Masterson EL, Ferracini R, Griffin AM et al. Capsular replacement with synthetic mesh: effectiveness in preventing postoperative dislocation after wide resection of proximal femoral tumors and prosthetic reconstruction. J Arthroplasty 1998; 13: 860–6.

26. Gottsauner-Wolf F, Egger EL, Giurea A et al. Biologic attachment of an allograft bone and tendon transplant to a titanium prosthesis. Clin Orthop 1999; 358: 101–10.

27. Sim FH, Frassica FJ, Chao EY. Orthopaedic management using new devices and prostheses. Clin Orthop 1995; 312: 160–72.

28. Unwin PS, Cannon SR, Grimer RJ et al. Aseptic loosening in cemented custom-made prosthetic replacements for bone tumours of the lower limb. J Bone Joint Surg Br 1996; 78: 5–13.

29. Hsu RW, Sim FH, Chao EY. Reoperation results after segmental prosthetic replacement of bone and joint for limb salvage. J Arthroplasty 1999; 14: 519–26.

30. Wirganowicz PZ, Eckardt JJ, Dorey FJ et al. Etiology and results of tumor endoprosthesis revision surgery in 64 patients. Clin Orthop 1999; 358: 64–74.

31. Shin DS, Weber KL, Chao EY et al. Reoperation for failed prosthetic replacement used for limb salvage. Clin Orthop 1999; 358: 53–63.

32. Chin HC, Frassica FJ, Hein TJ et al. Metastatic diaphyseal fractures of the shaft of the humerus. The structural strength evaluation of a new method of treatment with a segmental defect prosthesis. Clin Orthop 1989; 248: 231–9.

33. Fielding JW. Subtrochanteric fractures. Clin Orthop 1973; 92: 86–99.

34. Fielding JW, Magliato HJ. Subtrochanteric fractures. Surg Gynecol Obstet 1966; 122: 555–60.

35. Delepine G, Hernigou P, Goutallier D, Delepine N. Orthopedic results of 87 massive allografts in reconstructive surgery for bone cancers. In Aebi M, Regazzoni P (eds), Bone Transplantation. Springer-Verlag: Heidelberg, 1989: 331–2.

36. Linclau L, Dokter G. Osteosynthesis of pathologic fractures and prophylactic internal fixation of metastases in long bones. Acta Orthop Belg 1992; 58: 330–5.

37. Zickel RE, Mouradian WH. Intramedullary fixation of pathological fractures and lesions of the subtrochanteric region of the femur. J Bone Joint Surg Am 1976; 58: 1061–6.

38. Harrington KD, Sim FH, Enis JE et al. Methylmethacrylate as an adjunct in internal fixation of pathological fractures. Experience with three hundred and seventy-five cases. J Bone Joint Surg Am 1976; 58: 1047–55.

39. Jofe MH, Gebhardt MC, Tomford WW, Mankin HJ. Reconstruction for defects of the proximal part of the femur using allograft arthroplasty. J Bone Joint Surg Am 1988; 70: 507–16.

40. McGoveran BM, Davis AM, Gross AE, Bell RS. Evaluation of the allograft–prosthesis composite technique for proximal femoral reconstruction after resection of a primary bone tumour. Can J Surg 1999; 42: 37–45.

41. Kohles SS, Markel MD, Rock MG et al. Mechanical evaluation of six types of reconstruction following 25%, 50% and 75% resection of the proximal femur. J Orthop Res 1994; 12: 834–43.

42. Abudu A, Carter SR, Grimer RJ. The outcome and functional results of diaphyseal endoprostheses after tumour excision. J Bone Joint Surg Br 1996; 78: 652–7.

43. Malawer MM, Chou LB. Prosthetic survival and clinical results with use of large-segment replacements in the treatment of high-grade bone sarcomas. J Bone Joint Surg Am 1995; 77: 1154–65.

44. Steinbrink K, Engelbrecht E, Fenelon GC. The total femoral prosthesis. A preliminary report. J Bone Joint Surg Br 1982; 64: 305–12.

45. Ward WG, Dorey F, Eckardt JJ. Total femoral endoprosthetic reconstruction. Clin Orthop 1995; 316: 195–206.

46. Chao EY. A composite fixation principle for modular segmental defect replacement (SDR) prostheses. Orthop Clin North Am 1989; 20: 439–53.

47. Chao EY, Sim FH. Modular prosthetic system for segmental bone and joint replacement after tumor resection. Orthopedics 1985; 8: 641–51.

48. Chao EYS, Sim FH. Composite fixation of salvage prostheses for the hip and knee. Clin Orthop 1992; 276: 91–101.

49. Heck DA, Chao EY, Sim FH et al. Titanium fibermetal segmental replacement prostheses. A radiographic analysis and review of current status. Clin Orthop 1986; 204: 266–85.

50. Okada Y, Suka T, Sim FH et al. Comparison of replacement prostheses for segmental defects of bone. Different porous coatings for extracortical fixation. J Bone Joint Surg Am 1988; 70: 160–72.

51. Shin DS, Choong PF, Chao EY, Sim FH. Large tumor endoprostheses and extracortical bone-bridging: 28 patients followed 10–20 years. Acta Orthop Scand 2000; 71: 305–11.

52. Kawai A, Healey JH, Boland PJ et al. A rotating-hinge knee replacement for malignant tumors of the femur and tibia. J Arthroplasty 1999; 14: 187–96.

53. Kawai A, Muschler GF, Lane JM et al. Prosthetic knee replacement after resection of a malignant tumor of the distal part of the femur. Medium- to long-term results. J Bone Joint Surg Am 1998; 80: 636–47.

54. Grimer RJ, Carter SR, Tillman RM et al. Endoprosthetic replacement of the proximal tibia. J Bone Joint Surg Br 1999; 81: 488–94.

55. Malawer MM, McHale KA. Limb-sparing surgery for high-grade malignant tumors of the proximal tibia. Surgical technique and a method of extensor mechanism reconstruction. Clin Orthop 1989; 239: 231–48.

56. Petschnig R, Baron R, Kotz R et al. Muscle function after endoprosthetic replacement of the proximal tibia. Different techniques for extensor reconstruction in 17 tumor patients. Acta Orthop Scand 1995; 66: 266–70.

57. Lee SH, Kim HS, Park YB et al. Prosthetic reconstruction for tumours of the distal tibia and fibula. J Bone Joint Surg Br 1999; 81: 803–7.

58. Clain A. Secondary malignant disease of bone. Br J Cancer 1965; 19: 15–29.

59. Jaffe HL. Tumors and Tumorous Conditions of the Bones and Joints. Lea & Febiger: Philadelphia, 1958.

60. Bos G, Sim F, Pritchard D et al. Prosthetic replacement of the proximal humerus. Clin Orthop 1987; 224: 178–91.

61. Burrows HJ, Wilson JN, Scales JT. Excision of tumours of humerus and femur, with restoration by internal prostheses. J Bone Joint Surg Br 1975; 57: 148–59.

62. Jensen KL, Johnston JO. Proximal humeral reconstruction after excision of a primary sarcoma. Clin Orthop 1995; 311: 164–75.

63. Moeckel BH, Dines DM, Warren RF, Altchek DW. Modular hemiarthroplasty for fractures of the proximal part of the humerus. J Bone Joint Surg Am 1992; 74: 884–9.

64. O'Connor MI, Sim FH, Chao EY. Limb salvage for neoplasms of the shoulder girdle. Intermediate reconstructive and functional results. J Bone Joint Surg Am 1996; 78: 1872–88.

65. Ross AC, Wilson JN, Scales JT. Endoprosthetic replacement of the proximal humerus. J Bone Joint Surg Br 1987; 69: 656–61.

66. Wada T, Usui M, Isu K et al. Reconstruction and limb salvage after resection for malignant bone tumour of the proximal humerus. A sling procedure using a free vascularised fibular graft. J Bone Joint Surg Br 1999; 81: 808–13.

67. Getty PJ, Peabody TD. Complications and functional outcomes of reconstruction with an osteoarticular allograft after intra-articular resection of the proximal aspect of the humerus. J Bone Joint Surg Am 1999; 81: 1138–46.

68. Redmond BJ, Biermann JS, Blasier RB. Interlocking intramedullary nailing of pathological fractures of the shaft of the humerus. J Bone Joint Surg Am 1996; 78: 891–6.

69. Hughes RE, Schneeberger AG, An KN et al. Reduction of triceps muscle force after shortening of the distal humerus: a computational model. J Shoulder Elbow Surg 1997; 6: 444–8.

70. Frassica FJ, Sim FH, Chao EY. Primary malignant bone tumors of the shoulder girdle: surgical technique of resection and reconstruction. Am Surg 1987; 53: 264–9.

71. Damron TA, Sim FH, Shives TC et al. Intercalary spacers in the treatment of segmentally destructive diaphyseal humeral lesions in disseminated malignancies. Clin Orthop 1996; 324: 233–43.

72. Sperling JW, Pritchard DJ, Morrey BF. Total elbow arthroplasty after resection of tumors at the elbow. Clin Orthop 1999; 367: 256–61.

12

Osteosynthesis for Pathological Fractures in Long Bones

P. D. S. Dijkstra and A. H. M. Taminiau

Leiden University Medical Centre, Leiden, The Netherlands

GENERAL INTRODUCTION

Skeletal metastases are the most common form of malignant bone tumours and have probably occurred for many thousands of years [1]. It was probably Wiseman in 1676 who first described "rotting the bones under them" as the effects of skeletal metastases [2]. In 1824 Cooper described several cases of breast cancer with bone metastasis and development of actual pathological fractures [3]. In three-quarters of patients with skeletal metastases the primary tumour is breast, bronchus, prostate and kidney carcinoma [4,5]. The incidence increases due to prolonged survival as a result of more effective treatment of the primary tumours [6,7].

Post mortem examination of various carcinomas has shown skeletal metastases in 27% of patients [8]. In patients with disseminated breast cancer, radiographic evidence of bone metastases can be found in 30–60%; about 80% have bone metastases at post mortem [8–10]. Most bone metastases are located in the axial skeleton: spine, pelvis, ribs, sacrum, skull, scapula and sternum [10,11]. The femur is the most common site in the peripheral skeleton, followed by the humerus [12]. Tibia, foot and radius are less commonly involved, and metastases of the ulna or hand are rare [13]. The proximal parts of the long bones are the most likely to be affected.

Actual pathological fractures occur in 1–2% of all patients with a malignant disease [14,15]. Furthermore, metastases of the long bones progress to pathological fractures in about 25%, but this risk is much higher in the proximal femur (40–60%), where mechanical load is high [16–18]. The mean age of cancer patients with a pathological fracture is 61 years, the female:male ratio is 4:1, and in 6% a bilateral fracture should be surgically treated. Survival analysis of various cancer patients with an actual pathological fracture of the tibia, femur and humerus showed half of the patients alive after 16.5, 9 and 4.5 months, respectively [19]. Peripheral bone metastases can be asymptomatic, particularly in prostatic cancer. If they are symptomatic, pain, usually at night or during physical stress, is the main clinical sign in about 75% of patients [20,21].

Pathological fractures of the long bones are not life-threatening but can greatly influence the patient's quality of life. The goals of palliative treatment are to achieve rapid relief of pain, reduce anxiety and depression in these already sick patients, facilitate nursing care, and restore the function of the limb. Rigid fixation with adjuvant bone cement for immediate stability and pain relief, even in the face of extensive and widespread bone destruction, is valuable [16,22–26]. In addition, impending pathological fractures can be predicted and treated prophylactically [16–19,27–30].

Although there are improved surgical, radiological and chemotherapeutic techniques in the management of secondary neoplastic deposits in the long bones, the problem arises of whether and when prophylactic internal fixation should be carried out. The benefits of surgical treatment of an impending pathological fracture of the long bones had already been confirmed

Textbook of Bone Metastases. Edited by C. Jasmin, R. E. Coleman, L. R. Coia, R. Capanna and G. Saillant
© 2005 John Wiley & Sons Ltd: ISBN 0 471 87742 5

by Griesmann and Schüttemeyer in 1947, long before guidelines to prophylactic surgical treatment were developed [31]. The survival of these surgically treated patients is highly variable [32,33]. However, after surgical treatment of pathological fracture in patients with a variety of skeletal metastases in the extremities the survival rate at 1 year is one-third [34].

BIOCHEMICAL CONSIDERATIONS

Considerable forces and moments act in many different ways on the long bones and the adjacent joints during a variety of physical activities [35]. In these physically compromised patients with bone metastases in the long bones, a pathological fracture can occur spontaneously or after a minor trauma [36]. During physical activities in this specific patient group, the axial and bending loading of the femur is less significant than torsional loading [37].

Concerning a cortical defect in the long bone, the influence of torsion loads increases compared to axial and bending loads, especially when the velocity of torque is reduced [38,39]. Frankel and Burstein reported that a single saw-cut one-fifth of the length of embalmed tibiae decreased the maximal 70% energy absorption in the 12 pairs tested. Increasing the width of these saw-cuts to one-half and full bone diameter did not cause further weakening [40]. These results are in close agreement with our recent findings [37]. If a longitudinal cortical defect is larger than the bone diameter, a sudden increase in strength reduction occurred in torsional loading; this is called an "open-section effect" (Figure 12.1) [41]. But these measured strength reductions due to the open-section effect are less dramatic than those described in the engineering literature.

Cortical defects smaller than the bone diameter are described as "stress riser lesions" (Figure 12.2) [42]. In these smaller defects, strength reduction is dependent on width and length, often found by a linear strength reduction to the diameter of the defect [43,44]. Burchardt et al. found no significant effect of the ratio of a very small defect, suggesting a critical size of the defect below which no large stress concentration occurs [45]. Besides the applied forces of the long bone, changes in structure and mechanical properties are also of particular importance. In intact long bones these changes are due to trabecular and cortical osteoporosis and different sizes and geometry of the bone [46,47]. Clark et al. found that oblong holes withstand more torque than rectangular holes with square corners [48]. Experimental studies reported a reduction of the torsion strength for a long period after irradiation of intact or fractured long bones [49,50].

Bone metastases of the long bones occur in a large variety of appearances; sharp and rough boundaries, partial cortical destruction, different geometries and local osteoporosis [51,52]. In daily life the femur will be subject to repetitive loads of various magnitudes in multiple directions [53,54]. In addition, fracture initiation is caused by gradual formation and/or growth of micro-cracks [55]. The clinical implications of the biomechanical studies briefly described above are still limited.

Recently, promising results have been achieved by combining CT scan data and finite element modelling in the prediction of strength reduction in long bones with metastasis-like defects [37,51,56,57]. It seems that both the width and the length of the cortical destruction influences the strength reduction, and this

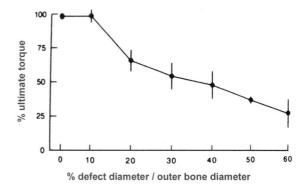

Figure 12.2. Changes in strength in torsional loading of femora with cortical holes of different diameters in percentage of intact bone. Edgerton et al. showed that there is a critical cortical circular defect between 10% and 20% of the outer bone diameter at which a sharp drop in strength reduction occurred. From Edgerton BC, An K, Morrey BF [44] Torsional strength reduction due to cortical defects in bone. J Orthop Res 1990; 8: 851–5

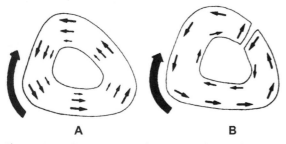

Figure 12.1. Stress pattern in open-section and closed-section in long bone during torsional loading. (A) In closed-section all shear stress resists the applied torque. (B) The concept of an open-section cortical lesion. A smaller area of bone (only the outer bone area) is able to resist the shear stress distribution to the applied torque, resulting in a high reduction of load to failure. From Frankel VH, Burstein AH [41]. Orthopaedic Biomechanics. Lea & Febiger, Philadelphia, PA, 1970

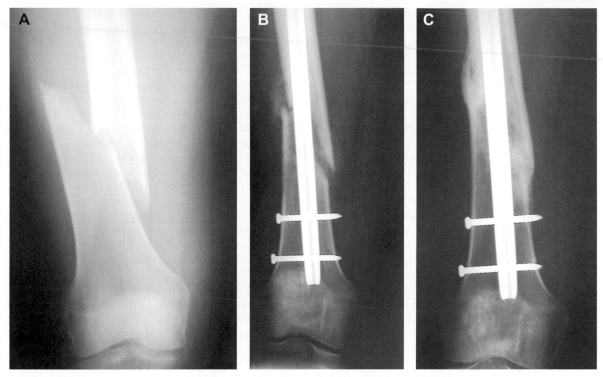

Figure 12.3. Anteroposterior roentgenogram (A) of the right knee in a 66 year-old women with metastatic breast carcinoma. A permeative bone destruction at the distal junction diaphysis to supracondylar region with an oblique actual pathological fracture. On screening no other lesion was detected at this limb. A reamed nail with bipolar fixation and postoperative irradiation was performed. Two months after surgery there was marginal bone reaction (B), but one year post-operatively full union was obtained (C)

could provide a good additional method of predicting the risk of fracture of a cortical lesion in the near future.

PROPHYLACTIC TREATMENT

Nowadays, prophylactic treatment of impending pathological fractures is generally preferred instead of treatment of actual fractures. Treatment additional to surgery can be radiotherapy, humoral therapy or chemotherapy.

Radiotherapy is the treatment of choice in patients with localised pain due to proven metastases. The response to irradiation in terms of pain relief, decrease of size and bone remodelling was studied in 1016 patients, of whom 759 had bone metastases. After irradiation (20–40 Gy) slight pain relief was found in 90% and complete relief in 54% [58]. However, it should be stressed that if consolidation of a lytic metastatic defect after irradiation therapy occurs, this

usually takes several months [59–61]. Also, radio-insensitive tumours are not uncommon [60]. One-third of patients with different sizes of metastatic lesions in the long bones who are irradiated subsequently fractured within a period of 6 months, which is related to the dose of irradiation [30,62]. It should be borne in mind that irradiation gives transient local osteoporosis during the second week after initiation, and irradiation suppresses the chondrogenetic phase of secondary ossification [60,63]. The effect of radiotherapy on preventing fractures is uncertain, and is dependent on several factors, such as site of the metastasis and life expectancy. The administration of radiation (single dose and multiple fractions, width of irradiation field) after surgical fixation and the expected response remains unclear [64]. Despite these caveats, irradiation of impending or actual pathological fractures is generally considered standard therapy after surgical fixation, starting 1 week after surgery (Figure 12.3) [65,66]. After intramedullary fixation the entire long bone should be irradiated. In the follow-up after surgical fixation, irradiation therapy to the treated long bone should be given when there is local progression of tumour adjacent to the device, with or without pain [37].

Systemic administration of strontium-89 (^{89}Sr) should be considered in patients without a predominantly painful site, as a first-line therapy [67]

Another prophylactic treatment of pathological fractures due to bone metastasis could be the use of bisphosphonates, which inhibits bone resorption. Long-term administration of this drug showed reduction of the occurrence of fractures and of bone pain [68].

Prophylactic surgery of impending pathological fractures is generally preferred, because of important advantages; quick relief of pain, earlier mobility, decreased hospital stay and reduction of operative complications [19,69]. Modern anaesthesia makes surgery possible in these patients with often poor general condition [70]. Because of the weakened bone, while positioning the anaesthetised patient or during the procedure particular care must be taken to avoid producing a fracture.

Although there is much contradiction in the guidelines to prophylactic surgery of the long bones, there are four main indications for surgery used in clinical practice [17,27,29,30,71–74]: (a) a lytic lesion of 25 mm or larger; (b) circumferential cortical destruction of 50% or more; (c) an osteolytic lesion (including permeative lesions); (d) persistent pain on weight-bearing or local progression after irradiation, humoral therapy or chemotherapy.

These guidelines have arisen from several, often small, retrospective clinical studies (Table 12.1). The first study in the early 1960s, conducted by Beals et al., looked at 19 pathological fractures of the femur due to breast metastases. They noted that 58% of these fractures were predictable when there was a well-defined cortical lesion of 2.5 cm in diameter or when a lesion of this size was painful, regardless of its bony location [17]. However, in another clinical study using these criteria, no differences were found between fracture and non-fracture patients who were receiving radiation therapy [79]. The guideline of 50% cortical destruction was originally defined after a retrospective study by Parrish and Murray, based on only four patients who were considered to have an impending fracture [72]. Fidler also reported that the risk of fracture correlated with the degree of circumferential cortical destruction [29]. Several years later he reviewed 66 patients with 100 consecutive metastases in long bones [71]. If less than 50% of the circumferential cortex was destroyed, the risk fracture was unlikely. A sudden rise in fracture incidence occurred when ≥50% of the cortex of a long bone was involved, resulting in a fracture incidence of 3.7% when 25–50% of the cortex was involved and 61% when the degree of involvement was 50–75%.

For lesions difficult to measure, a tube of paper was used to represent diameter of the bone and the outline of the lesion was drawn on the tube. After unrolling the tube the percentage of cortical involvement expressed as the perimeter of bone lesion was divided by the periosteal perimeter. The accuracy of this method is unclear. Nowadays, CT imaging may be of help in assessing the degree of bone destruction. Zickel and Mouradian attempted to identify a lesion at risk in the subtrochanteric region of the femur in 34 patients with metastatic disease [75]. They concluded that the size of the lesion did not correlate with the likelihood of fracture; even small parts of cortical destruction in the subtrochanteric region places the femur at high risk

Table 12.1. Literature review of femoral bone lesions at risk of fracturing. [a]Despite radiotherapy; [b]including pathological humerus

Reference	Lesions (actual fractures)	Pain	Radiographic lytic aspect	Circumferential bone destruction (%)	Size of cortical lesion (mm)	Longitudinal cortical destruction (mm)
Parrish [72]	108 (104)[b]	↑	+	+ ≥50		
Beals [17]	60 (19)	+			+ ≥25	
Zickel [75]	46 (35)	↑	+		+ ≥?	
Fidler [71]	87 (32)		+	+ ≥50	+ ≥25	
Miller [76]	136 (15)		+	+ ≥25	+ ≥20	
Keene [77]	516 (26)	−		−		+ ≥?
Menck [74]	69 (69)	−	+	+ ≥50		+ ≥30
Mirels [30]	78 (27)[b]	↑		+ ≥67		
Yazawa [16]	120 (71)	+	+	+ ≥50		
Dijkstra [78]	54 (19)	↑				+ ≥38

for fracture and warrants prophylactic fixations. Based on clinical and experimental studies, Dijkstra et al. produced criteria for prophylactic treatment for lytic lesion in the subtrochanteric region: (a) increasing local pain despite analgesics and/or radiotherapy; (b) a ratio of maximal longitudinal cortex destruction to bone width exceeding 1 [37]. In addition, longitudinal cortical destruction of more than 3 cm diameter is a reliable predictive value of metastatic femoral lesions, as described by Menck et al. in accurate measurements of 69 actual femur fractures [74]. Several investigators have considered the difficulty of accurate measurements of these long bone lesions [73,77]. Errors of as much as 100% can occur when measuring very simple diaphyseal defects from plain radiographs [80]. In general, the literature demonstrates that 45–60% of the metastatic lesions of the long bones are visible by using radiographs [16,77,78]. Furthermore, Keene et al. analysed 516 metastatic lesions of the proximal femur in patients with breast carcinoma [77]. They found no consistent relationship between the size of a measurable lesion on anteroposterior X-ray and their propensity to fracture; pre-fracture pain was not a reliable sign, and there was no difference in outcome among lytic, mixed or blastic lesions.

Because there are major limitations in the predictive capabilities of pain and measurable destruction by the tumour on radiographs, Mirels proposed a weighted scoring system to quantify the risk of sustaining a pathological fracture in a long bone [30]. The system is based on a retrospective study of 78 irradiated metastatic bone lesions; it assigned points to the following four variables (Table 12.2); (a) the location of the lesion; (b) the degree of pain caused by the lesion; (c) the type of lesion; (d) the degree of cortical involvement by the lesion. Mirels' data indicated that on a scale of 12 points, a score of ≤7 is a low-risk lesion. A score of 8 is associated with a 15% risk for fracture, while the fracture risk is 33% in patients with a score of 9. Mirels concluded that a score of 8 or more is an indication for prophylactic fixation.

PREOPERATIVE WORK-UP

In patients with known primary tumours and suspicion of bone metastasis, the diagnosis should be confirmed by cytology, core- or open biopsy [81]. In skeletal lesions without a known primary tumour, oncological work-up (scintigraphy/MRI) should precede the biopsy. A number of ancillary techniques have been developed over recent years (immunohistochemistry, cytogenetics and molecular genetic techniques) that will unravel tumour-specific features and are helpful in confirming the diagnosis.

An impending or actual pathological fracture can be the first sign of malignancy. In general, in cases of unknown primary tumours screening is limited to carcinoma of the breast, lung, renal, prostate and thyroid [19]. Prior to intramedullary stabilisation or reaming, an intramedullary biopsy should be performed [82,83]. In cases of plate osteosynthesis or hemiarthoplasty with curettage of the lesion, tissue sampling is easily performed [24].

For clinical evaluation of a metastatic lesion in a long bone, anteroposterior and lateral radiographs of the entire affected bone should be made. Special attention should be given to the perpendicularity of the two directions, otherwise an accurate cortical assessment is impossible. In metastatic bone disease, the pattern of bone destruction is related to the aggressiveness of the tumour growth. Slowly growing metastases have well-defined lytic areas of geographic destruction, whereas aggressive lesions have a more permeative or "moth-eaten" destructive pattern. Skeletal metastases may present as osteolytic (majority), osteoblastic or mixed osteolytic/osteoblastic lesions. It should be noted that only one-third of impending and actual pathological fractures are solitary at the affected bone. The remaining parts of the lesions appear to be diffuse and/or multiple. Radiographs may deliver useful information about site, extent, periosteal reaction and presence or absence of mineralisation. Radiography is helpful in a symptomatic patient but

Table 12.2. Mirel's scoring system for fracture risk of pathological lesion of the long bones

Variable	Risk score		
	1	2	3
Site	Upper limb	Lower limb	Intertrochanteric region
Pain	Mild	Moderate	On weight-bearing
Lesion	Blastic	Mixed	Lytic
Size related to bone diameter	<1/3	1/3–2/3	>2/3

From Mirels H [30] Metastatic disease in long bones: a proposed scoring system for diagnosing impending pathologic fractures. Clin Orthop 1989; 14: 513–25

ineffective as a screening method, because a normal X-ray does not exclude presence of metastasis. To detect metastases by plain X-ray, more than 50% destruction of the trabecular bone is needed [84]. In cortical metastatic involvement, the amount of destruction is much smaller and requires a more sensitive technique to detect it. The use of radiographs is limited in several ways; no standard radiograph or mutual perpendicular projection is performed, variable effects of geometry and destruction of the bone lesion on radiographical detection occur, margins of the lesion are poorly defined and cause error in the accurate measurement of the involved cortical bone, and the different locations of the lesions and the degree of bone density are variable [30,36,78,85].

If the geometry of the cortical defect cannot adequately be determined, a computed tomography (CT) scan examination can be additionally performed [12,86]. Radiographic and CT scan examinations have a large interobserver variability, so they should be interpreted with caution [37,85].

Magnetic resonance imaging (MRI) examination can be used to evaluate an unknown bone lesion, but should not be used to predict risk of fracture while the amount of cortical destruction is inadequately visualised [87].

Radionuclide scanning with technetium-99m (^{99m}Tc) is a very sensitive modality for identification of associated bone lesions, and should be used to determine whether a metastatic lesion is single or whether multiple sites are involved [5,88]. In a patient with a known primary carcinoma and local skeletal pain normal radiographs should be followed by scintigraphy and if not conclusive by MRI [89]. In a similar patient but with diffuse pain, scintigraphy comes first.

Occasional metastases, particularly those from renal carcinoma and myeloma, may be highly vascular and surgery may be associated with excessive blood loss; pre-operative angiography or MRI with gadolinium (Gd)-enhancement is advised to establish the vascularity of the lesion. Pre-operative embolisation of the lesion, within 1 week before operation, will facilitate surgery and decreases the risk of extended blood loss [90]. (Figure 12.4E).

SURGICAL MANAGEMENT

The surgical treatment of metastatic lesions in the long bones presents unique challenges. For optimal surgical treatment, the following items should be taken into account.

First, appropriate patient selection is important. The estimated life expectancy should be longer than the time to recover from surgery (Table 12.3). Survival depends on multiple factors and should be estimated by a multidisciplinary team. Surgery should only be performed if it improves quality of life. The success of fixation depends on the site, on the extent of destruction caused by the bone lesion and on the fixation device used. An ideal construction should be stable and durable. The different types of operative techniques used for the treatment of pathological fractures should all allow direct loading of the affected limb. The additional use of polymethyl methacrylate (PMMA) is essential in achieving this function. We are more concerned about direct biomechanical stability than about bone healing. Healing of pathological fractures cannot be relied on because of impaired healing due to effects of the metastatic tumour and radiation therapy [91]. The planned reconstruction should address all areas of destroyed bone at operation as well as all locations likely to be weakened subsequently. Post-operative radiation therapy should be considered. Finally, it is important that in each case the surgical treatment should be individualised. It should be stressed that heroic attempts to fix pathological fractures internally are likely to fail, especially in the proximal femur [92].

Table 12.3. Probable survival time of patients with their primary tumours

Survival time in years	Primary tumour
< 1 year	Unknown
	Melanoma
	Lung
	Pancreas
	Thyroid
	Stomach
1–2 years	Colon
	Breast (not responding to adjuvants)
	Liver
	Uterus
>2 years	Thyroid (differentiated)
	Myeloma
	Lyphoma
	Breast (responding to adjuvants)
	Rectum
	Prostate
	Kidney

From Capanna R [139] The treatment of metastases in bone. In Jakob R (ed.), Eur Instruc Course Lect, vol 4. London; the British Editorial Society of Bone and Joint Surgery: London, 1999: 24–34

There are many different surgical techniques for treatment of metastatic lesions of long bones. As already described by Griesmann and Schüttemeyer in 1947, *nailing* is nowadays a surgical fixation that is performed frequently [31]. The advantages of nailing are reduced blood loss and lower local complication rate because the fracture site and majority of the soft tissue remain untouched [93,94]. Furthermore, compared to plate fixation, intramedullary nailing can create stabilisation of the whole bone [95]. In cases of multiple metastases, special attention should be given to prevent (re-) fracturing during operation. Nail fixation without bipolar static locking resulted in a high incidence of failure of fixation. In general, if a nail is the treatment of choice, we recommend a reamed nail fixation with bipolar static locking (Figure 12.3). This can be performed by anterograde or retrograde nailing; the latter has no higher local recurrence rate [96]. Hoare showed in 1968 that tumour cells can be detected in the blood at the time of intramedullary nailing in pathological fractures [97]. This could raise the issue of possible dissemination of systemic metastasis during the operation. However, because of the short survival time of these patients, this appears not to influence the disease outcome [16,17]. Furthermore, experiments by Bouma have shown that nailing of impending pathological fractures does not increase dissemination of tumour cells, whereas nailing in actual pathological fractures can increase spread of tumour cells appreciably [98].

In the last decades the use of *plates* has been reduced because of the wide exposure required, high local complication rate, high blood loss, improved nail design, and less invasive stabilisation of the entire bone by nailing [92,95,99]. However, in pathological fractures of the humeral shaft we were unable to find a significant difference in clinical outcome between plating or nailing [96]. In biomechanical tests, two orthogonal plates with bone cement had a higher failure of loading compared to a nail with PMMA [100].

The additional effect of the use of *bone cement* to provide immediate stability, and tumour necrosis caused by hyperthermia or by toxicological effect should be considered [101,102]. Not only the ability to walk post-operatively but also the amount of pain relief is significantly improved by the use of PMMA [103,104]. The reported side-effects of PMMA are cardiovascular depression during intramedullary insertion and non-union [26]. After reposition, the normal bone above and below the lesion is fixed to the implant and, after curettage, the defect is filled with cement. When the cement has hardened, additional screws are sometimes necessary. Injection of PMMA around the screw also improves proximal and distal stability. The operative working time of PMMA can be prolonged by cooling the liquid monomer. In an impending fracture with widely diffuse metastases of the long bones, a closed reamed nailing technique with supplementary low-viscosity bone cement can be used [25,105–107]. Additional use of bone cement after curettage of the bone lesion improves bone strength three-fold [108,109]. To prevent additional local tumour growth, recent studies have indicated that methotrexate-loaded bone cement may have an important role as part of this management [110]. For some solitary diaphyseal lesions, an intercalary reconstruction with an allograft can be performed. Sometimes, in a solitary and extended lesion in the proximal humerus or femur with a long-term prognosis, an allograft in combination with a cemented hemi-arthroplasty can be used (Figure 12.5).

If indicated, a cemented *endoprosthesis* is the favoured device at the proximal femur site. Quick relief of pain, early mobilisation and low complication rate are several benefits of the cemented hemi-arthroplasty. In two studies, both including nearly 200 patients, reconstruction by endoprostheses showed the lowest failure rate (2–9%) as compared with osteosynthetic devices (12–14%) [19,111]. Megaprostheses and modular prostheses, used when the entire proximal femur is destroyed, are not frequently necessary. Endoreconstruction nails consist of a proximal femoral prosthesis with the distal end like a reconstruction nail, with interlocking capability. These new devices have some interesting advantages compared to the more well-known devices.

FEMORAL HEAD AND NECK

Pathological fractures of the femoral neck have a high risk of non-union, irrespective of the method of internal fixation [76,92]. Incidence of 12–33% of failure of fixation after treatment with internal fixation of the femoral neck is reported [16,19,112]. Endoprosthetic replacement is usually the treatment of choice, regardless of the degree of displacement of the head [113] (Figure 12.6). Lane et al. reported excellent results in 167 patients who had endoprosthetic replacement as treatment for pathological fractures about the hip [114]. Within a median survival time of 5.6 months, there were no dislocations, loosening or failure of the devices. It is also prudent to treat this type of fracture with a long-stemmed total hip replacement, as there is a

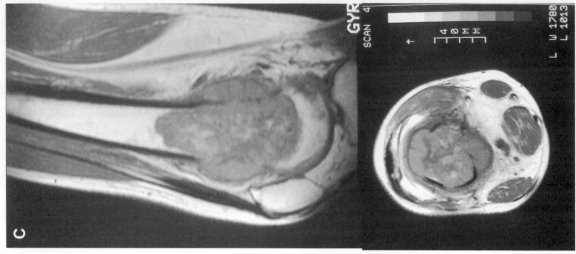

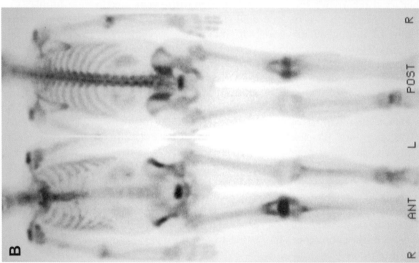

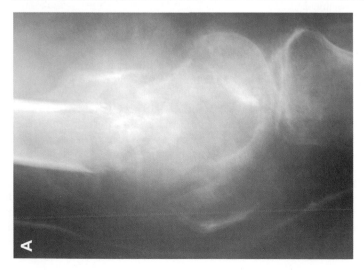

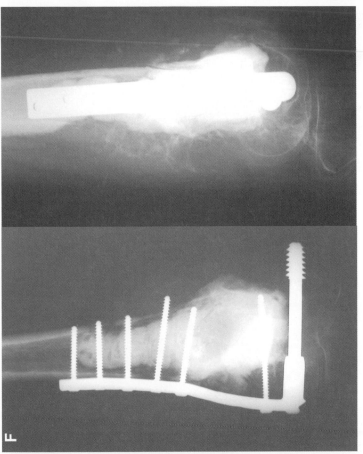

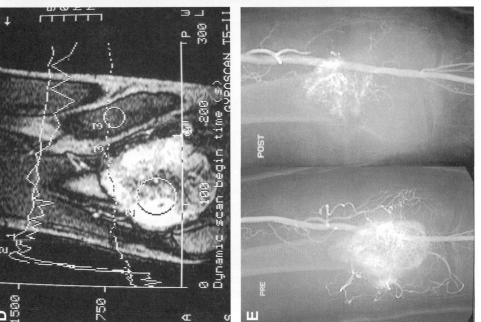

Figure 12.4. Lateral roentgenogram (A) of the right distal femur in a 42 year-old men with metastatic kidney carcinoma. Technetium-99 bone scan with hot spot at the distal site of the femur (B). Lesion demonstrated on saggital magnetic resonance images, T1 weighted (C). Dynamic magnetic resonance images with gadolineum (GD-DPTA) intravenously demonstrates a sudden enhancement within 10 seconds after starting. The superimposed time-intensity curves show the enhancement pattern of tumour (1), muscle (3) in relation to arterial enhancement (2). The earliest enhancing part of the tumour (1) shows some wash-out of GD-DPTA shortly after the maximal signal intensity. This pattern of dynamic enhancement is highly suggestive for malignancy like kidney carcinoma (D). Angiography showed successfully pre-operative embolisation (E). Anteroposterior and lateral roentgenogram of cemented 90° angled screw side plate (F)

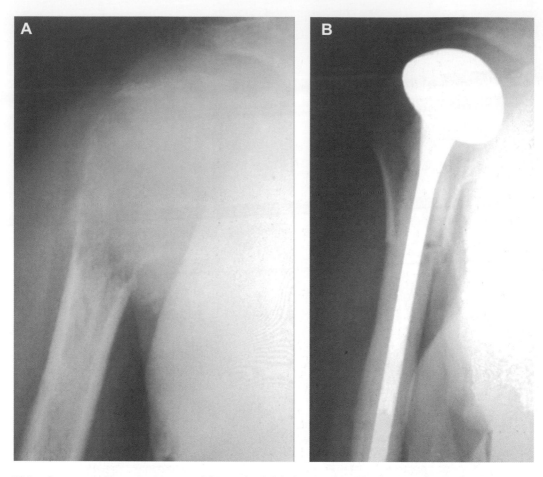

Figure 12.5. Anteroposterior roentgenogram of the proximal right humerus in a 57 year-old patient with breast cancer (A). The extended proximal humeral lesion was treated with an allograft in combination with a cemented hemi-arthroplasty (B)

significant risk of more distal femoral metastases. In practice, the tip of the femoral stem should bypass the destroyed cortex for a distance of at least twice the bone diameter. Because cemented long-stemmed hip prostheses are associated with an increased risk of embolisation and cardiac arrest, they should be used only on indication [115].

The advantages of cementation of the femoral stem and/or acetabulum in patients with a limited lifespan make non-cemented devices of little use. A calcar replacement prosthesis is recommended in cases of extensive destruction in the base of the neck. In cases of large metastatic involvement of the proximal femur, custom-made or modular devices can be used to bridge the defect and restore hip function [113,116,117].

Hemi-arthroplasty with double or floating cup is prudent only when the acetabulum is intact or with involvement of the acetabulum but an intact subchondral plate. Pre-operative unrecognised (minimal) involvement of the acetabulum occurs frequently, as reported by Haberman et al., but has not been shown to lead to more complications or persistent pain; we recommended hemi-arthroplasty in this setting [118,119]. Although not often necessary, total hip replacement gives good results, if several facts are taken into account; degree of tumour involvement, acetabular involvement and more distal lesions in the femoral shaft. If there is extensive involvement of the acetabulum, pelvic reconstruction may be required at the time of arthroplasty. In cases where restoration is inappropriate, special devices for the pelvis can be

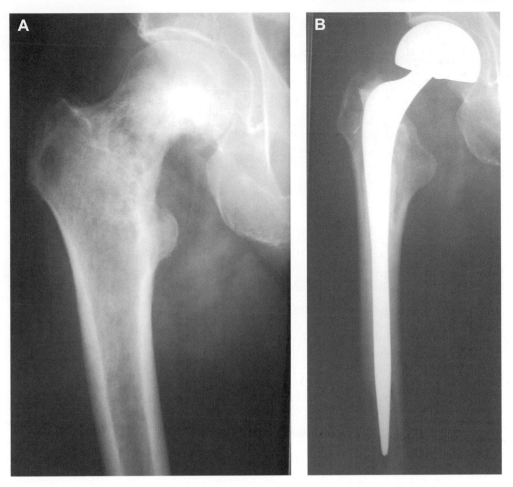

Figure 12.6. Anteroposterior roentgenogram of the proximal right femur in a 52 year-old patient with renal cancer (A). Endoprosthetic replacement with a long stem and additional PMMA was performed (B)

achieved using allografts, custom-built devices or saddle prostheses to solve the problem of the loss of bone stock [116,120].

Intertrochanteric Region

Intertrochanteric fractures may demand the same approach as fractures of the femoral neck [121], but if there is limited tumour extension, conventional stabilisation devices augmented with PMMA might be used, such as the Zickel nail [75], gamma nail (Strijker-Howmedica) (Figure 12.7) [95,122] and dynamic hip screw (Figure 12.8) [16,19]. In more extensive involvement of the proximal femur, an endoprosthesis with a long stem is recommended [113]. Good results are

obtained with the use of calcar replacement endoprosthesis [119]. The advantages of this device are immediately full weight-bearing and protection of the entire bone, and modularity allows improved equalisation of limb length and improved hip stability.

Before the revival of intramedullary fixation, the dynamic hip screw, with complete filling of the defect with bone cement, was used for internal fixation. The advantages of this technique are the width spread experienced by surgeons, better control in removing tumour tissue and easier filling of the defect with PMMA compared to nailing. This known surgical technique needs some modifications for optimal use: curettage of the tumour tissue through the created defect in the lateral cortex after using the calibrated reamer that follows the inserted guide pin. After

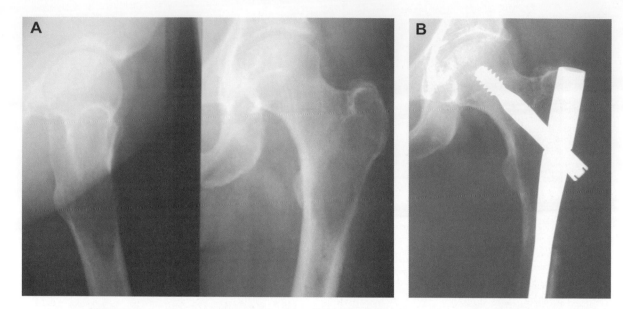

Figure 12.7. Anteroposterior and lateral roentgenogram of the proximal right femur in a 62 year-old patient with breast cancer (A). The impending fracture was treated with a long Gamma nail and distal locking without additional PMMA (B). No bone cement filling of this large cortical lesion was obtained resulting in a high risk of implant failure and persistent pain

placing the sliding screw and side plate, the side plate is again removed and the defect is injected with liquid bone cement with a gun, and manual pressure is applied to avoid cement extrusion. A wet half-cute plastic tube is often used to pressurise. Before the bone cement cures, the side plate is reapplied and fixed. The major disadvantages are the limited region of the bone protected by a sliding plate, and a high complication rate due to biomechanical limitations. Comparisons of the reconstruction nail showed that non-pathological fractures fixed with this device are 80% stiffer in torsion and 40% in bending than the dynamic hip screw [123].

The current generation of devices are available with extended long femoral stems, enabling protection of the entire femoral shaft [94]. The most useful device has been the long intramedullary hip screw, and in our experience the gamma nail is an excellent device [124].

Enders nails are not recommended because more than one-third of patients developed complications due to fixation [28]. In contrast, recent studies with a rather short follow-up reported no complications after reconstruction nail fixation [93]. Proper proximal and distal locking should be performed to achieve rigid internal fixation.

Short intramedullary hip screws should not be used, as they are associated with a higher complication rate,

due to fracturing at the nail tip and limited bone protection. Refractures at the distal end of plate or an endoprosthesis may be managed by an additional plate with PMMA. Alternatively, in such cases a retrograde reamed femoral nail can be used and, depending on the locking sites, with augmentation of PMMA (Figure 12.8).

Subtrochanteric Region

Metastatic lesions of the subtrochanteric region are best suited for intramedullary fixation. Compared to a laterally applied plate, a nail device allows better load sharing and resistance to bending stresses.

The dynamic hip screw is of limited use because of restricted prophylactic fixed cortex and the high prevalence of failure (Figure 12.9) [92]. We recommended a reamed reconstruction nail of the second (Russell-Taylor nail; Smith & Nephew) or third generation (gamma nail; Howmedica). In a recent multicentre study of 110 pathological femoral fractures treated with the long gamma nail, only 5% had a technical failure at follow-up [122]. Special attention must be paid to the technique of the interlocking reconstruction nail. Before introducing the reamed nail, the lateral cortex is exposed at the level of the

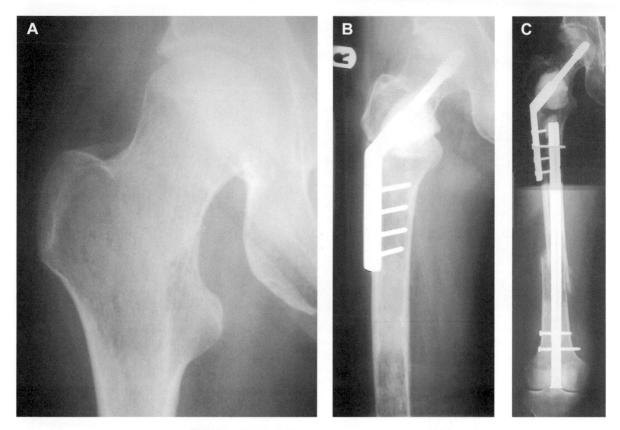

Figure 12.8. Anteroposterior roentgenogram of the proximal right femur in a 50 year-old patient with multiple myeloma (A). Cemented dynamic hip screw with short side plate is placed (B). This situation is insufficient because the entire long bone should be prophylactically stabilised specially in multiple myeloma. One year after surgery an actual pathological fracture of the distal diaphysis was sustained. A retrograde reamed nail with bipolar fixation is performed, proximally the nail is fixed at the level of the side plate to reduce stress risers and to protect the entire femur (C)

fracture, and the tumour tissue can be easily curetted. An intramedullary nail of appropriate length is chosen that should be approximately 2 mm smaller in (shaft) diameter than the last reamer used. If there is a large cortical defect, the interlocking screw(s) are placed in the femoral neck, and the defect is separately filled with bone cement by use of a cement gun. The window of the defect is patched by a wet glove or split plastic tube as the cement cures. In cases of a defect smaller than the bone diameter or an impending fracture, the intramedullary device is introduced as in non-pathological fracture treatment, with minimal soft tissue exposure. If a gamma nail is used, the proximally set (anti-rotation) screw is placed proximally as far as possible; this prevents proximal loss of bone cement during filling the defect by cement through the sliding hole in the nail, followed by introducing the dynamic hip screw (lag screw).

Using reconstruction nails as fixation prior to fracture provides better early results than after fracture occurrence [28]. The need for PMMA with these nails, especially in impending pathological fractures, has not been established. The unreamed third-generation nails (UFN, Synthes) have failed to create a proper proximal fixation with the spiral blade, as reported in biomechanical testing and clinical usage [126,127]. However, recent reports have shown good results with a low device failure rate [128]. If long-term survival is expected and internal fixation is not possible because of extensive destruction, a resection of the tumour and reconstruction with an allograft or megaprosthesis have to be considered.

To prevent dislocation, a megaprosthesis should be, if possible, placed without an acetabulum component [92]. Smaller lesions distal to this region should be fixed with a cemented long intramedullary stem. If the

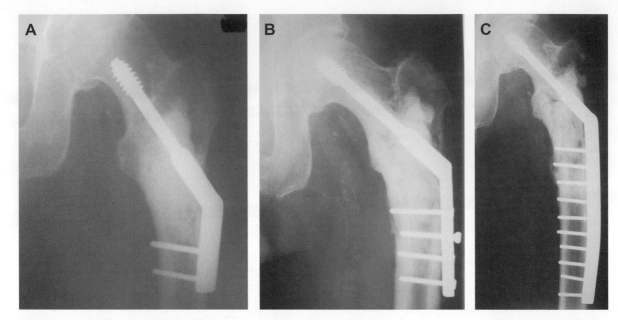

Figure 12.9. Anteroposterior roentgenogram (A) of the left hip in a 73 year-old man with carcinoma of the kidney. The impending intertrochanteric fracture was after preoperative embolisation fixed with dynamic hip screw and the bone defect was filled with PMMA. No other lesion in the affected femur was detected. Six months postoperative the too small placed side plate and compression screw were broken. After revision with a longer slide plate and compression screw this failure occurred within half a year (B). A long slide plate was placed with additional bone cement (C)

trochanter major cannot reinsert to the proximal prosthesis, the remaining abductor muscles are reefed down to the vastus lateralis or tratus iliotibialis. We recommend using bipolar cups with a mega- or modular cemented endoprosthesis. The disadvantages of a mega- or endoprosthesis are the cost, the extended surgical exposure required, with higher intra-operative and post-operative complication rates, and weak abductor muscles. In a clinical study by Sim et al., the overall rate of complications in the use of proximal replacement prostheses was high; 38/82 patients [117].

An alternative to the use of megaprostheses is described by Voggenreiter et al., who have used total hip replacement combined with anterograde cemented intramedullary nailing [129].

Shaft Region

Although (AO) plates provide excellent rigid fixation in experimental and clinical studies, we recommend an interlocking nail, with or without bone cement, as the most effective surgical treatment in femoral shaft lesions. In general, shaft lesions of a long bone are treated with an interlocking nail, with rigid proximal and distal fixation, and if necessary with bone cement.

In lesions larger than the bone diameter, we recommend a separate open procedure with curettage and after internal fixation filling the defect with PMMA. Usually a standard lateral approach is used. We advocate second and third reamed reconstruction nails if a locking nail is used, because it is important to prevent refracturing of the treated long bone. When intramedullary fixation of only the shaft was used, 1/6 treated patients are reported to have sustained an (impending) pathological fracture of the proximal femur in follow-up [95].

In an impending fracture or an actual fracture with small lesion(s), the use of PMMA in closed nailing is still controversial. Although augmentation with PMMA increased the bone strength, clinically this is not superior to locking nail fixation without bone cement [122,128]. If closed nailing is used in combination with low-viscosity PMMA without opening the fracture site, the liquid cement is injected before placing the nail, or through a hollow nail, resulting in retrograde filling of the medullary space, or after placement of the nail with separate anterograde and retrograde (auxiliary drill hole) insertion of cement [130].

In rare cases, there is a need for AO plates placed 90° to each other. Sometimes, when extended bone destruction results in segmental bone loss, the involved diaphyseal bone is resected and an intercalary allograft with nail or plate fixation is performed.

Supracondylar and Condylar Region

The most common treatment of the distal femur is a lateral approach, an open reduction, curettage of the lesion, 90° screw-plate or blade-plate or AO supracondylar plates, and finally bone cement (Figure 12.4). We have had some promising but limited experience with retrograde nailing in impending pathological fractures in this region. In a small lesion at the supracondylar region, closed techniques should be used, while such a defect at the condylar region is simply filled with PMMA [131]. If extended destruction of the condyle(s) exist, no heroic attempts should be made [130]. In these cases we recommend cemented constrained total knee prosthesis. Sometimes the destroyed bone can be resected and reconstructed using an allograft, followed by an endoprosthetic replacement.

HUMERUS

The humerus has a relatively small cortical mass. This, together with specific biomechanics of the humeral bone in response to torsional loading, results in fractures of the middle third of the humeral shaft in 50% of patients [41,96,132].

Pathological fractures of the humeral shaft are better managed with a functional cast brace if the patient has a limited life expectancy of a few weeks [133]. However, poor results of non-operative treatment of pathological fractures of the humerus have been reported [134,135]. Patients expected to survive longer than several weeks, and/or patients who depend on the support of the arms for walking, or patients with bilateral involvement of the upper extremities, require internal fixation to ensure pain relief, restore function or avoid subsequent fracture [96]. The vast majority of pathological fractures of the humerus are better fixed by intramedullary nailing to provide mobility and rapid pain relief [136,137]. A major pitfall of the anterograde use of interlocking nail fixation is impingement of the acromion during abduction (Figure 12.10). It is essential that the nail tip protrudes deep into the humeral cortical head. The technique of retrograde humeral nailing via a distal

entrance portal in the humerus avoids complications to the rotator cuff region and will achieve adequate fixation. Adequate stabilisation will result in 90% good restoration of function. Unstable fixation requires methyl methacrylate augmentation, usually performed by a separate incision and after curettage of the metastasis. Hyperthermia about the radial nerve by polymerisation of PMMA should be avoided [96].

An (extended) anterolateral approach is used for lesions in the mid-one-third of the humerus, and a deltopectoral approach for proximal humeral lesions. If plate osteosynthesis is performed, in the proximal humerus a T plate or 4.5 mm dynamic compression (DC) plate, and for midshaft humeral lesions a 4.5 mm DC plate is recommended (Figure 12.11). Although better rigidity is obtained by using two DC plates at 90° to each other, we have seen no failure of fixation

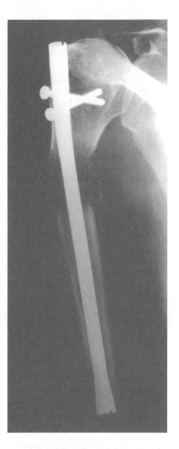

Figure 12.10. Seldel nail failure 3 months post operatively in a patient with disseminated breast cancer. Three most frequent failures are shown; humeral varisation due to the large cortical defect without filling it with bone cement, rotation instability, and subacromional impingement due to proximal tip of the nail

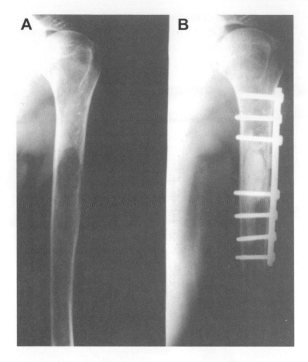

Figure 12.11. Anteroposterior roentgenogram of the left humeral shaft with an impending fracture in a 58 year-old patient with breast cancer (A). dynamic compression plate with adjunctive PMMA is placed (B)

with one DC plate [96]. It is more important to fix cortical bone with a plate over an extended region.

In an impending fracture with extensive destruction of the humerus, a closed reamed nailing technique with low-viscosity PMMA has been suggested [105]. If PMMA stabilisation of the entire bone is necessary, venting by a drill bit placed in the anterolateral cortex can be beneficial. Alternatively, in patients with a solitary lesion and a prognosis of prolonged survival, resection and shortening of the humeral shaft may be chosen if the lesion is smaller than 4 cm in length. It is still not clear which fixation method, plating or nailing, should be advocated in the surgical treatment of pathological fractures of the humeral shaft [96].

Extended fractures or tumour involvement of the proximal humerus usually require replacement hemiarthroplasty with long stem [117]. In selected patients where prolonged survival is anticipated, a custom-made prosthesis or an allograft–prosthesis composite is used (Figure 12.5). When using a massive proximal humeral prosthesis, special attention should be made to prevent migration and dislocation of the humeral component.

Lesions in the distal one-third of the humerus can often not be rodded, because the distal locking screws do not achieve adequate fixation, despite augmentation by PMMA. In these cases we prefer a posterior approach, curettage of the metastasis, filling the defect with PMMA and 4.5 mm DC plate fixation. In the distal metaphyseal humerus, a combination of a 3.5 mm DC plate and a pelvic reconstruction plate with PMMA is recommended. Olecranon osteotomy should be avoided, as there is a high non-union rate. In extensive lesions around the elbow, a cemented long-stemmed total elbow can be used.

TIBIA

The tibia is an infrequent site of involvement and only rarely is it a surgical problem [105]. The majority of pathological fractures involve the metaphysis of the tibia. In those patients who survive more than a few weeks, these fractures can sometimes unite by conservative care [138]. We consider that metastatic involvement of the proximal tibia of more than half of the epiphyseal or metaphyseal circumferential cortical bone should be treated by resection and reconstruction, using a cemented tumour-prosthesis [139]. If there is less than 50% cortical bone involvement in this area, we use two T plates, PMMA and, depending on articular destruction, a total knee arthroplasty (Figure 12.12).

Anterograde interlocking nailing and augmentation with methyl methacrylate is advised for actual diaphyseal fracture; this treatment may restore immediate weight-bearing ability. When nailing an impending fracture, the use of PMMA depends on the amount of cortical destruction and the quality of the bone stock at the site of locking. The preference of type of nailing, reamed or unreamed, is still controversial in treatment of these pathological fractures.

In fixation by plating of the lesion at shaft and/or distal metaphysis, after wide curettage the lesion is filled with polymethylmethacrylate and fixed with a 4.5 mm DC plate, with three or more cortical screws on both sites of the defect [19]. With plating of the diaphyseal tibia, good clinical results are obtained, even with regard to prolonged survival, compared to pathological fractures of the humerus (50% died in 16.5 months vs. 4.5 months, respectively) [19]. An anterolateral approach is used, and the DC plate is placed at the tibia laterally. Care of the soft tissue is mandatory.

Rehabilitation of the distal tibia and ankle reconstructions can be time-consuming; alternatively,

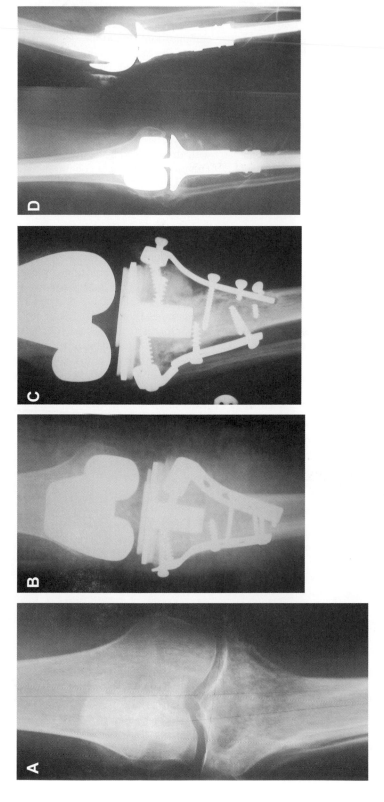

Figure 12.12. Anteroposterior roentgenogram of extended metastatic lesion at the proximal right femur in a 63 year-old patient with carcinoma of the breast (A). First reconstructed with an allograft, two side L plates and posterior stabilised total knee prosthesis with bone cement (B). Two year post-operative complicated by collapse of the allograft with loosening of the osteosynthesis (C). Distal femur and proximal tibia were reconstructed with proximal tibial segmental replacement and hinge cemented total knee (D)

amputation is a valid option, allowing quick relief of pain and early return of function [140]. If a reconstruction of this region by internal fixation or arthrodesis is performed, postoperative radiation should be avoided.

RADIUS AND/OR ULNA

Ulna and radius metastases are rare and can occasionally be handled by intramedullary rodding (Rush rods) or plate osteosynthesis, with or without cementation [141]. In case of prolonged survival and intra-articular involvement of the wrist, an allograft or arthrodesis is performed and postoperative radiation is avoided.

COMPLICATIONS

These debilitated patients have many operative and post-operative complications. In patients with an actual pathological fracture of the long bone, the overall complication rate can be as high as 52% [99]. Cardiac and pulmonary problems are systemic complications, with a wide occurrence rate (3–18%) Thromboembolic complication occurs in 2% [16,19]. The most common local complication is deep wound infection (3%). In these compromised patients antibiotic prophylaxis is mandatory [99]. Attention should

be directed to preventing deep wound haematomas. If the expected operative blood loss is high, pre-operative embolisation should be considered. The recurrence rate of the metastasis in the soft tissue adjacent to the surgically treated bone is very low. The local and systemic spread of tumour cells secondary to surgical fixation are infrequently of clinical significance.

Impairment of the function of peripheral nerves can occur, but are usually transient. Hyperthermia caused by polymerisation of bone cement could be associated with destructive effects on the nerve. We pay special attention to adequate cooling of the bone cement, or protect the soft tissue with a plastic layer if necessary.

The failure of implant rate after surgical treatment depends mainly on the loading capacity of the implant and the cortex. This is greatly influenced by size, location, progression of the metastatic defect and actual or impending fracture.

Resection of the entire metastasis, as done before implantation of an endoprosthesis, increases the likelihood of good fixation if compared to osteosynthesis. The complications (9%) after endoprosthesis compare favourably with the results for the treatment of non-pathological femoral neck fractures [142]. Failure of internal fixation of a lower extremity occurs in 1/8 patients. Of particular concern is long-term failure caused by fatigue breaking, loosening of the device, penetration of the femoral head by the plate, and

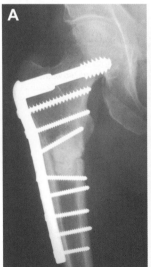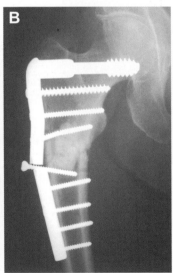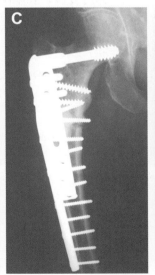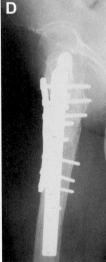

Figure 12.13. Anteroposterior roentgenogram of the proximal femur after treatment of a pathological subtrochanteric fracture with internal fixation by a 90° compression screw and side plate, and adjunctive use of bone cement (A). Four months after surgery two screws of the side plate were broken without a trauma (B). The angled compression screw plate was changed for a larger one, and an additional AO femur plate with bone cement was used. Anteroposterior and lateral roentgenogram demonstrated union one year after the latter surgery (C,D)

refracturing of bone at the distal end of the angled blade plate. The majority of failed fixations are in the subtrochanteric region. The reported failure in this region is up to 23%, mainly due to eccentric loadsharing of the proximal angled blade plate screw holes (Figure 12.13) [16,19]. The torque and shear forces on the plate at the subtrochanteric region cannot entirely be relieved by the pressure of PMMA bone cement within the medullary canal. By inserting a new longer plate, one can treat fatigue breaks after plating. Angled plates are nowadays seldom placed. The use of second- and third-generation reconstruction nails is advocated.

REFERENCES

1. Strouhal E. Tumors in the remains of the ancient Egyptians. Am J Phys Anthrop 1976; 45: 613–20.
2. Wiseman R. Several Chirurgical Treatises. Royston: London, 1676.
3. Cooper A. Lectures on diseases of the breast. Lancet 1824; 2: 710–25.
4. Fitts WT, Roberts B, Ravdin IS. Fractures in metastatic carcinoma. Am J Surg 1953; 85: 282–7.
5. Galasko CSB. Skeletal Metastases. Butterworth: Cambridge, 1986; 14–27.
6. Albright JA, Gillspie TE, Butaud TR. Treatment of bone metastases. Semin Oncol 1980; 7: 418–34.
7. Friedlaender GE, Johnson RM, Brand RA et al. Treatment of pathological fractures. Conn Med 1975; 39: 765–72.
8. Abrahams HL, Spiro R, Goldstein N. Metastases in carcinoma. Analysis of 1000 autopsied cases. Cancer 1950; 3: 74–85.
9. The Netherlands Cancer Registry. Incidence of Cancer in the Netherlands 1994. ISBN 90-72175-17-4.
10. Galasko C. Pathological fracture. In Peckham M, Pinedo H, Veronesi U et al. (eds), Oxford Textbook of Oncology, 1st edn. Oxford University Press: Oxford, 1995; 19.7: 2286–95.
11. Coleman RE, Rubens RD. The clinical course of bone metastases from breast cancer. Br J Cancer 1987; 55: 61–6.
12. Lenz M, Freid JR. Metastases to the skeleton, brain and spinal cord from cancer of the breast and the effects of radiotherapy. Ann Surg 1931; 93: 278–93.
13. Leeson MC, Makley JT, Carter JR. Metastatic skeletal disease: distal to elbow and knee. Clin Orthop 1986; 206: 94–9.
14. Galasko CSB. Skeletal metastases and mammary cancer. Ann R Coll Surg Engl 1972; 50: 3–28.
15. Johnston AD. Pathology of metastatic tumors in bone. Clin Orthop 1970; 73: 8–12.
16. Yazawa Y, Frassica FJ, Chao EYS et al. Metastatic bone disease: a study of surgical treatment of 166 pathologic humeral and femoral fractures. Clin Orthop 1990; 251: 213–19.
17. Beals RK, Lawton GD, Snell WE. Prophylactic internal fixation in metastatic breast cancer. Cancer 1971; 28: 1350–4.
18. Clain A. Secondary malignant disease of bone. Br J Cancer 1965; 19: 15–29.
19. Dijkstra PDS, Wiggers T, van Geel AN, Boxma H. Treatment of impending and actual pathological fractures in patients with bone metastases of the long bones. Eur J Surg 1994; 160: 535–42.
20. Front D, Schenck SO, Frankel A, Robinson E. Bone metastases and bone pain in breast cancer. Are they closely associated? J Am Med Assoc 1979; 242: 1747–8.
21. Sherry HS, Levy RN, Siffert RS. Metastatic disease of bone in orthopedic surgery. Clin Orthop 1982; 169: 44–52.
22. Douglass JO. Treatment of pathological fracture of long bones excluding those due to breast cancer. J Bone Joint Surg 1976; 58A: 1055–60.
23. Friedl W. Indication, management and results of surgical therapy for pathological fractures in patients with bone metastases. Eur J Surg Oncol 1990; 16: 380–96.
24. Harrington KD, Sim FH, Enis JE et al. Methylmethacrylate as an adjunct in internal fixation of pathological fractures. J Bone Joint Surg 1976; 58A: 1047–54.
25. Lewallen RP, Pritchard DJ, Sim FH. Treatment of pathologic fractures or impending fractures of the humerus with Rush rods and methylmethacrylate: experience with 55 cases in 54 patients, 1968–1977. Clin Orthop 1982; 166: 193–8.
26. Sim FH, Daugherty TW, Ivins JC. The adjunctive use of methylmethacrylate in fixation of pathological fractures. J Bone Joint Surg 1974; 56A: 40–8.
27. Francis KC. Prophylactic internal fixation of metastatic osseous lesions. Cancer 1960; 13: 75–6.
28. Ward WG, Spang J, Howe D, Gordan S. Femoral reconstruction nails for metastatic disease: indications, technique, and results. Am J Orthop 2000; 29(suppl 9): 34–42.
29. Fidler M. Prophylactic internal fixation of secondary neoplastic deposits in long bones. Br Med J 1973; 1: 341–3.
30. Mirels H. Metastatic disease in long bones: a proposed scoring system for diagnosing impending pathologic fractures. Clin Orthop 1989; 14: 513–25.
31. Griesmann H, Schüttemeyer W. Weitere Erfahrungen mit der Marknagelung nach Kuntscher an der Chirurgischen Universitatsklinik Kiel. Chirurg 1947; April: 17–18.
32. Henderson IC. Breast cancer. N Eng J Med 1980; 302: 78–90.
33. Marcove RC, Yang DJ. Survival times after treatment of pathologic fractures. Cancer 1967; 20: 2154–8.
34. Bauer HCF, Wedin R. Survival after surgery for spinal and extremity metastases. Acad Orthop Scand 1995; 66: 143–6.
35. Simon SR, Alaranta H, An K et al. Kinesiology. In Simon SR (ed.), Orthopaedic Basic Science. American Academy of Orthopedic Surgeons: Rosemont, IL, 1994: 582–4.
36. Springfield D, Jennings C. Pathologic fractures. In Rockwood CA, Green DP (eds), Fractures in Adults, vol 1. Lippincott-Raven: New York, 1996: 513–19.
37. Dijkstra PDS. Pathological fractures of the long bones due to bone metastases. Thesis, 1997.
38. Behiri JC, Bonfield W. Crack velocity and the longitudinal fracture in bone. J Mat Sci 1980; 15: 1841–9.
39. Bonfield W, Grynpas MD. Spiral fracture of cortical bone. J Biomech 1982; 15: 555–9.

40. Frankel VH, Burstein AH. Load capacity of tubular bone. In Kenedi RM (ed.), Biomechanics and Related Bioengineering Topics. 1965: 381–96.

41. Frankel VH, Burstein AH. Orthopaedic Biomechanics. Lea & Febiger: Philadelphia, PA, 1970.

42. Pugh J, Sherry HS, Futterman B, Frankel VH. Biomechanics of pathologic fractures. Clin Orthop 1982; 169: 109–14.

43. DeSouza ML, An KN, Morrey BF, Chao EYS. Strength reduction of rectangular cortical defects in diaphyseal bone. Trans Orthop Res Soc 1989; 14: 113.

44. Edgerton BC, An K, Morrey BF. Torsional strength reduction due to cortical defects in bone. J Orthop Res 1990; 8: 851–5.

45. Burchardt H, Busbee GA III, Enneking WF. Repair of experimental autologous grafts cortical bone. J Bone Joint Surg Am 1975; 57: 814–19.

46. Alho A, Hoiseth A, Husby T. Bone-mass distribution in the femur. A cadaver study on the relations of structure and strength. Acta Orthop Scand 1989; 60: 101–6.

47. Kennedy JG, Carter DR. Long bone torsion: I. Effects of heterogeneity, anisotropy and irregularity. J Biomech Eng 1985; 107: 183–8.

48. Clark CR, Morgan C, Sonstegard DA, Matthews LS. The effect of biopsy hole shape and size on bone strength. J Bone Joint Surg Am 1977; 59(2): 213–17.

49. Brown RK, Pelker RR, Friedlaender GE et al. Post-fracture irradiation effects on biomechanical and histologic parameters of fracture healing. J Orthop Res 1991; 9: 876–82.

50. Widman RF, Pelker RR, Friedlaender GE et al. Effects of prefracture irradiation on biomechanical parameters of fracture healing. J Orthop Res 1993; 11: 422–8.

51. Hipp JA, McBroom RJ, Cheal EJ, Hayes WC. Structural consequences of endosteal metastatic lesions in long bones. J Orthop Res 1989; 7: 828–37.

52. Hipp JA, Rosenberg AE, Hayes WC. Mechanical properties of trabecular bone within and adjacent to osseous metastases. J Bone Min Res 1992; 7: 1165–71.

53. Williams JF. A force analysis of the hip joint. J Biomed Eng 1968; 3: 365–73.

54. Toridis TG. Stress analysis of the femur. J Biomech 1969; 2: 163–71.

55. Netz P. The diaphyseal bone under torque. Thesis, Stockholm. Sweden, 1979.

56. Keyak JH, Fourkas MG, Meagher JM, Skinner HB. Validation of an automated method of three-dimensional finite element modelling of bone. J Biomed Eng 1993; 15: 505–9.

57. McBroom RJ, Cheal EJ, Hayes WC. Strength reductions from metastatic cortical defects in long bones. J Orthop Res 1988; 6: 369–78.

58. Peabody T. Evaluation and management of carcinoma metastatic to bone. Curr Opin Orthop 1996; 7(VI): 75–9.

59. Behr JT, Dobozi WR, Badrinath K. The treatment of pathologic and impending pathologic fractures of the proximal femur in the elderly. Clin Orthop 1985; 198: 173–8.

60. Schocker JD, Brady LW. Radiation therapy for bone metastasis. Clin Orthop 1982: 169: 38–43.

61. Gainor BJ, Buchert P. Fracture healing in metastatic bone disease. Clin Orthop 1983; 178: 297–302.

62. Tong D, Gillick L, Hendrickson FR. The palliation of symptomatic osseous metastases: final results of the study by RTOG. Cancer 1982; 50: 893–9.

63. Howland WJ, Loeffler RK, Starchman DE et al. Postirradiation atrophic changes of bone and related complications. Ther Radiol 1975; 117: 677–85.

64. Poulsen HS, Nielsen OS, Klee M, Rorth M. Palliative irradiation of bone metastases. Cancer Treat Rev 1989; 16: 41–8.

65. Body JJ. Metastatic bone disease: clinical and therapeutic aspects. Bone 1992; 12(suppl 1): S52–62.

66. Townsend PW, Smalley SR, Cozad SC et al. Role of postoperative radiation therapy after stabilization of fractures caused by metastatic disease. Int J Radiat Oncol Biol Phys 1995; 31: 43–9.

67. Porter AT, Reddy SM. Strontium 89 in the treatment of metastatic prostate cancer. Adv Oncol 1995; 18: 19–22.

68. van Holten Verzantvoort AT, Bijvoet OL, Cleton FJ et al. Reduced morbidity from skeletal metastases in breast cancer patients during long-term biphosphonate (APD) treatment. Lancet 1987; 2: 983–5.

69. Harrington KD. Orthopaedic management of extremity and pelvic lesions. Clin Orthop 1995; 312: 136–47.

70. Pedersen T, Elias K, Henriksen E. A prospective study of mortality associated with anaesthesia and surgery: risk indicators of mortality in hospital. Acta Anaesth Scand 1990; 34: 176–82.

71. Fidler M. Incidence of fracture through metastases in long bones. Acta Orthop Scand 1981; 52: 623–7.

72. Parrish FF, Murray JA. Surgical treatment for secondary neoplastic fractures. J Bone Joint Surg Am 1970; 52: 665–86.

73. Harrington KD. New trends in the management of the lower extremity metastases. Clin Orthop 1982; 169: 53–61.

74. Menck H, Schulze S, Larsen E. Metastasis size in pathologic femoral fractures. Acta Orthop Scand 1988; 59: 151–4.

75. Zickel RE, Mouradian WH. Intramedullary fixation of pathological fractures and lesions of the subtrochanteric region of the femur. J Bone J Surg Am 1976; 58: 1061–6.

76. Miller F, Whitehill R. Carcinoma of the breast metastatic to the skeleton. Clin Orthop Rel Res 1984; 184: 121–7.

77. Keene JS, Sellinger DS, McBeath AA, Engber WD. Metastatic breast cancer in the femur. Clin Orthop Rel Res 1986; 203: 282–8.

78. Dijkstra PDS, Oudkerk M, Wiggers T. Prediction of pathological subtrochanteric fractures due to metastatic lesions 1997; 116: 221–4.

79. Cheng DS, Seitz CB, Harmon JE. Non-operative treatment of femoral, humeral and acetabular metastases in patients with breast carcinoma. Cancer 1980; 45: 1533–7.

80. Hipp JA, Katz G, Hayes WC. Local demineralization as a model for bone strength reductions in lytic transcortical metastatic defects. Invest Radiol 1991; 26: 934–8.

81. Simon MA. Biopsy of musculoskeletal tumors. J Bone Joint Surg Am 1982; 64: 1253–5.

82. Smith DG, Behr JT, Hall RF, Dobozi WR. Closed flexible intramedullary biopsy of metastatic carcinoma. Clin Orthop Rel Res 1988; 229: 162–5.

83. Herbert J, Couser J, Seligson D. Closed medullary biopsy of dissemenated malignancy. Clin Orthop Rel Res 1982; 163: 214–17.

84. Edelstyn GA, Gillespie PJ, Grebbel FS. The radiological demonstration of osseous metastases. Experimental observations. Clin Radiol 1967; 18: 158–62.

85. Hipp JA, Springfield DS, Hayes WC. Predicting pathologic fracture risk in the management of metastatic bone defects. Clin Orthop Rel Res 1995; 312: 120–35.

86. Rafii M, Firooznia H, Kramer E et al. The role of computed tomography in evaluation of skeletal metastases. J Comput Tomogr 1988; 12: 19–24.

87. Zimmer WD, Berquist TH, McLeod RA et al. Bone tumours: magnetic imaging vs. computed tomography. Radiology 1985: 155; 709–18.

88. Goris ML, Bretille J. Skeletal scintigraphy for the diagnosis of malignant metastatic disease to the bone. Radiother Oncol 1985; 3: 319–29.

89. Algra P, Bloem J. Magnetic resonance imaging in metastatic disease and multiple myeloma. In Bloem JL, Sartorius DJ (eds), MRI and CT of the Musculoskeletal System. Williams & Wilkins: Baltimore, MD, 1992; 218–35.

90. Roscoe MW, McBroom RJ, St. Louis E et al. Preoperative embolization in the treatment of osseous metastases from renal cell carcinoma. Clin Orthop Rel Res 1989; 238: 302–7.

91. Bonarigo BC, Rubin P. Non-union of pathologic fracture after radiation therapy. Radiology 1967; 88: 889–98.

92. Damron TA, Sim FH. Surgical treatment for metastatic disease of the pelvis and the proximal end of the femur. AAOS Instruct Course Lect 2000; 49: 461–70.

93. Weikert DR, Schwartz HS. Intramedullary nailing for impending pathological subtrochanteric fractures. J Bone Joint Surg 1991; 73B: 668–70.

94. Karachalios T, Atkins RM, Sarangi PP et al. Reconstruction nailing for pathological subtrochanteric fractures with coexisting femoral shaft metastases. J Bone Joint Surg Br 1993; 75: 119–22.

95. Hulst van der RRWJ, Wildenberg van der FAJM, Vroemen JPAM et al. Intramedullary nailing of pathologic fractures. J Trauma 1994; 36: 211–15.

96. Dijkstra PDS, Stapert JWJL, Boxma H, Wiggers T. Treatment of pathological fractures of the humeral shaft. A retrospective study among intramedullary nail and AO plate osteosynthesis with adjunctive bone cement. Eur J Surg Oncol 1996; 22: 621–6.

97. Hoare JR. Pathological fractures. In Proceedings of North-west Metropolitan Orthopaedic Club. J Bone Joint Surg 1968; 50B: 232.

98. Bouma WH, Mulder JH, Hop WC. The influence of intramedullary nailing upon the development of metastases in the treatment of an impending pathological fracture: an experimental study. Clin Exp Metast 1983; 1: 205–12.

99. Van Geffen E, Wobbes T, Veth RPH, Gelderman WAH. Operative management of impending pathological fractures: a critical analysis of therapy. J Surg Oncol 1997; 64: 190–4.

100. Anderson JT, Erickson JM, Thompson RC, Chao EY. Pathologic femoral shaft fractures comparing fixation techniques using cement. Clin Orthop Rel Res 1978; 131: 273–7.

101. Chan PYM, Norman A. Hyperthermia (HT) effects of methamethylacrylate (MM) in bone metastases. Proc Am Assoc Cancer Res 1979; 20: 299.

102. Cameron HU, Jacob CBR, Macnab I et al. Use of polymethylmethacrylate to enhance screw fixation in bone. J Bone Joint Surg 1975; 57A: 655–6.

103. Habermann ET, Lopez RA. Metastatic disease of bone and treatment of pathological fractures. Orthop Clin N Am 1989; 20: 469–86.

104. Bouma WH, Cech M. The surgical treatment of pathologic and impending fracture of the long bones. J Trauma 1980: 12; 1043–5.

105. Vandeweyer E, Gebhart M. Treatment of humeral pathological fractures by internal fixation and methylmethacrylate injection. Eur J Surg Oncol 1997; 23: 238–42.

106. Kunec JR, Lewis RJ. Closed intramedullary rodding of pathologic fractures with supplemental cement. Clin Orthop Rel Res 1984; 188: 183–6.

107. Miller GJ, van der Griend RA, Blake WP, Springfield DS. Performance evaluation of a cement-augmented intramedullary fixation system for pathologic lesions of the femoral shaft. Clin Orthop Rel Res 1987; 221: 246–54.

108. Ryan JR, Begeman PC. The effects of filling experimental large cortical defects with methylmethacrylate. Clin Orthop 1984; 185: 306–10.

109. Leggon RE, Lindsey RW, Panjabi MM. Strength reduction and the effects of treatment of long bones with diaphyseal defects involving 50% of the cortex. J Orthop Res 1988; 6: 540–6.

110. Wang HM, Galasko CS, Crank S et al. Methotrexate loaded acrylic cement in the management of skeletal metastases. Biomechanical, biological, and systemic effect. Clin Orthop Rel Res 1995; 312: 173–86.

111. Wedin R, Bauer HC, Wersall P. Failures after operation for skeletal metastatic lesions of long bones. Clin Orthop Rel Res 1999; 358: 128–39.

112. Levine A. Pathological fractures. In Browne B et al. (eds), Skeletal Trauma: Fractures, Dislocations, and Ligamentous Injuries. 1992: 401–41.

113. Aaron AD. Treatment of metastatic adenocarcinoma of the pelvis and the extremities. Review. J Bone Joint Surg Am 1997; 79: 917–32.

114. Lane JM, Sculco TP, Zolan S. Treatment of pathological fracture of the hip by endoprosthetic replacement. J Bone Joint Surg Am 1980; 62: 954–9.

115. Patterson BM, Healy JH, Cornell CN, Sharrock NE. Cardiac arrest during hip arthroplasty with a cemented long-stem component: a report of seven cases. J Bone Joint Surg Am 1991; 73: 271–7.

116. Allan D, Bell R, Davis A, Langer F. Complex acetabular reconstruction for metastatic tumor. J Arthoplasty 1995; 10: 301–6.

117. Sim FH, Frassica FJ, Chao EYS. Orthopaedic management using new devices and prosthesis. Clin Orthop 1995; 312: 160–72.

118. Habermann ET, Sachs R, Stern RE et al. The pathology and treatment of metastatic disease to the femur. Clin Orthop 1982; 169: 70–82.

119. Clarke HD, Damron TA, Sim FH. Head and neck replacement endoprotheses for pathological proximal femoral lesions. Clin Orthop 1998; 169: 210–17.

120. Abouliafa A, Buch R, Matthews J et al. Reconstruction using the saddle prosthesis following excision of primary and metastatic acetabular tumors. Clin Orthop Rel Res 1995; 314: 203–13.

121. Rompe J, Eysel P, Hopf C, Heine J. Metastatic instability at the proximal end of the femur: comparison of endoprosthetic replacement and plate osteosynthesis. Arch Orthop Trauma Surg 1994; 113: 260–4.

122. Van Doorn R, Stapert JW. Treatment of impending and actual pathological femoral fractures with the long gamma nail in The Netherlands. Eur J Surg 2000; 166(3): 247–54.

123. Russell TA, Dingman CA, Wisnewski P. Mechanical and clinical rationale for femoral neck fracture fixation with a cephalomedullary interlocking nail. Trans 38th Orthop Res Soc Meeting 1992; 17: 177.

124. Lefevre C, Yaacoub C, Dubrana F, Caro P. Abstract: Long gamma locking nails. Results of a prospective European multicentric study of 120 cases. J Bone Joint Surg Br 1997; 79: 28.

125. Tencer AF, Johnson KD, Johnston DWC, Gill K. A biomechanical comparison of various methods of stabilization of subtrochanteric fractures of the femur. J Orthop Res 1984; 2: 297–305.

126. Wheeler DL, Croy TJ, Woll TS et al. Comparison of reconstruction nails for high subtrochanteric femur fracture fixation. Clin Orthop 1997; 338: 231–9.

127. Broos PL, Reynders P, Vanderspeeten K. Mechanical complications associated with the use of unreamed AO femoral intramedullary nail with spiral blade: first experiences with thirty-five consecutive cases. J Orthop Trauma 1998; 12: 186–9.

128. Giannoudis PV, Bastawrous SS, Bunola JA et al. Unreamed intramedullary nailing for pathological femoral fractures. Good results in 30 cases. Acta Orthop Scand 1999; 70(1): 29–32.

129. Voggenreiter G, Assenmacher S, Klaes W et al. Pathological fractures of the proximal femur with impending shaft fractures treated by THR and cemented intramedullary nailing: a report of nine cases. J Bone Joint Surg Br 1996; 78(3): 400–3.

130. Peabody TD, Finn HA. Femoral diaphysis and distal femur. In Simon MA, Springfield D (eds), Surgery for Bone and Soft-Tissue Tumors. Lippincott-Raven: New York, 1998: 705–11.

131. Varriale PL, Evans PEL, Sallis JG. A modified technique for fixation of pathologic fractures in the lower femur. Clin Orthop 1985; 199; 256–60.

132. Katzner M, Schvingt E. Métastases osseuses des cancers du sein. Traitement chirurgical de 228 localisations aux membres. Chirurgie 1989; 115: 741–50.

133. McCormack R, Glass D, Lane J. Functional cast bracing of metastatic humeral shaft lesion. Orthop Trans 1985; 9: 50–1.

134. Fleming JE. Pathological fractures of the humerus. Clin Orthop 1996; 203: 258–60.

135. Lancaster JM, Koman LA, Gristina AG et al. Pathologic fractures of the humerus. South Med J 1988; 87: 38.

136. Redmond BJ, Bierman JS, Blasier RB. Interlocking intramedullary nailing in pathological fractures of the shaft of the humerus. J Bone Joint Surg Am 1996; 78: 891–6.81: 52–5.

137. Lewallen RP, Pritchard DJ, Sim FH. Treatment of pathologic fractures or impending fractures of the humerus with Rush rods and methylmethacrylate. Experience with 55 cases in 54 patients, 1969–1977. Clin Orthop Rel Res 1982; 166: 193–7.

138. Peabody T. Evaluation and management of carcinoma metastatic to bone. Curr Opin Orthop 1996; 7(VI): 75–9.

139. Capanna R. The treatment of metastases in bone. In Jakob R (ed.), Eur Instruc Course Lect, vol 4. London; the British Editorial Society of Bone and Joint Surgery: London, 1999: 24–34.

140. Francis KC. The role of amputation in the treatment of metastatic bone cancer, Clin Orthop 1970; 73: 61–3.

141. Leeson MC, Makley JT, Carter JR. Metastatic skeletal disease: distal to elbow and knee. Clin Orthop Rel Res 1986; 206: 94–9.

142. Johnston CE, Ripley LP, Bray CB et al. Primary endoprosthetic replacement for acute femoral neck fractures: a review of 150 cases. Clin Orthop 1982; 123–7.

13

Surgical Treatment of Pelvic Metastases

R. Windhager

University of Graz, Graz, Austria

INTRODUCTION

Although the pelvis, after the spine, represents the most commonly affected site in patients with bony metastasis, surgical interventions are necessary in only a few cases compared to metastases of the long bones, especially the proximal end of the femur. Nevertheless, with the still-increasing prognosis for the survival of patients suffering from metastatic cancer and a more aggressive approach to treat these patients surgically in order to preserve life quality, the number of interventions in the pelvic region will increase [1,2]. 5-Year survival data of the American Cancer Society [3] for patients treated between 1988 and 1992 indicate survival rates for prostate cancer of 90% for Whites and 75% for Blacks, for breast cancer of 86% for Whites and 70% for Blacks. Furthermore, estimates in this report suggest that 15% of new cancer cases diagnosed each year are at risk of developing bone metastases.

The risk of pathological fracture and loss of function has been decreased by the wide use of biphosphonates, which are able to attenuate the amount of bone destruction, resulting in a significant delay and reduced incidence of fractures in short-term trials. Thus, surgical intervention has to be considered more urgently in patients with progressive osteolysis, despite treatment with biphosphonates and adjuvant therapy. Estimation of individual prognosis is one of the key factors in treating these patients with limited life expectancy and thus indicating surgery at the appropriate time. Surgical therapy has to be tailor-made in this interdisciplinarily-treated group to fit individual patients' expectation and improvement of life quality. In the periacetabular region, the timing of surgical procedures is more important than in all other skeletal regions, as reconstruction of this force-transmitting area requires sufficient bone stock to provide satisfactory post-operative outcome. The early treatment of small lesions is a much less demanding procedure for both the patient and the surgeon than resection and reconstruction of a completely destroyed acetabulum, and the patient will have more benefit from the procedure the earlier it is carried out. The main goals of surgical intervention are restoration and maintenance of function and life quality, although the aspect of local recurrence has to be taken into account when planning the procedure. For most cases, a compromise has to be attempted between the aggressiveness of local treatment in order to prevent local recurrence and the burden to the patient, taking into account the stage of the disease and the possible peri-operative complications. Besides the oncological complications, the surgeon has to be aware of the special anatomical and technical aspects of reconstruction to manage metastatic disease of the pelvis. Numerous technological advances have simplified surgery of pelvic metastases during the last two decades, such as new off-the-shelf protrusion acetabulum ring devices for large acetabular reconstructions as well as custom-made endoprosthetic replacements to fit the largest defects. This planning is supported by the possibility of 3-D imaging, either on the screen or with a 3-D model, for the manufacture of endoprosthetic replacements.

Textbook of Bone Metastases. Edited by C. Jasmin, R. E. Coleman, L. R. Coia, R. Capanna and G. Saillant
© 2005 John Wiley & Sons Ltd: ISBN 0 471 87742 5

Despite these advances in imaging, surgical technique and reconstruction, the treating physician is challenged to choose the best type of treatment for these patients, who have a limited lifespan, against a background of increasing economic pressure to the medical system.

STAGING AND SURGICAL PLANNING

Oncological Staging

Exact estimation of the individual prognosis can only be achieved by thorough work-up of metastatic spread. Basic investigations include total skeletal technetium-99 (^{99m}Tc) nuclear bone scanning in the assessment of occult disease, as well as chest X-rays and computed tomography (CT) scan of the lung in cases of a negative plain X-ray. Serum markers should also be evaluated routinely, e.g. alkaline phosphatase, LDH, calcium and tumour-specific markers. A CT scan of the retroperitoneum may be useful in case of suspicious nodules detected by sonography.

Estimation of the prognosis can be achieved by different scoring systems. According to Bauer [4], no difference in survival rates could be detected between patients suffering from metastases of the spine or central region compared to the appendicular skeleton. In this system five prognostic parameters were defined by multiple regression analysis, including: no pathological fracture; no visceral metastasis; no cancer from the lung; singular bony lesion; and primary tumour arising from breast, kidney, myeloma or lymphoma. Depending on the number of parameters, estimates for 1 year survival range from 50% with four or five positive parameters, 25% with two or three positive parameters, and less than 6 months with zero or one positive parameter. In general, most of the patients requiring surgical treatment of pelvic metastasis suffer from thyroid, breast or prostate cancer, or hypernephroma.

Surgical Staging

Different staging systems should be applied to exactly define the location of the metastasis. For a description of pelvic involvement, the system proposed by Enneking [5,6] is widely used and allows for comparison of different results. In this system, PI describes involvement of the ileum, PII of the acetabulum, PIII of the pubis and ischium, and PIV of the lateral part of the sacrum. In metastatic diseases, but also in primary malignant tumours, more than one of the described areas is usually involved.

As metastatic destruction of the acetabulum (PII) with respect to reconstruction represents a more challenging problem than the other areas of the pelvis, these lesions should be classified more accurately. For this purpose, three main systems can be used to exactly define the lesion. The most widely used classification system has been described by Harrington [7] and also provides guidelines for treatment. In class I defects, the lateral cortices as well as the superior medial parts of the walls are structurally intact, representing cavitary and contained defects. In class II lesions, the medial part of the wall is deficient while the acetabular rim is intact. In class III defects the lateral cortices in the superior part of the wall are deficient, while class IV defects are defined as lesions requiring resection for cure. However, class IV defects should be treated only in cases of a solitary metastasis of the tumour with a good prognosis for survival.

A similar system was proposed by Levy et al. [8], in which "minor involvement" (100% of the acetabular globe is intact) describes an acetabulum that requires only curettage of small enough areas of tumour to represent large cement fixation studs, in addition to general preparation of the acetabulum. "Major involvement" is defined as either significant structural defect after tumour removal or mobility of the superior and inferior segment. Finally, "massive acetabular involvement" describes those cases in which no reasonable local bony support is available after tumour excision.

More accurate staging can be achieved with the classification system of the American Academy of Orthopedic Surgeons, which categorises the lesions into five types [9]. Type 1 describes segmental bone loss; type 2 cavitary defects; type 3 combined segmental and cavitary defects; type 4 pelvic discontinuity; and type 5 massive bone loss. This detailed system, although designed for description of bony defects after failed acetabular endoprosthetic replacement, is useful for evaluation purposes and comparisons between different series, especially if metastatic lesions are treated at an early stage with minor acetabular involvement.

For local staging and exact planning, radiographs are not regarded as sufficient. MRI and CT scans, or at least CT, should be performed to provide a clear impression of the full extent of the lesion. 3-D reconstruction of these cross-sectional images may be helpful. In the author's experience, a 3-D model in certain cases where a special reconstruction will be required provides more accurate and individual information during the procedure, taking the 3-D model as an individual template [10].

PREOPERATIVE EMBOLISATION

Embolisation of the feeding arteries should be performed in all lesions treated surgically, in order to decrease the amount of blood loss during curettage of the tumour. Especially highly vascularised lesions, such as metastases arising from hypernephroma or thyroid cancer, may even require a second embolisation if there is no pathological fracture necessitating acute surgery. Depending on the technique used, surgical intervention should be performed no later than 3 days after embolisation.

SURGICAL TECHNIQUE

After thorough oncological work-up and defining the indication for pelvic surgery, special preparations are necessary in order to prevent intra-operative and post-operative complications. Preparation of the bowel represents an important aspect to decrease infection in these high-risk patients; the bowel should be cleaned before surgery by liquid diet for at least 1 day and enema until clear on the night before surgery. A more aggressive bowel preparation by a wash-out is usually not required, unless there is a risk of opening the bowel during surgery in case of re-operations.

As the risk of pulmonary embolism is higher in patients with pelvic tumours, venograms of both legs should be performed shortly before surgery to rule out venous thrombi.

Sufficient blood units have to be prepared, especially in patients with a rare blood group. Furthermore, large central intravenous lines, as well as the possibility of a rapid infusion system, should be provided for the procedure. In cases of medial extension of the tumour, the patient should have not only a urinary catheter but also ureteral stents, which help in identifying the ureter during preparation. Epidural catheters provide pain relief, not only during the operation but mainly post-operatively for the first few days. All these aspects of pre-operative preparation seem to be self-evident; however, only the rigorous application of these steps guarantees a decrease in peri-operative risk of morbidity and mortality.

The patient is positioned on the table in a lateral decubitus position which is the standard for most types of pelvic resections. This can be achieved with a vacuumed bean bag, which provides a large contact area to the patient's body as well as secure fixation of the position of the patient. However, the author prefers a rather mobile position, where only the chest is fixed ventrally and dorsally, allowing the pelvis and legs to be rotated to both sides. Additionally, a heating mattress is positioned under the patient and the undraped areas of the body are covered with a heating blanket to prevent sinking of the patient's temperature, which might disturb blood coagulation and increase the risk of intra-operative bleeding.

For PIII resections, the patient is positioned in a supine position with both legs abducted and slightly flexed, each on a separate support. In order to allow manipulation of the leg, the operated leg is prepared and left unfixed. In cases where only the supra-acetabular part of the ileum is involved, a simple supine position is sufficient and provides satisfactory exposure for curettage and reconstruction with a protrusio acetabuli ring.

SURGICAL APPROACHES

Most resections can be done by an ilioinguinal incision, extending from the posterior iliac spine to the pubic tubercle (Figure 13.1A, B). Depending on the location of the metastasis, the dissection is performed more dorsally or ventrally. For exposure of the proximal part of the femur, the incision from the iliac crest is directed more laterally over the trochanteric region [11]. In cases where an ilioinguinal incision has already been performed, the approach to the trochanteric region can also be gained by a T-like elongation of the incision to the lateral part of the upper thigh. For PIII resections, the incision is placed from the anterior iliac spine over the inguinal region to the medial part of the thigh. A combined anterior and posterior approach is rarely necessary in resection of metastatic lesions. The skin flaps should be kept as thick as possible in order to prevent skin breakdown.

Iliac Resection (Type I, According to Enneking)

Independent of the type of resection or curettage, this region is easily approached by a standard ilioinguinal skin incision. In cases of curettage, the incision is placed exactly over the lesion and can be kept much smaller than in cases of resection. The ilium is directly approached and the lesion curetted and filled with methylmethacrylate in cases of a cavitary defect without discontinuity of the pelvic ring. If the resection is intralesional, within the bone, phenol is applied to the bone as a local adjuvant treatment after the metastasis has been curetted thoroughly. In extensive cases it might be necessary to use metallic augmenta-

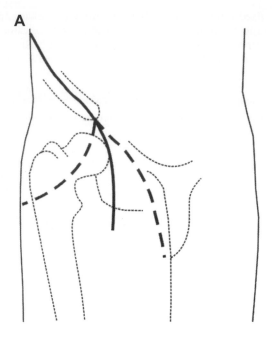

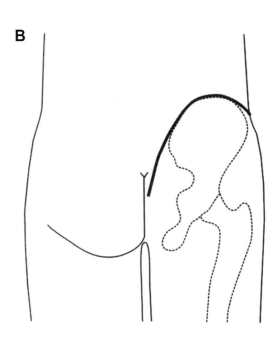

Figure 13.1. (A) Ilioinguinal approach from the ventral side; the skin incision may be placed more laterally to approach the acetabulum, or more medially to obtain access to the pubis. (B) Ilioinguinal skin incision from dorsally. The ilioinguinal skin incision can be extended over the posterior superior iliac spine to the lateral part of the sacrum to approach the sacroiliac joint

tion of the cement, such as screws or heavy Steinmann pins, which are inserted before cementation.

In cases of resection of the ilium, a wider exposure has to be performed. The abdominal wall musculature (external, internal, oblique and transverse abdominal muscles) is dissected carefully off the iliac crest, taking care of the lateral femoral cutanous nerve, which is kept medially together with the sartorius muscle. The internal iliac (hypogastric) vessels are identified, as well as the gluteal and obturator branches. The internal iliac artery and vein are ligated and dissected, even if these vessels have been occluded by preoperative embolisation. The author recommends this step, as manipulation during resection of the specimen might cause damage to these vessels and cause dangerous bleeding. Furthermore, the ureter is identified and marked with an elastic loop, and the same applies to the obturator vessels and nerves. The peritoneum is prepared bluntly and retracted to the medial side, after the inguinal ligament has been detached laterally from the anterior iliac spine, allowing preparation of the iliopsoas and femoral nerve as well as the retroperitoneal space. Care has to be taken in the inguinal region not to damage the spermatic cord in male patients, which should be dissected from medially to laterally and retracted. The femoral nerve is usually retracted medially, together with the psoas muscle, which is dissected from the iliac muscle; the latter is left on the specimen to achieve wide margins. Finally, the L4 and L5 nerve roots are identified medially to the sacroiliac joint and prepared distally to the sciatic notch. As a next step, the gluteal muscles are detached from the iliac wing to the sciatic notch from the lateral side and the sciatic nerve is exposed, taking care also to avoid the gluteal vessels and nerves. If wide margins are attempted, the gluteus minimus and part of the gluteus median muscle have to be left on the specimen. Retractors are inserted into the sciatic notch and the ilium is resected with an oscillating saw and chisels. In cases where the resection has to be carried out through the sacroiliac joint, the exposure in the dorsal area has to be extended, including detachment of the paravertebral muscles. The angle of the sacroiliac joint to the sagittal plane is in the range of 45–50° and has to been taken into account when doing the osteotomy parallel to this joint.

Reconstruction in these cases is usually done with a cement spacer, augmented with screws inserted into the first and second sacral vertebrae as well as into the ilium, ischium and possibly the pubis (Figure 13.2). Biological reconstruction should be avoided in these patients with limited life expectancy, and might be considered only in patients with thyroid cancer. If

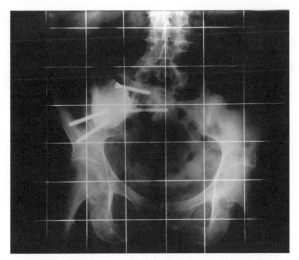

Figure 13.2. 71 year-old female patient suffering from metastases of an adenocarcinoma from an occult primary tumour. The destruction of the sacroiliac joint was treated by curettage and methylmethacrylate, fixed with screws to the sacrum and ilium

significant bleeding has occurred during the resection, reconstruction might be done in a second step; however, filling the defect with methylmethacrylate usually stops bleeding and prevents accumulation of haematoma in the defect. In general, the patients recover very quickly provided thorough reconstruction has been carried out connecting the abdominal wall musculature with the gluteal muscles. The entire iliac wing is usually not reconstructed, in order to allow for better wound closure (Figure 13.3A–D).

The patients are allowed only partial weight-bearing for the first 4 weeks, until the muscle reconstruction has healed, and they should use at least one cane for a longer period until complete recovery of the muscles. In some cases long-term use of a cane may be necessary.

Obturator Resections
(Type III, According to Enneking)

As mentioned above, the approach by an ilioinguinal incision is extended to the medial side of the thigh. Similar to the type I approach, the inguinal ligament is detached and the femoral neurovascular bundle is exposed and prepared proximally into the retroperitoneal space. The pectineus and the adductor muscles are detached from the pubic ramus and, depending on the extension of the lesion, the ischiocrural muscles are

dissected from the ischium. By putting the leg in flexion in the hip joint, the vessels can be elevated and preparation is extended retroperitoneally to the obturator foramen. The obturator artery and nerve are usually infiltrated by the metastasis and have to be resected, unless an intralesional resection has been chosen. The symphysis is identified and dissected after the urethra has been protected by retractors. If part of the acetabulum has to be resected, the capsule of the hip joint is incised in a T-shape manner and the femoral head is dislocated. The sciatic notch is prepared bluntly and retractors are inserted; the sacrotuberal and sacrospinal ligaments are identified and dissected. After osteotomy through the inferior part of the acetabulum, the remaining pelvic muscles are dissected before the specimen can be removed. Even with this extensive resection, ligation and dissection of the internal iliac artery and vein usually is not necessary, as flexion of the hip joint allows for sufficient retraction of these vascular structures. If the acetabulum can be spared, the hip capsule should not be opened, in order not to compromise the blood supply to the femoral head. In this case, retractors are inserted into the lesser sciatic notch and osteotomy is done either with a Gigli saw or with an oscillating saw.

If the acetabulum has not been touched, no major reconstruction is necessary in this type of resection. A resorbable mesh should be sutured between the remaining part of the symphysis, the pelvic muscles and the muscles of the abdominal wall, leaving space for the femoral artery and vein. If resection of the adductor muscles was too extensive, the resulting defect should be filled with viable tissue, for which the distally detached sartorius muscle offers an easy type of reconstruction and prevents haematoma and infection. Alternatively, the rectus abdominis muscle from the contralateral side may be used for larger defects. In cases where the inferior part of the acetabulum has been resected, either a protrusio ring, fixed with several long cancellous screws into the ileum, can be inserted or a saddle prosthesis is used to reconstruct the defect. However, a total hip replacement with the reconstructed acetabulum provides better results. Immobilisation in a plaster or splint for several weeks should be applied in both types of reconstruction, in order to prevent dislocation.

Acetabular Resection and Reconstruction
(Type II, According to Enneking)

Metastases in this location are treated by curettage and reconstruction rather than by resection and recon-

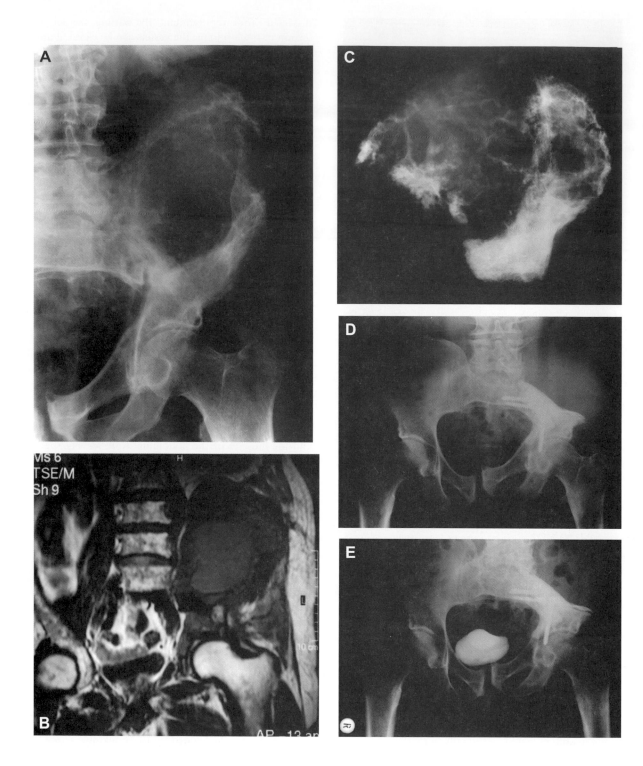

Figure 13.3.   *(Caption opposite)*

struction, as the latter requires a much more extensive approach, with a greater challenge of reconstruction, a higher loss of function even after successful reconstruction, and a higher risk of intra- and post-operative morbidity. The approach to curettage of the proximal part of the acetabulum is easily done by an antero-lateral approach, with a skin incision starting from the iliac crest and extending to the lateral thigh of the femur. From this approach both the iliac and ischial part of the acetabulum can be visualised sufficiently to enable curettage. As mentioned above, the areas involved were divided by Harrington into three classes, determining also the type of reconstruction.

Class I defects are cavitary contained defects with an intact periacetabular rim. In small lesions, even standard acetabular components can be cemented with a large amount of methylmethacrylate and the possible use of a fibre mesh to reinforce the medial wall. In tumours which are not responding well to post-operative radiation therapy, a more stable reconstruction with an acetabulum reinforcement ring and screw fixation into the ileum and ischium should be added (Figure 13.3E,F).

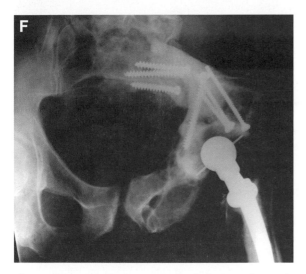

Figure 13.3. (A) Single metastasis of a hypernephroma in the left iliac wing of a 64 year-old male patient. (B) MRI shows the huge soft tissue expansion, reaching to the 3rd lumbar vertebra. (C) Resected specimen, including the entire ilium (Type I, according to Enneking). (D) Reconstruction with methylmethacrylate bridging the gap between the acetabulum and sacrum, fixed to the ischium and sacrum with cancellous screws. (E) Local recurrence after 1 year in the acetabulum and also in the pubis and ischium, which were unaffected pre-operatively. (F) After total hip replacement, with reinforcement of the cup anchorage by cortical screws connected to the cement of the previous operation, the patient was pain-free and ambulatory

In class II defects, where the medial part of the acetabular wall has been destroyed but the acetabulum and lateral cortices of the ileum, ischium and pubis are left intact, protrusio acetabuli rings are mandatory to transmit the stress of weight-bearing from the prosthetic socket onto the intact part of the acetabular rim and the ilium. In all these cases, the ring should be secured with screws into the ilium and ischium to provide sufficient stability for the remaining period of life.

Class III defects are defined as loss of structural continuity without sufficient bone stock in the inferior part of the acetabular rim to allow conventional protrusio acetabuli ring reinforcement. In these defects, the technique described by Harrington provides a stable reconstruction with sufficient durability for these patients with limited life expectancy. This type of reconstruction aims at transmission of the weight-bearing load to the intact bone of the ilium and sacrum. For this purpose, large (4.8 mm) threaded Steinmann pins are drilled into the healthy bone of the superior part of the ilium, and in most instances across the sacroiliac joint into the lateral mass of the sacrum. The orientation of the pins should be mainly along the longitudinal axes of weight-bearing, and positioning is controlled by putting the fingertip into the sciatic notch and protecting the sciatic nerve and gluteal vessels. Occasionally a Steinmann pin can also be positioned into the pubis. After positioning of the pins, their distal ends are cut as distal as possible but without interference to the normal positioning of the protrusio acetabuli ring and acetabular prosthetic component. Fibre mesh can be added medially to prevent cement dislocation. The pins should be left as long as possible to fill the cavity defect, which is then filled with methylmethacrylate before the acetabular component, and preferably a combination of protrusio acetabular cup and the polyethylene cup, are cemented to form a biomechanical continuum between socket, ring, pins and the intact bone superiorly.

Class IV lesions, according to the Harrington classification, describe solitary metastases suitable for resection. This may be applied to large singular metastatic lesions arising from hypernephroma that do not respond to radiation therapy, or to thyroid cancer, providing the best long-term survival of patients with metastatic bone disease. Even these lesions can be approached from an extensive ilio-inguinal incision, including preparation of the iliac and pubic part as described above. Alternatively, a double anterior–posterior approach can be used, in which the anterior incision is positioned over the iliofemoral neurovascular bundle and the dorsal over the sciatic nerve. This approach has been described in detail elsewhere and is applicable for tumours with extensive anteroposterior soft tissue extension [10].

A 3-D model has also proved successful in significantly minimising the risk of intralesional resection [10]. These models are usually made for designing and manufacturing custom-built endoprostheses, which are the most suitable to bridge these defects, especially if the entire ilium has to be resected together with the acetabulum. In cases where part of the ilium can be spared, a saddle prosthesis [12] offers a valuable modular type of reconstruction (Figure 13.4A,B). Resection without reconstruction, leaving the leg in a flail position, should be avoided in patients with metastatic disease, as functional recovery takes several months to >1 year. Also, biological reconstructions such as arthrodeses enlarge the procedure and are of inferior value in these patients, as they do not provide early restoration of function [6,13]. An alternative procedure was described by Winkelmann, who fixed the acetabulum to the lateral part of the sacrum and the remaining part of the ilium in cases of a type I and II resection [14]. With this procedure, a significant shortening of the leg and permanent use of a walking support, at least one cane, has to be taken into account. However, as a limp is also frequently seen after endoprosthetic reconstruction of the pelvis, this procedure provides an economic alternative to custom-made endoprosthetic replacement.

RESULTS

Results in the literature are rare and are difficult to compare, due to variability in classification as well as type of reconstructions [15–17].

The most extensive results on acetabular reconstruction in patients with metastatic disease has been reported by Harrington [7,18]. In 1981 he reported on 58 patients treated by hip replacement arthroplasty for pathological fractures and fracture dislocations of the acetabulum secondary to metastatic diseases; 11 patients had class I defects, 19 had class II defects, 25 class III defects and only three patients had resection for cure (class IV defects). With a mean survival time of 19 months, this group of patients differs from the general survival time of patients with metastatic bone disease, reflecting a selection bias for this challenging procedure. The patients were evaluated at 6 months and 2 years post-operatively for relief of pain, resumption of walking, stability of fixation of the prosthetic components, and survival without recurrence at the operative site. At 6 months 67% had

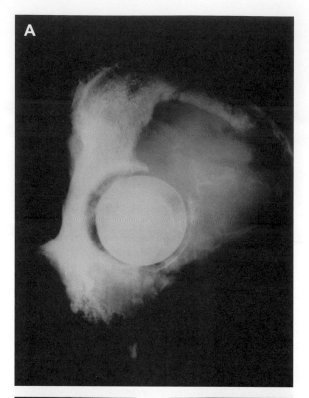

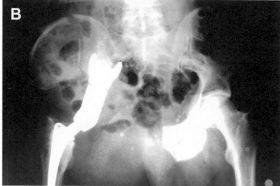

Figure 13.4. (A) Resected metastases of hypernephroma, including the ischium and pubis, acetabulum and part of the ilium (Types II, III and partially I, according to Enneking). (B) Reconstruction with a saddle prosthesis bridging the gap between the ilium and the femoral endoprothesis

excellent or good pain relief and 43% even at 2 years. 80% were ambulatory at 6 months and 45% kept their walking ability at 2 years. There were two perioperative deaths and five patients had loosening of the acetabular prosthetic components due to local tumour recurrence, despite adequate radiotherapy.

Levy et al. in 1982 [8] also described 58 cases with metastatic disease involving the area of the hip. Similar to Harrington's report, the majority of cases were metastases arising from breast carcinomas (38/58), followed by neoplasms of the haematopoetic system (10 cases). The average survival time was 14.5 months from the time of surgery and there were no immediate operative deaths. All patients in this series who were able to walk prior to fracture or the pain of an impending fracture lesion were able to regain comparable status after surgery. Also, patients who were unable to walk prior to the local hip problem nevertheless appeared to be greatly benefited. Exact data on the evaluation of these patients and the time of evaluation are lacking in this paper.

Algan and Horowitz [15], in their series of pathological hip lesions in patients with metastatic disease, included five cases treated with a protrusio acetabuli ring, of whom one patient required re-operation with open reduction and internal fixation after local recurrence. All patients were ambulatory and four had moderate and one severe pain; one regained walking after having been confined to wheelchair.

Vena et al. [19] published 21 patients with severe acetabular deficiency, with a mean post-operative survival of 14.5 months (± 4.0) and a period of independent living of 10.4 months (± 3.0). For the first time, the Musculoskeletal Tumour Society (MSTS) score has been applied for evaluation, and a mean post-operative score of 14.2 (of a total of 30) has been calculated. However, low scores were attributed to the patients' overall disease and the presence of a Trendelenburg limp. Apart from six patients with surgical complications, three died early post-operatively, due to poor pre-operative pulmonary function, there were two dislocations, one related to a late infection, one femoral and one peroneal nerve palsy. Nevertheless, there was statistically significant improvement in pain and mobility scores post-operatively.

Another series of 55 patients with metastatic disease of the acetabulum has been reported by Marco et al. [20], including mainly patients with breast carcinoma, followed by carcinoma of the kidney and prostate. The median survival time was 9 months, which may be explained by the high percentage of patients with multiple skeletal metastases (73%) and association with visceral metastases (33%). Again, patients with breast cancer had a significantly increased prognosis compared to other carcinomas. 54 of the hips were reconstructed with a protrusional cup (modified Harrington technique) and one patient had endoprosthetic reconstruction of the hemipelvis. 76% of the patients had relief of pain, determined by decreased use of narcotics. Nine of 18 patients unable to walk pre-operatively regained walking ability and another 14 patients regained full ambulatory status. At 6 months (33 patients available) 76% still had relief of pain and 58% were able to walk. Local progression was seen in 14/55 patients (25%), leading to failure of the fixation in five patients. The mean operative time was 290 ± 72 min, the mean estimated blood loss 2200 ± 1100 ml. Fourteen complications were observed in 12 patients (22%), including five deep vein thromboses, three superficial wound infections, one multidisseminated intravascular coagulation like coagulopathy, one sacral decubitus ulcer, one wound haematoma, one Sudeck dystrophy and one hip subluxation, requiring a revision of the acetabular component. One patient died in the early post-operative period. There were five late fixation failures after a median time of (12 ± 7) months.

Giurea et al. [21] in their retrospective analysis of 43 patients, compared 37 patients with intralesional to six patients with extralesional resection. The clinical evaluation was performed by the Karnovsky performance state [22], which showed significant improvement from 55% pre-operatively to 57% at 3 months and even 77% at 6 months ($p=0.0001$). Patients undergoing an intralesional resection had a median survival time of 13 months, a complication rate of 24% and a local recurrence rate of 19 months. In contrast, those undergoing an extralesional resection had a survival time of 16 months and no local recurrences; however, complications had to be accounted for in 3/6 patients. The high complication rate in the latter group may be attributed to the large types of resection performed, using saddle prostheses and endoprosthetic replacements for the reconstructive procedure.

A similar complication rate was reported in a series using saddle prostheses for acetabular reconstruction by Aboulafia et al. [23], which included nine patients with metastatic disease. None of the patients was able to walk without a walking support. Nevertheless, 17% were rated as excellent and good according to the MSTS score.

SUMMARY

Despite significant progress in imaging and surgical techniques, surgical treatment of pelvic metastases still has to be regarded as a challenging problem, especially if the acetabulum is involved. For proper indication, a thorough oncological work-up is necessary, as well as detailed preparation of the operation in order to decrease intra- and post-operative morbidity. Estimation of the individual prognosis of the patient and selection of the appropriate procedure are critical steps for successful treatment. Moreover, the extent of the surgical procedure has to be calculated in the light of adjuvant therapies in a multidisciplinary approach.

REFERENCES

1. Frassica FJ, Sim FH. Pathogenesis and prognosis. In Sim FH (ed.), Diagnosis and Management of Metastatic Bone Disease. Raven: New York, 1988: 1–6.
2. Sim FH. Lesions of the pelvis and hip. In Sim FH (ed.), Diagnosis and Management of Metastatic Bone Disease: a Multidisciplinary Approach. Raven: New York, 1988; 183–98.
3. American Cancer Society. Cancer Statistics. American Cancer Society: New York, 1998: 6–30 (Table 11).
4. Bauer HF, Wedin R. Survival after surgery for spinal and extremity metastases. Acta Orthop Scand 1995; 66(2): 143–6.
5. Enneking WF, Dunham WK. Resection and reconstruction for primary neoplasms involving the innominate bone. J Bone Joint Surg 1978; 60A: 731–46.
6. Enneking WF, Menendez LR. Functional evaluation of various reconstructions after periacetabular resection of iliac lesions. In Enneking WF (ed.), Limb Salvage in Musculoskeletal Oncology. Churchill Livingstone: New York, 1987: 117–35.
7. Harrington KD. The management of acetabular insufficiency secondary to metastatic malignant disease. J Bone Joint Surg 1981; 63-A: 653–64.
8. Levy RN, Sherry HS, Siffert RS. Surgical management of metastatic disease of bone and the hip. Clin Orthop 1982; 169: 62–9.
9. Brady OH, Masri BA, Garbuz DS, Duncan CP. Use of reconstruction rings for the management of acetabular bone loss during revision hip surgery. J Am Acad Orthop Surg 1999; 7: 1–7.
10. Windhager R, Karner J, Kutschera HP et al. Limb salvage in periacetabular sarcomas. Clin Ortho 1996; 331: 265–76.
11. Letournel E. La voie ilio-inguinale. In Meary R, Techniques Orthopediques 1978/9. Expansion Scientifique Paris 1978.
12. Nieder E, Elson RA, Engelbrecht E et al. The saddle prosthesis for salvage of the destroyed acetabulum. J Bone Joint Surg 1990; 72B: 1014–22.
13. Capanna R, Guernelli N, Ruggieri P et al. Periacetabular pelvic resections. In Enneking WF (ed.), Limb Salvage in Musculoskeletal Oncology. Churchill Livingstone: New York, 1987: 141–6.
14. Winkelmann W. Eine neue Operationsmethode bei malignen Tumoren des Darmbeins. Z Orthop 1988; 126: 671–4.
15. Algan SM, Horowitz SM. Surgical treatment of pathologic hip lesions in patients with metastatic disease. Clin Orthop 1996; 332: 223–31.
16. Johnson HTJ. Reconstruction of the pelvic ring following tumor resection. J Bone Joint Surg 1978; 60-A: 747–51.
17. Walker RH. Pelvic reconstruction/total hip arthroplasty for metastatic acetabular insufficiency. Clin Orthop 1993; 294: 170–5.
18. Harrington KD. Orthopaedic management of extremity and pelvic lesions. Clin Orthop 1995; 312: 136–47.
19. Vena VE, Hsu J, Rosier RN, O'Keefe RJ. Pelvic reconstruction for severe periacetabular metastatic disease. Clin Orthop 1999; 362: 171–80.
20. Marco RAW, Sheth DS, Boland PJ et al. Functional and oncological outcome of acetabular reconstruction for the treatment of metastatic disease. J Bone Joint Surg 2000; 82-A: 642–51.
21. Giurea A, Ritschl R, Windhager R et al. The benefits of surgery in the treatment of pelvic metastases. Int Orthop; (SICOT) 1997; 21: 343–8.
22. Karnofsky DA. Clinical evaluation of anticancer drugs. GANN Monograph 1967; 2: 223–31.
23. Aboulafia AJ, Buch R, Mathews J et al. Reconstruction using the saddle prosthesis following excision of primary and metastatic periacetabular tumors. Clin Ortho 1995; 314: 203–13.

14

Indications and Strategy for the Treatment of Spinal Metastases

E. A. Enkaoua

Hôpital de la Pitié-Salpêtrière, Paris, France

INTRODUCTION

The appearance of bone metastasis during the course of cancer represents a major turning point in the treatment strategy. Since metastatic dissemination to bone occurs essentially via the venous circulation, the vertebrae are common target sites because of the presence of the Batson venous plexus.

In the face of vertebral metastases, too many physicians tend to give up hope and abandon any form of antitumour therapy. This is not in the patients' best interest and in many centres multidisciplinary teams have been set up to help patients, as far as possible, preserve an acceptable quality of life and sometimes to increase their life expectancy.

The choice of treatment is difficult and depends to a large extent on the nature of the primary tumour, which essentially determines the prognosis. The vertebral location compounds the difficulty because of the neurological risk. Furthermore, carcinologically satisfactory surgery is almost impossible if ample margins are considered mandatory.

Roy-Camille [1] codified vertebral tumours that are "*en bloc*" removable according to the location of the affected vertebrae. Boriani et al. [2] refined the indication by providing a good description of the surgical technique.

Palliative surgery for vertebral metastasis can be recommended in most cases. The three goals of this surgery are relief of pain, reduction of neurological risk or deficit and mechanical destabilisation of the fracture.

There is no real therapeutic consensus regarding the optimal surgical approach to vertebral metastases. For many years some physicians, e.g. Kostuik et al. [3], have attempted to devise a treatment scoring system based on the vertebral location of the tumour. Others, such as Harrington [4], have defined a strategy based on the neurological state of the patient. Those scoring systems may help the surgeon to choose a technique, but they do not take into account the extent of the disease or the patients' general state of health. Indeed, according to their general condition, patients will respond differently to surgery and the results may be completely different even though the surgery was carried out by the same physician on a tumour located at the same place on the vertebra. For patients in poor general health, a carefully planned surgical approach is indispensable for an optimal result. Vertebral metastases have been analysed according to their location and to the neurological status of the patient, but such analyses do not take into account the primary aetiology of the cancer. Saillant et al. [5] in their report of metastases of thyroid origin emphasised the fact that the primary site is decisive. Indeed, the primary site is an essential parameter for determining the surgical outcome. This was confirmed by the SOFCOT [6] report on vertebral metastases in 1996 and later confirmed by Klekamp and Samii [7] in their study of 740 cases of vertebral tumours.

The treatment of vertebral metastases requires a global assessment of the status of the patient and the prognosis, which is why multidisciplinary teams have been set up in oncology centres.

Textbook of Bone Metastases. Edited by C. Jasmin, R. E. Coleman, L. R. Coia, R. Capanna and G. Saillant
© 2005 John Wiley & Sons Ltd: ISBN 0 471 87742 5

Tokuhashi et al. [8] were the first to devise a scoring system for vertebral metastases; it comprised six parameters reflecting the global status of the patient and of the disease and was a turning point in assessment of the therapeutic indications of vertebral metastasis. Unfortunately, it did not take account of the respective weights of the various parameters, which do not all have the same importance, as underlined in the 1996 SOFCOT [6] report, in which only four significant patient parameters (primary tumour site, general health status, presence of visceral metastasis, and neurological status) were validated. The Tokuhashi scoring can only be used if the entire patient history is available, which is not always the case when the patient is admitted to hospital as an emergency. Enkaoua et al. [9] demonstrated the problems of this scoring when metastases have been insufficiently investigated. Hence, a multidisciplinary team has attempted to create a new scoring system, taking into account the differently weighted parameters, the nature of the surgical emergency and the spinal and vertebral locations of the metastases.

A NEW SCORING SYSTEM TO ASSIST STRATEGIC TREATMENT

This system is designed to assist surgical and medical therapeutic decision making on local treatment of osteolytic or osteoblastic bone metastases. It was devised by an international multidisciplinary team comprising orthopaedic surgeons, neurosurgeons and chemotherapy, radiotherapy and neuroradiology specialists, and consists of four therapeutic classes, as described below.

Class I: Unique Metastases of Thyroid or Renal Origin that have Appeared 3 Years after the Primary Tumour

Treatment must be aggressive, comprising an *en bloc* resection (vertebrectomy), if possible combined with reconstruction by graft and fixation, according to the habit and experience of the surgeon (Figure 14.1). These two primary tumours were chosen because they generally have a good prognosis of long survival. The breast as a primary site was set aside because, as we routinely use a "full-spine MRI" this kind of metastasis is detected rarely for this cancer.

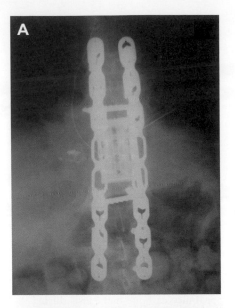

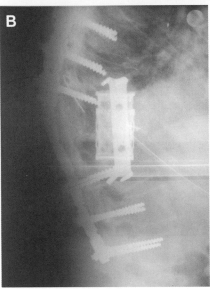

Figure 14.1. Vertebrectomy of T8 for a Schwannosarcoma metastasis with reconstruction by autograft with plate and cage by two approaches, posterior and anterior. (A) Anteroposterior view. (B) Lateral view

Class II: Neurological Metastasis

In most cases this is a surgical emergency. Location in the spine and the extent of the deficit (complete or partial) determine the therapeutic strategy. It is essential to prevent patients being subjected to neurological deficit, which is the result of a vascular lesion rather than mechanical compression, in which the tumour progressively compresses the medullar vessels. Even after complete liberation of the dura mater, when no mechanical compression remains, neurological recovery is rare. This class comprises only thoracic metastases (Figure 14.2) and some cervical tumours but never any lumbosacral metastases, since at this location there is no medulla so the only neurological risk is a root deficit.

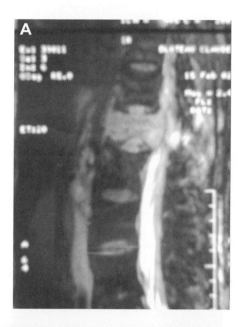

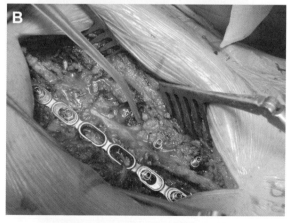

Figure 14.2. Thoracic metastasis causing a neurological deficit. (A) MRI of thoracic metastasis, with cord compression. (B) Perioperative view of metastasis resection, dura mater liberation and pedicular screw plate fixation

Partial Deficit

This is a surgical emergency whatever the location. The treatment must be a medullar decompression, which may or may not be associated with vertebral stabilisation of two possible types:

- Surgical, by fixation with various devices (plates and pedicular screws, stems and hooks, etc.).
- By vertebroplasty, i.e. the injection of cement into the vertebra by a percutaneous approach if surgical fixation is not possible because of major tumoral invasion.

Complete Deficit

- Spastic deficit: this is an acute surgical emergency which requires action within the 6 h period following the appearance of the deficit. The surgery comprises decompression and/or stabilisation and the degree of neurological recovery depends on the rapidity of deficit development. Recovery will be more difficult if the deficit developed within 24 h than in cases in which the deficit appeared progressively.
- Flaccid deficit: if this has been present for more than 6 h and if it appeared in less than 24 h, surgery has little chance of success. If the general status of the patient is poor, surgery should be avoided as the risk is too major for so uncertain a result.

Class III: Metastasis Presenting a Neurological or Destabilisation Risk

For this class no treatment consensus exists, although this is the most common case. The treatment strategy varies according to four parameters, as set out below. Each parameter has a score that is balanced according to its importance; the higher the score, the more surgery is indicated.

Cancer Prognosis

- <1 year survival: score 1
- Survival 1–2 years: score 3
- Survival >2 years: score 6

The prognosis depends on the primary tumour but does not take into account the status of the disease, e.g. a generally good breast cancer prognosis (>2 years, score 6) can be reduced to score 1 if the patient has multiple metastases and a very poor general status.

One must therefore balance the prognosis of the primary tumour against other parameters:

- Alteration in the general status of the patient, using Karnofski index <70%.
- Presence of visceral metastasis.
- Presence of multiple bone metastasis.

If two of these parameters are present, the length of survival regresses by one stage of the scoring system (6 to 3, or 3 to 1). If three of these parameters are present, survival cannot exceed 1 year, hence score 1. The higher the possibility of survival, the more surgery is indicated.

Spinal Location

The neurological risk varies with the location in the spine:

- Cervical spine (wide vertebral canal): score 2.
- Thoracic spine (most important neurological risk): score 3.
- Lumbo-sacral spine (no medullar risk): score 1.

The higher the neurological risk, the more surgery is indicated.

Vertebral Location

The vertebra is divided in three parts: anterior, middle and posterior, according to Denis [10].

- If one part is invaded: score 1.
- If two parts are invaded: score 2.
- If three parts are invaded (total vertebra; Figure 14.3): score 3.

The more the vertebra is invaded, the more surgery is indicated.

Efficiency of Adjuvant Treatment of the Vertebral Metastasis

- If the adjuvant treatment is efficient (radiotherapy, chemotherapy): score 0.
- If the adjuvant treatment is not efficient: score 3.

The more inefficient the adjuvant treatment, the more surgery is indicated.

Once these four parameters are defined, they are added to obtain a global score (minimum 3, maximum 15) which assists in determining treatment strategy:

- If the score is 3–6, surgery is not indicated.

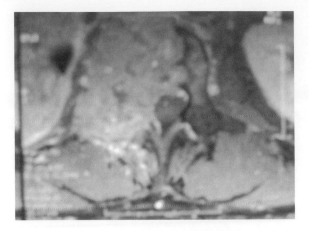

Figure 14.3. CT scan of an example of lumbar metastasis invading the three parts of the vertebra

- If the score is 7–11, palliative surgery is indicated, comprising neurological liberation and/or vertebral stabilisation (Figure 14.4).
- If the score is 12–15, aggressive surgery is indicated if the survival prognosis is good; otherwise, palliative surgery must be chosen.
- If Karnofski scoring is less than 50%, the prognosis for surgery is hazardous.

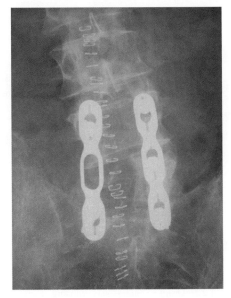

Figure 14.4. Metastasis of L5 from kidney: palliative surgery with pedicular screw plating and neural liberation, anteroposterior view

Class IV:
Multiple Metastasis Without any Neurological or Mechanical Risks

This class does not require surgery and requires only adjuvant treatment with radiotherapy or chemotherapy or a percutaneous vertebroplasty.

CONCLUSION

The treatment of vertebral metastases is difficult because of the anatomical location, the neurological risk, and the uncertain outcome of any cancer treatment. The ISBM scoring system is a useful tool for strategic decision making and can be used in all clinical situations, even if the physician treating a neurological emergency does not have the entire history of the patient at his/her disposal. The first clinical results depending on this system are encouraging and will be published soon.

REFERENCES

1. Roy-Camille R. Tumeurs du rachis. Conf d'Enseign 1989; 34: 137–60.

2. Boriani S, Biagini R, De Iure F et al. Resection surgery in the treatment of vertebral tumors. Chir Organi Mov 1998; 83(1–2): 53–64.

3. Kostuik JP, Errico TJ, Gleason TF, Errico CC. Spinal stabilization of vertebral column tumors. Spine 1988; 13(3): 250–6.

4. Harrington KD. The use of methylmethacrylate for vertebral body replacement and anterior stabilization of pathological fracture dislocations of the spine due to metastatic malignant disease. J Bone Joint Surg Am 1981; 63(1): 36–46.

5. Saillant G, Enkaoua EA, Aimard T et al Métastases rachidiennes d'origine thyroïdiennes. A propos d'une série de 37 cas. Rev Chir Orthop 1995; 81: 672–81.

6. SOFCOT (Société Française de Chirurgie Orthopédique et Traumatologique). Vertebral Metastasis Report. SOFCOT: Paris, 1996.

7. Klekamp J, Samii H. Surgical results for spinal metastases. Acta Neurochir (Wien) 1998; 140(9): 957–67.

8. Tokuhashi Y, Matsuzaki H, Toriyama S et al. Scoring system for the pre-operative evaluation of spinal metastasis tumor progression. Cancer 1990; 15: 1110–13.

9. Enkaoua EA, Doursounian L, Chatellier G et al. A critical appreciation of the preprative prognostic Tokuashi score in a series of 71 cases. Spine 1997; 22: 2293–8.

10. Denis F. Spinal instability as defined by the three-column spine concept in acute spinal trauma. Clin Orthop 1984; 189: 65–76.

15

Surgical Techniques for the Treatment of Bone Metastases of the Spine

Stefano Boriani, Alessandro Gasbarrini, Stefano Bandiera, Giovanni Barbanti Bròdano, Stefania Paderni and Silvia Terzi

Ospedale Maggiore, Bologna, Italy

INTRODUCTION

Surgery in metastatic disease is always palliative and its aim is to allow the patient a better quality of life and to support chemo-, radiation or hormonal therapy by reducing or excising the tumour mass. The increasing survival of patients affected by primary tumours makes it increasingly important to establish appropriate treatment for spinal bone metastases responsible for severe functional impairment.

Since metastasis is a systemic disease, curative eradication of the metastatic lesion (*en bloc* resection, vertebrectomy, spondylectomy) seems to be unnecessary, particularly in the spine, due to anatomic constraints and related morbidity. The results obtained after *en bloc* resection vs. curettage combined with radiation therapy seem to be similar in terms of local control and survival [1]. Morbidity [2,3] and the cost:effectiveness ratio must be weighed against the choice of *en bloc* surgery. However, small size and favourable location, making vertebrectomy or spondylectomy possible, combined with good prognosis of the primary disease, make the choice of *en bloc* surgery feasible in some selected cases. This is particularly true in cases such as metastases from renal cell carcinoma, which have a high risk of recurrence after intralesional excision even if combined with radiation therapy [4]. Indeed, the worst results after curettage are achieved in those cases in which such excision is not complete and radiation therapy is not able to eradicate the lesion:

this confirms that intralesional excision must be complete ("extracapsular") in partially or totally radio-resistant tumours, frequently requiring double-approach surgery.

Palliative surgery is considered to allow a rate of neurological improvement (expressed by quality of life) comparable to curettage at short-term follow-up, but the mid-term survival rate is shorter in patients treated by simple decompression and stabilisation. However, it must be remembered that patients treated with palliative surgery are usually of poorer health status than those submitted to curettage.

Our aim is to review the surgical treatment options and techniques for bone metastases of the spine.

SURGICAL TECHNIQUES

The rationale for any surgical choice must include:

- The best decompression.
- The most effective stabilisation.
- The most complete and oncologically appropriate tumour removal, when a direct approach to the tumour is indicated.

Surgical treatment of spinal bone metastatic disease no longer includes laminectomy, as its results are comparable to those of radiation alone [5,6], further submitting the spine to the risk of worsening instability with neurological deterioration [7].

Textbook of Bone Metastases. Edited by C. Jasmin, R. E. Coleman, L. R. Coia, R. Capanna and G. Saillant
© 2005 John Wiley & Sons Ltd: ISBN 0 471 87742 5

The surgical options considered are:

1. Decompression and stabilisation (Figure 15.1).
2. Intralesional excision (tumour debulking) and reconstruction (Figures 15.2 and 15.3).
3. *En bloc* resection (Figure 15.4).

Decompression and Stabilisation

This is the shortest and least aggressive surgical procedure, aiming to decompress the spinal cord and to stabilise the spine in the thoracic and lumbar regions. The procedure does not necessarily include a direct approach to the tumour.

Indications

Pathological fracture or impending collapse in the thoracic and/or lumbar spine at two opposed extremities of the spectrum of spine metastases:

● Highly radio-sensitive conditions (lymphoma, plasmacytoma) or known sensitivity to hormonotherapy (some metastases from breast carcinoma), regardless of neurological encroachment.
● Patients with poor life expectancy, to save neurological function and spine stability as long as possible. The longitudinal extension of the instrumentation can cover multiple tumour sites until

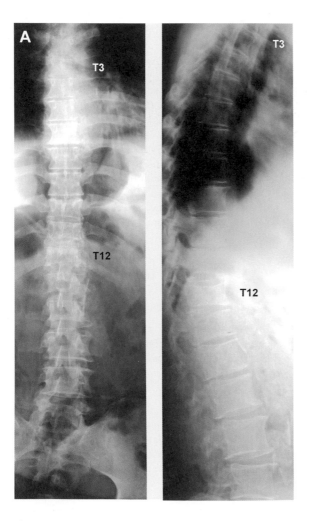
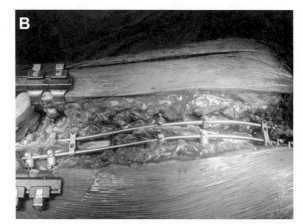
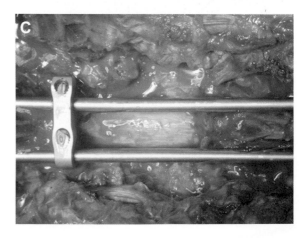

Figure 15.1A–C *(Caption opposite)*

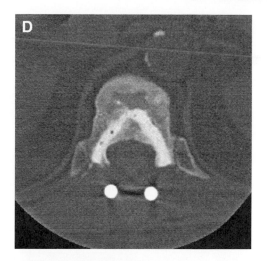

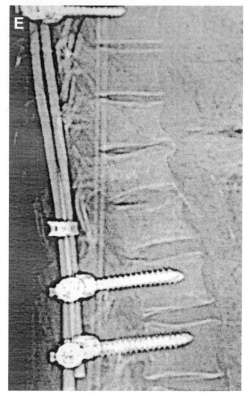

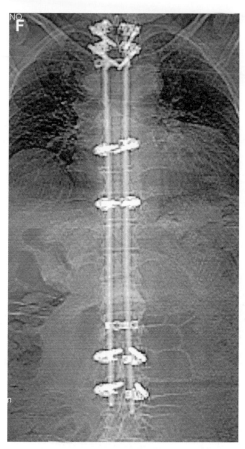

Figure 15.1. Patient 61 years old affected by metastatic disease of T3 and T12 from a prostatic cancer. The patient had a good response to the chemotherapy and thus underwent posterior decompression and stabilisation from T2 to L4. (A) Pre-operative anteroposterior and left lateral radiographs, showing the osteolysis in T3 and T12. (B) Intra-operative. enlarged view of the operating field, showing the long transpedicular stabilisation from T2 to L4 by means of titanium instrumentation. (C) Intra-operative: detail of the circumferential decompression in T2. (D) Post-operative CT scan, showing the introduction of transpedicular acrylic cement, bilaterally, to reinforce vertebra T12 (vertebroplasty) after removal of the tumour inside. (E,F) Anteroposterior and left lateral radiographs at the 7 month follow-up

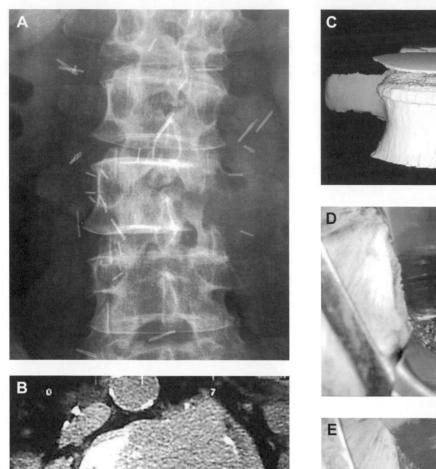

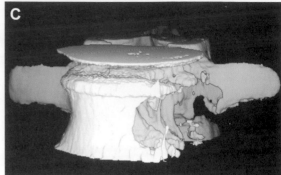

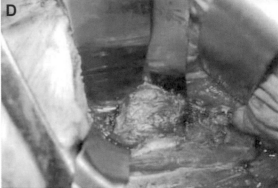

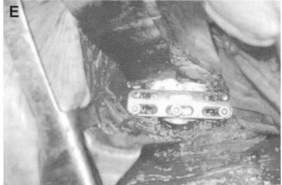

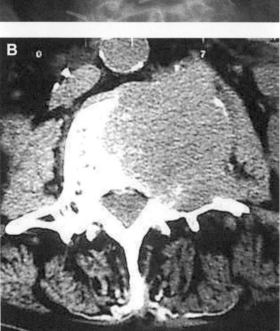

Figure 15.2A–E. *(Caption opposite)*

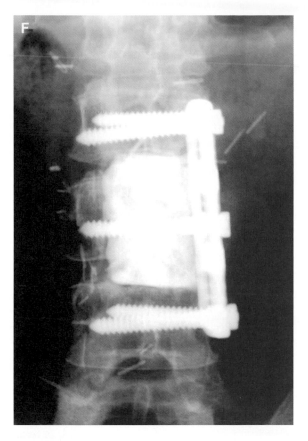

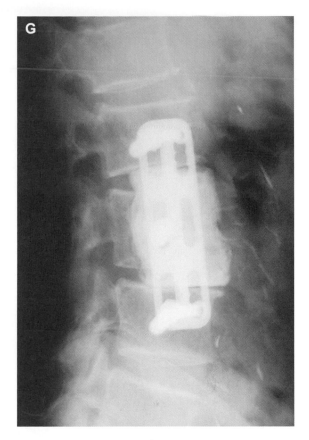

Figure 15.2. Patient 70 years old affected by an isolated metastasis from a hypernephroma of the left half of the L3 posterior body. Hemivertebrectomy was performed by an anterior approach, with reconstruction of the vertebral body with cement and stabilisation by an anterior plate. (A) Anteroposterior radiograph: osteolysis of L3 with disappearance of the right pedicle. (B) Pre-operative CT scan, showing the neoplastic replacement of the hemisome. (C) 3-D CT scan reconstruction. (D) Intra-operative: retroperitoneal approach and isolation of L3. (E) Intra-operative: after complete curettage, the vertebra was reconstructed with PMMA, fixed with a plate to the adjacent vertebrae. (F,G) Post-operative anteroposterior and left lateral radiographs

stability is obtained. The advantages and risks of surgical stabilisation must be weighed against palliative medical treatment, mostly precluding ambulatory activities. We do not believe it is ethical to query the economic aspects of performing expensive surgery in poor life-expectancy patients, but we must be reasonably sure that this surgery will allow better neurological and static function and pain relief not achievable by other techniques.

This procedure is not highly technically demanding, only a basic knowledge of spine posterior fixation being required.

Surgical Technique

A prone position is needed, with hips and knees flexed. A careful check should be made of soft supports on the shoulder and iliac regions to avoid skin, vascular and nerve damage and to prevent any compression to the abdomen and chest wall.

A longitudinal midline approach is performed, detaching the paravertebral muscles from the posterior arches at least two levels above and below the affected vertebra or vertebrae, as far as the sacrum for L4 and L5 tumours. Pedicular screws and/or hooks can be implanted at this time, before laminectomy, to make rapid closure of the procedure possible in the event of

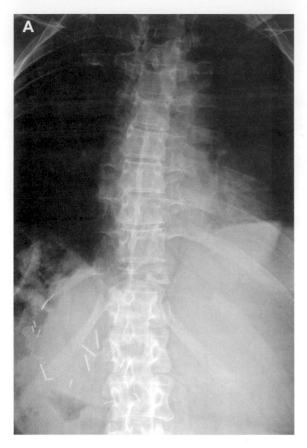
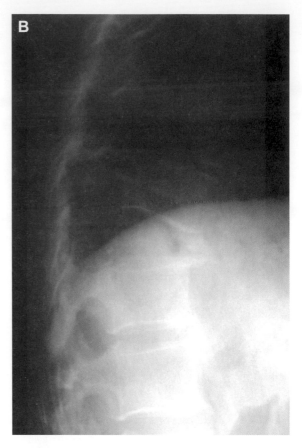

Figure 15.3. Patient 44 years old affected by metastatic disease of T11 and the lungs from a bile duct cancer. Complete vertebrectomy of T11, decompression and stabilisation from T6 to L2 by posterior approach. The reconstruction of the vertebral body was made with titanium mesh. (A,B) Anteroposterior and left lateral radiographs showing the neoplastic involvement of T11. (C) Pre-operative CT scan, showing the pathological fracture and the intra-canal compression of the neoplastic mass. (D,E) Anteroposterior and left lateral radiographs after circumferential decompression by means of intralesional vertebrectomy. Titanium cage and transpedicular instrumentation from T6 to L2, all by the posterior approach. (F) Post-operative CT scan

severe bleeding. The pre-operative planning for reconstruction must aim to achieve stability: a typical construction based on two levels (at least) above and below the level of the metastatic lesion must therefore be considered in most cases, with the following suggestions:

- The only role of palliative posterior stabilisation in the cervical spine is for C1 and C2 tumours: in these cases occipito-cervical fixation can be performed by special devices [8].
- When the tumour occurs in the high thoracic spine (T1–T3), fixation to the cervical spine must be considered. The stabilisation system can be a couple of plates or double diameter rods,

connected to pedicle screws inferiorly and to lateral mass screws or hooks superiorly.

- The construction should never be stopped at the apex of the kyphotic curve (T4–T6) or at T12, to prevent loosening and further kyphotic deformity.
- In the thoracic spine (T4–T10), hooks or pedicles can be chosen according to personal experience and approach. The great advantage of screws is that, once implanted, connection or disconnection to the rods is easy and fast whenever necessary, according to oncologic needs.
- At the thoraco-lumbar junction (T11–L2), the advantages of pedicle screws are outstanding from a mechanical point of view.

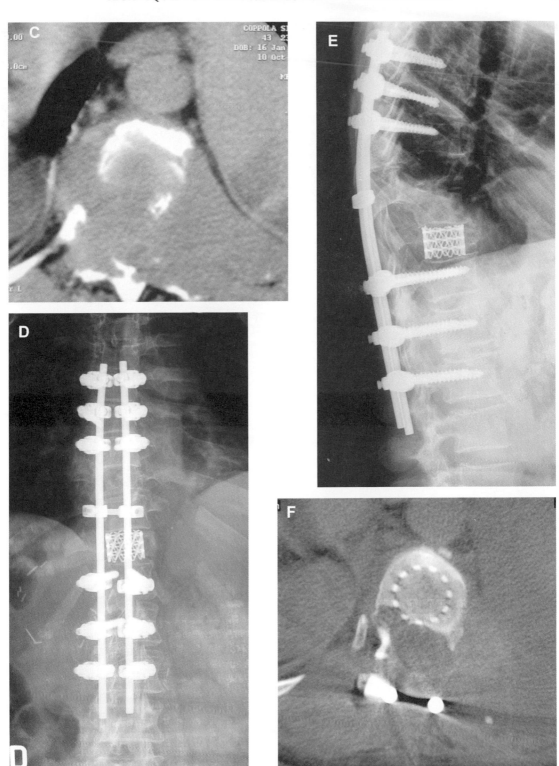

Figure 15.3C–F *(Caption opposite)*

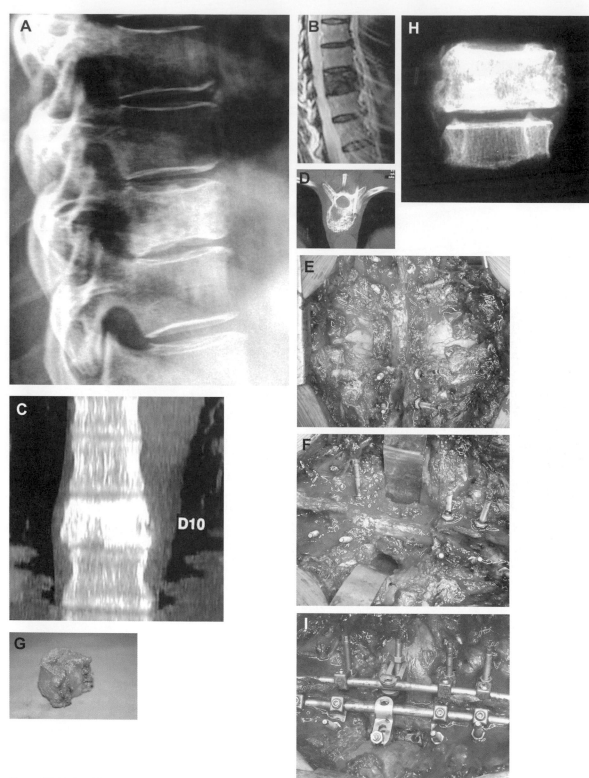

Figure 15.4A–I *(Caption opposite)*

- In the lumbar spine: for tumours located only in L3, a simple one level above and one level below implant is sufficiently strong provided that the anterior column is not destroyed, while for L4 and for L5 fixation to the sacrum is mandatory.
- Since the surgery is palliative, there is no point in talking about "short fixations": the patient's expectation is stability without pain: when a doubt arises about the possibility of further metastatic involvement, that vertebra should be included in the fusion area.
- A graft for fusion purposes seems useless and the bleeding from decorticated area is harmful.

A complete laminectomy can be performed as a second step, usually removing all the posterior elements, pedicles included, to achieve complete posterior decompression. Rongeurs can be used, as well as a Tomita saw, but this is more technically demanding. Complete circumferential decompression can be obtained by excising the tumour mass anterior to the cord [9]. If the planned procedure is a simple extralesional decompression, the construction can be completed according to the chosen system—mainly a pair of rods with transverse connectors.

Intralesional Excision (Tumour Debulking) and Reconstruction

Under this term we can include both direct aggressive treatment of the tumour mass by curettage of the lesion and partial excision of the tumour for decompression purposes. This kind of procedure seems the

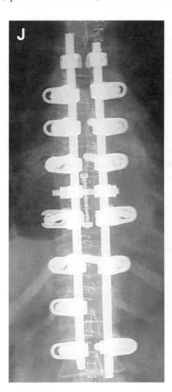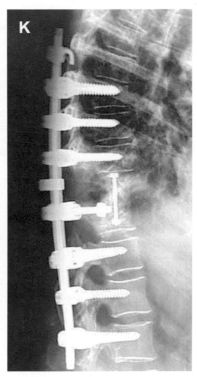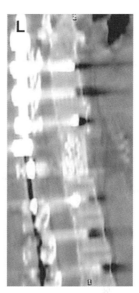

Figure 15.4. Patient 56 years old affected by an isolated metastasis of T10 body from thyroid cancer. Vertebrectomy of T10 and superior hemivertebrectomy of T11 were performed by a posterior approach, reconstruction of the vertebral body by BBT prosthesis and posterior spinal instrumentation from T7 to L2. (A) Left lateral radiograph showing the thickening of T10. (B) Pre-operative MRI. (C) Pre-operative 2-D CT scan reconstruction. (D) Transpedicular needle biopsy under CT control with a local anaesthetic. (E) Intra-operative: removal of the posterior arch and bilateral T10 T11 costotransversectomy after positioning of the pedicular screws. (F) Intra-operative: isolation of the vertebra by a posterior approach. (G–H) En bloc removal of the affected vertebra with the overlying disc and the superior hemivertebra of T11. (I) Intra-operative: instrumentation completed with a carbon prosthesis filled with autoplastic grafts, connected to the posterior instrumentation, which replaces the removed vertebrae. (J,K) Post-operative anteroposterior and left lateral radiographic control. (L) 2-D sagittal CT scan reconstruction control, 12 months after the operation, showing integration of the graft inside the carbon prosthesis

most appropriate, from an oncological point of view, to treat systemic disease such as metastases, and must be included in a multidisciplinary approach. Treatment should include selective arterial embolisation [11,12] to reduce bleeding (which can sometimes be life-threatening) and surgical planning to correctly perform excision and reconstruction.

Indications

Intralesional excision is the procedure of choice for metastases in the cervical spine, as the anterior approach allows easy and direct access to the tumour mass and better biomechanical reconstruction. Further, the posterior approach in the cervical spine is ineffective for both tumour removal (almost all cervical metastases occur in the vertebral body, which is not accessible posteriorly) and for reconstruction. Intralesional excision can also be considered in the case of:

- Cord compression by the tumour mass in radio-resistant metastases.
- Pathological fracture in radio-resistant metastases.
- The need to reduce the tumour mass ("debulking") for chemotherapy purposes.

Surgical Technique

The surgical technique for intralesional excision depends on the site and location of the tumour. In the cervical spine the approach is always anterior; in the thoracic and lumbar spine a subtotal excision can also be performed by a posterior approach alone.

The anterior approach to the cervical spine (C3–T1) is well known [13]. The approach to C1 and C2 can be performed by a trans-oral [14] or extra-oral approach [15]. The trans-oral approach is believed to be burdened by a high risk of local problems (infection and device loosening) [16] and does not make it possible to perform an extracapsular curettage. An extension of this approach is the trans-mandibular approach [17] which requires a highly aggressive technique. The vertebral arteries are a problem in the circumferential approach [18]. The anterior approach alone in the low cervical area is suggested for small metastatic deposits (sectors 4–9).

Whenever the tumour is growing posteriorly, completely invading at least one articular mass, a double approach is safest, not only for complete tumour excision but for reconstruction purposes overall. Circumferential reconstruction, especially in the cervical spine, allows good function and painless stability, which are the goals of surgical treatment for metastases.

The seated position can sometimes be useful in lesions presumed to be profusely bleeding [19]. Selective arterial embolisation is sometimes very useful in reducing bleeding [10].

Metastases in the thoracic spine can be submitted to complete excision by thoracotomy through the classic anterolateral approach, technically demanding only at the cervico-thoracic junction [20]. Thoracoscopy has recently been reported as a possible surgical technique for intracapsular excision [21].

Complete extracapsular excision requires a double approach. Excision for decompression and debulking purposes can be performed by a posterior approach alone [22]. Extending the procedure by a costotransversectomy makes it possible to maintain better oncological margins in the anterior structures of the spine.

In the lumbar spine anterior approach with decompression, instrumentation and fusion seem to be the best treatment for anteriorly located lesions. The posterior approach to this site often requires the sacrifice of one or more nerve roots; the functional value of the nerve roots to be sectioned will be obviously considered and informed consent obtained from the patient. Possible sequelae include persistent pain syndrome, motor loss and cord ischaemia.

En Bloc Resection

The techniques of *en bloc* resection in the thoracic and lumbar spine were described—from an appropriate oncological viewpoint—in the 1970s by Stener [23] and Roy Camille et al. [24]. Tomita [25] more recently reported a similar technique of vertebrectomy by a posterior approach especially conceived for metastases. The most interesting feature of Stener's work [23], never found in papers published later, is the concept that to achieve an appropriate *en bloc* excision, each tumour extension must be carefully evaluated and the surgical resection must be "personalised". Our attitude has been to further develop this philosophy by setting up a surgical staging (the so-called "WBB system" [26]) for planning the surgical procedure in each tumour.

Indications

En bloc excisions have been developed and performed with the main purpose of achieving an appropriate oncological margin that is a continuous shell of healthy tissue all around the tumour mass, the width of which (*marginal*=only the tumour pseudocapsule; *wide*=a coverage of healthy tissue such as muscle or fascia or a layer such as pleura) depends on the oncological stage of the tumour [27].

Surgical Technique: Vertebrectomy (en bloc resection of the vertebral body)

Planning. *En bloc* resection of the vertebral body is oncologically appropriate only by a posterior approach [24,25] and only for tumours contained within the vertebral body (no invasion of layer A in the WBB system [26]). The *en bloc* resection of thoracic and lumbar vertebral bodies described here is the same as proposed by Roy Camille et al. [24] for the lumbar spine, with some minor modifications. Two stages, to be performed in the same operation, are suggested: first, a posterior approach in the prone position, then a simultaneous posterior and anterior approach in the lateral position.

Posterior Stage. The aim is to excise the posterior healthy elements, in order to separate the dura from the tumour and begin the excision of the posterior wall. It ends with the implant of the posterior construct. If one pedicle is involved, the anterior approach will be performed from this side.

Anterior Stage. A thoracotomy (through intercostal spaces 4–10), a thoraco-lumbar trans-diaphragm approach or a retroperitoneal approach is performed, according to the level affected by a posterolateral skin incision. The tumour is found and dissected from the neighbouring tissues, and the posterior incision is re-opened. At this point, the surgeon can visualise two-thirds of the vertebral body surface, as well as the posterior vertebral wall. It is now possible to complete the resection by chisel if performed through the bone, or by knife or scissors if performed through the disc.

Reconstruction. Considering the long-term positive results of the combined treatments, the target of the reconstruction must be both immediate stability and long-term painless fusion [29,30]. The Stackable Cage system (DePuy-AcroMed®), a carbon fibre modular system including octagonal thoracic and lumbar size cages, combined with the posterior system (6.35 mm ISOLA®, MOSS-MIAMI® rods, or with VSP®) seems to allow immediate weight-bearing after corpectomy and vertebrectomy, promoting fast bone fusion

(through the hypertrophic evolution of small chips of autogenous bone) and a long-term satisfying functional result. Radiographic evolution of 80% of our cases demonstrated hypertrophy of such small chips of bone inside the substance [31].

Alternative reconstructive devices include: titanium cages [32]; allografts, the oldest and perhaps the most used spacers in oncological surgery as a whole [33]; stainless steel spacers [34]; madreporic spacers [35]; and acrylic cement [28,36].

The biomechanical features of carbon fibre-reinforced implants allow immediate stability (the patient is immediately verticalised, without or with a light orthosis); the early fusion of the chips of autogenous bone allow long-term stability and a complete fusion of the instrumented anterior column. A review of the literature reports only one case of mechanical failure of a carbon fibre implant, secondary to septic non-union [37]. Further, the advantage of a modular system is to give the surgeon the opportunity to intra-operatively reconstruct any unanticipated loss of spinal substance resulting from unexpected enlargement of the resection.

Post-operative Care. The patient can begin standing exercises without support or with a simple three-point orthosis a few days after discharge from the intensive care unit. At the 3 month follow-up, initial bone bridging through the carbon cages will be noted and the orthosis will be useless.

Surgical Technique; Sagittal Resection

Planning. The criteria for achieving an oncologically appropriate margin include: no extension to layer D in the WBB system [26], or limited extension with cleavage between the tumour pseudocapsule and the dura.

Posterior Stage. Position, positioning care, skin incision, approach and screw implantation are as for vertebrectomy. A complete excision of all the posterior healthy elements is then performed, always remaining at a distance from the tumour. The dura must be exposed cephalad and caudad to the tumour mass. The tumour mass must then be dissected from the muscles of the thoracic and abdominal wall. In the thoracic spine, one rib above and one below the tumour mass are prepared for excision.

Anterior Stage. The patient is placed in the lateral position (90°) with four solid fixations. The posterior approach is re-opened and is enlarged by a transverse incision, starting at 90° over the projection of the lesional level, thus obtaining a T-shaped incision. The dural sac is carefully displaced and protected; a wide chisel is introduced against the posterior vertebral wall and hammered in the sagittal plane as far as the anterior surface of the vertebral body, where the malleable retractor is still positioned to protect the vessels and viscera. Once the sagittal osteotomy has been completed, two transverse hemi-cylindrical osteotomies are performed above and below the lesion, making *en bloc* tumour removal possible. Profuse bleeding during the chiselling is to be expected.

Reconstruction. The posterior stabilisation is performed following the criteria previously discussed, depending on the sectors resected: Brantigan cages [37], autogenous grafts (rib or iliac crest), allografts, titanium cages (small size) and special stackable cages are the possible options.

Surgical Technique: Posterior Resection

Planning. According to the WBB system [26], the criteria for achieving an oncologically appropriate margin include: sectors 4 and 9 free from tumour; no extension to layer D, or limited extension with cleavage between the tumour pseudocapsule and the dura.

Posterior Stage. A classic approach is performed. The whole approach must be extended more laterally than the transverse processes in the lumbar spine and over the rib angles in the thoracic spine. The pedicles must be sectioned, whichever technique is used.

Reconstruction. Posterior instrumentation and fusion are finally performed, mostly by pedicular screws and rods fixating at least two levels above and below the resection area. The possibility must be considered of performing an interbody fusion (by posterior approach in the same session, or later by an anterior approach), to reduce the stress on the posterior rods.

Complications. The morbidity of these procedures is very high. Vertebrectomy and sagittal resections combine all the risks and complications of anterior surgery [3] with all the possible problems connected with a long and difficult posterior approach, with possible careful dissection of the dura, sometimes closely adherent to the tumour. The complications related to procedures of long duration must be also considered [2]. The risks of damaging large vessels are increased by the need to leave healthy tissues around the tumour. Obviously, if previous surgery has been performed, scar dissection will expose neighbouring structures (ureter, cisterna magna, segmental vessels, nerve roots, and so on) to lesions. Among late complications, infection is particularly threatening, due to the extensive exposure required and the reduced immunocompetence of these patients. Posterior resection is a shorter procedure; its possible complications are connected with dura dissection from the tumour and with possible damage of vessels and viscera by posterior dissection of the tumoural mass.

CONCLUSIONS

The topic is extremely difficult to discuss, due to the complexity of the matter and the intrinsic difficulty in comparing lesions which are only apparently similar. A few years ago a metastatic deposit in the spine was correctly considered a terminal event; now it is a severe complication endangering the risk of severe functional derangement, but the prognosis (and, consequently, metastasis treatment) is related to the primary tumour and its spread.

En bloc resection, which is the appropriate surgical technique for stage 3 benign and stage 1 primary malignant tumours [27], can be considered as indicated for a few selected cases of solitary metastases from long life expectancy primary tumours (teratoma and hypernephroma are the clearest examples).

Indications for surgical treatment must be based on a complete survey of the tumoural spread and of the general condition of the patient. The life expectancy of the patient must be discussed with the oncologist and the pathologist.

We can conclude by affirming that the surgical indications in the case of metastatic disease of the spine must be the result of a multidisciplinary approach to the patient, and not an individual decision by the surgeon, radiotherapist or oncologist, even if they are considerably experienced. Specific care should be devoted to the combination of surgery and radiation therapy, as the experience of many centres [38,39], and our own, shows that the rate of complications of tumour surgery of the spine is higher in patients previously treated by radiation therapy.

Knowledge of the biological behaviour of the different tumour types is mandatory in deciding which is the most appropriate surgical margin for any tumour, and therefore in deciding the extent of surgical *en bloc* or intralesional excision. To popularise this concept, the Enneking staging system was set up

[27]. A surgical staging system is also required for planning the surgical procedure in order to achieve such margins [26]. The combination of Enneking staging [27] and WBB staging [26] should aim to:

- Avoid high-morbidity surgery when it is not necessary (e.g. in stage 2 benign or metastatic tumours).
- Achieve the appropriate margin by correctly performed *en bloc* resections in selected cases.
- Increase the knowledge of these tumours by comparing uniform reports on the outcomes of homogeneously treated series.

The advantages of *en bloc* surgery in terms of eradication of local disease should be compared with the results achieved by less morbid intralesional surgery combined with adjuvants such as radiotherapy and/or chemotherapy and/or hormonotherapy, according to different primary tumours. Many biases prevent significant results from being achieved in this study: the small number of appropriate cases, different primary tumours, different treatment of the primary tumour, involvement of other organs, and elements which make it difficult to create a homogeneous series. Further, one should consider that a vertebrectomy requires 100–120% blood mass substitution [2] with all subsequent morbidity, including reduction of immunocompetence and a long hospitalisation (at least 3–4 weeks, if no complications occur). We must also consider the possibility of discovering another previously undetected bone metastasis a few months after discharge. The decision-making process for treating metastases of the spine has been widely investigated in the recent literature [40–43].

ACKNOWLEDGEMENTS

We are indebted to Professor M. Campanacci, our unforgettable teacher, and to B. Stener and R. Roy Camille, the pioneers of this surgery. Further, S.B. must thank C. Mazel, who gave him the first practical suggestions and followed him during his initial experiences, and Jim Weinstein for the considerable work on staging, for helping him to organise ideas and to select cases, and for his friendship. Special thanks to Gigliola Gamberini and Carlo Piovani, from the Rizzoli Istitute "Scuola di Disegno Anatomico", and to Anna Viganò, from the Rizzoli Institute Library, for her invaluable help in the literature review. Also the authors wish to acknowledge Associazione per la Ricerca in Medicina.

REFERENCES

1. Jacobs WB, Perrin RG. Evaluation and treatment of spinal metastases: an overview. Neurosurg Focus 2001; 11(6).

2. Di Fiore M, Lari S, Boriani S et al. Chirurgia vertebrale "maggiore": problemi anestesiologici intra e post-operatori. Chir Org Mov 1998; 83: 53–66.

3. Faciszawski T, Winter RB, Lonstein JE et al. The surgical and medical perioperative complications of anterior spinal fusion surgery in the thoracic and lumbar spine in adults: a review of 1223 procedures. Spine 1995; 20: 1592–99.

4. Kim RY, Smith JW, Spencer SA et al. Malignant epidural spinal cord compression associated with a paravertebral mass: its radiotherapeutic outcome on radiosensitivity. Int J Radiat Oncol Biol Phys 1993; 27: 1079–83.

5. Sorensen S, Borgesen E, Rhode K et al. Metastatic epidural spinal cord compression. Results of treatment and survival. Cancer 1990; 65: 1502–8.

6. Young F, Post EM, King GA. Treatment of spinal epidural metastases. Randomized prospective comparison of laminectomy and radiotherapy. J Neurosurg 1980; 53: 741–8.

7. Hall AJ, Mackay NN. The results of laminectomy for compression of the cord and cauda equina by extradural malignant tumour. J Bone Joint Surg Br 1973; 55: 497–505.

8. Hertlein H, Mittlmeier T, Schurmann M, Lob G. Posterior stabilization of C2 metastases by combination of atlantoaxial screw fixation and hook plate. Eur Spine J 1994; 3(1): 52–5.

9. Gokaslan ZL, York JE, Walsh GL. Transthoracic vertebrectomy for metastatic spinal tumors. J Neurosurg 1998; 89: 599–609.

10. Gellad FE, Sadato N, Numaguchi Y, Levine AM. Vascular metastatic lesion of the spine: pre-operative embolization. Radiology 1990; 176: 683–6.

11. Hess T, Kraman B, Schmidt E, Rupp S. Use of preoperative vascular embolization in spinal metastases resection. Arch Orthop Trauma Surg 1997; 116(5): 279–82.

12. Roscoe MW, McBroom RJ, St Louis E et al. Preoperative embolization in the treatment of osseous metastases from renal cell carcinoma. Clin Orthop 1989; (238): 302–7.

13. Mcafee PC. Anterior surgical approaches to the lower and upper cervical spine. In Sherk HH (ed.), The Cervical Spine: an Atlas of Surgical Procedures. Lippincott: Philadelphia, PA, 1994: 37–70.

14. Louis R. Surgery of the Spine. Berlin, Springer-Verlag: 1983.

15. McAfee PC, Bohlman HH, Riley LH et al. Anterior retropharyngeal approach to the upper part of the cervical spine. J Bone Joint Surg Am 1987; 69: 1371–83.

16. Jones DC, Hayter JP, Vaughan ED, Findlay GF. Oropharyngeal morbidity following transoral approaches to the upper cervical spine. Int J Oral Maxillofac Surg 1998; 27(4): 295–8.

17. Shah JP, Shaha AR. Transmandibular approaches to the upper cervical spine. In Sundaresan SN, Schmidek HH, Schiller AR, Rosenthal DI (eds), Tumors of the Spine: Diagnosis and Clinical Management. WB Saunders: Philadelphia, PA, 1990: 329–35.

18. Harms, J: 360° Treatment of cervical spine tumors. In Proceedings of the 18th annual meeting of the Cervical Spine Research Society (Paris June 13–14, 2002), page114.

19. Matjasko J, Petrozza P, Cohen M, Steinberg P. Anesthesia and surgery in the seated position: analysis of 554 cases. Neurosurgery 1985; 17: 695–9.

20. Kurz LT, Brower RS, Herokwitz HN, Pursel SE. Surgical approaches to the cervico-thoracic junction. In Sherk HH (ed.), The Cervical Spine: an Atlas of Surgical Procedures. Lippincott: Philadelphia, PA, 1994.

21. McLain RF. Spinal cord decompression: an endoscopically assisted approach for metastatic tumors. Spinal Cord 2001; 39(9): 482–7.

22. Magerl F, Coscia MF. Total posterior vertebrectomy of the thoracic and lumbar spine. Clin Orthop 1988; 232: 62–9.

23. Stener B. Complete removal of vertebrae for extirpation of tumors. Clin Orthop Rel Res 1989; 245: 72–82.

24. Roy-Camille R, Mazel Ch, Saillant G, Lapresle Ph. Treatment of malignant tumors of the spine with posterior instrumentation. In Sundaresan N, Schmidek HH, Schiller AL, Rosenthal DI (eds), Tumors of the Spine. Diagnosis and Clinical Management. WB Saunders: Philadelphia, PA, 1990: 473–92.

25. Tomita K, Kawahara N, Baba H et al. Total *en bloc* spondylectomy for solitary spinal metastases. Int Orthop (SICOT) 1994; 18: 291–8.

26. Boriani S, Weinstein JN, Biagini R. Spine update. Primary bone tumors of the spine: terminology and surgical staging. Spine 1997; 22: 1036–44.

27. Enneking WF. Clinical Musculoskeletal Pathology. Florida University Press: Boca Raton, FL, 1990.

28. Kanayama M, Ng JTW, Cunningham BW et al. Biomechanical analysis of anterior vs. circumferential spinal reconstruction for various anatomic stages of tumor lesions. Spine 1999; 24(5): 445–50.

29. Gurr KR, McAfee PC, Shih Chi-Ming. Biomechanical analysis of anterior and posterior instrumentation systems after corpectomy. A calf-spine model. J Bone Joint Surg Am 1988; 70(8): 1182–91.

30. Oda I, Cunningham BW, Abumi K et al. The stability of reconstruction methods after thoracolumbar total spondylectomy. Spine 1999; 24: 1634–8.

31. Boriani S, Biagini R, Bandiera S et al. The reconstruction of the anterior column of the thoracic and lumbar spine with the carbon fiber stackable cage system. Orthopedics 2002; 25(1): 37–42.

32. Simmons ED. Anterior reconstruction for metastatic thoracic and lumbar spine disease. In Bridwell KH, DeWald RL (eds), The Textbook of Spinal Surgery, 2nd edn. Lippincott-Raven: Philadelphia, PA, 1997: 2057–70.

33. Scoville WB, Palmer AH, Samra K, Chong G. The use of acrylic plastic for vertebral replacement and fixation in metastatic disease of the spine. A technical note. J Neurosurg 1967; 27: 274–81.

34. Rezaian SM. Rezaian spinal fixator for management of fractures of the thoracolumbar spine. J Neurol Orthop Surg 1991; 12: 307–14.

35. Kaneda K, Takeda N. Reconstruction with a ceramic vertebral prosthesis and Kaneda device following subtotal or total vertebrectomy in metastatic thoracic and lumbar spine. In Bridwell KH, DeWald RL (eds), The Textbook of Spinal Surgery, 2nd edn. Lippincott-Raven: Philadelphia, PA, 1997: 2071–87.

36. Harrington KD. The use of methylmethacrylate for vertebral body replacement and anterior stabilization of pathologic fracture-dislocations of the spine due to metastatic malignant disease. J Bone Joint Surg Am 1981; 63: 36–48.

37. Brantigan JW, Steffee AD. A carbon fiber implant to aid interbody lumbar fusion. Two year clinical results in the first 26 patients. Spine 1993; 18: 2106–17.

38. McPhee IB, Williams RP, Swanson CE. Factors influencing wound healing after surgery for metastatic disease of the spine. Spine 1998; 23: 726–33.

39. Ghogawala Z, Mansfield FL, Borges LF. Spinal radiation before surgical decompression adversely affects oucomes of surgery for symptomatic metastatic spinal cord compression. Spine 2001; 26: 818–24.

40. Cooper PR, Errico TJ, Martin R. A systematic approach to spinal reconstruction after anterior decompression for neoplastic disease of the thoracic and lumbar spine. Neurosurgery 1993; 32: 1–9.

41. Sundaresan N, Steinberger AA, Moore R. Indications and results of combined anterior–posterior approaches for spine tumor surgery. J Neurosurg 1996; 85: 438–45.

42. Sundaresan N, Krol G, Steinberger A, Moore F. Management of tumors of the thoracolumbar spine. Neurosurg Clin N Am 1997; 8: 541–52.

43. Tokuhashi Y, Matsuzaki H, Toriyama S, Kawano H, Ohsaka S. Scoring system for the preoperative evaluation of metastatic spine tumor prognosis. Spine 1990; 15: 1110–3.

16

Total *En Bloc* Spondylectomy for Spinal Metastases

Norio Kawahara, Katsuro Tomita, Hideki Murakami, Tomoyuki Akamaru, Koshi Nanbu, Yasuhiro Ueda and Mohamed E. Abdel-Wanis

Kanazawa University, Kanazawa, Japan

INTRODUCTION

Conventionally, due to the difficulty in surgical approach and the anatomical proximity of major vessels to the vertebra or vertebrae involved, curettage and resection of vertebral tumours have been commonly practised, including the removal of malignant tissue in a piecemeal fashion. The disadvantages of these conventional approaches are clear and include a high possibility of tumour cell contamination of the surrounding structures. If the expected survival period is >2 years, piecemeal excision can lead to local recurrence in most patients with spinal metastases. Therefore, it becomes necessary to take oncological concepts [1] into consideration to achieve successful local control of the spine lesion within the patient's remaining lifespan.

To reduce local recurrence as far as possible, we have developed a new surgical technique of spondylectomy (vertebrectomy) called total *en bloc* spondylectomy (TES) [2–6]. We describe here the indications and technique for total *en bloc* spondylectomy in spinal metastases.

SURGICAL INDICATIONS FOR SPINAL METASTASES

Surgical Strategy for Spinal Metastases [7] (Figure 16.1)

A new scoring system for spinal metastases consists of three prognostic factors: (a) grade of malignancy (slow growth, 1 point; moderate growth, 2 points; rapid growth, 4 points); (b) visceral metastases (no metastasis, 0 points; treatable, 2 points; untreatable, 4 points); (c) bone metastases (solitary or isolated), 1 point; multiple, 2 points). These three factors are added together to give a prognostic score of 2 (minimum)–10 (maximum). The treatment goal for each patient is set according to this prognostic score. The surgical strategy for spinal metastases of each patient is decided along with the treatment goal: a prognostic score of 2 or 3 points suggests a wide or marginal excision for long-term local control (3 years or more); 4 or 5 points indicate marginal or intralesional excision for middle-term local control (around 2 years); 6 or 7 points justify palliative surgery for short-term palliation (1 year or less); 8, 9 or 10 points indicate non-operative supportive care. The extent of the spinal metastases is stratified using the surgical classification of spinal tumours and technically appropriate and feasible surgery is employed, such as *en bloc* spondylectomy, piecemeal thorough excision, curettage or palliative surgery.

Surgical Classification of Spinal Tumours [3,4] (SCST)

Surgical classification of spinal tumours has already been reported in several studies. The anatomical site of the tumour has been classified as one of the following:

Textbook of Bone Metastases. Edited by C. Jasmin, R. E. Coleman, L. R. Coia, R. Capanna and G. Saillant
© 2005 John Wiley & Sons Ltd: ISBN 0 471 87742 5

Scoring system

Point	Prognostic factors: Primary tumour	Visceral metastases	Bone metastases
1	Slow growth (breast, thyroid, etc.)		Solitary or isolated
2	Moderate growth (kidney, uterus, etc.)	Treatable	Multiple
4	Rapid growth (lung, stomach, etc.)	Untreatable	

Prognostic score	Treatment goal	Surgical strategy
2 3	Long-term local control	Wide or marginal excision
4 5	Middle-term local control	Marginal or intralesional excision
6 7	Short-term palliation	Palliative surgery
8 9 10	Terminal care	Supportive care

Figure 16.1. Surgical strategy for spinal metastases. *No visceral metastases = 0 points. **Bone metastases, including spinal metastases

1, vertebral body; 2, pedicle; 3, lamina and spinous process; 4, spinal canal (epidural space); or 5, paravertebral area (Figure 16.2). The numbers used to denote the anatomical sites reflect the common sequence of tumour progession. The numbers assigned to the anatomical sites are also related to the surgical classification, and the new Surgical Classification of the Spinal Tumors, was devised [3,4] (Figure 16.3). For example, a type 3 lesion in our classification involves the vertebral body (anatomical site 1), the pedicle (anatomical site 2) and the lamina (anatomical site 3). The authors of the present study considered types 1, 2 and 3 lesions as intracompartmental, whereas types 4, 5 and 6 were considered extracompartmental. A type 7 tumour is a multiple-skip lesion.

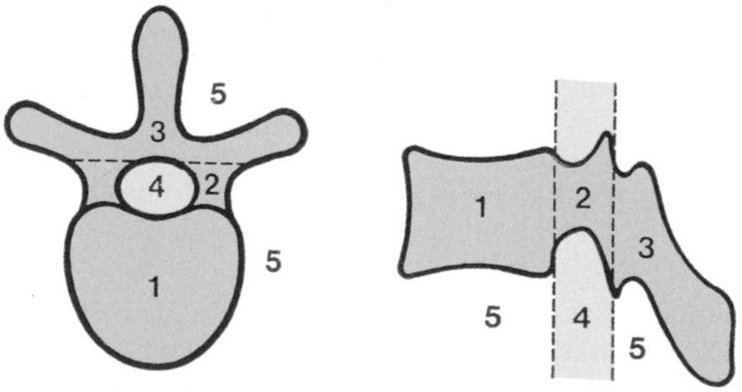

Figure 16.2. Definitions of different anatomical sites of the vertebra. 1, vertebral body; 2, pedicle; 3, lamina, transverse and spinous processes; 4, spinal canal (epidural space); 5, paravertebral area

The surgical procedure is decided for each patient, based on the surgical strategy for spinal metastases and the surgical classification of spinal tumours. Total *en bloc* spondylectomy is recommended for types 2, 3, 4 and 5 lesions, and relatively indicated for types 1 and 6 lesions among the patients recommended for wide or marginal excision, based on the surgical strategy (prognostic score 2, 3 and 4). TES is not recommended (or contraindicated) for type 7 lesions [7].

SURGICAL TECHNIQUE

The TES technique consists of two steps, including *en bloc* resection of the posterior element and *en bloc* resection of the anterior column. The following is a description of each step.

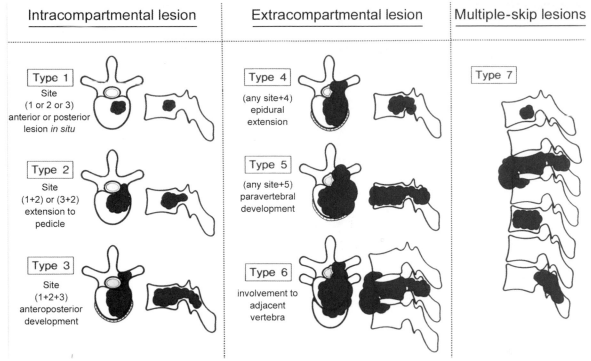

Figure 16.3. Schematic diagram of the surgical classification of vertebral tumours

Step 1: *En bloc* Laminectomy (Resection of the Whole Posterior Element of the Vertebra)

Exposure

The patient is placed prone over a Relton-Hall four-poster frame to avoid compression to the vena cava. A straight vertical midline incision is made over the spinous processes and is extended three vertebrae above and below the involved segment(s). The para-spinal muscles are dissected from the spinous processes and the laminae, and then retracted laterally. If the patient has undergone posterior route biopsy, the tracts are carefully resected in a manner similar to that used in a limb-salvaging procedure. After a careful dissection of the area around the facet joints, a large retractor called an articulated spinal retractor, having a uniaxial joint in each limb and designed for this surgery, is applied. By spreading the retractor and detaching the muscles around the facet joints, a wider exposure is then obtained. The operative field must be wide enough on both sides to allow dissection under the surface of the transverse processes. In the thoracic spine, the ribs on the affected level are transected 3–4 cm lateral to the costotransverse joint, and the pleura is bluntly separated from the vertebra.

To expose the superior articular process of the uppermost vertebra, the spinous and the inferior articular processes of the neighbouring vertebrae are osteotomised and removed, with dissection of the attached soft tissues, including the ligamentum flavum.

Introduction of the T-saw Guide

To make an exit for the T-saw guide through the nerve root canal, the soft tissue attached to the inferior aspect of the pars interarticularis is dissected and removed, using utmost care so as not to damage the corresponding nerve root. A C-curved malleable T-saw guide is then introduced through the intervertebral foramen in a cephalocaudal direction. In this procedure, the tip of the T-saw guide should be introduced along the medial cortex of the lamina and the pedicle, so as not to injure the spinal cord and the nerve root (Figure 16.4). After passing the T-saw guide, its tip at the exit of the nerve root canal can be found beneath the inferior border of the pars interarticularis. In the next step, a threadwire saw (T-saw®; flexible multi-filament threadwire saw, 0.54 mm in diameter [8], DePuy Motech, Warsaw, IN) is passed through the

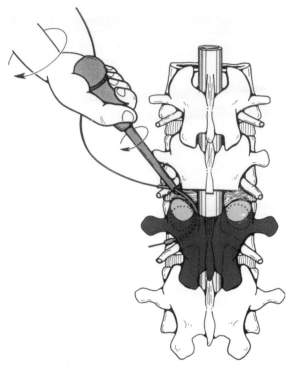

Figure 16.4. Operative schema of introducing the T-saw guide

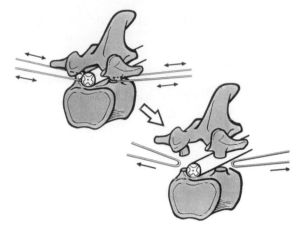

Figure 16.5. Operative schema of the pediclotomy

hole in the wire guide and is clamped with a T-saw holder at each end. The T-saw guide is removed and tension on the T-saw is maintained. When two or three vertebrae are resected, the T-saw is inserted into a thin polyethylene catheter (T-saw catheter) and both are passed under the lamina. This procedure is also applied to the contralateral side.

Cutting the Pedicles and Resection of the Posterior Element

While tension is maintained, the T-saw is placed beneath the superior articular and transverse processes with a specially designed T-saw manipulator. With this procedure, the T-saw placed around the lamina is wrapped around the pedicle. With a reciprocating motion of the T-saw, the pedicles are cut and then the whole posterior element of the spine (the spinous process, the superior and inferior articular processes, the transverse process, and the pedicle) is removed in one piece (Figure 16.5). The cut surface of the pedicle is sealed with bone wax to reduce bleeding and to minimise contamination by tumour cells. To maintain

stability after segmental resection of the anterior column, a temporary posterior instrumentation is performed. When one vertebra is resected, two above and two below segmental fixation is recommended. However, if two or three vertebrae are resected, more than two above and two below segmental fixation is mandatory.

Step 2: *En Bloc* Corpectomy (Resection of the Anterior Column of the Vertebra)

Blunt Dissection around the Vertebral Body

At the beginning of the second step, the segmental arteries must be identified bilaterally. The spinal branch of the segmental artery, which runs along the nerve root, is ligated and divided. This procedure exposes the segmental artery, which appears just lateral to the cut edge of the pedicle. In the thoracic spine, the nerve root is cut on the side from which the affected vertebra is removed. The blunt dissection is done on both sides through the plane between the pleura (or the iliopsoas muscle) and the vertebral body (Figures 16.6, 16.7A,B). Usually, the lateral aspect of the body is easily dissected with a curved vertebral spatula. Then the segmental artery should be dissected from the vertebral body. By continuing dissection of both lateral sides of the vertebral body anteriorly, the aorta is carefully dissected posteriorly from the anterior aspect of the vertebral body with a spatula and the surgeon's fingers (Figure 16.7A,B). Vascular anatomy around the vertebral body should be thoroughly understood to avoid vascular damage.

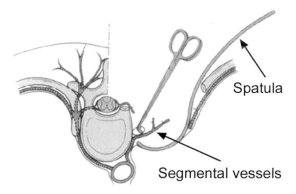

Figure 16.6. Operative schema of anterior dissection around the vertebral body

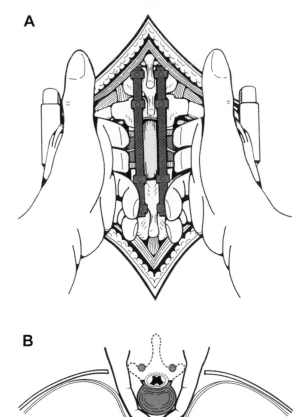

Figure 16.7. Operative schema of anterior finger dissection around the vertebral body. (A) Posterior view. (B) Axial view

When the surgeon's fingertips meet with each other anterior to the vertebral body, a series of spatulae, starting from the smallest size, are inserted sequentially to extend the dissection. A pair of the largest spatulae is kept in the dissection site to prevent the surrounding tissues and organs from iatrogenic injury and to make the surgical field wide enough for manipulating the anterior column.

In a patient in whom the segmental artery(ies) may adhere to, or to be involved by, the vertebral tumour, as in the case of surgical classification type 5, anterior management of vessels around the vertebral body, using thoracoscopy or a minimally open approach, should precede the total *en bloc* spondylectomy by a posterior approach. This is safer for the vessels around the vertebral body than TES by a single posterior approach.

Passage of the T-saw

T-saws are inserted at the proximal and distal cutting levels of the vertebral bodies, where grooves are made along the desired cutting line, using a V-notched osteotome after confirmation of the disc levels with needles.

Dissection of the Spinal Cord and Removal of the Vertebra

Using a cord spatula, the spinal cord is mobilised from the surrounding venous plexus and the ligamentous tissue. The teeth-cord protector, which has teeth on both edges to prevent the T-saw from slipping, is then applied. The anterior column of the vertebra is cut by the T-saw, together with the anterior and posterior

longitudinal ligaments (Figure 16.8). After cutting the anterior column, the mobility of the vertebra is again checked to ensure a complete corpectomy.

The freed anterior column is rotated around the spinal cord and removed carefully to avoid injury to the spinal cord. With this procedure, a complete anterior and posterior decompression of the spinal cord (circumspinal decompression) and total *en bloc* resection of the vertebral tumour are achieved.

Anterior Reconstruction and Posterior Instrumentation

Bleeding, mainly from the venous plexus within the spinal canal, should be exhaustively arrested. An anchor hole on the cut end of the remaining vertebra is made on each side to seat the graft. A vertebral

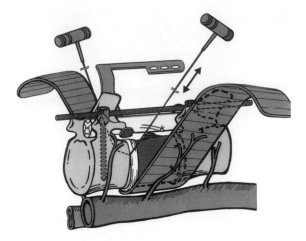

Figure 16.8. Operative schemes for cutting the anterior column. A pair of spatulae is kept around the affected vertebral body to prevent the surrounding tissues and organs from iatrogenic injury and to make the surgical field wide enough for manipulating the anterior column. The anterior column of the vertebra is cut by the T-saw, together with the anterior and posterior longitudinal ligaments. The teeth-cord protector, which has teeth on both edges to prevent the T-saw from slipping, is then applied

spacer, such as autograft, fresh and/or frozen allograft, and a titanium mesh cylinder (MOSS Miami, DePuy Motech, Warsaw, IN), is precisely inserted to the anchor holes within the remaining healthy vertebrae. After checking the appropriate position of the vertebral spacer radiographically, the posterior

instrumentation is adjusted to slightly compress the inserted vertebral spacer (Figure 16.9). If two or three vertebrae are resected, application of a connector device between the posterior rods and the anterior spacer is recommended. Finally, a Bard® Marlex® mesh (Bard, Billerica, MA, USA) covers the entire anterior and posterior reconstructed areas to establish the compartment for suppressing the bleeding.

Post-operative Management

Suction draining is preferred for 2–3 days after surgery, and the patient is allowed to start walking 1 week after surgery. The patient wears a thoraco-lumbo-sacral orthosis for 2–3 months, until bony union or incorporation of the artificial vertebral prosthesis is attained.

RESULTS

Twenty-eight patients were oncologically treated with wide or marginal excision from 1993 to 1996. Their mean prognostic score was 3.3 points (range, 2–5 points). Total *en bloc* spondylectomy was performed in 26 patients and *en bloc* corpectomy in two patients. Of these 28 patients, 19 patients had died and nine were alive at the time of the last follow-up. Mean length of survival of the 28 patients was 38.2 months (range,

spondylectomy reconstruction
(vertebrectomy) (shortening & locking)

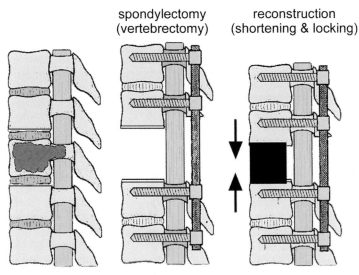

Figure 16.9. Operative schemes of spinal reconstruction. A vertebral spacer is properly inserted into the anchor holes within the remaining healthy vertebrae (middle). After checking the appropriate position of the vertebral spacer radiographically, the posterior instrumentation is adjusted to slightly compress the inserted vertebral spacer (right)

6–84 months); 26/28 patients had successful local control during their lifetime.

CASE HISTORY

A 67 year-old woman was hospitalised due to severe back pain. Seven years before admission, the patient was diagnosed with renal cell carcinoma, which was treated by left nephrectomy. Imaging work-up showed a tumour growth in the L3 vertebral body, right pedicle and part of lamina (surgical classification, type 3; Figure 16.10A,B). Whole-body CT scan and bone scintigram did not show any other metastatic lesion (prognostic score: 3 points). Total *en bloc* spondylectomy was performed at vertebra L3 (Figure 16.10C). Anterior reconstruction was carried out using an apatite–wollastonite glass–ceramic prosthesis (Lederle, Tokyo, Japan) with an allo-strutgraft. A Cotrel–Dubosset screw and rod arrangement was performed posteriorly between L1–L5 levels. Radiographs did not show any loosening of the implants anteriorly and posteriorly (Figure 16.10D). The patient has been well, without local recurrence for the last 9 post-operative years.

DISCUSSION

The ring-shaped bony structure of the vertebra, containing the spinal cord, hinders a wide surgical margin. There exist other obstacles, such as the thin surrounding soft tissues, major blood vessels and visceral organs neighbouring the involved vertebra. Thus, most operations were amenable to curettage or piecemeal resection. However, the intralesional procedure apparently leads to incomplete resection and to definite contamination by tumour cells.

Roy-Camille et al. [9,10], Stener [11–13], Stener et al. [14], Sundaresan et al. [15], and Boriani et al. [16,17] have described total spondylectomy for improving local curability, together with excellent clinical results. Different from these, our procedure involves the whole vertebra (both vertebral body and lamina), except for the pedicle, and the lesion is removed *en bloc*. Our TES technique minimises the risk of contamination compared with that described by the above authors.

The major risks in TES operation include: (a) mechanical damage to the adjacent neural structures during the excision of the pedicles; (b) possible contamination by tumour cells during pediculotomy; (c) injury of the major vessels during blunt dissection of the anterior aspect of the vertebral body; (d)

disturbance of spinal cord circulation at the level of surgery; and (e) excessive bleeding from the internal vertebral vein and epidural venous plexus during the second step of surgery. To reduce the risk of nerve root and spinal cord damage, we designed the T-saw [8]. It is made of multifilament twisted stainless steel wires and has a smooth surface to cut hard bony materials with minimal damage to the surrounding soft tissues. If the T-saw is properly passed into the nerve root canal and pulled posteriorly, it should not damage the nerve root. It is obvious that resection of the vertebra in one piece without cutting a certain point of the ring-shaped bony structure is impossible because of the encasement of the spinal cord within the vertebra. The pedicle is the best site for this purpose, since: (a) it is the narrowest portion connecting the posterior element with the anterior part, so that the intralesional cut surface will minimise the chance of contamination to a great extent; and (b) the spinal cord and the nerve root can easily be freed atraumatically. Pediculotomy is thus justified from the anatomical viewpoint. However, the pedicle does not always serve as a safe point for cutting, particularly when it is involved with the malignant process. Under such circumstances, the ipsilateral side of the lamina and contralateral part of the pedicle are cut together. These cutting levels may be considered separately in each case.

Blunt dissection of the anterior part of the vertebral body is another risky manoeuvre in the TES operation. The anatomical relationship between the vertebra, major vessels, and the visceral organs should be well understood [6,18,19]. Based on anatomical studies on cadavers, it is less likely to damage the thoracic aorta between T1 and T4. However, the artery must be carefully retracted anteriorly in areas caudal to T5, before manipulation of the affected vertebra(e). For a lesion at L1 and L2, the diaphragm and the first two lumbar arteries should be treated with utmost care.

Possible circulatory compromise after the ligation of the radicular artery is another concern. In the cat model, the authors [6] found that ligation of the Adamkiewicz artery reduced spinal cord blood flow by approximately 81% of the control value, and this decrementation did not affect spinal cord evoked potentials. Abundant arterial network around the dura mater and the spinal cord may completely compensate for the ligation of one or two radicular arteries. Actually there has been no neurological degradation in any of the 60 patients in our series who have undergone TES. Bleeding from the epidural venous plexus is often profuse. Haemostasis of tamponade in the epidural space, using Oxycell cotton®, Aviten® or fibrin glue, is mandatory. In

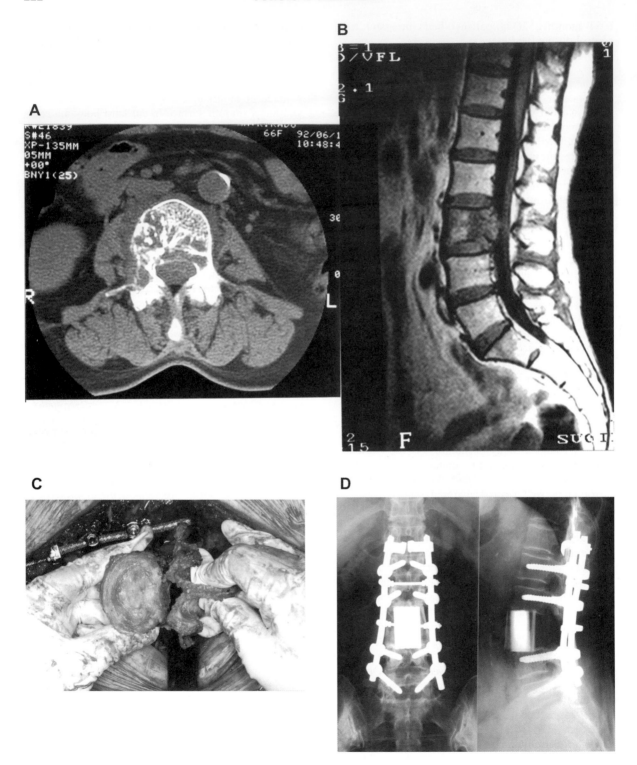

Figure 16.10. Illustrative patient presentation. (A) CT of vertebra L3. (B) T1-weighted sagittal MRI of the lumbar region. (C) Intra-operative photogram of the resected specimen of vertebra L3. (D) Post-operative X-ray

addition to hypotensive anaesthesia (systolic blood pressure, 60–80 mmHg), exhaustive management to arrest bleeding must be followed.

Roy-Camille et al. [9,10] suggested that the origins of the iliopsoas and iliac muscles from the lumbar spine make one-stage posterior total spondylectomy infeasible. They also stressed that the close proximity of major abdominal vessels to the anterior vertebral column in the lumbar spine enhances the risk in a patient with increased lumbar lordosis. For this reason, they recommended a two-stage operation to resect malignant vertebral neoplasms occurring between L2 and L4. Stener [13] reported total spondylectomy through a single-stage posterior approach for tumours at L3 or cephalad but denied the indication of this procedure at L4. He advocated a combined anteroposterior approach for a tumour at L4, based on the close contact of major vessels, especially the inferior vena cava with the L4 vertebral body, and interference by the iliac crest in accessing L4–5 and L5 posteriorly. The authors [3–6] agree with these two anatomical annoyances pointed out by Stener [13] but, for a case with an iliac wing positioned rather distal, they do not always disagree with single-stage posterior total *en bloc* spondylectomy for a solitary L4 vertebral tumour. For a tumour involving vertebra L5, it is undoubtedly necessary to use a two-stage anteroposterior approach because of additional difficulty of managing the common iliac and iliolumbar arteries and veins as well as the lumbosacral neural plexus.

A wide surgical margin, or at least a marginal margin, is achievable around the affected vertebra(e) when the lesion is intracompartmental (types 1, 2 or 3), particularly when the healthy part of the lamina or pedicle is cut. For a vertebral tumour extending into the spinal canal (type 4) or one invading the paravertebral areas (type 5), a marginal margin may be possible when the lesion is well encapsulated with a fibrous reactive membrane. In type 6 lesions, it is possible to obtain a wide margin at the proximal and caudal osteotomised sites of the vertebrae, but a paravertebral tumour sometimes adheres to or invades surrounding soft tissues, major vessels and visceral organs neighbouring the involved vertebra. In such an instance, anterior dissection followed by posterior TES operation is indicated. Thoracoscopy or a mini-open approach for anterior dissection is another option.

REFERENCES

1. Enneking WF, Spanier SS, Goodmann MA. A system for the surgical staging of musculoskeletal sarcoma. Clin Orthop 1980; 153: 106–20.

2. Kawahara N, Tomita K, Fujita T et al. Osteosarcoma of the thoracolumbar spine. Total *en bloc* spondylectomy. A case report. J Bone Joint Surg Am 1997; 79: 453–8.

3. Tomita K, Kawahara N, Baba H et al. Total *en bloc* spondylectomy for solitary spinal metastasis. Int Orthop 1994; 18: 291–8.

4. Tomita K, Kawahara N, Mizuno K et al. Total *en bloc* spondylectomy for primary malignant vertebral tumors. In Rao RS, Deo MG, Sanghri LD, Mittra I (eds), Proceedings of the 16th International Cancer Congress. Monduzzi Editore: Bologna, 1994: 2409–13.

5. Tomita K, Kawahara N, Kobayashi T et al. Surgical strategy for spinal metastases. Spine 2001; 26: 298–306.

6. Tomita K, Toribatake Y, Kawahara N et al. Total *en bloc* spondylectomy and circumspinal decompression for solitary spinal metastasis. Paraplegia 1994; 32: 36–46.

7. Tomita K, Kawahara N, Baba H et al. Total *en bloc* spondylectomy. A new surgical technique for primary malignant vertebral tumors. Spine 1997; 22: 324–33.

8. Tomita K, Kawahara N. The threadwire saw: a new device for cutting bone. J Bone Joint Surg Am 1996; 78: 1915–17.

9. Roy-Camille R, Mazel CH, Saillant G, Lapresle PH. Treatment of malignant tumor of the spine with posterior instrumentation. In Sundaresan N, Schmidek HH, Schiller AL, Rosenthal DI (eds), Tumor of the Spine. W.B. Saunders: Philadelphia, PA, 1990: 473–87.

10. Roy-Camille R, Saillant G, Bisserie M et al. Resection vertebrale totale dans la chirurgie tumorale au niveau du rachis dorsal par voie posterieure pure. Rev Chir Orthop 1981; 67: 421–30.

11. Stener B. Total spondylectomy in chondrosarcoma arising from the seventh thoracic vertebra. J Bone Joint Surg Br 1971; 53: 288–95.

12. Stener B. Complete removal of vertebrae for extirpation of tumors. Clin Orthop 1989; 245: 72–82.

13. Stener B. Technique of complete spondylectomy in the thoracic and lumbar spine. In Sundaresan N, Schmidek HH, Schiller AL, Rosenthal DI (eds), Tumor of the Spine. W.B. Saunders: Philadelphia, PA, 1990: 432–7.

14. Stener B, Johnsen OE. Complete removal of three vertebrae for giant cell tumour. J Bone Joint Surg Br 1971; 53: 278–87.

15. Sundaresan N, Rosen G, Huvos AG, Krol G. Combined treatment of osteosarcoma of the spine. Neurosurgery 1988; 23: 714–19.

16. Boriani S, Biagini R, De Iure F et al. Vertebrectomia lombare per neoplasia ossea: tecnica chirurgica. Chir Organi Mov 1994; 79: 163–73.

17. Boriani S, Chevalley F, Weinstein JN et al. Chordoma of the spine above the sacrum. Treatment and outcome in 21 cases. Spine 1996; 21: 1569–77.

18. Adachi B. Das Arteriensystem der Japaner. Maruzen: Kyoto Tokyo, 1928: 1–10.

19. Kawahara N, Tomita K, Baba H et al. Cadereric vascular anatomy for total *en bloc* spondylectomy in malignant vertebral tumors. Spine 1996; 21: 1401–7.

4

Local Treatments

Editor: Lawrence R. Coia

17

External Beam Radiation Therapy for the Treatment of Bone Metastases

Penny R. Anderson[1] and **Lawrence R. Coia**[2]

[1]*Fox Chase Cancer Center, Philadelphia, PA, USA*
[2]*Community Medical Center, Toms River, NJ, USA*

Over 100 000 new patients develop osseous metastases annually in the USA alone [1–3] and the prevalence of patients with bone metastases is estimated to be twice that [4]. Bone metastases occur in approximately 30–70% of patients with cancer [5]. The sites of the primary tumours most associated with bony metastases are breast (50%), prostate (17%) and lung (11%) [6]. Other primary tumours, viz. kidney, pancreas, rectum, colon, stomach, thyroid and ovary, are also associated with bony metastases. The most commonly involved skeletal sites are the vertebrae (69%), pelvis (41%), femur (25%) and skull (14%). The upper extremity is much less commonly involved, with a 10–15% incidence of bony metastasis occurring at this site [7].

It is well established that radiation therapy is an effective modality for palliative treatment of cancer that has metastasised to bone. Approximately 80–90% of treated patients will experience improvement in pain from their osseous metastases, with complete relief of pain established in about 50% of the treated patients [8,9]. Retrospective and randomised data have demonstrated conflicting evidence regarding the treatment of bony metastatic disease. The optimal treatment approach remains controversial, and an international consensus meeting on the treatment of bone metastases concluded that a relatively broad range of radiation dose fractionations were acceptable [10,11].

The American College of Radiology designed appropriateness criteria to serve as guidelines in the USA for the treatment of bone metastases [11]. Results were based on a survey of radiation oncologists regarding the management approach to a series of clinical vignettes (or variants). It was recommended that dose/fraction schemes of 2000 cGy/5 fractions, 3000 cGy/10 fractions, or 3500 cGy/14 fractions be utilised in most clinical situations for the initial treatment of metastatic bone disease. Higher dose schedules were only recommended in special situations, e.g. in a patient with a solitary metastasis and a long disease-free interval after initial diagnosis of breast cancer, or in a patient with a solitary melanoma metastasis presenting after a long disease-free interval. It was concluded that patient performance status and life expectancy are the factors that must be taken into consideration when determining optimal dose–fractionation schemes.

TREATMENT—LOCALISED EXTERNAL BEAM RADIATION THERAPY

The indications to treat bone metastases with radiation therapy include pain, risk of pathological fracture and spinal cord compression. The goals of radiation therapy in patients with bony metastases are to palliate pain, decrease the use of narcotic analgesics, improve ambulation and restore function, and prevent complications of pathological fracture and spinal cord compression. External beam radiation therapy has

Textbook of Bone Metastases. Edited by C. Jasmin, R. E. Coleman, L. R. Coia, R. Capanna and G. Saillant
© 2005 John Wiley & Sons Ltd: ISBN 0 471 87742 5

been well established as the standard of care for the palliative treatment of metastases to bone. Numerous series have reported results based on various radiation therapy dose/fractionation schedules.

The Radiation Therapy Oncology Group (RTOG) conducted a prospective randomised trial (RTOG 74-02) that consisted of a variety of radiation treatment schedules [12]. Patients were stratified according to whether they had a solitary site or multiple sites of bony metastases. Patients with solitary bone metastases were stratified by primary site, site of metastasis, use of internal fixation, and institution prior to randomisation to either 4050 cGy in 15 fractions over 3 weeks or 2000 cGy in five fractions over 1 week. Patients with multiple sites of bone metastases were stratified in a similar fashion prior to randomisation to one of four dose/fractionation schedules: 3000 cGy/10 fractions/2 weeks vs. 1500 cGy/5 fractions/1 week vs. 2000 cGy/5 fractions/1 week vs. 2500 cGy/5 fractions/1 week. In patients with solitary bone metastases, there was no significant difference in partial pain relief, complete pain relief, or the duration of pain relief between 2000 cGy using 4 Gy fractions compared with 4050 cGy delivered with 2.7 Gy fractions. Overall, minimal relief was obtained in 91% of patients, 83% experienced partial relief, and 57% of patients obtained complete relief. Recurrence of pain occurred in 57% of patients at a median of 15 weeks for each of the dose/fractionation schedules. In patients with multiple bony metastases, no difference was noted in the rates of pain relief or relapse of pain between the various treatment schedules. Overall, 89% of patients experienced minimal pain relief, 83% obtained partial relief, and 53% obtained complete relief. The incidence of relapsing pain was 54%. The median duration of pain control was 12 weeks for each of the dose/ fractionation schedules. These results indicated that the low-dose, short-course schedules were as effective as the more aggressive high-dose, protracted regimens. The only notable difference by treatment group was in the solitary metastasis group, with an 18% rate of fracture in those patients receiving 4050 cGy/15 fractions compared to a 4% fracture rate after treatment with 2000 cGy/5 fractions.

Blitzer [13] reanalysed the RTOG 74-02 data, using logistic regression multivariate analysis, grouping solitary and multiple bony mestastases, and using the endpoint of pain relief, taking into account narcotic score and retreatment. The author demonstrated that the protracted fractionation schedules (4050 cGy/15 fractions/3 weeks and 3000 cGy/10 fractions/2 weeks) were more effective in producing significantly improved pain relief than the shorter fractionation schedules. Blitzer found, on logistic regression analysis, that the number of fractions was significantly associated with complete combined pain relief. Complete combined pain relief was obtained in 55% of patients with solitary bone metastases who were treated with 4050 cGy/15 fractions compared to 37% in those patients who received 2000 cGy/5 fractions. In the patients with multiple bony metastases, 46% of patients treated with 3000 cGy/10 fractions achieved complete pain relief compared to 28% of patients who received 2500 cGy/5 fractions.

There have been numerous prospective randomised trials, particularly from Europe, that have evaluated different dose/fractionation schemes without demonstrating any significant differences in results (Table 17.1). In addition, a radiation dose–response for the treatment of bone metastases has not been adequately defined. Niewald et al. randomised 100 patients with painful bony metastases to receive either 20 Gy in 4 Gy daily fractions in 1 week or 30 Gy in 2 Gy daily fractions over 3 weeks [14]. No significant differences were noted in frequency or duration of pain relief, improvement of mobility, recalcification of bone, frequency of pathological fractures, or survival. The 1 year survival rate was 28% in the 20 Gy arm and 37% in the 30 Gy arm (NS). Overall survival was influenced by primary tumour site, Karnofsky performance status, age, response to radiation therapy, and the biological equivalent dose (BED). Rasmusson et al. performed a prospective randomised trial comparing 217 breast cancer patients with bone metastases who received 30 Gy in 10 daily fractions over 2 weeks vs. 15 Gy in three fractions over 2 weeks [15]. At 3 months, relief of pain was similar in both treatment arms, with 80% and 75% of patients experiencing pain relief in the 30 Gy and 15 Gy arms, respectively. In addition, no statistically significant difference was noted in the use of analgesics between the two treatment groups. Price et al. from the Royal Marsden Hospital randomised 288 patients with metastatic bone pain to receive either a single radiation fraction of 8 Gy or 30 Gy in 10 daily fractions over 2 weeks [16]. No significant differences were noted between the two treatment groups in the onset of pain relief, duration of response or incidence of response according to initial pain score. The incidence of a complete response was 45% with 8 Gy in a single fraction compared to 28% with 30 Gy over 2 weeks, but this difference was not statistically significant. In patients who survived more than 1 year from initial treatment, 57% of those responding to a single fraction and 59% of those responding to multiple fractions obtained durable pain relief. There was no increased acute morbidity observed with the

Table 17.1. Randomised trials evaluating various dose/fractionation schemes of local-field radiation therapy for treatment of bone metastases

Reference	Number of patients	Dose (Gy)/No. of fractions	Response pain relief (%)	Significance	Comments
Tong et al. (RTOG 74-02) [12]	1016	*20/5	53	NS	No difference between fractionation schedules
		*40.5/15	61		
		**15/5	49	NS	Only difference noted in S group (18% fracture rate with 40.5 Gy vs. 4% with 20 Gy)
		**20/5	56		
		**25/5	49		
		**30/10	57		
Blitzer (re-analysis of RTOG 74-02) [13]	759	*20/5	37	$p=0.0003$	Logistic regression analysis demonstrated number of fractions as only signif-
		*40.5/15	55		
		**15/5	36	$p=0.0003$	cant variable associated with complete combined pain relief
		**20/5	40		
		**25/5	28		
		**30/10	46		
Niewald et al. [14]	100	20/5	68	NS	No significant differences between arms in pain relief, pathological fracture rate, or survival
		30/15	83		
Rasmusson et al. [15]	217	15/3	75	NS	No difference in pain relief or analgesic use
		30/10	80		
Price et al. [16]	288	8/1	45	NS	No difference between arms in onset of pain relief, duration of response, or toxicity
		30/10	28		
Madsen [17]	57	20/2	48	NS	Similar pain control and toxicity in both treatment groups
		24/6	48		
Okawa et al. [18]	80	30/15	76	NS	Pain control similar in all three groups
		22.5/5	75		
		20/10 b.i.d.	78		

*Solitary metastasis; **Multiple metastases.

larger fractionation size. Madsen prospectively randomised 57 patients with bony metastases to receive 24 Gy in six fractions delivering two fractions/week or 20 Gy in two fractions delivering one fraction/week [17]. Both treatment groups responded similarly, with 48% satisfactory pain control. No differences were observed in toxicity according to dose/fractionation or field size. Okawa et al. randomised 80 patients with bone metastases to receive 30 Gy/15 fractions/20–22 days or 22.5 Gy/5 fractions/14–16 days or 20 Gy/10 fractions b.i.d./5–7 days. Pain control was the same in all three treatment groups, with approximately 75% pain relief achieved in each group [18].

Upon careful analysis of the numerous randomised trials evaluating dose/fractionation schemes for treatment of bony metastases, no optimal radiotherapy schedule or dose seems to exist. Protracted courses of treatment to higher total doses using smaller fraction sizes remain the most commonly used schedules in the USA. The Patterns of Care Study survey of the use of palliative radiation in 1984–1985 in the treatment of bone metastases, brain metastases and locally advanced lung cancer demonstrated that the most commonly practised radiation therapy schedule was 30 Gy in 10 daily fractions over 15 days [1]. Weight-bearing and non-weight-bearing bones were the predominate sites for palliative radiotherapy. 40 Gy in 20 fractions was the most commonly used schedule for weight-bearing bones, while non-weight-bearing bones were most often treated with shorter courses of radiation. Despite evidence that demonstrates similar effectiveness between shorter and longer fractionation schedules, many radiation oncologists in the USA prefer protracted treatment schemes in some clinical situations.

Because good dose–response data have not been defined and long-term prognosis is poor for many patients with metastatic disease to bone, single-fraction radiotherapy has been advocated as a cost-effective way to palliate bony metastases. Single-fraction radiation has the advantages of decreased visits to the radiation department and decreased cost in terms of treatment. Hoskin et al. prospectively evaluated 270 patients with painful bony metastatic disease receiving either 4 Gy or 8 Gy in a single fraction [19] (Table 17.2). The overall response rate was significantly higher in the 8 Gy group (69% at 4 weeks vs. 44% in the 4 Gy group), but complete response rate, duration of response and survival rates were similar in both treatment groups. Retreatment was needed more frequently in the 4 Gy group (20% vs. 9%). A more recent trial by Jeremic et al. [20] compared three single dose radiation therapy regimens for treatment of metastatic bone pain that consisted of either 4 Gy × one fraction, 6 Gy × one fraction or 8 Gy × one fraction. Patients in the 6 Gy and the 8 Gy groups had significantly higher overall response rates (73% and 78%) compared to the 4 Gy group (59%). Patients who received 8 Gy × one fraction had the shortest time to the occurrence of pain relief. No difference between the duration of response and retreatment rate was observed between the three groups.

As mentioned previously, Price et al. demonstrated similar effectiveness with 8 Gy in a single fraction compared to 30 Gy in 10 daily fractions [16]. Cole et al. randomised patients to 24 Gy in six fractions over 2–3 weeks vs. 8 Gy in a single fraction [21]. There was no difference in response to radiotherapy regarding pain relief between the two groups. However, 25% of patients who received 8 Gy in a single fraction required retreatment. Similar findings were noted by the Dutch Bone Metastasis Study [22], which demonstrated no significant difference in pain response, analgesics consumption, side-effects during treatment or quality of life between 8 Gy × one fraction vs. 4 Gy × six fractions. There was a 25% retreatment rate vs. a 7% retreatment rate between the single-fraction group and the multi-fraction group, respectively. However, there were indications that the physicians were more willing to retreat the patients in the single-fraction group because the time to retreatment was significantly shorter in this group and the preceding pain score was lower. Nielsen et al. [23] demonstrated no significant difference in analgesic consumption, performance status, degree of pain or quality of life between 8 Gy × one fraction vs. 5 Gy × four fractions, as evaluated 4, 8, 12 and 20 weeks after treatment. The authors also reported no difference in the duration of pain relief, the number of new painful sites and the need for re-irradiation.

The Bone Pain Trial Working Party conducted a randomised comparison of 8 Gy single fractionation vs. a multi-fraction regimen (20 Gy/5 fractions or 30 Gy/10 fractions) [24]. No differences were noted in the time to first improvement in pain, time to complete pain relief or in time to first increase in pain up to 12 months post-treatment. Retreatment was twice as common after the single course of 8 Gy than after the multi-fraction regimens (23% vs. 10%). It is speculated that the rate of retreatment in the single fraction group reflects the willingness of physicians to prescribe further radiation therapy after a single fraction, rather than the actual need for re-irradiation.

In a prospective randomised trial performed by Koswig et al. [25], 107 patients with bony metastases were randomised to 8 Gy in one fraction vs. 30 Gy in 10 fractions. Pain relief and recalcification of bone was evaluated following the two fractionation schemes. Pain relief was assessed using pain score, analgesic use and subjective perception of pain. Recalcification was measured using computed tomography (CT). There was no significant difference in overall and complete pain response. However, there was a significant difference in recalcification between the two groups,

Table 17.2. Randomised trials evaluating single-fraction local field radiotherapy

Reference	Number of patients	Dose (Gy)	Response (%)	Comments
Jeremic et al. [20]	327	4	59	6 Gy and 8 Gy provide significantly higher overall response rates compared to 4 Gy. 8 Gy provides shortest time to occurrence of pain relief
		6	73	
		8	78	
Hoskin et al. [19]	270	8	69	Increased pain relief with 8 Gy ($p < 0.001$), but no difference in duration of response and survival. Decreased probability of retreatment with 8 Gy (9% vs. 20%)
		4	44	
Price et al. [16]	288	8/1 fraction	45	No difference between arms in onset of pain relief, duration of response or toxicity
		30/10 fractions	28	
Cole [21]	29	8/1 fractions	90	No difference in pain relief response, but 25% of patients in 8 Gy arm required retreatment
		24/6 fractions	86	

with the fractionated group having improved recalcification rates of 17.3% vs. 12.0% in the single-dose group ($p < 0.0001$). Therefore, these data suggest that it may be reasonable to offer a protracted radiotherapy course for better stabilisation of bone in patients with bony metastatic disease with a prolonged life-expectancy.

A Canadian trial reported by Kirkbride et al. randomized 398 patients to 20 Gy in five fractions over 1 week or 8 Gy as a single fraction [26]. The primary endpoint was clinically significant pain relief at 3 months after treatment, defined as a reduction in pain score at the treated site with reduced analgesics or a pain score of zero at the treated site at 3 months without an increase in analgesics; 46% of patients who received fractionated treatment achieved significant pain relief, as compared to 32% of patients treated with a single fraction ($p=0.03$). Over a quarter of patients entered onto the study were not evaluable, mostly due to death occurring before 3 months after treatment. As a criterion for entry onto the study, the estimated survival was greater than 4 months, thus indicating how poor physicians are in estimating survival in patients with metastatic disease.

The literature generally supports the efficacy of single fractions or shorter courses of radiation therapy in the palliative treatment of bony metastatic disease. These accelerated regimens may be appropriate in certain clinical settings, e.g. expected survival that is less than 3 months, inability of the patient to return for daily radiation treatments, or rapid progression of tumour. A protracted course of irradiation may be more appropriate in patients with indolent disease, good performance status, life expectancy > 3 months or a solitary bone metastasis with a controlled primary tumour [27,28].

IMPENDING PATHOLOGICAL FRACTURES

Weight-bearing bones are one of the most predominant sites for palliative radiation therapy, comprising 51% of the palliative sites compared to non-weight-bearing bones, which comprise 13% [1]. Patients with lytic lesions in weight-bearing bones causing > 50% destruction of the cortex of tubular bone or a lesion measuring $\geqslant 2.5$ cm are considered at high risk for pathological fracture [29]. These patients should undergo orthopaedic evaluation for consideration of prophylactic fixation. Following fixation, patients should receive palliative irradiation to the involved area. It is generally advocated that intramedullary or other fixation devices should be included in the radiation portal in order to encompass any microscopic tumour that may have been dislodged during surgery. Adjacent joints should be spared unless there is tumour involvement.

HEMI-BODY IRRADIATION

Hemi-body irradiation (HBI) or wide-field radiation therapy has been advocated for two clinical situations: as primary palliative therapy for widespread extensive bony metastases, or as adjuvant therapy to local-field irradiation to reduce the development of occult metastases and progression of existing metastases and to reduce the need for retreatment. Single-dose HBI for the palliation of multiple bone metastases relieved pain in 73% of patients in a large prospective trial by the RTOG [30] (Table 17.3). In 20% of the patients, complete pain relief was achieved. The response was dramatic, with approximately 50% of all responders doing so within 48 h and 80% within 1 week from HBI treatment. The RTOG demonstrated that the most effective and safest doses of HBI to be delivered in a single fraction are 600 cGy and 800 cGy for upper and lower HBI, respectively.

In a separate study, the RTOG randomised 499 patients to receive either "adjuvant" HBI or no further treatment following completion of standard palliative local-field radiation therapy of 3000 cGy in 10 fractions [31]. HBI given with local-field radiation compared with local irradiation alone resulted in a decrease in the percentage of patients with progression of symptoms at 1 year (35% vs. 46%), percentage of patients with new disease in the targeted hemi-body at 1 year (50% vs. 68%), and median time-to-new disease within the targeted HBI area (12.6 months vs. 6.3 months). The need for retreatment within the hemi-body region was also reduced from 76% to 60% with the addition of HBI to local-field irradiation.

Zelefsky et al., from the Memorial Sloan-Kettering Cancer Center, evaluated fractionated HBI therapy in 15 patients with hormone-refractory prostate cancer receiving 25–30 Gy in nine or 10 fractions [32]. The results in this group were compared to a group of 14 patients who received single doses of 600 cGy upper or 800 cGy lower HBI. The complete response rate at 1 month was approximately 80% in both treatment groups. A slower time to response of 1–2 weeks was noted in the fractionated scheme compared to a 1–2 day response with the single fraction scheme. However, the median duration of pain relief was longer in the fractionated group vs. the single-dose group, with 8.5

Table 17.3. Results of hemi-body irradiation as palliative treatment

Reference	Number of patients	Hemi-body RT	Response (%)	Comments
Salazar et al. (RTOG 78-10) [30]	168	Single-dose	73	Complete pain relief in 20% of patients. Demonstrated 600 cGy for UHBI and 800 cGy for LHBI most effective and safest doses
Poulter et al. (RTOG 82-06) [31]	499		Time to disease progression:	HBI delayed time to disease progression and median time to new disease within HBI area (12.6 vs. 6.3 months)
		Local-field (30 Gy)	46	
		Local-field + HBI	35	
Zelefsky et al. [32]	29	Single-dose HBI (600 cGy or 800 cGy)	76	Complete response rates similar between two groups, but median duration of pain relief was longer in the fractionated group (8.5 vs. 2.8 months). Retreatment was required more often in the single-dose group (71% vs. 13%)
		Fractionated HBI (25–30 Gy/ 9–10 fractions)	86	
Scarantino et al. (RTOG 88-22) [33]	144	Local field (30 Gy) plus HBI in 2.5 Gy/fraction:	Time to new disease in HBI area:	No differences in the time to new disease or additional treatment in treated field. Maximum tolerated dose of fractionated HBI was found to be 17.5 Gy
		10 Gy HBI	19	
		12.5 Gy HBI	9	
		15 Gy HBI	17	
		17.5 Gy HBI	19	
		20 Gy HBI	13	

months vs. 2.8 months, respectively. Retreatment was required in 71% of the patients in the single-dose arm compared to 13% in the fractionated arm.

The RTOG performed a Phase I/II study to determine the maximum tolerable total dose that can be delivered by fractionated HBI [33]. A total of 144 patients with symptomatic bony metastases were entered and all patients initially received 30 Gy/10 fractions to the painful bony site, followed by HBI in 2.5 Gy fractions to doses of 10–20 Gy. The maximum tolerated dose of fractionated HBI was found to be 17.5 Gy, with the major dose-limiting toxicity being myelosuppression (primarily leukopenia and thrombocytopenia).

HBI (6–8 Gy) is an effective treatment that may be considered for patients with diffuse bone metastases. The acute side-effects which may be associated with HBI, viz. nausea, vomiting, diarrhoea and pneumonitis, are tolerable with appropriate pre-radiation medications. In addition, there is the potential risk of severe haematological toxicity, which may also result in decreased ability to use subsequent chemotherapy if warranted in the future. This concern regarding the permanent effects on bone marrow reserve, coupled

with the lesser duration of palliation, are significant reasons why HBI is not routinely used in the management of diffuse bone metastases in the USA. However, in the patient with multiple bony metastases and poor Karnofsky performance status, it can offer rapid and effective palliation.

Clinical trials evaluating the use of radiation therapy for the treatment of bone metastases have yielded important information regarding response to radiation therapy, yet leave many questions unanswered. Future studies should also examine the role of promising cointerventions, such as the use of pamidronate when palliating pain from bone metastases. For example, initial results of a study by Yavux et al. indicate that no significant differences were detected in the changes of pain and analgesia, performance, quality of life or tumour markers between patients who received radiation and pamidronate vs. pamidronate alone [34]. However, in the combined modality group, the median time to progression of pain within the irradiated field was 26 weeks without pamidronate and 68 weeks with pamidronate ($p=0.05$). In addition, the median time to new bone metastases was 23 weeks without pamidronate and 59 weeks with pamidronate ($p=0.05$).

CLINICAL TRIAL DESIGN

There are multiple study-design elements that must be taken into account when interpreting a clinical trial for patients treated with radiation for palliation of symptoms of bone metastases [35]. First, the eligibility criteria should be examined for the histological types of malignancies allowed, whether or not there is a minimal pain score, the performance status of the patient, the life expectancy of the patient and whether or not co-interventions have occurred during or prior to treatment. Pain assessment variables include the scale used, which pain is assessed (i.e. overall pain or local site pain), who assesses the pain and whether a body diagram is used as part of the assessment. An important analgesic assessment variable is the method of scoring of analgesic use (visual scale, numerical scale, scale gradation). The endpoint definition variables include the definition of complete and partial response and whether pain score alone or pain plus analgesics scores would be used in addition to the time that the endpoint is evaluated. Follow-up variables include whether a questionnaire is used or the visit is done in person, and the frequency of follow-up (daily, weekly or monthly), as well as the overall duration of follow-up. The description of how the radiation is to be delivered is perhaps less important than in definitive treatment trials; however, there should be some guidelines for the treatment volume, whether or not a simulation will be used and what methods of quality assurance would be utilised to determine that the appropriate treatment volume was being treated (e.g. the use of port or verification films). One should establish whether re-irradiation is an endpoint as well as the definition of what qualifies for re-irradiation. The clinical trial endpoints may be reported by intent to treat, actuarial analysis, or crude analysis at fixed times. Toxicity, such as nausea and vomiting, and quality of life, as well as the occurrence of spinal cord compression or pathological fractures, may be recorded. Considering all of the design elements, it is easy to see that keeping such a study simple may be difficult to achieve, but nonetheless simplicity in design must be a goal. An international consensus on endpoints to be used in clinical trials of the treatment of bone metastases with radiation is currently in development [36].

Critical analysis of clinical trials of local-field irradiation trials indicates that care practices need to be improved [26]. In many patients complete relief of pain has not been achieved and for most of those who did have relief, the duration of relief was less than their period of survival after treatment.

ONGOING RANDOMISED TRIALS

In an attempt to further define the most effective radiotherapy dose/fractionation schedule, the RTOG has recently begun enrolment onto a new trial (RTOG 97-14), which randomises patients with painful bone metastases from a breast or prostate primary to receive either 3000 cGy in 10 fractions or 800 cGy in a single fraction of radiation therapy. One goal of the trial is to assess palliative pain response between the two treatment arms. Response will be determined by follow-up questionnaires filled out by the patients as well as phone call interviews. This method of assessing pain relief according to the patient is in contrast to the prior RTOG 74-02 study, in which response to treatment was assessed by the physician. In addition, the effect on quality of life measures for the two treatment groups will be analysed in the new trial. Another component of this trial is a cost-effectiveness analysis between the two treatment schemes. Previous palliative radiotherapy trials for bony metastases have not included an evaluation of the economic impact of treatment. Given the current cost-conscious health-care environment, this trial should provide important information regarding the costs of palliative radiotherapy, as well as defining the optimal dose/fractionation treatment schedule for patients with bone metastases.

The Trans-Tasman Radiation Oncology Group (TROG) is conducting a randomised trial for patients with neuropathic bone pain. The term "neuropathic pain" refers to pain or dysaesthesia with a radiating superficial component due to compression or irritation of nerves. The study began in 1998 and randomises patients to a single 8 Gy fraction vs. 20 Gy in five fractions. Preliminary results indicate there is indeed a role for radiation in the treatment of neuropathic bone pain, with an overall response rate of 59% [37].

SUMMARY OF RADIATION THERAPY FOR BONE METASTASES

It is established that radiation therapy is an effective treatment modality in the palliation of bone metastases. Various treatment approaches are currently available, including external beam radiation therapy to local fields, hemi-body irradiation, and the administration of systemic radionuclides. For patients treated with local-field radiation, most, although not all, studies show little advantage to multi-fractionated radiation over single fractions [35,38]. However, there is reluctance to use single fractionated radiation in many countries [10,39]. The optimal treatment schedule requires further definition through the conduct of well-designed clinical trials.

REFERENCES

1. Coia L, Hanks G, Martz K et al. Practice patterns of palliative care for the United States, 1984–1985. Int J Radiat Oncol Biol Phys 1988; 14: 1261–9.
2. Landis S, Murray T, Bolden S, Wingo P. Cancer Statistics, 1998. CA Cancer J Clin 1999; 49: 1.
3. Hanks G. The crisis in health care cost in the United States: some implications for radiation oncology. Int J Radiat Oncol Biol Phys 1992; 23: 203–6.
4. Perez C. Principles and Practice of Radiation Oncology. Lippincott-Raven: Philadelphia, PA, 1998: 1583–5.
5. DeVita VT, Hellman S, Rosenberg S. Cancer: Principles and Practice of Oncology. Lippincott-Raven: Philadelphia, PA, 1997: 1331.
6. Arcangeli G, Micheli A, Arcangeli G et al. The responsiveness of bone metastasis to radiotherapy: the effect of site, histology and radiation dose on pain relief. Radiother Oncol 1989; 14: 95.
7. DeVita VT, Hellman S, Rosenberg S. Cancer: Principles and Practice of Oncology. Lippincott: Philadelphia, PA, 1993: 2225.
8. Bates T. A review of local radiotherapy in the treatment of bone metastases and cord compression. Int J Radiat Oncol Biol Phys 1992; 23: 217–21.
9. Maher E. The use of palliative radiotherapy in the management of breast cancer. Eur J Cancer 1992; 28: 706–10.
10. Maher E, Coia L, Duncan G, Lawton P. Treatment strategies in advanced and metastatic cancer: differences in attitude between the USA, Canada and Europe. Int J Radiat Oncol Biol Phys 1992; 23: 239–44.
11. Rose C, Kagan R. The final report of the expert panel for the radiation oncology bone metastasis work group of the American College of Radiology. Int J Radiat Oncol Biol Phys 1998; 40: 1117–24.
12. Tong D, Glick L, Hendrickson F. The palliation of osseous metastases—final results of the study by the Radiation Therapy Oncology Group. Cancer 1982; 50: 893–9.
13. Blitzer P. Reanalysis of the RTOG study of the palliation of symptomatic osseous metastasis. Cancer 1985; 55: 1468–72.
14. Niewald M, Tkocz H, Abel U et al. Rapid course radiation therapy vs. more standard treatment: a randomized trial for bone metastases. Int J Radiat Oncol Biol Phys 1996; 36: 1085–9.
15. Rasmusson B, Vejborg I, Jensen A et al. Irradiation of bone metastases in breast cancer patients: a randomized study with 1 year follow-up. Radiother Oncol 1995; 34: 179–84.
16. Price P, Hoskin P, Easton D et al. Prospective randomised trial of single and multifraction radiotherapy schedules in the treatment of painful bony metastases. Radiother Oncol 1986; 6: 247–5.
17. Madsen E. Painful bone metastasis: efficacy of radiotherapy assessed by the patients: a randomized trial comparing 4 Gy × 6 vs. 10 Gy × 2. Int J Radiat Oncol Biol Phys 1983; 9: 1775–9.
18. Okawa T, Kita M, Goto M et al. Randomized prospective clinical study of small, large and twice-a-day fraction radiotherapy for painful bone metastases. Radiother Oncol 1988; 13: 99–104.
19. Hoskin P, Price P, Easton D et al. A prospective randomised trial of 4 Gy or 8 Gy single doses in the treatment of metastatic bone pain. Radiother Oncol 1992; 23: 74–8.
20. Jeremic B, Shibamoto Y, Med D et al. A randomized trial of three single-dose radiation therapy regimens in the treatment of metastatic bone pain. Int J Radiat Oncol Biol Phys 1998; 42: 161–7.
21. Cole D. A randomized trial of a single treatment vs. conventional fractionation in the palliative radiotherapy of painful bone metastases. Clin Oncol 1989; 1: 59–62.
22. Steenland E, Leer J, Houwelingen H et al. The effect of a single fraction compared to multiple fractions on painful bone metastases: a global analysis of the Dutch Bone Metastasis Study. Radiother Oncol 1999; 52: 101–9.
23. Nielsen O, Bentzen S, Sandberg E et al. Randomized trial of single dose vs. fractionated palliative radiotherapy of bone metastases. Radiother Oncol 1998; 47: 233–40.
24. Yarnold JR. 8 Gy single fraction radiotherapy for the treatment of mestastatic skeletal pain: randomised comparison with a multifraction schedule over 12 months of patient follow-up. On behalf of the Bone Pain Trial Working Party. Radiother Oncol 1999; 52: 111–21.
25. Koswig S, Budach V. Remineralization and pain relief in bone metastases after different radiotherapy fractions (10 × 3 Gy vs. 1 × 8 Gy). A prospective study. Strahlentherap Onkol 1999; 175(10): 500–8.
26. Kirkbride P, Warde PP, Panzarella J et al. A randomized trial comparing the efficacy of a single radiation fraction with fractionated radiation therapy in the treatment of skeletal metastases. Int J Radiat Oncol Biol Phys 2000; 48: 185a.
27. Richter M, Coia L. Palliative radiation therapy. Semin Oncol 1985; 12: 375.
28. Ratanatharathorn V, Powers W, Moss W, Perez C. Bone metastasis: review and critical analysis of random allocation trials of local field treatment. Int J Radiat Oncol Biol Phys 1999; 44(1): 1–18.
29. Fidler M. Incidence of fracture through metastasis in long bones. Acta Orthop Scand 1981; 52: 623.
30. Salazar O, Rubin P, Hendrickson F et al. Single-dose half-body irradiation for palliation of multiple bone metastases from solid tumors. Cancer 1986; 58: 29–36.
31. Poulter C, Cosmatos D, Rubin P et al. A report of RTOG 8206: a phase III study of whether the addition of single dose hemibody irradiation to standard fractionated local field irradiation is more effective than local field irradiation alone in the treatment of symptomatic osseous metastases. Int J Radiat Oncol Biol Phys 1992; 23: 201–14.
32. Zelefsky M, Scher H, Forman J et al. Palliative hemiskeletal irradiation for widespread metastatic prostate cancer: a comparison of single dose and fractionated regimens. Int J Radiat Oncol Biol Phys 1989; 17: 1281–5.
33. Scarantino C, Caplan R, Rotman M et al. A phase I/II study to evaluate the effect of fractionated hemibody irradiation in the treatment of osseous metastases-RTOG 88-22. Int J Radiat Oncol Biol Phys 1996; 36: 37–48.

34. Yavux M, Yavux A, Cakibay H et al. Effects of pamidronate use on the palliative radiotherapy of bone metastases: a prospective randomized study. Int J Radiat Oncol Biol Phys 2000; 48: 185a.

35. Dawson R, Currow B, Stevens G et al. Radiotherapy for bone metastases: a critical appraisal of outcome measures. J Pain Sympt Manag 1999; 17(3); 208–18.

36. International Consensus Working Party. International bone metastases consensus on endpoint measurements for future clinical trials: proceedings of the first survey and meeting. Clin Oncol 2001 (in press).

37. Roos DE, O'Brien PC, Smith JG et al. A role for radiotherapy in neuropathic bone pain: preliminary response rates from a prospective trial (RTOG 96.05). Int J Radiat Oncol Biol Phys 2000; 46(4): 975–81.

38. Arcangeli G, Giovinazzo G, Saracino B et al. Radiation therapy in the management of symptomatic bone metastases; the effect of total dose and histology on pain relief and response duration. Int J Radiat Oncol Biol Phys 1998; 42(5): 1119–26.

39. Roos D. Continuing reluctance to use single fraction of radiotherapy for metastatic bone pain: an Australian and New Zealand practice survey and literature review. Radiother Oncol 2000; 56: 315–22.

18

Interventional Radiology
for Bone Metastases

J. Chiras, C. Adem, J. N. Vallée, D. Lo and M. Rose

Hôpital de la Pitié-Salpêtrière, Paris, France

INTRODUCTION

Interventional radiology has been largely developed for the treatment of vascular malformations, haemorrhagic syndromes and hepatic tumours, and to improve the possibilities of surgical removal in many carcinological situations. Initially limited to the preoperative embolisation of highly vascular masses, especially spinal or pelvic, during the past 10 years, its field is largely widening for the treatment of metastases by development of new endovascular or percutaneous techniques. New percutaneous (cimentoplasty) or endovascular (local infusion) techniques are demonstrating their usefulness in the treatment of bone metastases and play an increasing part in multidisciplinary approaches to bone metastases.

Each of these techniques has its own indications in cases of either carcinological or palliative treatment and their indication should be discussed in a multidisciplinary approach, including orthopaedic surgeons, interventional radiologists, radiotherapists and oncologists. In a palliative intervention, therapeutic protocol depends also on the clinical status of the patient, life expectancy and, essentially, on the clinical goal: bone stabilisation and reinforcement and/or pain relief.

ENDOVASCULAR TECHNIQUES

Endovascular embolisation was developed during the past 20 years to reduce blood loss during surgical removal of tumours (Figure 18.1) [1,2]. Concomitantly some authors have outlined its potential to induce tumour necrosis, diminish tumour size and relieve tumoral pain (Figure 18.2). Following the success of embolisation, local infusion of anti-mitotic drugs (so-called "intraarterial chemotherapy") and chemoembolisation (a combination of intraarterial chemotherapy and selective embolisation) have been developed.

Endovascular Embolisation

Technique

This consists in selective injection of embolic material into the arteries, feeding the tumour as distally as possible, to obtain tumoral devascularisation followed by tumour necrosis.

Using gelfoam powder, Nagata and colleagues [3] showed that embolisation induced necrosis in $62 \pm 22\%$ of the tumour, compared to the control group, in whom tumour necrosis was $19 \pm 7\%$. The procedure is usually realised by the femoral route, rarely the brachial route, and requires neuroleptanalgesia, as injection of the embolic agent is usually painful.

Different types of embolic agent have been used over the years: particles are most frequently employed and in some cases liquid agents, such as absolute alcohol (ethanol); tissue adhesives (e.g. Bucrylate) can be used, but they require hyperselective injection to prevent adjacent tissue necrosis [4].

Textbook of Bone Metastases. Edited by C. Jasmin, R. E. Coleman, L. R. Coia, R. Capanna and G. Saillant
© 2005 John Wiley & Sons Ltd: ISBN 0 471 87742 5

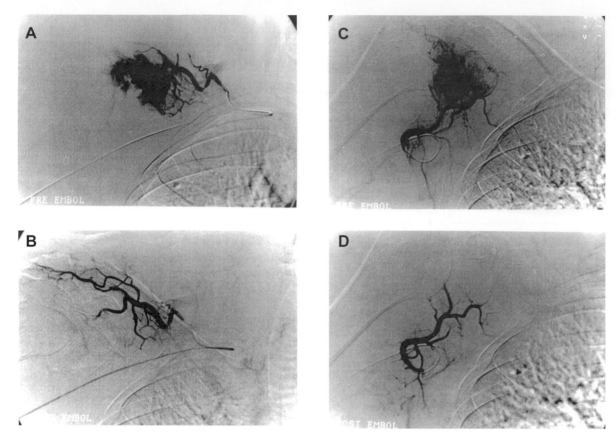

Figure 18.1. Metastasis of the scapula from thyroid carcinoma. Pre-operative embolisation. Huge hypervascularisation of the lesion. Embolisation gives a large devascularisation of the lesion, extremely useful for surgical removal. (A,B) Suprascapular artery before (A) and after embolisation (B). (C,D) Subscapular branch before (C) and after embolisation (D)

For that reason particles are most often employed, as they follow the blood flow and can reach the tumour site while sparing the normal adjacent tissues. Different particulate material can be used, e.g. gelfoam powder, polyvinyl alcohol (PVA), gelatine sponges. The size and calibration of particles is an important point to consider: the efficacy of tumoral necrosis is higher with small particles ($100\,\mu$m) but the risk of necrosis of the surrounding normal soft tissue (cutaneous or mucosal necrosis, nerve palsy due to arterial ischaemia) is higher with such small-sized particles, particularly in previously irradiated patients.

Liquid agents can also be used, but they need to be delivered in close contact with the tumour, as the risk of acute necrosis of normal adjacent tissues is very high. In this class of embolic agents, absolute alcohol or adhesive glue (Bucrylate) are the most commonly employed.

Embolisation usually gives rapid relief of pain, but in some cases it can induce an increase of pain for a few days, due to tumour necrosis; in large masses, a post embolisation syndrome (pain, nausea, fever) can be observed after embolisation. This syndrome is considered to be due to tumour necrosis and disappears in < 2 weeks [4].

Complications are rare and probably more frequent with embolic agents that induce acute tumour necrosis, such as gelfoam powder, Bucrylate or alcohol. They can consist of skin necrosis or ischaemic ulcer but also nerve palsy, which can remain permanent [4,5]; the risk of complication is higher in patients who have been previously treated by irradiation.

Indications and Results

Embolisation is used to obtain temporary or definitive devascularisation or necrosis of the tumour pre-operatively or to relieve local pain in lesions uncontrolled by more usual treatment.

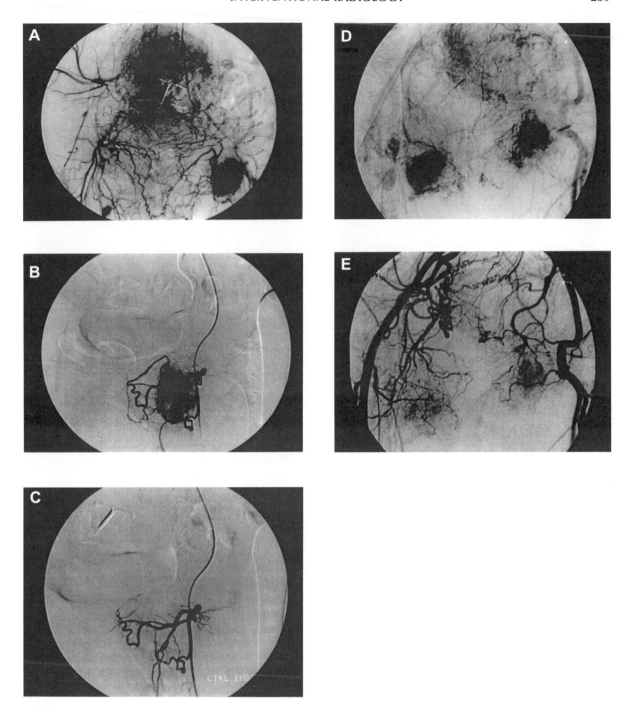

Figure 18.2. Palliative embolisation of pelvic girdle metastasis from thyroid carcinoma. (A) Pre-embolisation angiography shows hypervascularisation in the left ischium. (B,C) Pre- and post-embolisation of one of the feeders. (D) Angiographic control 2 years later: recurrence of hypervascularisation and concomitant pain on walking. (E) Control angiogram 1 year later (asymptomatic patient): slight recurrence of hypervascularisation. This embolisation allows control of pain and tumoral progression for 5 years

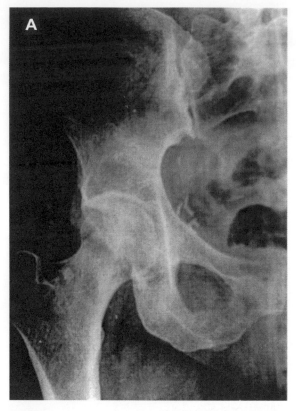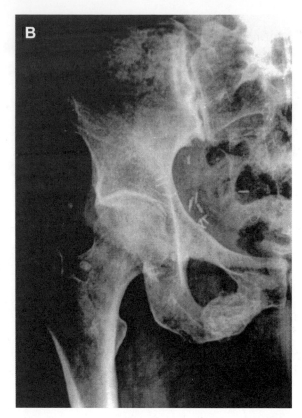

Figure 18.3. Local pain from breast metastasis involving pubic and ischio-pubic branch. (A) Plain film before chemoembolisation. (B) Plain film 3 months after one session of chemoembolisation (paraplatinium 150 mg, pirarubicine 5 mg). Complete disappearance of pain with re-ossification of the lesion and disappearance of the extension into the soft tissues

Pre-operative Embolisation. Embolisation performed before surgical removal is known to be effective in reducing blood loss during surgery and improving the post-operative period in tumours involving the spine or pelvic girdle [5–7]. The effectiveness of such a technique appears greater in highly vascularised lesions, such as metastases from kidney or thyroid cancer [1] (Figure 18.1). It is also very useful in deeply located tumours, where it allows complete surgical removal, which in most cases was not feasible before embolisation [5].

According to the literature, no significant difference in pre-operative embolisation quality was found concerning the choice of the embolic agent: PVA, tissue adhesive or ethanol. As ethanol or Bucrylate tremendously increase the complication rate [6], it appears to be more appropriate to use calibrated PVA particles for pre-operative treatment. In some cases, it can be necessary to occlude the origin of the main vessels feeding the lesion by coils, and preventing an

intractable haemorrhage if a surgical wound to the artery were to occur.

Some authors have discussed the delay between embolisation and surgical removal. Usually a delay of 1–3 days [1–8] is recommended, especially in highly vascular lesions. In poorly vascularised lesions, a longer delay, up to 15 days, can be allowed.

Palliative Embolisation. Different reports have emphasised the role of palliative embolisation to reduce pain in patients presenting with chemoresistant and unoperable bone metastases [3,5,6,9,10]. Pain relief for 3 weeks–8 months has been observed following embolisation, independent of the embolic material used [7]. In most circumstances the result is obtained during the 2 days following the embolisation. Different success factors can be outlined: a complete embolisation gives a longer pain sedation than a partial one. The use of ethanol or Bucrylate may induce longer pain relief, but conversely, the risk of neurological or

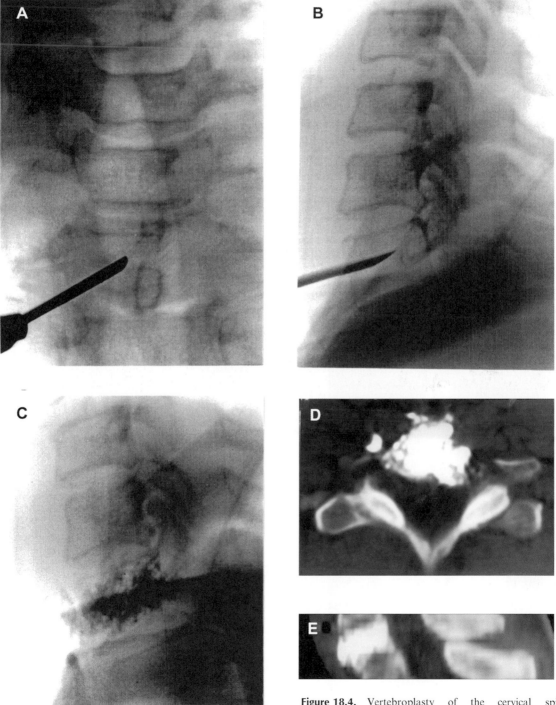

Figure 18.4. Vertebroplasty of the cervical spine: anterolateral approach of the vertebral body. (A) Front view. (B) Lateral view of the needle position. (C) Plain film after cement injection. (D,E) CT control performed immediately after the vertebroplasty. Slight extravertebral issue of cement along the route of the needle.

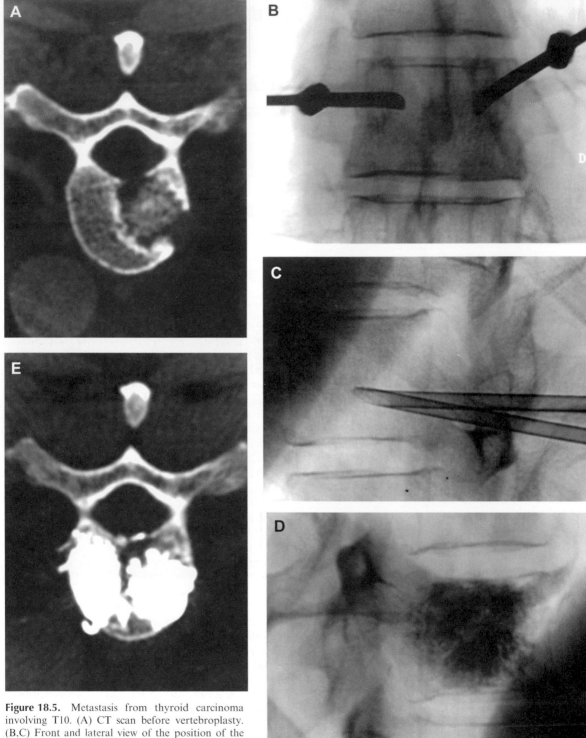

Figure 18.5. Metastasis from thyroid carcinoma involving T10. (A) CT scan before vertebroplasty. (B,C) Front and lateral view of the position of the needle in the vertebral body during vertebroplasty. (D,E) Plain film and CT control after vertebroplasty

skin complications appears higher [2,7,10]. Consequently, these agents should not be used in arteries feeding nerves or in superficial territories.

The result is largely influenced by the aggressiveness of the metastasis. Longer benefit can be expected in metastases from thyroid carcinoma [5] (Figure 18.2), whose progression time is slow, but in most cases early recurrence of pain necessitates iterative embolisation. Usually efficacy declines after iterative embolisation compared to the first procedure [7].

Currently, chemoembolisation, comprising embolisation in association with anti-neoplastic drugs, seems to be more effective and we use palliative embolisation only in chemoresistant tumours, such as thyroid carcinoma or malignant phaeochromocytoma metastases.

Selective Chemotherapy

The rationale for local intraarterial infusion chemotherapy is to deliver a higher concentration of drug into a tumour. By this means, a higher carcinolytic effect is obtained according to the so-called "first pass effect", i.e. high drug extraction during the first contact with the tumour. This effect directly depends on drug concentration in the tumoral artery and can be greatly increased by selective catheterisation. Anderson and associates [11] showed that local drug administration increases the uptake sixfold. Its usefulness depends also on drug pharmacokinetic factors, but most antineoplastic drugs have a response curve depending on the concentration level in the artery [12]. Conversely, this technique increases local drug toxicity, especially causing necrosis in cutaneous arterial territories.

Nevertheless, this technique should be useful in case of poorly chemosensitive tumours where it can improve the response. Conversely, although it increases local efficacy, it does not prevent the development of other metastases. Its indications should therefore be very restrictive in bone metastases, as its analgesic effect does not seem to be clearly significant.

Chemoembolisation

This approach is a combination of tumoral intraarterial infusion of chemotherapeutic agents and vascular supply embolisation. It was first proposed by Kato et al. [13], who used ethylcellulose microencapsulated with mitomycin. In addition to the direct effect of ischaemia on the neoplasm, the decreasing blood flow through the tumoral vascular bed increases tumour–

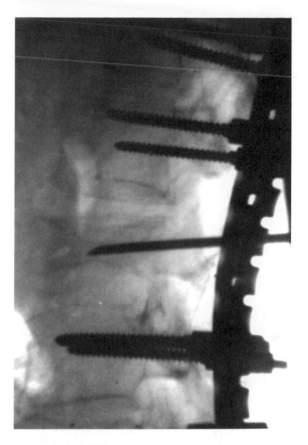

Figure 18.6. Posterolateral approach in a patient with previous surgery for cord compression

drug contact time and, theoretically, local drug uptake. The cytotoxic result affects not only the neoplasm but the embolised and infused vessels, producing vasculitis and occlusion. Other trials have been carried out in bone metastases [13–14] using cisplatinium.

In our experience with paraplatine and pirarubicine, this approach should be promising, as it can induce lasting tumoral regression (Figure 18.3).

PERCUTANEOUS TECHNIQUES

Percutaneous techniques have been developed more recently to induce tumour necrosis or to reinforce bone structure (vertebroplasty [15], or acrylic cementation of the hip joint [16]).

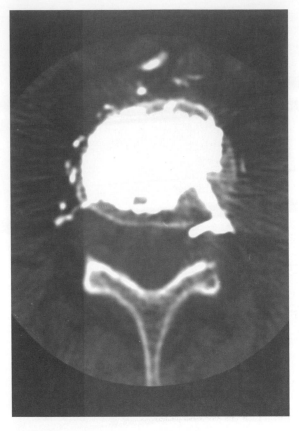

Figure 18.7. Posterolateral approach: issue of cement along the route of the needle, in close contact with the nerve root, which can induce radicular pain

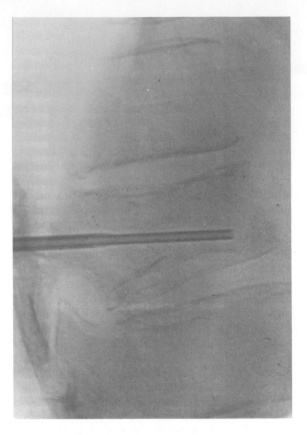

Figure 18.8. Coaxial biopsy by a transpedicular approach, realised with a 10G needle. The biopsy is taken with a 15G bone biopsy needle

Vertebroplasty

This technique strengthens the vertebra by a percutaneous approach, without open surgery: a needle is placed under fluoroscopic control into the involved vertebra, through which polymerising cement is injected into the vertebral body to obtain a satisfactory cast of the lesion.

Polymerisation of the cement induces stabilisation of the vertebra and subsequent relief of pain in most cases [17].

Technique

The approach to the vertebral body is realised under fluoroscopic control on a digital angiography (DSA) neurovascular system with front and lateral view. This procedure does not necessitate general anaesthesia, but local anaesthesia and neuroleptanalgesia are required. The approach depends on the vertebra involved, according to techniques described for percutaneous biopsy under imaging control [18–20].

Cervical Spine. The patient is in the supine position. The needle is introduced by an anterolateral approach (Figure 18.4). A unilateral approach is usually sufficient to allow a satisfactory filling of the vertebra.

Thoracic and Lumbar Spine. The patient is in the prone position. The needle is introduced by a pedicular approach under fluoroscopic control (Figure 18.5). Usually a bilateral approach is necessary to obtain adequate filling of the vertebra, and it reduces the risk of extravertebral issue of cement.

When the pedicle is not satisfactorily evaluable by fluoroscopy (posterior arch involvement or previous

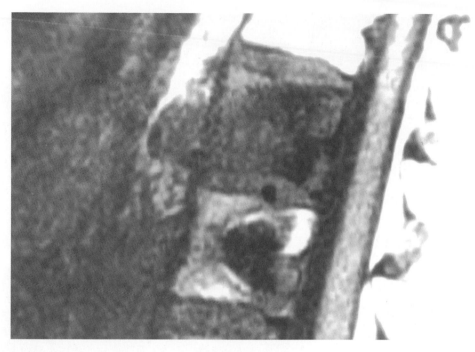

Figure 18.9. MRI: metastases treated by vertebroplasty. The vertebroplasty was adequate and induced necrosis, shown by a hypersignal surrounding the cement on T1 sequences

surgical approach), a posterolateral approach can be used (Figure 18.6). In this case, a unilateral approach is usually sufficient but this increases the risk of leakage of cement along the nerve root, inducing radicular pain (Figure 18.7). For this reason, in all cases where it is feasible we prefer the pedicular route.

Usually the size of the needle (10G) is sufficient to allow a coaxial biopsy (Figure 18.8), using a bone biopsy needle.

Injection of the cement is controlled under fluoroscopy and immediate radiographic control is realised (front and lateral views and CT scan with reformatted slices: Figure 18.4).

Indications

Vertebroplasty is a part of the palliative treatment for metastatic vertebrae, but recently it has been shown that it can also induce necrosis of the metastasis at the site of the injection (Figure 18.9). As previously suggested by Radin [21], this probably explains the prolonged pain relief observed after vertebroplasty in the great majority of patients, as well as stabilisation of progression of the metastases. Initially vertebroplasty was only used to treat recurrence of pain after local

treatment, but its importance is increasingly recognised in the treatment of bone metastases at an early stage in association with general treatment.

Its effectiveness can be related to three phenomena: first, the reinforcement of the vertebra due to the cement, which reduces the mechanical pain due to the metastasis; second, the destruction of metastatic cells; and third, probable destruction of nervous ramification in the vertebra which could be responsible for tumoral pain. Nevertheless, its effect is limited to the vertebra and it has no efficiency on perivertebral metastatic involvement and this is one limitation for this technique.

Vertebroplasty can be useful in three main clinical situations:

1. Recurrence or persistent pain after local treatment, including radiotherapy and/or surgery: in such cases the pain is usually mechanical in origin and vertebroplasty, allowing consolidation of the vertebra, induces relief of pain in most cases (Figures 18.10, 18.11).
2. Spinal metastases not previously treated: vertebroplasty is used as a local treatment in the same way as radiotherapy. These two techniques can be used in association or independently. Vertebroplasty has

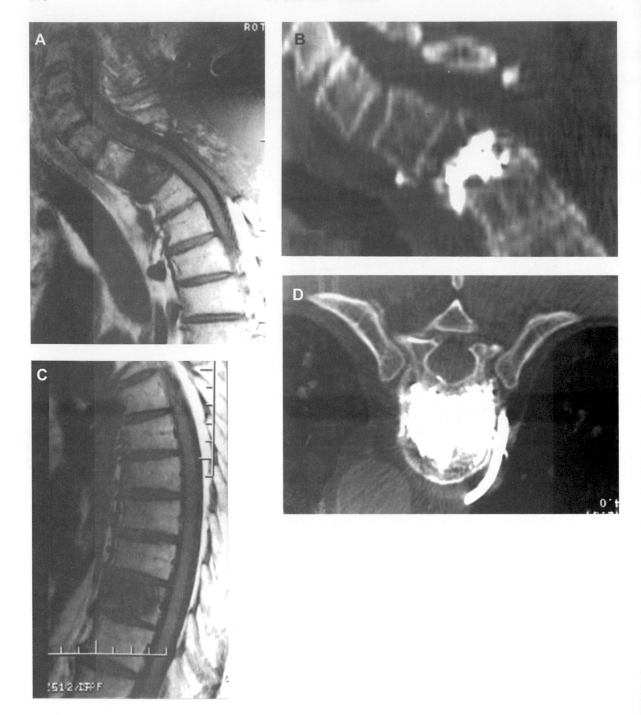

Figure 18.10. Renal carcinoma from T3. There was a surgical posterior approach to remove spinal compression. The vertebroplasty was done to consolidate vertebra T3. (A) Post-operative MRI. (B) Post-vertebroplasty CT control: satisfactory consolidation of the vertebra. (C,D) Vertebroplasty at T10 to reinforce the vertebra and obtain an antalgic effect

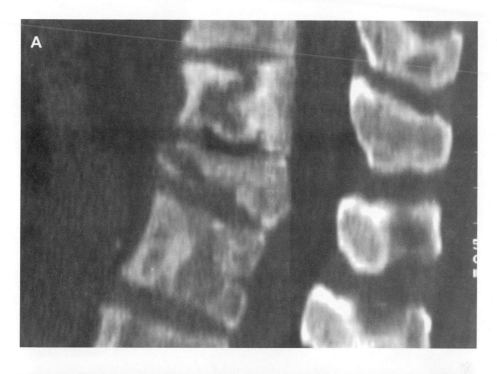

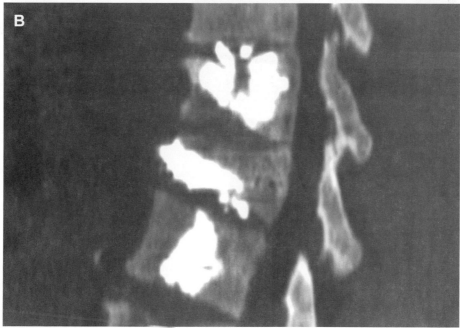

Figure 18.11. Mixed osteosclerotic and osteolytic metastasis from prostate cancer, previously treated by irradiation: very good pain relief following vertebroplasty. (A) CT scan before vertebroplasty. (B) CT control after vertebroplasty

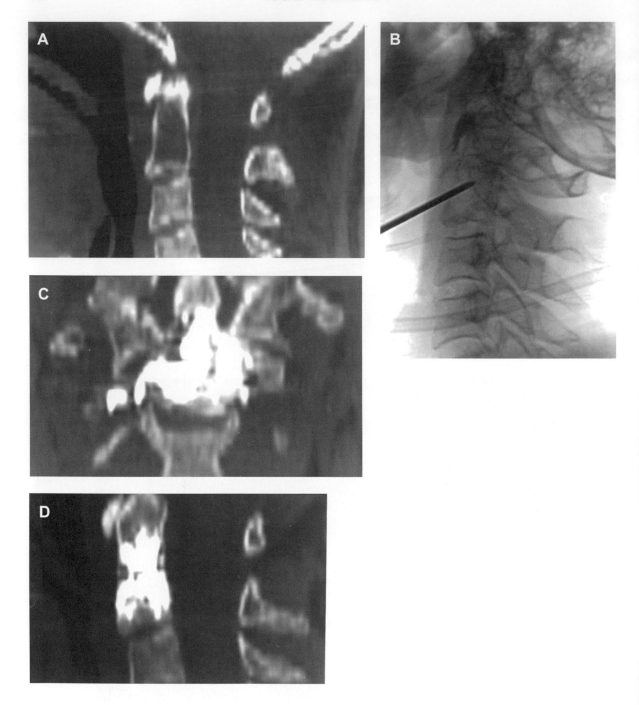

Figure 18.12. Malignant phaeochromocytoma: unstable metastasis involving C2. (A) CT scan before vertebroplasty. (B) Anterolateral approach to the vertebral body of C2. (C,D) Reformatted CT scan post-vertebroplasty

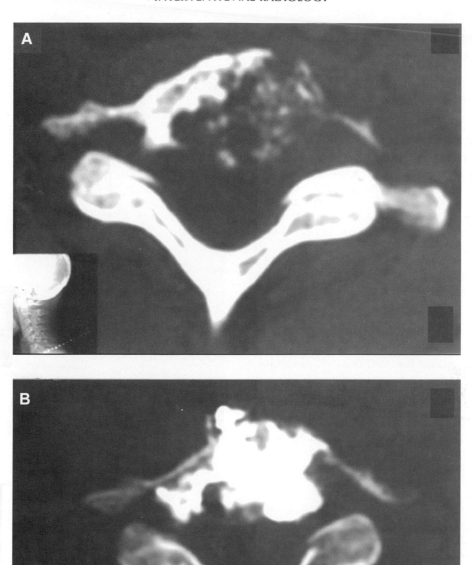

Figure 18.13. Unstable metastasis C7 from breast cancer: pre-irradiation stabilisation by vertebroplasty. (A) CT before vertebroplasty (B) CT after vertebroplasty

the advantage of giving very rapid pain relief (within days of the procedure). It stabilises the vertebra and is particularly indicated in cases of unstable (Figure 18.12) or hyperalgic metastases. In such cases, it can replace the surgical approach when there is no spinal cord compression or when the lesion is limited to the vertebral body. It has been demonstrated that there is no antagonism between acrylic cementation and radiotherapy [22] and both techniques can be applied (Figure 18.13), especially for lesions that are poorly responsive to chemotherapy. On the other hand, when the chemosensitivity of the lesion is high, vertebroplasty can replace radiation therapy, which should be reserved for later recurrence of the disease (Figure 18.14).

3. Metastases causing neurological impairment: in most cases, neurological symptoms are due to epiduritis, which requires emergency treatment by surgery or radiation therapy. In these cases, vertebroplasty has no place in the first step of the treatment but can be useful after surgery to consolidate the vertebral body and prevent secondary deterioration of the stabilisation (Figure 18.10).

Results

The clinical result is obtained very rapidly, but rarely there is an increase of pain, considered to be caused by an inflammatory reaction to the cement, which disappears rapidly under appropriate treatment [17,23,24,25].

Pain relief had been reported by various authors; it is approximately 70–90%, with complete relief of pain obtained in about 70% of cases [17].

The stabilisation and pain relief usually allows an important reduction of antalgic drugs, improves the ability to stand and walk and hence greatly improves the quality of life. While such satisfactory results are observed in osteolytic lesions, in painful mixed or osteosclerotic metastases, vertebroplasty also gives satisfactorily relief of pain in about 70% of cases (Figures 18.11, 18.15).

Complications are rare [26], most often relate to the clinical status of patients and are essentially due to pulmonary embolism in invalid patients. The global complication rate is estimated at 1.5%. Exceptional pulmonary embolism caused by the cement had been reported [27]. Local complications are directly caused by extravertebral migration of cement into the vertebral plexus, perivertebral veins, intervertebral discs or soft tissue. Most of these migrations are

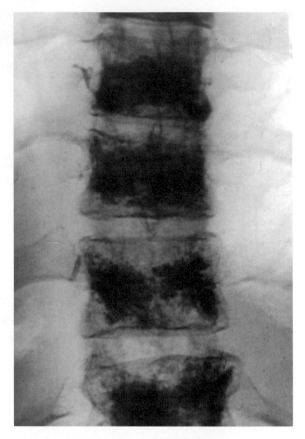

Figure 18.14. Young woman aged 31 years. Multi-focal bone metastases from breast cancer under chemotherapy. Vertebroplasty at different levels induced very good pain relief

asymptomatic (especially in the intervertebral discs, perivertebral veins and perivertebral soft tissue) but intraspinal migration can be responsible for neurological complications. Although cord compression is very exceptional under standard quality fluoroscopic control, radicular pain can be observed in about 3.5% of cases; its rate diminish with the experience of the operator. Some radiculalgias disappear spontaneously but in some cases local treatment (anaesthetic local infiltration, or surgical removal of part of the cement) may be necessary and residual pain after appropriate treatment is exceptional.

According to a previous report, involvement of the posterior wall of the vertebral body does not contraindicate vertebroplasty if there is no neurological impairment and does not increase significantly the rate of local complications [17].

Pain relief is often prolonged and probably this is due to tumoral necrosis induced by the cement, as

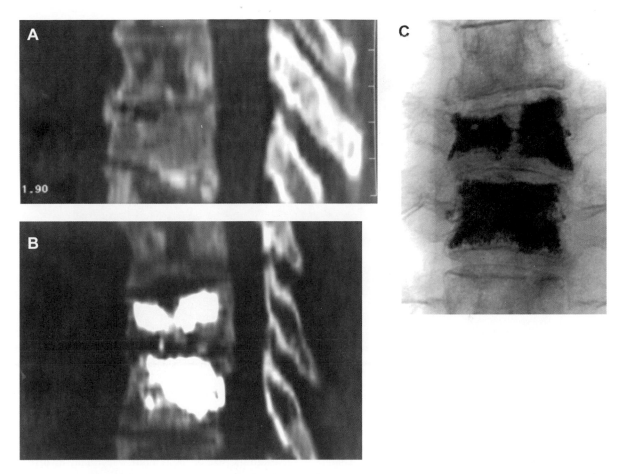

Figure 18.15. Mixed osteosclerotic and osteolytic metastases from breast cancer. Local pain. Very satisfactory result after vertebroplasty. (A,B) CT scan before and after vertebroplasty. (C) Plain film front view: complete pain relief after vertebroplasty

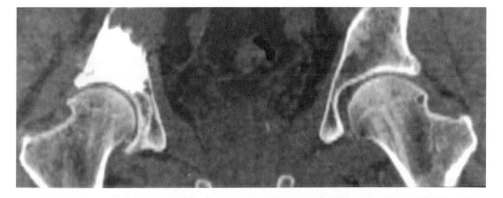

Figure 18.16. Acetabular lesion due to thyroid cancer: consolidation of the vertebra with complete pain relief

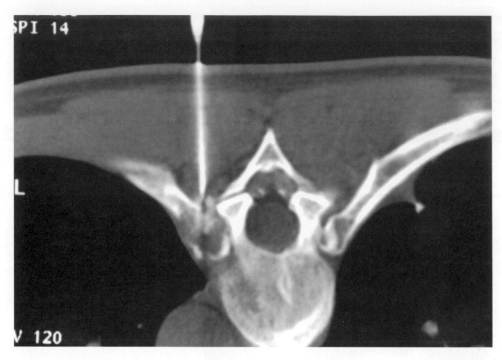

Figure 18.17. Patient presenting multiple metastases from thyroid cancer. Osteolytic lesion of the costovertebral joint. Injection of alcohol with good pain relief

previously suggested by Radin et al. [21], and San Millan Ruiz et al. [28] reported that in post mortem specimens cement induced tumoral necrosis 5 mm around the cement cast. This is probably responsible for the stabilisation of lesions when the vertebra has been sufficiently filled with cement, hence recurrence of pain is not usually observed during the years following vertebroplasty treatment for metastasis.

Acrylic Cementation on Other Sites

Acrylic cementation can be helpful in stabilising metastatic lesions involving spongious bones in other anatomical sites, such as the pelvic girdle and bony extremities. In particular, it has been used for consolidation of the acetabulum [16–29].

Acetabular Cementation

Encouraged by the results of vertebroplasty, various authors have developed acrylic cementation for treatment of metastases involving the hip joint. This technique gives also satisfactory results concerning

pain and stabilisation of the hip joint (Figure 18.16), but there is a lower rate of good results (70%). This relates to the size of the tumour, which may involve a large part of the iliac bone, with soft tissue diffusion.

Probably the outcome would be better if the treatment was instigated at an earlier stage in the development of the metastasis, while the lesion remains enclosed within the bone.

Other Anatomical Sites

Due to the mechanical effects of cement, this technique should be restricted to metastases involving spongious bone, especially in extremities such as the upper humerus or shoulder. In long bones, however, it does not diminish the risk of fracture.

PERCUTANEOUS EMBOLISATION

Percutaneous embolisation was developed to induce tumour necrosis when endovascular embolisation or acrylic cementation are not feasible. Such an eventuality is observed where there are large metastases invading soft tissues. Injection of absolute alcohol can induce a partial necrosis of the lesion and reduce local pain. The approach is usually realised under CT scan using small needles; injection of pure alcohol made radio-opaque by contrast medium can produce partial necrosis of the lesion. Pain relief is usually temporary and does not exceed 3 months but the procedure can be repeated (Figure 18.17) [30].

CONCLUSION

Interventional radiology by way of endovascular techniques and the percutaneous approach can participate beneficially in the improvement of quality of life in patients suffering from bone metastases.

REFERENCES

1. Chiras J, Gaston A, Gaveau T et al. Embolization pré-opératoire en pathologie rachidienne. J Radiol 1983; 64: 397.
2. Keller FS, Rösch J, Bird CB. Percutaneous embolization with tissue adhesive. Radiology 1983; 147: 21–7.
3. Nagata Y, Mitsumori M, Okajima K et al. Transcatheter arterial embolization for malignant osseous and soft tissue sarcomas. II. Clinical results. Cardiovasc Intervent Radiol 1998; 21: 208–13.
4. Hemingway AP, Allison DJ. Complications of embolization: analysis of 410 procedures. Radiology 1988; 166: 669–72.
5. Cormier E, Chiras J, Bories J. Artériographie et embolization des tumeurs lombo-sacrées: à propos de 41 cas. VIIIèmes Journées d'Orthopédie de la Pitié. Masson: Paris, 1992: 19–26.
6. Barton P, Waneck R, Karnal J et al. Embolization of bone metastases. JVIR 1996; 7: 81–8.
7. Layalle I, Flandroy P, Trotteur G et al. Arterial embolization of bone metastases: is it worthwhile? JBR-BTR 1998; 81: 223–5.
8. Rowe DM, Becker GK, Rabe FE et al. Osseous metastases from renal cell carcinoma: embolization and surgery for restoration of function. Radiology 1984; 150: 673–6.
9. Chuang VP, Wallace S, Swanson D et al. Arterial occlusion in the management of pain from metastatic renal carcinoma. Radiology 1979; 133: 611–14.
10. Wallace S, Granmayeh M, De Santos LA et al. Arterial occlusion of pelvic bone tumors. Cancer 1979; 43: 322–8.
11. Anderson JH, Gianturco C, Wallace S. Experimental transcatheter intra-arterial infusion occlusion chemotherapy. Invest Radiol 1981; 16: 496–500.
12. Frei E III. Effects of dose and schedule of response. In Holland JR, Frei E III (eds), Cancer Medicine. Lea & Febiger: Philadelphia, PA, 1973: 717–30.
13. Kato TI, Nemoto R, Mori H et al. Arterial chemoembolization with microencapsulated anticancer drug. J Am Med Assoc 1981; 245: 1123–7.
14. Courtheoux P, Alachkar F, Casasco A et al. Chemoembolization of lumbar spine metastases: a preliminary study. J Neuroradiol 1985; 12: 151–62.
15. Deramond H, Darrason R, Galibert P. La vertébroplastie acrylique dans le traitement des hémangiomes vertébraux agressifs. Rachis 1989; 1: 143–53.
16. Cotten A, Deprez X, Migaud H et al. Malignant acetabular osteolysis: percutaneous injection of acrylic bone cement. Radiology 1995; 197: 307–10.
17. Weill A, Chiras J, Simon JM. Spinal metastases: indications for and results of percutaneous injection of acrylic surgical cement. Radiology 1996; 199: 241–7.
18. Laredo JD, Bard M, Leblanc G et al. Technique et résultats de la ponction-biopsie transcutanée radioguidée du rachis dorsal. Rev Rhum 1985; 52(4): 283–7.
19. McCollister M, Evarts C. Diagnostic techniques: closed biopsy of bone. Clin Orthop Rel Res 1975; 107: 100–11.
20. Ottolenghi CE, Schajowicz F, Deschant FA. Aspiration biopsy of the cervical spine. Technique and results in thirty-four cases. J Bone Joint Surg 1964; 46-A: 715–33.
21. Radin EL, Rubin CT, Thrasher EL et al. Changes in the bone cement interface after total hip replacement. J Bone Joint Surg 1982; 64: 1188–200.
22. Murray JA, Bruels MC, Lindberg R. Irradiation of polymethylacrylate. J Bone Joint Surg 1974; 56: 311–12.
23. Deramond H, Depriester C, Galibert P. Percutaneous vertebroplasty. In Wilson D (ed.), Intervention Radiology of the Musculoskeletal System. Edward Arnold: London, 1995; 133–42.
24. Cotten A, Dewatre F, Cortet B, Assaker R et al. Percutaneous vertebroplasty for osteolytic metastases and myeloma: effects of the percentage of lesion filling and the leakage of methylmetacrylate at clinical follow-up. Radiology 1996; 200(2): 525–30.
25. Kaemmerlen P, Thiesse P, Jonas P et al. Percutaneous injection of orthopedic cement in metastatic vertebral lesions. N Engl J Med 1989; 321: 121.
26. Chiras J, Deramond H. Complications des vertébroplasties. In Saillant G, Laville C (eds), Echecs et Complications de la Chirurgie du Rachis. Chirurgie de reprise. Sauramps Médical: Paris, 1995; 149–53.
27. Padovani B, Kasriel O, Brunner Ph. Pulmonary embolism caused by acrylic cement: a rare complication of percutaneous vertebroplasty. Am J Neuroradiol 1999; 20: 375–7.
28. San Millan Ruiz D, Burkhardt K, Jean B et al. Pathology findings with acrylic implants. Bone 1999; 25(2): 85–90S.
29. Weill A, Kobaiter H, Chiras J. Acetabulum malignancies: technique and impact on pain of percutaneous injection of acrylic surgical cement. Eur Radiol 1998; 8: 123–9.
30. Gangi A, Kastler BA, Klinkert A et al. Percutaneous injection of ethanol: a new method for pain therapy in bone metastasis. Radiology 1992; 185: 195.

19

Percutaneous Injection of Ethanol

A. Cotten[1] and L. Ceugnart[2]

[1]*Hôpital Roger Salengro, Lille, France*
[2]*Centre Oscar Lambret 3, Lille, France*

INTRODUCTION

Patients with osteolytic metastases and myeloma usually experience severe pain and disability. Surgery is usually not undertaken because of the multifocal nature of the disease. Percutaneous injection of ethanol is a palliative procedure that may be helpful in these patients, as it may provide early and frequently striking pain relief, especially when the initial pain is considerable. Indeed, ethanol is an efficient sclerosing agent that may cause tumour destruction and marked reduction of the vascularity in the tumour.

INDICATIONS

Ethanol injection is indicated in patients suffering from malignant osteolyses and who are unable to tolerate surgery. This palliative procedure may be performed prior to radiation therapy, which complements its action due to similar but delayed effects on pain, or after radiation therapy that has failed to relieve pain, or in cases of local recurrence. It has also been suggested that ethanol injection can have a value in treating bone metastases from thyroid carcinoma that do not respond to radioiodine [1].

As ethanol injection results in minimal and delayed (2–4 months) bone strengthening, pain relief is the sole object of the procedure. Consequently, ethanol injection is indicated when osteolysis does not involve the weight-bearing part of the bone, or when bone destruction is extensive. Owing to the mechanical properties of bone cement, which hardens as polymerisation occurs, injection of methyl methacrylate is preferred when osteolysis involves the weight-bearing part of the bone, but only when bone destruction is not too extensive and the cement may be expected to produce a mechanical effect. Ethanol and methyl methacrylate injections may be performed together if both weight-bearing and non-weight-bearing parts of a bone are involved or extensive soft tissue involvement is associated.

Ethanol injection may also result in reduction in tumour volume, especially when extensive soft tissue involvement is present and when repeat ethanol injections are peformed. Associated soft tissue involvement consequently also represents an excellent indication for ethanol injection.

TECHNIQUE

Radiography and CT scan must be performed prior to the procedure to assess the location and extent of the lytic process, the presence of cortical destruction or fracture, and the presence of soft tissue involvement. This procedure is performed under strict sterile conditions in patients under diazananalgesia, neuroleptanalgesia or general anaesthesia, as excruciating pain may be experienced during ethanol injection.

CT guidance is usually performed for both needle positioning and the injection itself, because this modality allows precise assessment of the bone and soft tissue involvement (Figure 19.1), but fluoroscopic guidance can be used in the appendicular skeleton, especially for the femur (Figure 19.2) [2,3]. Ultrasound

Textbook of Bone Metastases. Edited by C. Jasmin, R. E. Coleman, L. R. Coia, R. Capanna and G. Saillant
© 2005 John Wiley & Sons Ltd: ISBN 0 471 87742 5

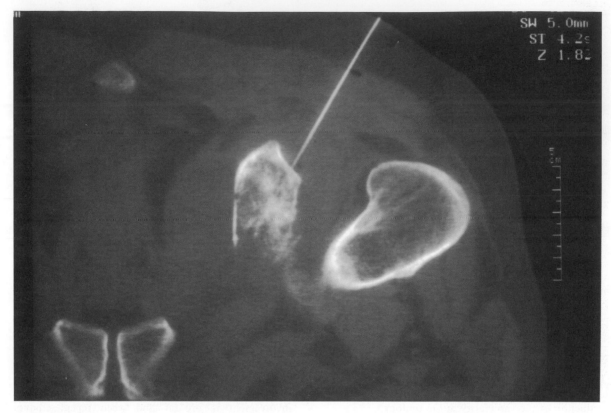

Figure 19.1.   Ethanol injection in a metastasis of the ischium after radiation therapy that had failed to relieve pain

guidance has also been reported for skull and sternum metastases [1,4]. This percutaneous procedure is easy to perform. A thin (20–22 gauge) needle is inserted into the lesion, and a mixture of lidocaine (1%) and contrast material is injected first, to assess the expected distribution of ethanol and decrease the pain produced by the ethanol injection. If leakage of contrast media is detected, especially into the joint space, the needle is repositioned and a second test injection is performed. If no contrast material is visualised, the needle has been positioned intravascularly and needs to be repositioned.

Next, a solution of 95% ethanol is injected slowly. Injection volume depends on lesion size and diffusion of the contrast material. A volume of 1–4 ml is usually sufficient for osteolytic lesions, but in patients with extensive soft tissue involvement, the volume can reach 20–30 ml. One or more injections may be performed at different sites on the same day, especially in bulky lesions. In such cases, repeat injections performed over the ensuing weeks may improve pain relief and decrease tumour size.

CONTRAINDICATIONS

There are no contraindications for percutaneous ethanol injection. Fracture or destruction of the articular cortex must prompt the use of extreme caution during the procedure to prevent leakage into the joint space. The thin needle used for the injection allows injections to be performed, albeit cautiously, in patients with coagulation disorders.

SIDE-EFFECTS AND COMPLICATIONS

A transitory worsening in pain may occur secondary to inflammatory reaction in the hours following injection [2,4,5]. This pain resolves spontaneously within days following the procedure. To minimise this side-effect, non-steroidal antiinflammatory drugs may be administered during this time. Few complications of this procedure have been described in the literature. Skin necrosis requiring reconstruction has been reported, as

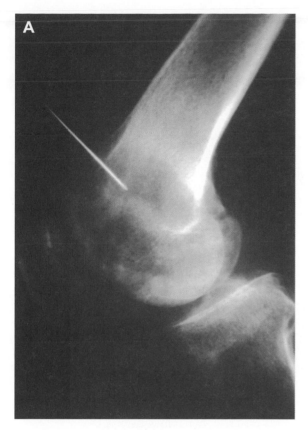
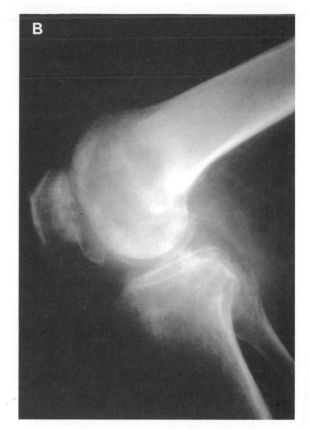

Figure 19.2. (A) Ethanol injection into a femoral metastasis. Due to the extent of the osteolysis, a mechanical effect of a cement injection could not be expected in this patient and the sole object of the procedure was pain relief. (B) Control radiograph 4 months later

well as gastrointestinal bleeding within 2 days of the ethanol injection [5]. Potential complications include vascular injury, nervous injury, infection and leaks of ethanol. Intraarticular leaks may produce potential chondrolysis, and intramuscular leaks may produce necrosis. Neuropathic pain may also occur secondary to a leak of ethanol adjacent to a nerve.

CLINICAL EFFECT

The principal effect of percutaneous injection of ethanol is early (within 6–48 h) and frequently striking pain relief, especially when the initial pain is considerable. This pain relief is probably attributable to tumour necrosis and destruction of sensitive nerve endings in the surrounding tissue. Owing to the rapid onset of clinical improvement, hospitalisation time is short, which is important in patients with a short life expectancy. Repeat ethanol injections may be

performed, increasing pain relief and in some cases reducing tumour volume, especially in extensive lesions [1–3].

OUR EXPERIENCE

Ethanol injection was performed in 39 patients (39 lesions), including 23 men and 16 women aged 45–78 years (mean, 55 years). The cause of the lesions was metastasis in 36 patients [lung ($n=14$), breast ($n=9$), colon ($n=4$), larynx ($n=2$), thyroid ($n=1$), pancreas ($n=1$), bladder ($n=1$), stomach ($n=1$), melanoma ($n=1$), unknown ($n=2$)] and myeloma in three patients. The bone involved by the osteolytic lesion was the pelvis ($n=30$), the posterior arch of a vertebra ($n=5$), the vertebral body ($n=2$) or the femur ($n=2$). Eleven patients had previous radiation therapy that had failed to relieve pain ($n=5$) or who had local recurrence (four patients). Marked or moderate pain relief was obtained in 40% and 30%, respectively, of the patients (80% of pain relief in patients with previous radiation therapy) within 6–48 hours. A second ethanol injection was performed in 22 patients with absent or moderate pain relief after the first injection. Marked or a moderate pain relief was obtained in 10% and 40% of these patients, respectively. A second ethanol injection was also performed in three patients with initial marked pain relief that progressively decreased. Marked and moderate pain relief was obtained in two and one patients, respectively. The mid-term follow-up was quite difficult to assess in our patients because of the associated radiation therapy in 75% of them and the similar effects of the latter on pain. In our patients with previous radiation therapy, pain relief could persist for at least 6 months.

Ethanol and methyl methacrylate injections were performed together in four patients with metastases with successful pain relief. No complication was observed in these patients.

CONCLUSION

Percutaneous injection of ethanol is a palliative procedure that may be helpful in the treatment of bone metastases and myeloma, as this procedure may provide early and frequently striking pain relief, tumour necrosis and, in some cases, reduction in size of the lesion. This procedure is easy to perform and can be safe if the test with contrast media and a slow injection of ethanol are performed with caution.

REFERENCES

1. Nakada K, Kasai K, Watanabe Y et al. Treatment of radioiodine-negative bone metastasis from papillary thyroid carcinoma with percutaneous ethanol injection therapy. Ann Nucl Med 1996; 10: 441–4.
2. Cotten A, Demondion X, Boutry N et al. Therapeutic percutaneous injections in the treatment of malignant acetabular osteolyses. RadioGraphics 1999; 19: 647–53.
3. Gangi A, Dietemann J-L, Schultz A et al. Interventional radiologic procedures with CT guidance in pain management. RadioGraphics 1996; 16: 1289–304.
4. Isaka T, Yoshimine T, Fujimoto K et al. Direct ethanol injection for skull metastasis from hepatocellular carcinoma. The techniques and consequences of a therapeutic trial. Neurol Res 1998; 20: 737–41.
5. Uflacker R, Paolini RM, Nobrega M. Ablation of tumor and inflammatory tissue with absolute ethanol. Acta Radiol Diagn (Stockh) 1986; 27: 131–8.

5

Systemic Treatments

Editor: Claude Jasmin

20

Chemotherapy

Marjorie C. Green and Gabriel N. Hortobagyi

The University of Texas M. D. Anderson Cancer Center, Houston, TX, USA

INTRODUCTION

Despite multiple advances in the surgical and medical management of cancer, many patients will develop distant and ultimately fatal metastases. Over 1 million new cases of invasive cancer were estimated to be diagnosed in the USA during the year 2004 [1]. During this same period of time it was predicted that 563 700 people would die from their cancer and that a significant proportion of patients would have bone metastases at the time of their death. Cancers that commonly metastasise or involve the bone include breast and prostate cancer as well as multiple myeloma. The development of bony disease from these cancers is a significant cause of morbidity. Pain, pathological fracture, nerve and spinal cord compression, as well as hypercalcaemia, all are possible consequences from bone metastases that adversely affect many patients' quality of life.

For the majority of patients, metastatic cancer is incurable. Some patients with metastatic cancer to the bone have a limited survival. For example, the median survival for patients with metastatic non-small-cell lung cancer who receive the best therapy available today is less than 1 year. However, patients with breast cancer or prostate cancer metastatic to bone can live much longer. Metastatic breast cancer involves bone for 50–70% of women with advanced disease and is confined to bone in approximately 25% of patients [2]. For patients with bone-only metastases, median survival is 36 months, with approximately 20% of patients remaining alive at 5 years [3].

Patients with metastatic prostate cancer have an even higher incidence of bony metastases; 80–100% of patients with metastatic prostate cancer have bony involvement and the majority of patients have bone-only disease [4]. The median survival for patients with bony metastases from prostate cancer is 30–35 months. Given the long period of time that many cancer patients live with their metastatic disease, the likelihood of adverse sequelae from bone metastases increases. Systemic treatment with chemotherapy can prolong survival for most cancers and palliate symptoms resulting from metastases throughout the body, including the bone.

EVALUATION OF METASTASES: PRESENCE OF AND RESPONSE TO THERAPY

Metastases result from systemic spread of disease. It is reasonable, therefore, that systemic therapy would be a component of appropriate therapy for most tumours. Historically, however, it has been difficult to determine the response rate of bony metastases to systemic therapy based upon the varied staging methods used to evaluate response. Any method used to evaluate tumour metastatic to bone only indirectly assesses the extent of tumour involvement. Therefore, assessing response to therapy is problematic—all methods used to evaluate response are indirect measurements and do not reflect the actual change in tumour volume. The inability to measure tumour burden directly in bone produces a delay in observing or documenting a response in bone when compared to evaluation of soft tissue or visceral lesions (directly visible by examination or radiographs). This delay is often manifested as the common occurrence of stable disease in bone after treatment with chemotherapy, while other sites may reflect decreasing tumour volume

Textbook of Bone Metastases. Edited by C. Jasmin, R. E. Coleman, L. R. Coia, R. Capanna and G. Saillant
© 2005 John Wiley & Sons Ltd: ISBN 0 471 87742 5

Adding to the difficulty in evaluating the response of bone metastases to therapy is the common practice of excluding bone metastases as measurable disease in clinical trial evaluation of new therapies. Earlier studies attempted to quantify changes in bone for evaluation of response. Given the technical limitations in assessing response to therapy, chemotherapy for metastatic disease to bone was often believed to be less effective than for disease located in other sites. In general, careful analysis has proved this to be untrue. For example, a retrospective study conducted at the M. D. Anderson Cancer Center evaluated the response of systemic (non-osseous) vs. osseous breast cancer metastases to systemic therapy with fluorouracil + doxorubicin + cyclophosphamide (FAC), utilising previously determined criteria for response in bone [5]. The overall response rate seen in non-osseous sites was 76%, with a 91% concordance between bone radiograph response and other systemic sites of disease. The investigators found, however, that changes seen on bone scan with therapy corresponded with non-osseous changes in only 57% of cases. The variability in responses seen by different radiographic techniques illustrates the difficulty in determining response to therapy. Based upon the evaluation chosen, an effective therapy can mistakenly be seen as inferior.

Radiographs

Multiple radiographic studies are used to assess both the extent of tumour-associated changes in bone and response to therapy. The tests used to detect the presence of a tumour are not always the same as those used to evaluate response to therapy. As described below, each test has advantages and disadvantages in its ability to detect the presence of disease and response to therapy. The judicious use of radiographs based upon the expected changes seen with therapy is essential to clarify and not confuse treatment-associated changes, so that appropriate treatment decisions may be made.

Bone Scan

Bone scans are valuable in defining the location and extent of osseous metastases for most tumours. For this study, labelled diphosphonates are injected intravenously and are then disseminated through the circulation to the bone and other sites. In areas of increased osteoblastic activity, the diphosphonates are chemoadsorbed onto the calcium of hydroxyapatite in bone. Osteoblastic activity reflects active bone healing, and its bone scan appearance is similar after a fracture, resolving infection or healing after any other type of insult. In the case of cancer, uptake is dependent upon the osteoblastic activity and skeletal vascularity associated with bone metastases. Tumours resulting in purely lytic disease (multiple myeloma) are poorly visualised by bone scans, due to the lack of osteoblastic activity. Many solid tumours that are associated with lytic activity often have a component of increased osteoblastic activity in most metastatic lesions, allowing visualisation with bone scans [6]. Bone scans are highly sensitive for alterations of bone architecture. Because of this, other "benign" processes can cause abnormal bone scans. The use of single-photon emission computed tomography (SPECT) scans increases the specificity of bone scans for the detection of metastases. These scans are still highly sensitive for bone abnormality and also warrant further evaluation with other radiographic tests. As a general rule, abnormal bone scans should be used in conjunction with other radiographic studies for evaluation of the presence of bony metastases.

While providing a sensitive baseline evaluation for the detection of bony metastases, variable changes on bone scan can be seen with effective therapy of cancer. Breast, lung and prostate cancer have been associated with temporary increase of bone scan activity after initiation of systemic therapy. These changes of new bone formation, or "flare", include increased intensity of previously visualised lesions or the appearance of lesions not previously seen on bone scan [6–8]. The bone scan flare can be associated with a temporary increase in pain; however, this is not universally true. Clinically silent changes of bone scans should therefore be examined with suspicion during the first 3–6 months after initiating therapy, so that an effective treatment is not prematurely discontinued. Bone scans may normalise with healing of bony lesions. However, as a single test, the bone scan is not specific for evaluation of response to therapy.

Bone Radiographs

Bone scans have superb ability to detect early abnormalities in bone. Radiographs are less sensitive. Approximately 50% of cortical bone must be destroyed before clinically evident lesions are detected by radiographs [9]. Different cancers result in variable patterns seen on radiographs, due to each tumour's ability to stimulate bone to increase osteoclast (lytic changes) and/or osteoblast (sclerotic changes) activity.

Pure lytic disease ⟶ Rim of sclerosis ⟶ Increasing calcification ⟶ Pure blastic lesion ⟶ Fading of lesion

Figure 20.1.   Progression of radiographic changes seen with healing of metastases

For example, breast cancer may appear as lytic lesions, blastic lesions or mixed (both lytic and blastic), while prostate cancer results in primarily blastic lesions. Whatever the initial appearance of bone metastastis by radiograph, tumours have a specific pattern of healing which can be systematically followed while patients are receiving therapy (Figure 20.1). Patients who present with purely blastic metastases follow the same pattern of response seen with lytic/mixed osseous lesions: gradual fading and resolution of radiographic change. The evaluation of response for patients with pure blastic disease is more difficult, given the length of time remodelling of bone takes. When possible, other studies are used in conjunction with plain radiographs for patients with blastic disease. Overall, however, plain radiographs are easily obtained and these tests are commonly used for both the initial evaluation of the presence of metastases and for evaluation of response to therapy.

Both the International Union Against Cancer (IUCC) and the World Health Organisation (WHO) classify progressive disease of breast cancer partly based upon the appearance of new lesions [10]. Progression of disease is similarly defined for other cancers, including prostate cancer and myeloma. Visible new lesions do not always signify progressive disease, however. Researchers have found that, when used as the sole determinant of response, radiographs identified 33% of lesions seen as progressive disease, when the same lesions viewed in the context of earlier bone scans were actually previously visible on the nuclear medicine test [11]. The lesions had developed increased sclerosis/healing and had therefore become visible. Radiographs are easily obtained, provide insight into overall bone architecture and are relatively inexpensive. Technical aspects of bone radiographs, including film exposure and overlying tissue/bowel gas, can hinder the specificity of studies. As with bone scans, they should be used in context with other tests as well as the clinical picture in judgement of response to therapy.

Computed Tomography (CT) and Magnetic Resonance Imaging (MRI)

Bone scans and radiographs are the most common methods of evaluating bony metastases. However, as seen, there are difficulties in evaluating disease presence and/or response of bone metastases in some circumstances. CT and MRI can be useful in identifying the presence of metastatic disease. CT evaluates cortex and marrow changes from metastases, as well as evaluating areas such as the sacrum, sternum and scapulae with greater detail than can be provided from plain radiographs. CT used with clinical information often allows discrimination between malignant and benign processes [12,13]. MRI evaluates changes in marrow intensity, allowing differentiation between benign and malignant processes as well as identifying lesions not seen on bone scan. One study found that vertebral metastases were more accurately diagnosed by MRI than by bone scan [14]. It is possible that MRI may detect marrow replacement prior to the induction of osteoblastic response. Since this increased osteoblastic activity is required for an abnormal bone scan, the MRI might lead to earlier detection of bone metastases. The expense and time required to perform the study have limited the widespread use of MRI for the detection of metastatic disease and, as with CT scans, MRI complements other studies.

CT and MRI also can be used to assist in the assessment of response to therapy. Quantitative CT scan can evaluate the recalcification of osteolytic metastases during therapy earlier than visualised by conventional radiographs [15]. One study found that the response to therapy was seen up to 8 weeks earlier on quantitative CT when compared to conventional radiographs [16]. Earlier detection could possibly allow a patient with a questioned response to therapy to remain on an active treatment. Likewise, MRI can evaluate response to therapy by evaluating changes in tumour volume or by changes in size and number [17]. Documentation of earlier response to therapy has not been found to prolong survival. However, as with CT, MRI could possibly protect patients from premature discontinuation of therapy that is effective. In general, these tests are more commonly used in the evaluation of the presence of metastases, particularly to complement other studies where the results are questioned. If a tumour is visualised by other methods, then these tests are not routinely used for evaluation of response to therapy.

Tumour Markers

Given the difficulty in assessing the response of bone metastases with radiological studies, investigators have studied multiple serological markers of bone metabolism and tumour cells to assist in determination of changes with therapy. When used in conjunction with radiographs and clinical picture, these tests can assist in the determination of response to chemotherapy. Haematological malignancies, such as multiple myeloma, have several well-established serological tests that can guide therapeutic decision (serum and urine protein electrophoresis, β2-microglobulin, lactate dehydrogenase). The use of tests for evaluation of the progression of solid tumours has only recently become widespread. While still considered experimental in most settings, there are several well-described markers of tumours and bone metabolism, which can assist in the management of patients with metastatic disease.

Prostate-specific Antigen (PSA)

One of the best-studied tumour-associated proteins studied in solid tumors, PSA is a glycoprotein that is found primarily in neoplastic and normal prostate tissue. As it is specific for prostate tissue and not necessarily prostate cancer, PSA may be elevated from non-malignant causes. PSA is, however, elevated in the majority of patients with metastatic prostate cancer. Considering that prostate cancer induces an osteoblastic reaction when metastatic to the bone, response to therapy is often difficult to quantify by radiographs alone. PSA levels are dependent upon the volume of tumour as well as the degree of tumour differentiation [18]. PSA has been studied extensively as a surrogate endpoint for evaluation of tumour response in the treatment of prostate cancer; decline of PSA (50% or greater) correlates with prolonged survival in several studies [19,20]. While encouraging, prolongation of survival with decreasing PSA has not been shown to be universally true [21]. In addition, benefit from therapy has been observed from treatment of prostate cancer without correlation between PSA decline and survival [22].

To complicate the use of PSA measurements in the evaluation of response to therapy, alterations in PSA have occurred with therapies that do not correspond with clinical findings. For example, in a model of prostate cancer evaluating suramin, researchers found that PSA decreased even though the volume of disease continued to increase [23]. Despite these possible confounding factors, response guidelines have been proposed for evaluating tumour response in clinical trials based upon PSA changes [24] (Table 20.1). The authors of these proposed guidelines stress that PSA

Table 20.1. Evaluation of PSA response to therapy

PSA normalisation	PSA < 0.2 ng/ml
PSA response	Serial decline of PSA confirmed by second PSA, 4 or more weeks after initial decline
PSA response duration	Time from first 50% decrease response in PSA to 50% increase from nadir
PSA progression	PSA increase 25% over baseline or progressive increase in absolute value of PSA by at least 5 ng/ml

PSA response is based upon serial measurements from established baseline. PSA response is used in context with other measurements and clinical picture. Based on [24].

evaluation is complementary to other studies and should be evaluated in the context of clinical and radiographic evaluation of disease.

CA 15-3 and CA 27-29

As with prostate cancer, researchers have searched for tumour-associated markers to aid in the detection and therapy of breast cancer. Recently two tumour-associated markers have become increasingly used in clinical investigation: CA 15-3 and CA 27-29. These tests are actually immunoassays using different monoclonal antibodies to detect epitopes of the mucin glycoprotein product of the MUC1 gene [25]. The product of the MUC1 gene is a membrane-associated mucin that exists in two forms. This mucin glycoprotein is not specific for breast cancer and has been associated with other malignancies. An underglycosylated form is associated with adenocarcinoma of the breast and is shed into the circulation. This protein is the target for the CA 15-3 and CA 27-29 immunoassays [26]. Both markers have been shown to be more sensitive for the determination of metastases from breast cancer when compared with carcinoembryonic antigen (CEA) (overall positivity in patients with metastatic breast cancer: CA 15-3, 79%; CA 27-29, 70%; CEA, 35%). These markers are most sensitive for the detection of liver and bone metastases. When compared to CEA, both markers also display improved sensitivity in reflecting response to therapy (CEA, 40%; CA 27-29 and CA 15-3, 81%) [27].

All patients with metastatic breast cancer do not uniformly express these tumour-associated markers. However, there are suggestions that CA 27-29 is elevated in more patients than CA 15-3. Both markers have been evaluated as surrogate markers of disease response. To illustrate, a 20% change of CA 27-29 has a published sensitivity of 75% and specificity of 77% in detecting a change in disease status. CA 27-29 has been approved by the United States Food and Drug Administration (US FDA) for monitoring disease in patients with metastatic breast cancer [26]. For patients whose tumours produce detectable mucin, these markers can assist in the evaluation of response to therapy.

Markers of Bone Metabolism

Multiple serologic tests have been developed to assess changes in bone metabolism. These markers can be utilised in the evaluation of response to cytotoxic therapy and the management of bone metastases. Normal bone continuously undergoes remodelling, with bone formation (by osteoblasts) and resorption (by osteoclasts). This process is tightly controlled throughout most of life. Synthesis of cytokines allows metastatic cancer cells to alter this process via indirect effects on osteoblasts/osteoclasts. With alteration of the normal bone microenvironment, biochemical markers of bone formation and/or breakdown can be elevated compared to normal values. With therapy, it is possible that the levels of these markers can normalise, thereby augmenting the evaluation of response to treatment. An advantage of these biomarkers is that changes can occur within a few weeks after the initiation of therapy, while radiographs often require longer periods of time to assess changes in bone mass. Specific markers of bone metabolism are extensively reviewed elsewhere in this book (see Section 2). Several studies specifically evaluate changes of markers with therapy and will be presented here.

Markers of Bone Resorption

The majority of published studies assessing response of bone-related markers to therapy evaluate markers of bone resorption. Several tested markers are non-reducible cross-links of mature Type I and II collagen, including pyridinoline (Pyr) and deoxypyridinoline (D-Pyr). These markers can be measured either directly in urine/serum or indirectly via antibodies directed against peptides in the cross-links (N-telopeptide and C-telopeptide) [28]. One study evaluating the possible use of bone resorption markers as an alternative to serial plain radiographs for the assessment of response to therapy with pamidronate found that N-telopeptide, hydroxyproline and urinary calcium levels did not alter significantly in patients with

no change or partial response to therapy [29]. Rise in N-telopeptide was predictive of disease progression, however.

Another study confirmed the ability of Pyr and D-Pyr to predict progression of disease a median of 2 months ahead of changes visible by radiographs. However, for these women with breast cancer being treated with hormonal therapy, neither marker of bone resorption was able to predict response to therapy [30].

While the previous two studies confirmed the concordance of increasing markers of bone resorption with progression of disease, they did not confirm the ability of these markers to predict response to therapy. One study evaluating pamidronate found that normalisation of N-telopeptide levels was associated with a significant decrease in fractures and progression of disease when compared with patients whose N-telopeptide levels did not normalise [31]. While not specific for predicting response to therapy, this study demonstrates that decreases in markers of bone resorption are predictive of benefit for patients receiving therapy. Additional studies are ongoing to evaluate the role of these markers in assessing treatment response, specifically in the context of cytotoxic therapies.

CHEMOTHERAPY FOR BONE METASTASES

Treatment of bone metastases should be based upon a multidisciplinary approach to patient care. Consultation from radiation oncologists and orthopaedic surgeons can assist the medical oncologist in determining the best appropriate local therapy for bone metastases, as well as the thoughtful combination of, or sequential use of, therapies (chemotherapy, hormonal therapy, bone-seeking radionuclides, orthopaedic surgery, physical therapy, analgesics). Unless bone metastases are a direct threat to mechanical structure or nerve function, a systemic approach to therapy is reasonable and can often prolong survival.

Breast Cancer

Over 217 000 cases of invasive breast cancer were predicted to be diagnosed in the USA during the year 2004 [1]. Advances in the adjuvant therapy of breast cancer have prolonged survival for a significant proportion of women. Unfortunately, approximately one-third of these patients will present with, or eventually develop, fatal metastases from their breast cancer. Bone is the most common first site of metastasis for the majority of patients and systemic therapy should be designed as therapy of all sites of disease. The biological course of breast cancer is variable. Patients with bone-only metastases from breast cancer live longer than women with extensive involvement of visceral organs. Choice of initial therapy for metastatic disease should be guided by several factors, including location of disease and hormone receptor status of the tumour. Patients with life-threatening visceral metastases should receive cytotoxic chemotherapy to obtain rapid tumour cyto-reduction. Patients with bone-only metastases or low-volume systemic disease should be evaluated for hormonal therapy as initial treatment if they have hormone-responsive tumours (oestrogen receptor-positive). For patients with hormone-insensitive tumours, or whose tumors become resistant to hormonal therapy, systemic cytotoxic chemotherapy is indicated.

Bony metastases respond well to systemic chemo-therapy for metastastic breast cancer; however, this therapy in general is not curative. Nevertheless, a small percentage of patients may obtain long-term remission of their cancer with chemotherapy. One study found that 17% of patients who obtained a complete remission (3.1% of all patients) remained in complete remission at 5 years. This included patients with osseous metastases [32]. In addition to significantly prolonging survival, cytotoxic therapy has been shown to improve quality of life for patients with metastatic breast cancer. Improvement of quality of life is directly related to the ability of a therapy to induce a response [33]. The choice of initial chemotherapeutic regimen should be based upon similar criteria that would guide choice of therapy for other sites of disease. Multiple agents have *in vivo* activity against breast cancer (Table 20.2).

Single-agent anthracyclines, such as doxorubicin, achieve response rates of 40–65% in areas of measur-able disease. Meta-analyses have shown that the combination of chemotherapeutics is superior to single agents and that anthracycline-containing regi-mens are superior to non-anthracycline-containing regimens in the adjuvant setting [34]. In the metastatic setting, anthracycline-containing regimens have also been shown to be superior to non-anthracycline-containing regimens. Fossati *et al.* [35] found, in meta-analysis, that polychemotherapies containing doxorubicin were associated with improved response and a trend towards improved survival when compared with other polychemotherapy regimens. Another analysis published in 1993 [36] compared anthracycline-containing regimens,

Table 20.2. Commonly used chemotherapeutics in the treatment of breast cancer

Doxorubicin
Epirubicin
Cyclophosphamide
5-Fluorouracil
Paclitaxel
Docetaxel
Methotrexate
Capecitabine
Gemcitabine
Vinorelbine

primarily cyclophosphamide + adriamycin + 5-fluoro-uracil (CAF) with cyclophosphamide + methotrexate + 5-fluorouracil (CMF) or its variants. As in other meta-analyses, benefit in response rates, failure-free survival and, in this review, overall survival were seen for patients receiving doxorubicin-based therapy. Com-monly used anthracycline-containing regimens include FAC, CAF, fluorouracil–epirubicin–cyclophospha-mide (FEC) and doxorubicin-cyclophosphamide (AC).

Very few studies evaluate anthracycline-containing therapy for bone-only metastases, making assessments regarding generalisation of response rates and overall survival for patients with bone-only disease difficult. Early studies of FAC, AC and CAF provide conflict-ing evidence regarding the response rate of bony metastases. Some studies reported response rates of osseous metastases in the range 0–43%—all signifi-cantly less than response rates seen for other disease sites [37–39]. These studies called for objective response on bone radiographs for evaluation of response data and these rates are artificially low due to the poor ability to measure bony disease. Other studies, however, have shown the efficacy of anthracy-cline-containing regimens to be similar for bony disease as for non-osseous sites of metastases (Table 20.3). One study conducted at the M. D. Anderson Cancer Center specifically examined the response rate of therapy with FAC for patients with bone-only metastases. Researchers found that the overall response rate was 59%, with 7% of patients obtaining a complete remission [3]. Despite concerns that therapy of bony metastases from breast cancer with che-motherapy results in inferior response rates, in general the responses in osseous vs. non-osseous sites appear equivalent. Given that most clinical trials evaluate very few patients with bone-only metastases, survival for this select group is often difficult to determine.

The taxanes paclitaxel and docetaxel have significant activity against breast cancer. These agents are used as

Table 20.3. Concordant osseous response to anthracycline-containing regimens—breast cancer

Regimen	Overall systemic response rate (CR + PR) (%)	Overall osseous response rate (CR + PR) (%)	Reference
AC	50	44	[39]
CAF	85	86	[38]
FAC	76	69	[5]
AC	80	84	[73]

second-line treatment after progression of disease with an anthracycline-containing regimen or first-line treatment for patients previously treated with anthracyclines in the adjuvant setting. Paclitaxel and docetaxel promote formation of unusually stable microtubules, inhibiting the normal dynamic reorganisation of the microtubular nework required for mitosis and cell proliferation. These agents have undergone extensive evaluation as treatment of metastatic disease during the past 10 years.

The activity of paclitaxel against bone metastases is difficult to elucidate from published clinical trials. The majority of Phase II and III studies evaluating this agent allowed patients with osseous metastases; however, patients were usually required to have measurable disease. When included in assessment of response, bone metastases had, in general, similar response rates when compared to other sites of disease (Table 20.4). To illustrate, a Phase II trial conducted by the National Cancer Institute evaluated the efficacy of paclitaxel (175 mg/m^2 over 24 h, administered every 21 days) against heavily pretreated breast cancer.

Response rates for bone and measurable disease were similar (20% vs. 23%) [40]. While not all studies demonstrate equivalent efficacy of chemotherapy against osseous metastases when compared to the results obtained in visceral metastases, it is important to recognise that researchers commonly used the WHO classification of response. The WHO response criteria require recalcification and radiographic resolution of visible bone lesions for changes to be classified as a complete response. As these radiographic changes are an indirect reflection of changes in tumour bulk, it is reasonable that the time delay necessary for the physiological response of healing could be translated into a decreased observed response rate. Because of this, decreased response rates found against bony metastases should be viewed with scepticism. As with studies evaluating anthracycline-containing regimens, little specific information regarding survival for patients with bone-only metastases can be obtained from these studies.

Docetaxel likewise has significant activity against breast cancer when used in the metastatic setting. The current widely utilised application for docetaxel is as therapy of anthracycline-resistant metastatic breast cancer. This indication stems from several Phase II and III studies evaluating docetaxel in this setting. When used as treatment of anthracycline-resistant breast cancer, docetaxel gives response rates of 30–43% [41]. When compared with single-agent doxorubicin, docetaxel gave a significantly higher response rate (48% vs. 33%; $p = 0.008$) without a significant improvement in overall survival. From Phase II and III studies, response rates seen in osseous metastases are similar to those seen in other sites. There is no indication that

Table 20.4. Efficacy of paclitaxel and paclitaxel combinations against osseous metastases—breast cancer

Regimen	Percentage of patients with dominant osseous metastases (%)	Overall response (%)	Osseous response (%)	Reference
Paclitaxel, 250 mg/m^2 or 200 mg/m^2 (based upon prior therapy) as 24 h continuous infusion q 3 weeks	32	32.8	24	[60]
Paclitaxel, 175 mg/m^2 as 24 h continuous infusion q 3 weeks		23	20	[40]
Paclitaxel, 200 mg/m^2 as 3 h infusion q 3 weeks	16	25	14	[74]
Paclitaxel, 210 mg/m^2 as 3 h infusion q 3 weeks	11	35.6	0	[75]
Paclitaxel, 85 mg/m^2 with cisplatin 40 mg/m^2 (weekly dose)	30	81	62.5—patients with bone-only disease	[76]

patients with osseous metastases performed worse compared to patients with non-osseous disease. For example, one study evaluating the use of docetaxel as front-line therapy against metastatic breast cancer (75 mg/m^2 q 3 weeks) found that of the 55% of patients who obtained an objective response, the most frequent site of tumour response seen was in bone [42]. Another study evaluating docetaxel confirms equivalent efficacy against osseous metastases compared with other sites (response rates: overall, 68.9%; osseous metastases, 56%) [43]. As with other chemotherapeutic agents, some studies have suggested relative chemoresistance of osseous metastases. One study investigating docetaxel illustrates the difficulty in evaluating response to therapy. This Phase II study evaluated two doses of docetaxel as therapy of advanced or recurrent breast cancer. The overall response rate seen was 44.4%. However, of the patients who had evaluable response in bone, the onset of visible response was delayed when compared to response in visceral or other sites (bone, after the third cycle; liver/lungs, after the second cycle). The duration of response was similar for the osseous metastases when compared with other sites [44].

The antitumour activity of docetaxel and paclitaxel is dependent upon the phase of cellular growth that an individual tumour cell is in. Both agents continue to undergo evaluation in different schedules in efforts to increase efficacy and decrease toxicity as well as to help define the optimal dose/schedule in the metastatic setting.

Recently combinations of anthracyclines and taxanes have been investigated as treatment of metastatic breast cancer. Taxanes and anthracyclines are the most effective agents used against breast cancer. The combination of these non-cross-resistant cytotoxic therapies does result in superior response rates. As with other studies evaluating therapy of metastatic breast cancer, a significant proportion of patients had bone metastases (38–60%), although the changes in bone were not measurable/reported. Unfortunately, the taxane/doxorubicin regimens are associated with a high incidence of neutropenia (75–100%) and febrile neutropenia (11–38%) [45]. While these combinations are attractive options for patients requiring rapid response to therapy (significant visceral disease), the role for patients with bone-only metastases is less well defined. The activity of these combinations should result in significant reduction of osseous metastatic burden; however, until studies confirm survival benefit for these regimens, there is no compelling evidence to use taxane/doxorubicin combinations as initial therapy of bone metastases.

Trastuzumab (herceptin) is not a classic cytotoxic agent but rather a humanised monoclonal antibody directed against the gene product of HER-2/*neu*. For patients whose tumours overexpress the gene product of HER-2/*neu*, trastuzumab has proved to be an effective therapy, both as a single agent and in combination with chemotherapeutic agents. Studies examining the efficacy of trastuzumab in the metastatic setting do not, in general, evaluate the effect of this therapy on bone metastases. As a single agent, trastuzumab has a reported response rate of 15% (measurable disease) [46].

The combination of trastuzumab and chemotherapy has proved to be of even greater benefit. In 1998, results of a clinical trial evaluating the benefit of trastuzumab administered in combination with chemotherapy vs. chemotherapy alone was presented at the American Society of Clinical Oncology annual meeting. Four hundred and sixty-nine patients with overexpression of HER-2 were given chemotherapy based on previous treatment exposure. The combination of chemotherapy and trastuzumab was shown to be superior to chemotherapy alone in terms of time to progression and response rate [47]. Updated information (with a median follow-up of 25 months) revealed that patients receiving the combination of chemotherapy and herceptin had a superior overall survival (25.4 months) when compared to patients receiving chemotherapy alone (20.9 months) [48]. The efficacy of trastuzumab against bony metastases from breast cancer is uncertain. Given the improved responses seen in measurable disease, it is reasonable to expect similar results from osseous disease.

Many other cytotoxic agents have activity against breast cancer and have potential roles as therapy of osseous metastases. Capecitabine is an orally active prodrug of 5-fluorouracil. This drug has preferential metabolism in neoplastic tissue, allowing higher intralesional concentrations of 5-fluorouracil than can be systemically administered. Capecitabine is indicated as third-line therapy for patients with metastatic breast cancer who have failed anthracyclines and taxanes. When tested in this population, the reported overall response rate is 20%. A similar response occurs in patients with non-measurable disease. Median survival for these patients was reported to be greater than 1 year, a significant period of time for the patient population studied. In addition to the response rate of 20%, an additional 40% of patients had stable disease—survival for this group was similar for those who obtained objective response to therapy [49]. This treatment is generally well tolerated and has the advantage of an oral formulation, allowing administration at home.

As patients with primary osseous metastases may have a relatively indolent course of disease progression, the opportunity for fourth-line or fifth-line therapy exists. Gemcitabine and vinorelbine both have activity against breast cancer and may be used as treatment after progression of disease. As with many of the recent studies evaluating cytotoxic therapy of breast cancer, most studies evaluating vinorelbine and gemcitabine report activity in terms of measurable disease and do not address the specific response of bone metastases. Vinorelbine is a semi-synthetic vinca alkaloid that has proven activity against breast cancer. As first-line therapy, vinorelbine has response rates in the range 38–50%. While active, the antitumour activity as first-line treatment is not comparable to anthracycline-containing regimens. In addition, when administered as a weekly regimen, vinorelbine is associated with dose-limiting granulocytopenia, which limits goal dose density delivery [50]. Vinorelbine has reported activity up to 25% as treatment of breast cancer in patients who have progressed after anthracyclines and taxanes [51]. As with other agents, vinorelbine has similar efficacy against osseous metastases when compared with other sites of disease (Table 20.5). Survival benefits have not been as dramatic as those seen with capecitabine and vinorelbine is reserved for patients with good performance status who have progressed through multiple chemotherapeutic regimens.

Gemcitabine is a nucleoside analogue with unique pharmacokinetics that allow higher concentrations and prolonged duration of exposure in tumour cells when compared with other nucleoside analogues. In a Phase II trial evaluating the efficacy of gemcitabine against breast cancer in patients who have received one or no prior chemotherapy regimens, gemcitabine produced an overall response rate of 25%, with an overall survival of 11.5 months [52]. For patients who responded to therapy, survival was 18.6 months. This medication is well tolerated with little associated infection or alopecia. This agent, as well as vinorelbine,

is appropriate palliative therapy for patients with good performance status who have failed other regimens.

Prostate Cancer

Prostate cancer affects millions of men worldwide and was expected to be the most common diagnosis of cancer in men (USA) during the year 2004. Over 230 000 men were expected to be diagnosed with prostate cancer and almost 30 000 were expected to die from this prevalent disease [1]. Similarly to breast cancer, prostate cancer commonly spreads to bone. Approximately 90–100% of patients with metastatic disease have osseous metastases. Unlike patients with breast cancer, however, only a small proportion of patients with prostate cancer have visceral disease (15–20%). The high incidence of bone-only disease creates difficulty in determining objective measurable response to therapy in clinical trials and clinical practice. In addition, patients with prostate cancer often have purely blastic metastases. Radiographic evaluation of response to therapy is difficult unless there is obvious progression of disease, with new lesions or clear fading of lesions over time. Often bone scans are used to augment the evaluation of response to therapy. Bone scans for these patients are problematic, due to the phenomenon of "flare" described above; however, in the appropriate clinical setting, obvious new lesions seen or the disappearance of lesions seen on bone scan can assist in the evaluation of response to therapy.

Due to difficulty found with radiographic evaluation for response of osseous metastases from prostate cancer, other surrogate markers of response are used as endpoints in clinical trials. PSA, quality of life assessments, survival, time to progression and radiographic response are commonly all chosen as evaluable endpoints for patients with prostate cancer [53].

Initial management of metastatic prostate cancer is treatment with hormonal ablation. Eventually most

Table 20.5. Efficacy of vinorelbine against osseous metastases—breast cancer

Regimen	Patients with dominant osseous metastases (%)	Overall response (%)	Osseous response (%)	Reference
Vinorelbine 30 mg/m², days 1 and 8	46	47	31	[77]
Vinorelbine, 30 mg/m²/week	31	46	0 (stable disease 44.5)	[78]
Vinorelbine, 30 mg/m²/week	67	41	30	[79]
Vinorelbine, 30 mg/m²/week	49	41	33	[80]

prostate cancers become hormone-refractory, i.e. the growth of cancer becomes independent of external hormonal influence. Once patients have progressed to this stage, their overall survival is usually limited, with a median survival of approximately 1 year. To improve survival and symptoms related to bone metastases, multiple chemotherapeutic agents are undergoing evaluation as treatment of metastatic prostate cancer.

Initial studies evaluating chemotherapy for prostate cancer were disappointing, with single-agent treatments having low response rates and no impact on survival. The development of different endpoints for clinical trials proved that several chemotherapy regimens have clinical benefit and, for some patients, improvement in survival. One of the first trials to show clinical benefit for patients with metastatic prostate cancer examined mitoxantrone with prednisone alone [22]. This Phase III trial evaluated the effect of chemotherapy in patients who had progressed after standard hormonal therapy but had not yet received other therapies. Patients were maintained on androgen ablation and randomised to receive mitoxantrone $12 \, mg/m^2$ every 21 days with daily prednisone (5 mg/day), or prednisone alone. Multiple endpoints were chosen for evaluation of response, including pain relief, analgesic requirement, duration of palliative response and survival. Palliative response was seen in 29% of patients receiving chemotherapy compared with 12% of patients receiving prednisone only ($p=0.01$). The duration of response was also longer for the chemotherapy arm (43 vs. 18 weeks; $p < 0.0001$). Overall, there was no survival advantage seen for the chemotherapy arm; however, 22% of patients assigned to prednisone alone also received mitoxantrone after progression of their disease. Mitoxantrone has been approved by the US FDA as treatment for palliation of symptoms in patients with hormone-refractory prostate cancer.

One agent that has had renewed interest in the past 10 years is estramustine, which is a conjugate of 17β-estradiol and the carbamate of nitrogen mustard. This agent blocks mitosis through interference with microtubule-associated proteins. These proteins are required for microtubule stabilisation after assembly. As a single agent against prostate cancer, estramustine obtains objective response rates of 20–30% [54,55]. The main toxicities associated with this medicine include gastrointestinal changes (nausea/vomiting/diarrhoea) as well as cardiac complications and risk of arterial/venous thrombosis. Estramustine's mechanism of action, combined with its ability to induce an objective response against prostate cancer, makes this agent a perfect candidate for combination therapy with other medications that affect microtubule assembly.

The taxanes (paclitaxel and docetaxel) have been investigated as monotherapy for the treatment of metastatic prostate cancer. Due to their mechanism of action, they have also been studied in combination with estramustine. Paclitaxel and docetaxel promote the formation of excessive abnormally functioning microtubules. Paclitaxel has other non-mitotic effects (antiangiogenesis, Bcl-2 phosphorylation), which also enhance its activity. As a single agent, paclitaxel achieves PSA responses (> 50% reduction in PSA) in 16–39% of patients without significant improvement in overall survival (9–13.5 months) [56,57]. In combination with estramustine, improved PSA response rates can be seen. In one study, the PSA response (> 50% reduction in PSA) for a 96-h infusion of paclitaxel was 53.1%. Survival for the group is estimated at 69 weeks—significantly longer than the historic survival for these patients [58]. The objective response rate for measurable disease was concordant with the PSA response: 44.4%. As predicted, the combination of the two antimicrotubule agents provides superior efficacy, as measured by survival and PSA response, than either agent alone.

Docetaxel possibly has greater *in vivo* activity against prostate cancer than either estramustine or paclitaxel. One study reported a PSA response with docetaxel of 46% and objective response rate (measurable disease) of 28% from treatment of patients with hormone-refractory prostate cancer [59]. The median overall survival seen in this study was 27 months—longer than most other single-agent trials in this patient population. Given the high response rate seen with single-agent docetaxel, investigators combined this taxane with estramustine in numerous Phase I/II trials. Preliminary reports from these studies suggest that the combination of docetaxel and estramustine provides superior response rates (Table 20.6). Data from these small Phase II trials are too preliminary to draw long-term conclusions regarding any survival advantage for these combinations, although results are encouraging. Estramustine does increase the toxicity of these regimens, with the serious potential for circulatory compromise from thrombosis. Larger Phase III trials will hopefully elucidate the best combination of these agents as treatment of metastatic prostate cancer.

Another chemotherapeutic with antimicrotubular activity is vinblastine. A Phase III study comparing vinblastine vs. the combination of vinblastine and estramustine found improved PSA response for the combination therapy (25.2% vs. 3.2%) [86]. Despite an improvement in time to progression seen with the

Table 20.6. Efficacy of docetaxel–estramustine combinations against prostate cancer: Phase I/II trials

Dose	PSA response (%)	Objective response (%)	Survival	Reference
Estramustine, 280 mg p.o. t.i.d. × 5 days Docetaxel, 40–80 mg/m^2 day 2: Phase I	63	28	Not reached	[81]
Estramustine, 280 mg p.o. t.i.d. × 5 days Docetaxel 70 mg/m^2 day 2: Phase II	74	57	77% 1-year	[82]
Estramustine, 10 mg/kg/day—divided into three doses p.o. t.i.d. × 5 days Docetaxel, 70 mg/m^2 day 2: Phase II	69	23	Not reached	[83]
Estramustine, 140 mg p.o. days 1–5 Docetaxel, 43 mg/m^2 day 2: Phase II	58	20	Not reached	[84]
Estramustine, 280 mg p.o. t.i.d. × five doses Docetaxel, 70 mg/m^2 12 h after first dose of estramustine: Phase II	38—study ongoing	25	Not reached	[85]

combination, overall survival was equivalent between both groups. A second study confirms activity of this combination, with a PSA response of 64% and objective response rate of 40% [60]. As with the taxanes, the combination of vinblastine and estramustine provides activity against hormone-refractory patients. Larger randomised trials will hopefully elucidate the best treatment regimen from these alternatives.

In addition to being combined with antimicrotubular agents, estramustine has been combined with anthracyclines in clinical trials. Both epirubicin and doxorubicin have been evaluated as single agents as treatment of hormone-refractory metastatic prostate cancer. Doxorubicin initially was believed to have minimal activity against hormone-refractory prostate cancer, with objective response rates of 5–7% [61,62]. Doxorubicin combinations with other agents have significantly higher activity. A commonly administered regimen utilises weekly doxorubicin administered with ketoconazole. A Phase II study conducted at the M. D. Anderson Cancer Center found a PSA response rate of 55%, with an objective response of measurable disease of 58% [63]. This combination does result in frequent adrenal insufficiency, necessitating routine use of corticosteroid replacement. The combination of estramustine and doxorubicin is equally efficacious, with a PSA response rate of 58% and an objective rate of 45% [64].

Multiple variations of the above chemotherapeutics continue to undergo investigation as treatment of metastatic prostate cancer. With newer endpoints as surrogate markers of disease response, it has become evident that chemotherapy can provide palliative support and possibly improved survival for patients with bone metastases. Evaluation of PSA, performance status and radiographic evidence of bone metastases should be used in combination to determine the most efficacious treatment plan for each individual. Currently there is no "standard" chemotherapeutic regimen for metastatic prostate cancer. The high response rates seen with docetaxel/estramustine combinations are encouraging and are undergoing continued investigation.

Other Solid Tumours

Many other solid tumours metastasise to bone, such as lung cancer and renal cell carcinoma, and also result in significant morbidity. Other tumours less commonly spread to bone, including ovarian, colon, pancreatic and gastric cancer. In general, patients with bone metastases from these tumours have expected survival of less than 1 year. Treatment addressing bone-only metastases from these sites is not well studied. As with breast and prostate cancer, therapy for metastases from other solid tumours is based upon a multidisciplinary approach, with the combination of systemic cytotoxic therapy as well as necessary radiation/surgical procedures performed to optimise palliation and survival.

Multiple Myeloma

Multiple myeloma is a haematological malignancy of monoclonal plasma cells that extensively involves bone. While less common than either prostate or breast cancer, myeloma was projected to cause almost 11 000 deaths in the USA in the year 2004 [1]. Approximately

70% of patients with multiple myeloma will have lytic bone metastases at the time of their diagnosis. Similarly to other malignancies, the abnormal plasma cells in the bone marrow disrupt the normal bone remodelling sequence, enhancing osteoclast activity by production of numerous cytokines. In addition to causing osteolytic lesions, the plasma cells of myeloma can cause diffuse osteopenia [65]. For most patients with osteolytic disease or osteopenia, myeloma is a generalised disease and treatment consists of systemic therapy.

Multiple myeloma is easily treatable initially but is rarely curable. Response to therapy is measured in several different ways. Bone scans are usually not helpful, given the primarily lytic nature of bone metastases. Bone radiographs, however, as well as spinal MRI can be useful in documenting initial staging as well as response to therapy. In general, these studies are not used for the primary determination of response to therapy. The appearance of new lytic lesions, however, can assist with the determination of progression of disease. Radiographic studies, such as MRI, can also assist with documentation of impending cord compression, thereby helping to direct therapy.

Several tumour-related abnormalities can be followed during therapy as surrogate markers of disease response and are more commonly used than plain radiographs. These include serum/urine protein electrophoresis, lactate dehydrogenase (LDH) and β2-microglobulin. The clonal population of myeloma cells produces abnormal proteins discernible by these serum and urine tests. The quantitative changes seen in the abnormal protein produced by myeloma cells can be used to assess response to therapy. Other parameters followed for evaluation of response to therapy include haemoglobin and the percentage of abnormal cells obtained via bone marrow biopsy.

Several regimens exist as treatment of multiple myeloma (Table 20.7). The majority of regimens contain steroids with a chemotherapeutic agent such as melphalan, vincristine or doxorubicin. The mainstay of therapy for multiple myeloma remains the combination of melphalan and prednisone (MP). Multiple studies have evaluated MP combinations compared with other chemotherapeutic regimens. In general, the MP combination results in response rates of 33–82% (median response rate 53.2%) with a median survival of 3 years [66].

As stated above, response rates are usually measured based upon changes in myeloma protein production (SPEP, etc.). Other regimens do result in superior response rates compared with those obtained from MP. For example, in one study the combination of

Table 20.7. Combination therapies used as treatment of multiple myeloma

Melphalan/prednisone (MP)
Vincristine/doxorubicin/dexamethasone (VAD)
Vincristine/carmustine/melphalan/cyclophosphamide/
    prednisone (VBMCP)
Vincristine/melphalan/cyclophosphamide/prednisone
    alternating with vincristine/carmustine/doxorubicin/
    prednisone (VMCP/VBAP)
Cyclophosphamide/prednisone

vincristine, doxorubicin, and dexamethasone (VAD) achieved a partial response of 62% of patients (stages IIA–IIIB) treated, with a complete response seen in an additional 5% [67]. A recent meta-analysis, however, has shown no significant improvement in overall survival or response duration when polychemotherapy regimens are compared with the MP combination [66]. Other standard chemotherapeutic agents are currently undergoing investigation as treatment options for patients with multiple myeloma, including paclitaxel and topotecan [68,69]. Also under investigation are novel therapies such as thalidomide and immunotherapy [70].

The current available therapies for multiple myeloma are, in general not curative. Patients who obtain remission with MP or other regimens almost invariably relapse, and the length of remission obtained with each successive therapy becomes shorter. Efforts to improve length of remission and, ultimately, to obtain cure have stimulated investigation of high-dose chemotherapy followed by stem cell transplantation (bone marrow or peripheral stem cells). Initially, transplantation was associated with high mortality (median age of multiple myeloma patients, 65). With improved techniques, transplant mortality has decreased to less than 5%. Evidence exists that there is a dose–response curve seen with increasing doses of melphalan, resulting in improved response rate. The use of stem cell transplantation has allowed increasing doses of melphalan to be administered, leading to increasing numbers of complete responses to therapy [71].

The knowledge that most patients will relapse from their myeloma has placed the timing of transplantation for these patients under investigation. When used as front-line therapy, the overall response rate of high-dose therapy and transplantation is 81% (22% complete remission), with improved survival compared to standard therapy [72]. It is important to recognise that the patients in this study were younger than the median age of most myeloma patients (65 years), possibly influencing their ability to tolerate therapy. Many investigators favouur transplantation as initial therapy for multiple myeloma. With increasing doses of melphalan, collection of adequate stem cells becomes more difficult. In addition, patients at a younger age and with improved performance status have less toxicity with transplantation therapy. This therapy remains experimental and patients with extensive disease should be considered for transplantation study protocols early after diagnosis.

SUMMARY

The presence of metastases to the bone is a common part of the natural history of most malignancies. The length of time patients live with their bone metastases correlates with their risk of morbidity, including pathological fractures, fractures from osteoporosis (breast, myeloma and prostate cancer) and possible nerve compression/damage. Chemotherapy produces amenorrhoea in most women with breast cancer aged > 35 years, placing these women at risk for osteoporosis. In men, prolonged administration of androgen blockade also leads to osteoporosis. In addition, both hormonal and chemotherapy of prostate cancer can result in erectile dysfunction. These therapies affect patients' lives and agents such as bisphosphonates, as well as education about possible side-effects of therapy, should be used to manage these patients.

Systemic chemotherapy in general produces similar responses in bone metastases as seen in other measurable disease. The response of bone metastases to systemic therapy is often difficult to determine, secondary to current technical limitations in imaging. Novel methods of imaging, including increasing use of PET scans as well as improved MRI techniques, will hopefully improve detection of cancer as well as the evaluation of response to therapy. The treatment of bony metastases often involves multiple approaches, with systemic chemotherapy, bisphosphonates and hormonal therapy working to control disease. A multidisciplinary approach to bone metastases will help decrease the risk of complications from bone metastases and hopefully improve patients' quality of life.

REFERENCES

1. Jemal A, Tiwari RC, Murray T, et al. Cancer Statistics, 2004. CA J Clin 2004; 54: 8–29.
2. Coleman RE, Rubens RD. Bone metastases and breast cancer. Cancer Treat Rev 1985; 12: 251–7.
3. Scheid V, Buzdar AU, Smith TL, Hortobagyi GN. Clinical course of breast cancer patients with osseous metastasis treated with combination chemotherapy. Cancer 1986; 58: 2589–93.
4. Whitmore WF. Natural history and staging of prostate cancer. Urol Clin N Am 1984; 11: 209–20.
5. Hortobagyi GN, Libshitz HI, Seabold JE. Osseous metastases of breast cancer. Cancer 1984; 53(3): 577–82.
6. Cook GJR, Fogelman I. Skeletal metastases from breast cancer: imaging with nuclear medicine. Semin Nucl Med 1999; 29(1): 69–79.
7. Pollen JJ, Witztum KF, Ashburn WL. The flare phenomenon on radionucleotide bone scan in metastatic prostate cancer. Am J Radiol 1984; 142(4): 773–6.
8. Cosolo W, Morstyn G, Arkles B et al. Flare responses in small cell carcinoma of the lung. Clin Nucl Med 1988; 13(1): 13–16.
9. Theriault RL, Hortobagyi GN. Bone metastasis in breast cancer. Anti-Cancer Drugs 1992; 3: 455–62.
10. Hayward JL, Carbone PP, Heusen JC et al. Assessment of response to therapy in advanced breast cancer. Br J Cancer 1977; 35(3): 292–8.
11. Ciray I, Astrom G, Andreasson I et al. Evaluation of new sclerotic bone metastases in breast cancer patients during treatment. Acta Radiol 2000; 41(2): 178–82.
12. Ciray I, Astrom G, Sundstrom C et al. Assessment of suspected bone metastases. CT with and without clinical information compared to CT-guided bone biopsy. Acta Radiol 1997; 38(5): 890–5.
13. Yoshida K, Akimoto M. Computed tomographic evaluation of bone metastases in prostatic cancer patients. Adv Exp Med Biol 1992; 324: 197–204.
14. Gosfield E, Alavi A, Kneeland B. Comparison of radionuclide bone scans and magnetic resonance imaging in detecting spinal metastases. J Nucl Med 1993; 34: 2191–8.
15. Vandemark RM, Shpall EJ, Affronti ML. Bone metastases from breast cancer: value of CT bone windows. J Comput Assist Tomogr 1992; 16(4): 608–14.
16. Crone-Munzebrock W, Carl UM. Dual-energy CT-scan quantification of recalcification in osteolysis of the vertebral body due to mammary carcinomas in the course of antineoplastic treatment. Clin Exp Metast 1990; 8(2): 173–9.
17. Saip P, Tenekeci N, Aydiner A et al. Response evaluation of bone metastases in breast cancer: value of magnetic resonance imaging. Cancer Invest 1999; 17(8): 575–80.
18. Partin AW, Carter HB, Chan DW et al. Prostate-specific antigen in the staging of localized prostate cancer: influence of tumor differentiation, tumor volume and benign hyperplasia. J Urol 1990; 143(4): 747–52.
19. Kelly WK, Scher HI, Mazumdar M et al. Prostate specific antigen as a measure of disease outcome in metastatic hormone-refractory prostate cancer: a Canadian randomized trial with palliative endpoints. J Clin Oncol 1993; 11(4): 607–15.
20. Smith DC, Dunn RL, Stawderman MS, Pienta KJ. Change in serum prostate-specific antigen as a marker of response to cytotoxic therapy for hormone-refractory prostate cancer. J Clin Oncol 1998; 16: 1835–43.
21. Bauer KS, Figg WD, Hamilton JM et al. A pharmacokinetically guided Phase II study of carboxyamido–triazole in androgen-independent prostate cancer. Clin Cancer Res 1999; 5(9): 2324–9.
22. Tannock IF, Osoba D, Stockler MR et al. Chemotherapy with mitoxantrone plus prednisone or prednisone alone

for symptomatic hormone-resistant prostate cancer: a Canadian randomized trial with palliative end points. J Clin Oncol 1996; 14: 1756–64.

23. Thalmann GN, Sikes RA, Chang SM et al. Suramin induced decrease in prostate-specific antigen expression with no effect on tumor growth in the LNCaP model of human prostate cancer. J Natl Cancer Inst 1996; 88: 794–801.

24. Bubley GJ, Carducci M, Dahut W et al. Eligibility and response guidelines for Phase II clinical trials in androgen-independent prostate cancer: recommendations from the prostate-specific antigen working group. J Clin Oncol 1999; 17(11): 3461–7.

25. Price MR, Rye PD, Petrakou E et al. Summary report on the ISOBM TD-4 workshop: analysis of 56 monoclonal antibodies against the MUC1 mucin. Tumor Biol 1998; 19(S1): 1–20.

26. Beveridge RA. Review of clinical studies of CA 27.29 in breast cancer management. Int J Biol Markers 1999; 14: 36–9.

27. Lauro S, Trasatti L, Bordin F et al. Comparison of CEA, MCA, CA 15-3 and CA 27-29 in follow-up and monitoring therapeutic response in breast cancer patients. Anticancer Res 1999; 19: 3511–16.

28. Fontana A, Delmas PD. Markers of bone turnover in bone metastases. Cancer 2000; 88(12): 2952–60.

29. Vinholes J, Coleman R, Lacombe D et al. Assessment of bone response to systemic therapy in an EORTC trial: preliminary experience with the use of collagen cross-link excretion. Br J Cancer 1999; 80(1/2): 221–8.

30. Walls J, Assiri A, Howell A et al. Measurement of urinary collagen cross-links indicate response to therapy in patients with breast cancer and bone metastases. Br J Cancer 1999; 80(8): 1265–70.

31. Lipton A, Demers L, Curley E et al. Markers of bone resorption in patients treated with pamidronate. Eur J Cancer 1998; 34(13): 2021–6.

32. Greenberg PAC, Hortobagyi GN, Smith TL et al. Long-term follow-up of patients with complete remission following combination chemotherapy for metastatic breast cancer. J Clin Oncol 1996; 14(8): 2197–205.

33. Carlson RW. Quality of life issues in the treatment of metastatic breast cancer. Oncology 1998; 12(3, S4): 27–31.

34. Early Breast Cancer Trialists' Collaborative Group. Polychemotherapy for early breast cancer: an overview of the randomized trials. Lancet 1998; 352: 930–42.

35. Fossati R, Confalonieri C, Ghislandi E et al. Cytotoxic and hormonal treatment for metastatic breast cancer. A 20-year analysis of published randomized trials. Proc Am Soc Clin Oncol 1998: 441.

36. A'Hern R, Smith I, Ebbs S. Chemotherapy and survival in advanced breast cancer: the inclusion of doxorubicin in Cooper-type regimens. Br J Cancer 1993; 67: 801–5.

37. Abeloff MD, Ettinger DS. Treatment of metastatic breast cancer with adriamycin–cyclophosphamide induction followed by alternating combination therapy. Cancer Treat Rep 1977; 61(9): 1685–9.

38. Smalley RV, Carpenter J, Bartolucci A et al. A comparison of cyclophosphamide, adriamycin, 5-fluorouracil (CAF) and cyclophosphamide, methotrexate, 5-fluorouracil, vincristine, prednisone (CMFVP) in

patients with metastatic breast cancer: a Southwestern Cancer Study Group project. Cancer 1977; 40(2): 625–32.

39. Kennealey GT, Boston B, Mitchell MS et al. Combination chemotherapy for advanced breast cancer—two regimens containing adriamycin. Cancer 1978; 42: 27–33.

40. Abrams JS, Vena DA, Baltz J et al. Paclitaxel activity in heavily pretreated breast cancer: a National Cancer Institute Treatment Referral Center trial. J Clin Oncol 1995; 13(8): 2056–65.

41. Burris HA. Single-agent docetaxel (Taxotere) in randomised phase III trials. Semin Oncol 1999; 26(S9): 1–6.

42. Trudeau ME, Eisenhauer EA, Higgins BP et al. Docetaxel in patients with metastatic breast cancer: a Phase II study of the National Cancer Institute of Canada clinical trials group. J Clin Oncol 1996; 14(2): 422–8.

43. Alexopoulos CG, Rigatos G, Efermidis AP et al. A Phase II study of the effectiveness of docetaxel (Taxotere) in women with advanced breast cancer previously treated with polychemotherapy. Cancer Chemother Pharmacol 1999; 44: 253–8.

44. Adachi I, Watanabe T, Takashima S et al. A late Phase II study of RP56976 (docetaxel) in patients with advanced or metastatic breast cancer. Br J Cancer 1996; 73(2): 210–16.

45. Nabholtz JM. Docetaxel (Taxotere) plus doxorubicin-based combinations: the evidence of activity in breast cancer. Semin Oncol 1999; 26(3S9): 7–13.

46. Cobleigh MA, Vogel CL, Tripathy D. Efficacy and safety of herceptin (humanized anti-HER2 antibody) as a single agent in 222 women with HER2 overexpression who had relapsed following chemotherapy for metastatic breast cancer. Proc Am Soc Clin Oncol 1998; 376.

47. Slamon D, Leyland-Jones B, Shak S. Addition of herceptin (humanized anti-HER2 antibody) to first line chemotherapy for HER2 overexpressing metastatic breast cancer (HER2$^+$/MBC) markedly increases anticancer activity: a randomized, multinational controlled Phase III trial. Proc Am Soc Clin Oncol 1998: 377.

48. Norton L, Slamon D, Leyland-Jones B. Overall survival (OS) advantage to simultaneous chemotherapy (CRx) plus the humanized anti-HER2 monoclonal antibody herceptin (H) in HER2 overexpressing (HER2 +) metastatic breast cancer (MBC). Proc Am Soc Clin Oncol 1999: 483.

49. Blum JL, Jones SE, Buzdar AU et al. Multicenter Phase II study of capecitabine in paclitaxel-refractory metastatic breast cancer. J Clin Oncol 1999; 17(2): 485–93.

50. Vogel C, O'Rourke M, Winer E et al. Vinorelbine as first-line chemotherapy for advanced breast cancer in women 60 years of age or older. Ann Oncol 1999; 10: 397–402.

51. Livingston RB, Ellis GK, Gralow JR et al. Dose-intensive vinorelbine with concurrent granulocyte colony-stimulating factor support in paclitaxel-refractory metastatic breast cancer. J Clin Oncol 1997; 15(4): 1395–400.

52. Carmichael J, Possinger K, Phillip P et al. Advanced breast cancer: a Phase II trial with gemcitabine. J Clin Oncol 1995; 13(11): 2731–6.

53. Dawson NA. Response criteria in prostatic cancer. Semin Oncol 1999; 26(2): 174–84.

54. Hauser AR, Merryman R. Estramustine phosphate sodium. Drug Intell Clin Pharm 1984; 18(5): 368–74.

55. Mittleman A, Shukla SK, Welvaart K, Murphy GP. Oral estramustine phosphate (NSC-89199) in the treatment of

advanced (stage D) carcinoma of the prostate. Cancer Chemother Rep 1975; 59(1): 219–23.

56. Roth BJ, Yeap BY, Wilding G et al. Taxol in advanced, hormone-refractory carcinoma of the prostate. A Phase II trial of the Eastern Cooperative Oncology Group. Cancer 1993; 72(8): 2457–60.

57. Trivedi C, Redman B, Flaherty LE et al. Weekly 1-hour infusion of paclitaxel. Cancer 2000; 89(2): 431–6.

58. Hudes GR, Nathan F, Khater C et al. Phase II trial of 96-hour paclitaxel plus oral estramustine phosphate in metastatic hormone-refractory prostate cancer. J Clin Oncol 1997; 15(9): 3156–63.

59. Picus J, Schultz M. Docetaxel (Taxotere) as monotherapy in the treatment of hormone-refractory prostate cancer: preliminary results. Semin Oncol 1999; 26(5, S17): 14–18.

60. Seidman AD, Scher HI, Petrylak D et al. Estramustine and vinblastine: use of prostate specific antigen as a clinical trial end point for hormone refractory prostate cancer. J Urol 1992; 147(3, Pt 2): 931–4.

61. Scher H, Yagoda A, Watson RC et al. Phase II trial of doxorubicin in bidimensionally measurable prostatic carcinoma. J Urol 1984; 131(6): 1099–102.

62. Torti FM, Shortliffe LD, Carter SK et al. A randomized study of doxorubicin vs. doxorubicin plus cisplatin in endocrine-unresponsive metastatic prostatic carcinoma. Cancer 1985; 56(11): 2580–6.

63. Sella A, Kilbourn R, Amato R et al. Phase II study of ketoconazole combined with weekly doxorubicin in patients with androgen-independent prostate cancer. J Clin Oncol 1994; 12(4): 683–8.

64. Culine S, Kattan J, Zanetta S et al. Evaluation of estramustine phosphate combined with weekly doxorubicin in patients with androgen-independent prostate cancer. Am J Clin Oncol 1998; 21(5): 470–4.

65. Mariette X, Khalifa P, Ravaud P et al. Bone densitometry in patients with multiple myeloma. Am J Med 1992; 93: 592–8.

66. Myeloma Trialists' Collaborative Group. Combination chemotherapy vs. melphalan plus prednisone as treatment for multiple myeloma: an overview of 6633 patients from 27 randomized trials. J Clin Oncol 1998; 16: 3832–42.

67. Segeren CM, Sonneveld P, van der Holt B et al. Vincristine doxorubicin and dexamethasone (VAD) administered as rapid infusion for first-line treatment in untreated multiple myeloma. Br J Haematol 1998; 105: 127–30.

68. Miller HJ, Leong T, Khandekar JD et al. Paclitaxel as the initial treatment of multiple myeloma; an Eastern Cooperative Oncology Group Study. (E1A93). Am J Clin Oncol 1998; 21(6): 553–6.

69. Kraut EH, Crowley JJ, Wade JL et al. Evaluation of topotecan in resistant and relapsing multiple myeloma: a Southwestern Oncology Group study. J Clin Oncol 1998; 16(2): 589–92.

70. Ludwig H, Meran J, Zojer N. Multiple myeloma: an update on biology and treatment. Ann Oncol 1999; 10(S 6): S31–43.

71. Selby PJ, McElwain TJ, Nandi AC et al. Multiple myeloma treated with high dose intravenous melphalan. Br J Haematol 1987; 66(1): 55–62.

72. Attal M, Harousseau JL, Stoppa AM et al. A prospective, randomized trial of autologous bone marrow transplantation and chemotherapy in multiple myeloma. Intergroupe Français du Myélome. N Engl J Med 1996; 335(2): 91–7.

73. Jones SE, Durie BG, Salmon SE. Combination chemotherapy with adriamycin and cyclophosphamide for advanced breast cancer. Cancer 1975; 36(1): 90–7.

74. Paridaens R, Biganzoli L, Bruning P et al. Paclitaxel vs. doxorubicin as first-line single-agent chemotherapy for metastatic breast cancer: a European organization for research and treatment of cancer randomized study with cross-over. J Clin Oncol 2000; 18(4): 724–33.

75. Ito Y, Horikoshi N, Watanabe T et al. Phase II study of paclitaxel (BMS-181339) intravenously infused over 3 hours for advanced or metastatic breast cancer in Japan. Invest New Drugs 1998; 16(2): 183–90.

76. Frasci G, Comella P, D'Aiuto G et al. Weekly paclitaxel–cisplatin administration with G-CSF support in advanced breast cancer. A Phase II study. Breast Cancer Res Treat 1998; 49: 13–26.

77. Terenziani M, Demiceli R, Brambilla C et al. Vinorelbine: an active, non cross-resistant drug. I. Advanced breast cancer. Results from a Phase II study. Breast Cancer Res Treatm 1996; 39(3): 285–91.

78. Canobbio L, Boccardo F, Pastorino G et al. Phase II study of Navelbine in advanced breast cancer. Semin Oncol 1989; 16(2, suppl 4): 33–6.

79. Fumoleau P, Delgado FM, Delozier T et al. Phase II trial of weekly intravenous vinorelbine in first-line advanced breast cancer chemotherapy. J Clin Oncol 1993; 11(7): 1245–52.

80. Romero A, Rabinovich MG, Vallejo CT et al. Vinorelbine as first-line chemotherapy for metastatic breast cancer. J Clin Oncol 1994; 12(2): 336–41.

81. Petrylak DP, Macarthur RB, O'Connor J et al. Phase I trial of docetaxel with estramustine in androgen-independent prostate cancer. J Clin Oncol 1999; 17(3): 958–67.

82. Petrylak DP, Shelton GB, England-Owen C et al. Response and preliminary survival results of a Phase II study of docetaxel (D) + estramustine (E) in patients with androgen-independent prostate cancer (AIPC). Proc Am Soc Clin Oncol 2000: abstr 1312.

83. Savarese D, Taplin ME, Halabi S et al. A Phase II study of docetaxel (Taxotere), estramustine and low-dose hydrocortisone in men with hormone-refractory prostate cancer: preliminary results of Cancer and Leukemia Group B Trial 9780. Semin Oncol 1999; 26(5, S17): 39–44.

84. Krosty MP, Ferreira A, Bryntesen T, Grossman J. Weekly docetaxel and low-dose estramustine phosphate in hormone refractory prostate cancer: a Phase II study. Proc Am Soc Clin Oncol 2000: abstr 1442.

85. Sinibaldi VJW, Carducci M, Laufer M et al. Preliminary evaluation of a short course of estramustine phosphate and docetaxel (Taxotere) in the treatment of hormone-refractory prostate cancer. 1999; 26(5, S17): 45–8.

86. Hudes G, Einhorn L, Ross E et al. Vinblastine vs. vinblastine plus oral estramustine phosphate for patients with hormone-refractory prostate cancer: a Hoosier Oncology Group and Fox Chase Network Phase II trial. J Clin Oncol 1999; 17(10): 3160–6.

21

Endocrine Treatment of Bone Metastases

Sophia Agelaki and Vassilis Georgoulias

University General Hospital of Heraklion, Crete, Greece

INTRODUCTION

Frequency of Bone Metastases

Metastatic cancer often involves the skeleton. Carcinomas of the breast, prostate, lung, kidney and thyroid possess a great tendency to metastasise to bone [1]. This is most evident in breast and prostate cancer, in which bone metastases are detected in nearly all patients by the time of death. Indeed, in an autopsy study of 358 patients who died of cancer between 1927 and 1941 it was shown that bone is the third most common metastatic site after lung and liver and that breast and prostate carcinomas metastasise to bone most frequently [2]. In that report 64% of 186 breast cancer patients had bone metastases at autopsy. Two more recent studies reported that 62% of 1060 and 69% of 587 patients who died of breast cancer had bone disease [3,4], suggesting that the introduction of chemotherapy has not changed the predilection of cancer cells to metastasise to bone. Up to 80% of patients dying from prostate cancer have bone metastases [5]. Most other primary tumours, such as lung, endometrium, cervix, bladder and gastrointestinal tract malignancies, metastasise to bone but these sites account for less than 20% of patients with bone disease.

Prognosis

Although the overall prognosis is rather poor, a significant proportion of patients will survive long enough to require active treatment because of morbidity related to bone disease. Patients with metastatic breast cancer survive an average of 34 months once the first metastasis is detected (range 1–90 months) [6], whereas median survival of patients with metastatic prostate cancer and lung cancer averages 24 and 12 months, respectively [7].

Classification

When solid tumours metastasise to the skeleton, they cause a variety of alterations in bone function which are characterised as "lytic", "sclerotic", or "mixed", according to the radiographic appearance of the lesions. The most common is the osteolytic lesion, in which bone resorption predominates, with little new bone formation. Lytic metastases are more commonly seen in lung, breast, renal, thyroid, adrenal and gastrointestinal malignancies. Less commonly, new bone formation exceeds bone destruction and the lesions appear sclerotic. Prostate cancer especially but also bronchial carcinoid and medulloblastoma tumours give rise to sclerotic lesions. However, in the majority of skeletal metastases, new bone formation develops simultaneously with bone destruction and this may be evident on the radiograph as a mixed lesion. Metastases from breast, lung, ovarian and cervical cancer often have mixed features.

MECHANISMS OF BONE METASTASIS

Metastasis is a multistep process involving a series of sequential interactions between cancer cells and the microenvironment at the metastatic site. Cancer cells metastasing to bone should have intrinsic properties that facilitate development of bone metastases. These include production of proteolytic enzymes, angiogenic factors, autocrine growth factors, expression or loss of cell adhesion molecules (CAMs), and ability to escape from host immune surveillance. Specific properties of the metastatic site are also critical in determining initial bone colonisation. It has been shown that endothelial cells in various organs preferentially adhere to tumour cells [8], suggesting a contributory role of sinus endothelial cells in "selecting" localisation of specific cells. Moreover, circulating tumour cells may respond to factors diffusing locally out of bone, which act chemotactically to attract the cells. Indeed, degradation products of normal bone resorption are chemotactic for tumour cells *in vitro* [9].

Once tumour cells invade the bone they are stimulated by a variety of cytokines and growth factors, such as transforming growth factor (TGF) β, heparin-binding fibroblast growth factors, platelet-derived growth factors and insulin-like growth factors I and II [10]. These growth factors secreted during bone formation are deposited in the bone matrix and are subsequently released into the marrow when the matrix is degraded during normal osteoclastic resorption [11]. The growth of tumour cells is further enhanced under the influence of cytokines and growth factors produced by stromal and haematopoietic tissue cells. Thus, it seems that the bone microenvironment provides a fertile soil on which metastatic cells can grow.

However, this alone cannot explain the osteotropism of certain primary tumours, since other metastatic cells passing through bone are exposed to the same influences. Clinical and experimental evidence suggests that tumour-produced parathyroid hormone-related protein (PTHrP) is an important agent for the development and progression of tumour metastases in bone. Indeed, patients with PTHrP-positive breast cancer more commonly develop bone metastases [12]. In addition, breast cancer cells metastatic to bone express PTHrP in 92% of cases compared with only 17% of metastases in non-bone sites [13], which suggests that the bone microenvironment may enhance PTHrP expression by tumour cells. It has been shown that growth factors present in bone, especially TGFβ, promote the expression of PTHrP by various tumour cells [14].

Thus, a vicious cycle exists in bone; once tumour cells invade the skeleton they grow under the influence of multiple growth factors and cytokines present in the bone microenvironment. These cytokines in turn promote PTHrP production by the tumour cells and subsequent osteoclastic bone resorption. So the bone microenvironment is even more enriched with growth factors, which further enhance tumour survival.

SKELETAL-RELATED EVENTS AND AIM OF TREATMENT

Bone metastases result in considerable morbidity. Pain is the dominant symptom in almost 75% of patients [15]. Pathological fractures have been reported in 8–30% of patients with bone metastases [16]. Hypercalcaemia occurs in about 10% [17] and spinal cord compression in about 5% [18] of patients. In two large randomised trials of patients with breast cancer receiving chemotherapy [19] or endocrine therapy [20], with and without biphosphonates, the mean skeletal morbidity rate (SMR), which has been defined as the number of skeletal complications occurring in a patient per year, was, in the arm without biphosphonates, 3.5 and 3.8, respectively. In a similar study in patients with multiple myeloma, the SMR was 2.0 [21].

The morbidity associated with bone metastases severely compromises the quality of life of patients with cancer. Treatment of bone disease is mainly palliative, aiming at pain relief, prevention of pathological fractures and improvement of patients' mobility and function. Furthermore, it should be of major importance to reduce the incidence of bone metastases and, if possible, to prolong the survival of patients with bone disease.

TREATMENT

Treatment of bone metastases requires a broad approach. The therapeutic options include both local treatment (surgery and/or radiotherapy) and systemic treatment. Systemic therapy for bone metastases may either reduce tumour cell proliferation and, as a consequence, the release of cytokines and growth factors, or block the effects of these products on osteoclasts. Chemotherapy, endocrine treatment and radioisotopes have direct effects on tumour cells, whereas agents such as biphosphonates and calcitonin inhibit osteoclast-mediated bone resorption.

The primary tumour plays a critical role in the selection of systemic antitumour treatment. If the primary is responsive to systemic manipulation, then hormonal or chemotherapeutic treatment is preferred. Endocrine therapy has few side-effects, making it the preferable palliative treatment modality in patients with hormone-responsive tumours, such as breast and prostate cancer. Moreover, the activity of at least some of the cytokines and growth factors present in the bone microenvironment can be regulated by oestrogens, so it is reasonable to suppose that antioestrogen and other hormonal therapies may be of special benefit against bone metastases. For example, it has been shown that PTHrP mRNA expression is significantly decreased in breast cancer tissue incubated for 24 h with medroxyprogesterone acetate (MPA) [22], which is particularly interesting given the intriguing role of PTHrP in the development of bone metastases.

ASSESSMENT OF RESPONSE

The accurate evaluation of bone response to treatment is of major importance for the determination of subsequent therapeutic interventions. Bone scan is more sensitive in detecting osseous metastases, whereas radiography is commonly used to evaluate symptomatic sites and to confirm findings on other imaging studies. Response assessment is based on the radiographic evaluation of a healing procedure or progression of a previously lytic metastasis; response is usually indicated as a sclerosis which tends to progress from the periphery towards the centre of the lesion [23]. However, changes in radiographs commonly become evident only when the whole sequence of events is reviewed from the baseline throughout the whole treatment, a process which is time-consuming and not often performed. Bone scans are not specific in assessing response to treatment, because decreased activity of an established lesion may imply either true improvement or lessened osteoblastic activity in response to a growing metastasis, whereas increased activity may signify improvement or worsening.

The response to treatment is classified as complete response, partial response, progressive disease or stable disease, according to the published criteria from the International Union Against Cancer (IUCC) [24]. Clinical trials in the treatment of breast cancer using the IUCC criteria have usually reported lower response rates for bone lesions than the overall response [25]. This could be true if bone metastases were relatively refractory to treatment, but it is more likely attributable to the insensitivity of the traditional methods used for the evaluation of response. Moreover, most authors consider bone metastases to be evaluable but not measurable; non-measurable disease cannot be assessed as being in partial response (only complete response, no change and progressive disease are possible outcomes), therefore this could have reduced the percentage of patients with objective remissions. Furthermore, bone scans and radiographs are poorly correlated with the clinical picture of the patient, since pain relief is commonly reported during treatment without any objective evidence of response. Therefore, one could suggest that traditional methods are of limited value in assessing the efficacy of palliative treatment of bone metastases.

In prostate cancer, the assessment of response is based on a combination of changes in radiography, bone scan, acid phosphatase, performance status and symptoms [26,27]. However, the validity and reproducibility of these criteria is questionable; the methods for evaluation of bone disease are inaccurate, patient-based symptom assessment has been undertaken in very few studies, and pre-treatment pain and/or quality of life has not been commonly measured [26]. Moreover, only a few studies provide sufficient documentation of the method of pain measurement and the degree of pain relief after treatment.

The physician should also bear in mind the tumour flare phenomenon in evaluating bone response. Tumour flare is commonly observed in breast cancer patients and has been defined as a transient worsening of the clinical picture, bone scan and/or specific or non-specific tumour markers, occurring within 2–21 days following the institution of a new hormonal treatment. Tumour flare has been reported most commonly following the administration of oestrogens (1%) [28], androgens (3%) [28] and tamoxifen (2.2%) [29]. In most cases flare is associated with hormone-sensitivity of the tumour and subsequent response to therapy [30]. However, some patients with possible tumour flare are prematurely removed off studies as progressors, while they might have benefited from continuation of treatment [31].

HORMONAL THERAPY

Breast Cancer

Hormonal therapies for metastatic breast cancer result in a 30–35% response rate in unselected patients [32,33]. Oestrogen receptor (ER) and progesterone receptor (PR) content of the tumour correlate with response; patients who are both ER- and PR-positive display response rates of approximately 70% compared to response rates of up to 20% in patients who are ER- and PR-negative [34]. Soft tissue or bony tumour sites are more likely to contain ER-positive cells [35], and patients with ER-positive tumours more commonly develop osseous metastases [36]. Phase II and III studies of different forms of endocrine therapy provide some information regarding the activity of endocrine treatment of bone metastases. However, there are no trials evaluating the efficacy of hormonal treatment in patients with bone-only disease.

Antioestrogens

Tamoxifen, a synthetic antioestrogen, has been the agent of choice for first-line endocrine treatment of breast cancer patients, based on its likelihood of response and favourable toxicity profile [37]. Tamoxifen was initially evaluated in postmenopausal women. Approximately one-third of the unselected patients achieve an objective response to tamoxifen therapy [38], while more than 50% of patients with ER-positive tumours obtain clinical benefit (complete response, plus partial response, plus stable disease for more than 24 weeks) [39–41].

There is a considerable variation on the reported skeletal response rates. Manni et al. [39] reported remissions in 19/35 (54%) patients in whom bone was the dominant site of involvement. In the study by Brule [42] only 4/75 (5%) patients with evaluable bone disease responded to tamoxifen, whereas in the study by Lerner et al. [43] 7/18 (39%) patients responded. In another trial, 8/42 (19%) patients with bone metastases experienced disease regression [44]. Generally, response rates for osseous metastases are lower than those reported for skin, nodal and other soft tissue lesions [44,45].

The clinical experience with tamoxifen in premenopausal women with advanced breast cancer has been limited. The responses in this setting ranged between 20% and 45%, with a mean response rate of approximately 31% [46]. Metastatic disease in soft tissue responded more favourably to tamoxifen therapy than did osseous or visceral disease [46]. Response rate correlated to steroid receptor status; no patients with ER-negative tumours had disease regression with tamoxifen [47]. For premenopausal women, response to tamoxifen is comparable to that of castration; indeed, randomised trials have reported no difference in overall response rate, duration of response or survival between tamoxifen and bilateral oophorectomy. In the trial by Ingle et al. [48] it appeared that tamoxifen was more effective than oophorectomy in patients with osseous disease; 1/5 (20%) and 4/7 (57%) patients with bone-dominant disease sites responded to oophorectomy and tamoxifen, respectively. However, the sample size was too small to draw any conclusions

and moreover, this was not observed in the trial by Buchanan et al. [49].

New antioestrogens with high affinity to the oestrogen receptor and pure antioestrogenic effects in the uterus are being evaluated in breast cancer patients. Toremifene (chlorotamoxifen), is a tamoxifen analogue which has been approved for the treatment of metastatic breast cancer. Phase II studies in previously untreated postmenopausal patients with metastatic disease reported response rates of 32.6–54.3% [50,51]. Phase III trials comparing two different doses of toremifene with tamoxifen administered in untreated, hormone receptor-positive or unknown, metastatic breast cancer patients have demonstrated no differences in response rates and tolerability [52–54]. Droloxifene (3-hydroxytamoxifen) has also been tested for the treatment of metastatic breast cancer, with response rates of 30–47% in postmenopausal women who had not received prior hormonal therapy [55]. Responses were also observed in patients with bone metastases, while the median pain score of patients decreased by nearly half within the first 2 weeks. Pure antioestrogens, such as the compound ICI 182 780, developed for the treatment of advanced breast cancer after failure of long-term adjuvant tamoxifen therapy, have been evaluated in clinical trials but data are limited. Howel et al. [56] reported a 37% response rate using ICI 182 780 in a group of 19 tamoxifen-resistant patients. Response to bone disease sites was observed in seven patients.

Progestins

Medroxyprogesterone acetate (MPA) and megoestrol acetate (MA), used mainly as second-line treatment in patients with metastatic breast cancer, resulted in response rates of 20–40%. MPA in daily low doses (< 500 mg/day) induced median objective remission rates of about 13% [57]. Doses of 500–1000 mg/day administered intramuscularly for 30 days, followed by a maintenance dose given weekly, have produced responses in 40% of treated patients [58]. Pannuti and colleagues demonstrated no difference in response or survival between doses of 1500 mg/day compared with 500 mg/day [59]. In the same study, objective response was noted in about 60% of patients with bone lesions without any statistically significant difference observed between the two arms. Moreover, pain was promptly relieved in about 80% of patients in both groups. MPA may also be given orally but it has low bioavailability at low doses [60].

Numerous trials have documented the efficacy and tolerability of MA, with responses of 25–45% in pretreated patients [61–64]. Response rates of osseous disease sites appear to differ considerably. Blackledge et al. [62] reported that none of 13 patients with evaluable bone disease had changes on X-ray sufficient to be characterised as a responder according to the IUCC criteria. However, seven patients experienced reduction in bone pain. Ross et al. [63] observed 12 responses (31%) in 39 evaluable patients, whereas in a study by Alexieva-Figusch [64] only one remission was recorded among 31 patients with osseous metastases as the dominant disease site. A randomised comparison of MA and MPA given orally as second-line treatment revealed no differences in clinical benefit, progression-free survival and overall survival between the two arms [65]. However, the response of skeletal lesions was seen more clearly in MPA- than MA-treated patients (45% of patients with bone-dominant disease site responded to MPA, compared to 12.5% on MA; $p < 0.05$).

It seems that there is a benefit for the use of MPA in comparison to tamoxifen for the treatment of bone disease. In an overview [66] of seven trials comparing the use of tamoxifen (at doses of 40 mg, 30 mg and 20 mg) and MPA (at varying doses of 500 mg–2 g/day), which included 801 patients, the frequency of overall response was 29% and 39%, respectively, in the tamoxifen and MPA-treated patients (odds ratio 1.5; 95% CI 1.1–2.0). Furthermore, the probability of response to MPA treatment was about three-fold higher than to tamoxifen in the subgroup with bone metastases (odds ratio 3.4; 95% CI 1.2–9.4). In the same analysis, combined data from four studies revealed no difference in the overall frequency of response or bone response rate between tamoxifen and MA.

Aromatase Inhibitors

Aminoglutethimide. Aminoglutethimide (AG), the first aromatase inhibitor to become available for the treatment of advanced breast cancer in postmenopausal women, has been predominantly evaluated as a second-line treatment. A review of the pooled Phase II data of this agent demonstrates that 296 (32%) of 929 postmenopausal patients achieved an objective response [67]. In a study by Harris et al. [68] a 23% response rate of bone tumour sites was reported in a group of 213 unselected, previously treated postmenopausal patients. Moreover, among 60 patients with progressive bone disease, 31.7% experienced reduction

of bone pain, often starting within 24 h of initiation of therapy. Smith and associates [69] observed a 53% bone response rate in pretreated breast cancer patients. In the study by Kaye et al. [70], although no responses at osseous sites were reported, nine of 30 patients with bone disease experienced marked pain relief. Cocconi and colleagues [71] reported a 38% bone response rate with AG given as first-line treatment.

Several randomised studies have shown that AG is as efficacious as tamoxifen as both initial [72,73] or secondary therapy [74]. However, it seemed that AG was particularly effective in the management of painful bone metastases and appeared better than tamoxifen in both relieving pain and achieving objective remissions. Indeed, Smith et al. [73] reported a 35% bone response rate and a further 26% subjective pain relief with AG compared to 17% objective response and a further 17% pain amelioration with tamoxifen, both given as first-line treatment. However, aminoglutethimide administration was associated with a greater incidence of side-effects (lethargy, depression and morbilliform skin rash), severe enough to necessitate treatment discontinuation in some patients. Similarly, Lipton et al. [74] noted a trend suggesting that AG compared to tamoxifen is more effective for the treatment of bone metastases (33% vs. 15% remission rate, $p=0.10$) and concluded that site of involvement may turn out to be an important factor in determining treatment selection.

AG has been also proved as efficacious as progestins for the treatment of breast cancer patients. In the study by Canney et al. [75] there were no statistically significant differences between AG and MPA regarding bone response (6/35 for MPA, 17%; and 6/24 for AG, 25%), while Lundgren et al. [76] in a randomised comparison of AG and MA demonstrated a significant difference in favour of AG (29.6% vs. 15.4%, $p < 0.05$).

Second-generation Inhibitors. AG inhibits the adrenal synthesis of both glucocorticoids and mineralocorticoids thus requiring the co-administration of hydrocortisone. This, together with the significant side-effects associated with the standard daily dose of 1000 mg, has severely limited its use. A second-generation, more selective, steroidal aromatase inhibitor, formestane (4-hydroxyandrostenodione), with a more favourable toxicity profile, became available. The overall response rate in Phase II trials testing this agent, usually in patients who had received one to three previous hormonal therapies, was 7–39% [77], with bone response rates of 18–27% [78,79]. In a randomised Phase III study comparing formestane with tamoxifen as first-line therapy in postmenopausal patients, equivalent efficacy in terms of response rate and response duration, as well as side-effects, was reported [80]. Patients with disease confined to bone had response rates of 19% and 27% for formestane and tamoxifen, respectively. Similarly, a randomised comparison of formestane with MA showed that both agents share similar antineoplastic activity as second-line hormonal treatment for advanced breast cancer, but formestane was better tolerated [81]. However, a substantially higher rate of progression in bones was observed in the formestane group (51/68) than in the MA group (25/53).

Formestane is administered intramuscularly and its use has been associated with injection-site reactions. Exemestane, a second-generation steroidal inhibitor, has the advantage over formestane of oral administration. In two Phase II studies, objective remission rates with exemestane as second-line therapy in postmeno-pausal women with advanced breast cancer were 22% and 28% [82,83]. When exemestane was used as third-line hormonal therapy, overall response rate was 26%, whereas in patients with bone predominant disease, it was 11% [84]. Exemestane proved superior to MA in prolonging overall survival, time to progression and time to treatment failure [85]. The response rate observed in patients with disease limited to bone was lower than the overall response reported.

Third-generation Inhibitors. Anastrozole, letrozole and fadrozole are non-steroidal selective aromatase inhibitors which cause irreversible inhibition of the enzyme. Two large randomised studies have compared anastrozole (1 and 10 mg daily) with MA as second-line therapy in postmenopausal women with advanced breast cancer, after tamoxifen failure [86]. A combined analysis of both studies demonstrated that anastrozole 1 mg confers a statistically significant survival advantage over MA, although there were no significant differences in terms of overall response and time to progression. Bone response rate was not mentioned in this trial but objective responses were observed in all disease sites. Anastrozole was demonstrated to be equivalent to tamoxifen in the first-line setting in terms of response rate and time to progression [87].

Letrozole has produced objective response rates of approximately 25–35% after failure of prior therapy [88,89]. A recent Phase III trial comparing letrozole (0.5 and 2.5 mg daily) with MA (160 mg daily) in postmenopausal women with advanced disease reported a better toxicity profile and a significant improvement in response rate, duration of response and time to treatment failure for letrozole over MA [90]. For patients with predominantly bone metastases

the objective response rate, averaging 15%, was similar in both groups. Letrozole 2.5 mg also proved superior to AG in terms of both time to progression and overall survival, although there were no significant differences in objective response [91]. As might be expected, significantly more patients on AG experienced drug-related adverse events. Letrozole also produced higher response rates in patients with predominant bone disease (17% vs. 9%, respectively). Preliminary data of a randomised comparison of letrozole with tamoxifen as first-line therapy in postmenopausal women with advanced breast cancer showed that letrozol is superior to tamoxifen in terms of overall response, time to progression and time to treatment failure [92]. Response to bone disease sites was observed in 32–146 (21.9%) patients treated with letrozol vs. 18/130 (13.8%) patients on tamoxifen (p=0.001).

Fadrozole compared to tamoxifen as first-line therapy was significantly better tolerated, in particular with respect to cardiovascular adverse events, but there were no differences in terms of antitumour efficacy [93]. Fadrozole has also been compared to MA in two large randomised trials with a total of 683 postmenopausal patients failing on antioestrogen therapy; no significant differences for objective response, time to progression, survival and incidence or severity of adverse events were shown [94]. Bone response rate was 12% and 21% for fadrozole and tamoxifen, respectively.

Overall, the results of previously mentioned randomised trials do not demonstrate augmented activity of the newer aromatase inhibitors regarding the response rate of bone metastases.

Oestrogens and Androgens

Oestrogens and androgens were the two main treatment options for postmenopausal women with advanced breast cancer until the mid 1980s. Although no longer widely used, oestrogens remain effective agents for postmenopausal patients, displaying response rates of 20–40% [95]. Ingle and co-workers [96] comparing diethylstilboestrol (DES) to tamoxifen in a randomised trial, reported equal antitumour efficacy for both drugs, whereas tamoxifen was associated with fewer side-effects. Regression rate in cases with osseous dominance was 35% and 20% for DES and tamoxifen, respectively (p=0.33). Similarly, the randomised comparison of ethinyl oestradiol to tamoxifen demonstrated equal response rates, durations of remission, and survival times for the two agents but less toxicity for tamoxifen [97]. In both studies it was concluded that tamoxifen was the drug of choice for postmenopausal women with advanced breast cancer.

Danazol, a synthetic steroid with partial androgen action that blocks pituitary gonadotropin secretion, has displayed response rates of 5–15% in previously treated patients [95]. Response rates to virilising androgens (testosterone, fluoxymesterone, testolactone and calusterone) have been noted in approximately 20% of patients [37]. These drugs are less commonly used because of their virilising side-effects (hirsutism, deepening of the voice, hair loss, acne and increased libido). Moreover, Westerberg [98]. randomised women to either fluoxymesterone or tamoxifen and found not only a higher response rate for tamoxifen-treated patients but also a significant time to treatment failure.

Overall, there are many effective endocrine therapies available for the treatment of metastatic breast cancer that have fewer side effects. Androgens should therefore be used as fourth- or fifth-line agents for patients who remain hormone sensitive.

Luteinising Hormone-releasing Hormone (LHRH) Agonists

LHRH agonists suppress ovarian production of oestradiol by desensitising pituitary LHRH receptors [60]. These drugs have optimal activity in premenopausal women but little efficacy in postmenopausal women, in whom ovarian oestrogen production is minimal. LHRH agonists, including leuprolide, bureselin and goreselin, have been associated with response rates approximating 35–40% in premenopausal women [37].

Goreselin, in a Phase II trial conducted in 118 evaluable, previously untreated premenopausal women with advanced disease, showed a 45% overall response rate [99]. Bone remission rate was 46.7%. A study enrolling 52 postmenopausal women demonstrated a 11% response rate, whereas responses occurred only in ER-positive patients with skin- or soft tissue-dominant disease [100]. Therefore, these agents should be considered for premenopausal patients responsive to prior endocrine therapy.

Combination Endocrine Therapy

Because sequential administration of various endocrine therapies can produce repeated tumour regressions, efforts have been made to increase the antitumour activity of hormonal treatment by giving various endocrine agents simultaneously with tamoxifen.

The combination of tamoxifen and fluoxymesterone compared to tamoxifen alone demonstrated similar response rates, duration of response and survival, whereas time to progression was better for the combination [101]. Response rate for tamoxifen and for tamoxifen plus fluoxymesterone in osseous dominant disease was 38% and 40%, respectively. These findings are similar to those published by Tormey and co-workers [102]. Powles et al. [103] treated patients with tamoxifen, aminoglutethimide, and danazol vs. tamoxifen alone; 43% of patients treated with the combination achieved a response to therapy compared with 31% responses in the tamoxifen-alone arm ($p=0.05$), with equal duration of remission and survival in both groups. There was a trend showing an increased response of bone metastases to the combination rather than to tamoxifen.

Smith et al. [104] found no difference between tamoxifen or aminoglutethimide administered alone vs. combination administration in terms of response rate and duration of response. Aminoglutethimide appeared superior to tamoxifen in the management of bone metastases, both in achieving objective evidence of response and in relieving pain. However, the combination of the two agents did not offer any advantage over aminoglutethimide alone. Similarly, no advantage of the combination was shown in the trials by Corkery et al. [105] and Ingle et al. [106]. A randomised comparison of tamoxifen, MA, or tamoxifen plus MA showed that the combination had no advantage over single agents used alone [107].

Overall, these studies suggest that combination endocrine treatment offers no advantage over sequential single-agent therapy. In addition, combination therapy is associated with additional toxicity.

Prostate Cancer

In metastatic prostate cancer, a wide range of response rates has been reported, primarily because of the poorly defined response criteria. Generally 70–80% of previously untreated patients can be expected to obtain pain relief after hormonal treatment [108,109], whereas an improvement in bone scan will be evident in 30–50% of cases [110]. Improvement in symptoms may occur within 24 h and, although difficult to assess, the median duration of response is approximately 12 months [23].

Oestrogens

Exogenous oestrogens were the first hormonal compounds to be used for metastatic prostate cancer, and for almost four decades they have been the standard hormonal treatment. Diethylstilboestrol (DES) has been used most extensively, producing objective bone responses ranging from 18% [111] to 30% [112], whereas in another trial subjective pain improvement was reported in 38% of the treated patients [113]. However, these agents have fallen out of favour because of the increased incidence of cardiovascular complications, consisting mainly of peripheral oedema and thromboembolic events.

Progestins

The progestational agents that have more commonly been evaluated in prostate cancer patients include cyproterone acetate (CPA) and medroxyprogesterone acetate. CPA is a synthetic 21-carbon hydroxyprogesterone derivative in which a 70% objective response rate, i.e. marked reduction in local disease, was reported in previously untreated patients [114]. CPA administration is also associated with serious adverse events, such as thrombophlebitis and fluid retention [115].

MPA has been used less extensively than CPA because it appears less potent. In a randomised comparison of CPA, MPA and DES, MPA was less efficacious than either CPA or DES when both time to progression and survival end points were measured [111]. When these end points were compared between CPA and DES, they were equivalent. MPA and CPA produced 3% and 13% bone response rates, respectively. There were no significant differences in the cardiovascular death rates among the three treatment groups.

LHRH Agonists

LHRH agonists were approved for the treatment of advanced prostate cancer on the basis of randomised comparisons showing equivalent antitumour effects to surgical castration, with response rates of around 85% [116,117]. Moreover, they demonstrated similar antitumour efficacy and fewer adverse events, particularly with respect to cardiovascular complications, in comparison to DES [118].

In the trial by Kaisary et al. [117] a 66% subjective response to treatment (based on improvement in urological symptoms, performance status, decrease in bone pain and/or analgesic requirement) with goreselin was reported. In another trial, 38% of patients treated with leuprolide reported subjective improvement of bone pain [113]. Caution is advised when administering these LHRH agonists to patients with symptomatic bone lesions, urinary obstuction, or impending spinal cord compression, because of the probability of tumour flare phenomena; LHRH analogues produce a transient stimulation in LH levels with consequent increase in the production of testosterone, which in turn may cause exacerbation of symptoms.

Antiandrogens

By analogy with the treatment of breast cancer, non-steroidal pure antiandrogens, such as nilutamide, flutamide and bicalutamide, have been developed that antagonise the action of androgens at the level of the androgen receptor. One use of the antiandrogens has been to suppress the flare in patients treated with LHRH agonists [119].

Nilutamide was the first pure antiandrogen to undergo large Phase III trials combined with either orchiectomy or the LHRH agonist, bureselin. Flutamide produced complete disappearance of pain in 40/52 (77%) patients with advanced prostatic carcinoma suffering from painful bone disease [120]. Bicalutamide demonstrated equivalent antitumour efficacy and an improved safety profile compared with flutamide [121].

Complete Androgen Blockade

A major use of antiandrogens has been the combination with LHRH analogues or orchiectomy to achieve complete androgen blockade (CAB). Both positive and negative trials and meta-analyses exist, raising much controversy regarding the efficacy of the combination vs. castration alone.

The NCI Intergroup Study 1 reported by Crawford et al. [122] which compared leuprolide plus flutamide to leuprolide alone, demonstrated an improved time to progression and overall survival for patients who received CAB. A statistically significant difference in pain relief was reported in favour of the combination. The addition of flutamide to bilateral orchiectomy did not result in clinically meaningful improvement in survival. Trials using a control group of orchiectomy alone, also reported a delay in time to progression and an improved overall survival with CAB [123–125]. In the trial by Janknegt et al. [123] significantly better bone response rate was reported for the CAB group. Indeed, 78% of the patients treated with nilutamide and orchiectomy experienced a decrease in pain and 52% had an improved bone scan vs. 65% and 39% in the control group, respectively. Similarly, Beland et al. [124] found a significant trend for better pain control in the group offered nilutamide plus surgical castration. However, in the Danish Prostate Cancer Group trial that used the same study design, no significant differences in time to progression, survival and subjective response to therapy, either in quality or duration, could be established [125].

A meta-analysis of the combination of surgical castration plus nilutamide showed a beneficial effect on objective response, time to disease progression, and possibly on survival [126]. Metastasis-related pain improved in a higher percentage of patients treated with the combination (48% vs. 34%, $p < 0.001$). However, the Prostate Cancer Trialists' Collaborative Group, in a systematic review of 22 studies with 5425 patients that compared castration (surgical or medical) with CAB, revealed a non-significant trend in favour of the combination therapy [127]. Nonetheless, the current standard approach is to offer combined androgen blockade in patients with advanced prostate cancer [128].

CONCLUSION

Bone metastases are a frequent clinical problem compromising the quality of life of cancer patients. Treatment of bone disease requires a broad approach, including both local and systemic treatment modalities Patients with hormone-sensitive tumours such as breast and prostate cancer are often treated with endocrine therapies. Although the evaluation of the response of bone lesions can be problematic, it is clear that endocrine treatment results in significant objective responses. Complete responses are rare but partial responses and disease stabilisation in bone are more common, conferring a significant clinical benefit to patients. However, despite initial response, the disease will progress. Breast cancer patients responsive to first-line endocrine treatment have a great chance for response to secondary therapy [129]. This is not true for prostate cancer, where second-line therapy is associated with modest results [130]. In any case, one should consider the addition of therapies that will slow down or prevent the progression of bone destruction in patients who are already offered

systemic antitumour treatment. Biphosphonates, agents that bind to the mineralised bone matrix, inhibiting osteoclast bone resorption, have been shown to reduce skeletal complications in patients with bone metastases [19,20]. Intravenous pamidronate is recommended in patients with metastatic breast cancer who have imaging evidence of lytic destruction of bone and who are receiving systemic hormonal therapy or chemotherapy [131]. Pamidronate use is also associated with pain relief in controlled trials, so it is recommended in women with pain due to osseous metastases from breast cancer [131]. Moreover, pamidronate was shown to reduce metastatic pain in a variety of other solid tumours, thus providing an important adjunct in the palliative care of patients with bone metastases [132].

REFERENCES

1. Rubens RD, Coleman RE. Bone metastases. In Abeloff MD, Armitage JO, Lichter AS, Niederhuber JE (eds), Clinical Oncology. Churchill Livingstone: New York, 1995: 643.
2. Walther HE. Krebsmetastasen. Bens Schwabe Verlag. Basel: Switzerland, 1948.
3. Weiss L. Comments on hematogenous metastatic patterns in humans as revealed by autopsy. Clin Exp Metast 1992; 10: 191.
4. Coleman RE, Rubens RD. The clinical course of bone metastases from breast cancer. Br J Cancer 1987; 55: 61.
5. Clinton K. Mortality rates by stage-at-diagnosis. Semin Surg Oncol 1994; 10: 7.
6. Scheid V, Buzdar AU, Smith TL et al. Clinical course of breast cancer patients with osseous metastases treated with combination chemotherapy. Cancer 1986; 58: 2589.
7. Lote K, Walloe A, Bjersand A. Bone metastasis. Prognosis, diagnosis and treatment. Acta Radiolol Oncol 1986; 25: 227.
8. Auerbach R, Lu WC, Pardon E et al. Specificity of adhesion between murine tumor cells and capillary endothelium: an *in vitro* correlate of preferential metastasis *in vivo*. Cancer Res 1987; 47: 1492.
9. Lam WC, Delicatny EJ, Orr FW et al. The chemotactic response of tumor cells: a model for cancer metastasis. Am J Pathol 1981; 104: 69.
10. Hauschka PV, Mavrakos AE, Iafrati MD et al. Growth factors in bone matrix. J Biol Chem 1986; 261: 12665.
11. Pfeilschifter J, Mundy GR. Modulation of transforming growth factor-β activity in bone cultures by osteotropic hormones. Proc Natl Acad Sci USA 1987; 84: 2024.
12. Bundred NJ, Walker RA, Ratcliffe WA et al. Parathyroid hormone related protein and skeletal morbidity in breast cancer. Eur J Cancer 1992; 28(2–3): 690.
13. Howell GJ, Southby J, Danks JA et al. Localization of parathyroid hormone-related protein in breast cancer metastasis: increased incidence in bone compared with other sites. Cancer Res 1991; 51: 3059.
14. Kiriyama T, Gillespie MT, Glatz JA et al. Transforming growth factor β stimulation of parathyroid hormone-

related protein (PTHrP): a paracrine regulator? Mol Cell Endocrinol 1992; 92: 55.

15. Wagner G. Frequency of pain in patients with cancer. Recent Results Cancer Res 1984; 89: 64.

16. Oda MAS, Schurman DJ. Monitoring of pathological fracture. In Stoll BA, Parbhoo S (eds), Bone Metastases: Monitoring and Treatment. Raven: New York, 1983.

17. Mundy GR. Bone resorption and turnover in health and disease. Bone 1987; 8(suppl 1): 9.

18. Rodriguez M, Dinapoli RP. Spinal cord compression with special reference to metastatic epidural tumors. Mayo Clin Proc 1980; 55: 442.

19. Hortobagyi GN, Theriault R, Porter L et al. Efficacy of pamidronate in reducing skeletal complications in patients with breast cancer and lytic bone metastases. N Engl J Med 1996; 335: 1785.

20. Lipton A, Theriault R, Leff R et al. Long-term reduction of skeletal complications in breast cancer patients with osteolytic bone metastases receiving hormone therapy, by monthly 90 mg pamidronate (Arredia™) infusions. Proc Am Soc Clin Oncol 1997; 16: 152a.

21. Berenson JR, Lichtenstein A, Porter L et al. Efficacy of pamidronate in reducing skeletal events in patients with advanced multiple myeloma. N Engl J Med 1996; 334: 488.

22. Sugimoto T, Shiba E, Watanabe T, Takai S. Suppression of parathyroid hormone-related protein messenger RNA expression by medroxyprogesterone acetate in breast cancer tissues. Breast Cancer Res Treat 1999; 56(1): 11.

23. Stoll BA. Hormonal therapy—pain relief and recalcification. In Stoll BA, Pabhoo S (eds), Bone Metastases: Monitoring and Treatment. Raven: New York, 1983; 321.

24. Miller AB, Hoogstraten B, Staquet M et al. Reporting results of cancer treatment. Cancer 1981; 47: 207.

25. Stewart J, King R, Hayward J, Rubens RD. Estrogen and progesterone receptors: correlation of response rates, site and timing of receptor analysis. Breast Cancer Res Treat 1982; 2: 242.

26. Aabo K. Prostate cancer: evaluation of response to treatment, response criteria, and need for standardization of the reporting results. Eur J Cancer Clin Oncol 1987; 23: 231.

27. Schroeder FH, EORTC GU-Group: treatment response criteria for prostate cancer. Prostate 1984; 5: 181.

28. Stoll BA. Endocrine Therapy in Malignant Disease. W. B. Saunders: London, 1972.

29. Patterson J, Furr B, Wakeling A, Battersby L. The biology and physiology of 'Nolvadex' (tamoxifen) in the treatment of breast cancer. Breast Cancer Res Treat 1982; 2: 363.

30. Hortobagyi GN. Bone metastases in breast cancer patients. Semin Oncol 1991; 18: 11.

31. Vogel CL, Schoenfelder J, Shemano I et al. Worsening bone scan in the evaluation of antitumor response during hormonal therapy of breast cancer. J Clin Oncol 1995; 13: 1123.

32. Muss HB. Endocrine therapy for advanced breast cancer: a review. Breast Cancer Res Treat 1992; 21: 15.

33. Santeen RJ, Manni A, Harvey H et al. Endocrine treatment of breast cancer in women. Endocr Rev 1990; 11: 221.

34. Pritchard KI, Sutherland DJA. Diagnosis and therapy of breast cancer: the use of endocrine therapy. Hematol Oncol Clin N Am 1989; 3: 765.

35. Allegra JC, Lippman ME, Thompson EB et al. Distribution, frequency, and quantitative analysis of estrogen, progesterone, androgen, and glucocorticoid receptors in human breast cancer. Cancer Res 1979; 39: 1447.

36. Stewart JF, King RJ, Sexton SA et al. Oestrogen receptors, sites of metastatic disease and survival in recurrent breast cancer. Eur J Cancer 1981; 17: 449.

37. Henderson IC. Endocrine therapy of metastatic breast cancer. In Harris JR, Hellman S, Henderson IC et al. (eds), Breast Diseases. Lippincott: Philadelphia, PA, 1991: 559.

38. Furr BA, Jordan VC. The pharmacology and clinical uses of tamoxifen. Pharmacol Ther 1984; 25: 127.

39. Manni A, Trujillo JE, Marshall JS et al. Antihormone treatment of stage IV breast cancer. Cancer 1979; 43: 444.

40. Rose C, Mouridsen HT. Treatment of advanced breast cancer with tamoxifen. Recent Results Cancer Res 1984; 91: 230.

41. Ingle JN, Mailliard JA, Schaid DJ et al. A double-blind trial of tamoxifen plus placebo in postmenopausal women with metastatic breast cancer. A collaborative trial of the North Central Cancer Treatment Group and Mayo Clinic. Cancer 1991; 68: 34.

42. Brule G. Co-operative clinical study of 178 patients treated with 'Nolvadex.' In The Hormonal Control of Breast Cancer. ICI Ltd, Pharmaceuticals Division: Ardsley Park, Macclesfeld, UK, 1978: 35.

43. Lerner HJ, Band PR, Israel L, Leung BS. Phase II study of tamoxifen: report of 74 patients with stage IV breast cancer. Cancer Treat Rep 1976; 60: 1431.

44. Kiang DT, Kennedy BJ. Tamoxifen (antiestrogen) therapy in advanced breast cancer. Ann Intern Med 1977; 87: 687.

45. Petru E, Schmahl D. On the role of additive hormone monotherapy with tamoxifen, medroxyprogesterone acetate and aminoglutethimide in advanced breast cancer. Klin Wochenschr 1987; 65: 959.

46. Sunderland MC, Osborne CK. Tamoxifen in premenopausal patients with metastatic breast cancer: a review. J Clin Oncol 1991; 9: 1283.

47. Margreiter R, Wiegele J. Tamoxifen (Nolvadex) for premenopausal patients with advanced breast cancer. Breast Cancer Res Treat 1984; 4: 45.

48. Ingle JN, Krook JE, Green SJ et al. Randomized trial of bilateral oophorectomy vs. tamoxifen in premenopausal women with metastatic breast cancer. J Clin Oncol 1986; 4: 178.

49. Buchanan RB, Blamey RW, Durrant KR et al. A randomized comparison of tamoxifen with surgical oophorectomy for premenopausal patients with advanced breast cancer. J Clin Oncol 1986; 4: 1326.

50. Hamm JT. Phase I and II studies of toremifene. Oncology 1997; 11(5, suppl 4): 19.

51. Valavaara R. Phase II trials with toremifene in advanced breast cancer: a review. Breast Cancer Res Treat 1990; 16(suppl): S31.

52. Hayes DF, Van Zyl JA, Hacking A et al. Randomized comparison of tamoxifen to two separate doses of toremifene in postmenopausal women with metastatic breast cancer. J Clin Oncol 1995; 13: 2556.

53. Gershanovich M, Garin A, Baltina D et al. Eastern European Study Group: a phase III comparison of two toremifene doses to tamoxifen in postmenopausal women with advanced breast cancer. Breast Cancer Res Treat 1997; 45(3): 251.

54. Pyrhonen S, Valavaara R, Mordig H. Comparison of toremifene and tamoxifen in postmenopausal patients with advanced breast cancer: a randomized double-blind, the Nordic phase III study. Br J Cancer 1997; 76(2): 270.

55. Rausching W, Pritchard KI. Droloxifene, a new anti-estrogen: its role in metastatic breast cancer. Breast Cancer Res Treat 1994; 31: 83.

56. Howel A, DeFriend D, Robertson J et al. Response to a specific antiestrogen (ICI 182,780) in tamoxifen-resistant breast cancer. Lancet 1995; 345: 29.

57. Muggia MF, Cassileth PA, Ochoa M et al. Treatment of breast cancer with medroxyprogesterone acetate. Ann Intern Med 1968; 68: 328.

58. Maatsson W. Current status of high dose progestin treatment in advanced breast cancer. Breast Cancer Res Treat 1983; 3: 231.

59. Pannuti F, Martoni A, Di Marco AR et al. Prospective randomized clinical trial of two different high dosages of medroxyprogesterone acetate (MPA) in the treatment of metastatic breast cancer. Eur J Cancer 1979; 15: 593.

60. Santeen RJ, Manni A, Harvey H et al. Endocrine treatment of breast cancer in women. Endocr Rev 1990; 11: 221.

61. Haller DG, Glick JH. Progestational agents in advanced breast cancer: an overview. Semin Oncol 1986; 13: 2.

62. Blackledge GRP, Latief T, Mould JJ et al. Phase II evaluation of megestrol acetate in previously treated patients with advanced breast cancer: relationship of response to previous treatment. Eur J Cancer Clin Oncol 1986; 22: 1091.

63. Ross MB, Buzdar AU, Blumenschien GR. Treatment of advanced breast cancer with megestrol acetate after therapy with tamoxifen. Cancer 1982; 49: 413.

64. Alexieva-Figusch J, Van Gilse HA, Hop WCJ et al. Progestin therapy in advanced breast cancer. Cancer 1980; 46: 2369.

65. Willemse P, Van Der Ploeg E, Sleijfer D et al. A randomized comparison of megestrol acetate (MA) and medroxyprogesterone acetate (MPA) in patients with advanced breast cancer. Eur J Cancer 1990; 26: 337.

66. Parazzini F, Colli E, Scatigna M, Tozzi L. Treatment with tamoxifen and progestins for metastatic breast cancer in postmenopausal women: a quantitative review of published randomized clinical trials. Oncology 1993; 50: 483.

67. Santen RJ. Suppression of estrogens with aminoglutethimide and hydrocortisone (medical adrenalectomy) as treatment of advanced breast carcinoma: a review. Breast Cancer Res Treat 1981; 1: 183.

68. Harris A, Powles T, Smith I. Aminoglutethimide in the treatment of advanced postmenopausal breast cancer. Cancer Res 1982; 42(suppl): 3405S.

69. Smith I, Fitzharris B, McKinna J et al. Aminoglutethimide in the treatment of metastatic breast carcinoma. Lancet 1978; 2: 646.

70. Kaye S, Woods R, Fox R et al. Use of aminoglutethimide as second-line endocrine therapy in metastatic breast cancer. Cancer Res 1992; 42(suppl): 3445S.

71. Cocconi G, Bisagni G, Ceci G et al. Low dose aminoglutethimide with and without hydrocortisone replacement as first-line endocrine treatment in advanced breast cancer: a prospective randomized trial of the Italian Oncology Group for Clinical Research. J Clin Oncol 1992; 10: 984.

72. Gale K, Andersen J, Tormey D et al. Hormonal treatment for metastatic breast cancer. An Eastern Cooperative Oncology Group Phase III trial comparing aminoglutethimide to tamoxifen. Cancer 1994; 73: 354.

73. Smith I, Harris A, Morgan M et al. Tamoxifen vs. aminoglutethimide in advanced breast carcinoma: a randomized cross-over trial. Br Med J 1981; 283: 1432.

74. Lipton A, Harvey H, Santen R et al. Randomized trial of aminoglutethimide vs. tamoxifen in metastatic breast cancer. Cancer Res 1982; 42(suppl): 3434S.

75. Canney PA, Priestman TJ, Griffiths T et al. Randomized trial comparing aminoglutethimide with high-dose medroxyprogesterone acetate in therapy for advanced breast carcinoma. J Natl Cancer Inst 1988; 80: 1147.

76. Lundgren S, Gundersen S, Klepp R et al. Megestrol acetate vs. aminoglutethimide for metastatic breast cancer. Breast Cancer Res Treat 1989; 14: 201.

77. Wiseman RL, McTavish D. Formestane: a review of its pharmacodynamic and pharmacokinetic properties and therapeutic potential in the management of breast cancer and prostate cancer. Drugs 1993; 45: 66.

78. Bajetta E, Zilembo N, Buzzoni R et al. Formestane: effective therapy in postmenopausal women with advanced breast cancer. Ann Oncol 1994; 5(suppl 7): S15.

79. Höffken K, Jonat W, Possinger K et al. Aromatase inhibition with 4-hydroxyandrostenodione in the treatment of postmenopausal patients with advanced breast cancer. J Clin Oncol 1990; 8: 875.

80. Perez Carrion R, Alberola Candel V, Calabresi F et al. Comparison of the selective aromatase inhibitor formestane with tamoxifen as first-line hormonal therapy in postmenopausal women with advanced breast cancer. Ann Oncol 1994; 5(suppl 7): 19.

81. Thürlimann B, Castiglione M, Hsu-Scmitz SF et al. Formestane vs. megestrol acetate in postmenopausal breast cancer patients after failure of tamoxifen: a phase III prospective randomized crossover trial of second-line hormonal treament (SAKK 20/90). Eur J Cancer 1997; 33: 1017.

82. Jones S, Belt R, Cooper B et al. A phase II study of antitumor efficacy and safety of exemestane (EXE) as second-line hormonal treatment of postmenopausal patients with metastatic breast cancer (MBC) refractory to tamoxifen (Tam). Breast Cancer Res Treat 1998; 50(abstr 436): 304.

83. Kvinnsland S, Anker G, Dirix LY et al. Activity of exemestane, an irreversible, oral, aromatase inhibitor in metastatic postmenopausal breast cancer patients (MBC) failing tamoxifen (TAM). Eur J Cancer 1998; 34(suppl 5, abstr 408): S91.

84. Thürlimann B, Paridaens R, Serin D et al. Third-line hormonal treatment with exemestane in postmenopausal patients with advanced breast cancer progressing on aminoglutethimide: a phase II multicentre multinational study. Eur J Cancer 1997; 33: 1767.

85. Kaufman M, Bajetta E, Dirix LY et al. Exemestane is superior to megestrol acetate after tamoxifen failure in postmenopausal women with advanced breast cancer:

results of a phase III randomized double-blind trial. J Clin Oncol 2000; 18: 1399.

86. Buzdar A, Jonat W, Howell A et al. Anastrozole vs. megestrol acetate in the treatment of postmenopausal women with advanced breast carcinoma: results of a survival update based on a combined analysis of data from two mature phase III trials. Cancer 1998; 83: 1142.

87. Robertson JF, Thürlimann B, Bonneterre J et al. Anastrozole (Arimidex) vs. tamoxifen as first-line therapy of advanced breast cancer in postmenopausal women—combined analysis from two identically designed multicenter trials. Proc Am Soc Clin Oncol 2000; 19(abstr): 609D.

88. Bisagni G, Cocconi G, Scaglione F et al. Letrozole, a new oral non-steroidal aromatase inhibitor in treating postmenopausal women with advanced breast cancer. A pilot study. Ann Oncol 1996; 7: 99.

89. Tominaga T, Ohashi Y, Abe R et al. Phase II trial of letrozole (a novel oral non-steroidal aromatase inhibitor) in postmenopausal patients with advanced or recurrent breast cancer. Eur J Cancer 1995; 31A: S81.

90. Dombernowsky P, Smith G, Falkson R et al. Letrozole, a new oral aromatase inhibitor for advanced breast cancer: double-blind randomized trial showing a dose effect and improved efficacy and tolerability compared with megestrol acetate. J Clin Oncol 1998; 16: 453.

91. Gershanovich M, Chaudri HA, Campos D et al. For the Letrozol International Group (AR/BC3). Letrozole, a new oral aromatase inhibitor: randomized trial comparing 2.5 mg daily, 0.5 mg daily and aminoglutethimide in postmenopausal women with advanced breast cancer. Ann Oncol 1998; 9: 639.

92. Mouridsen H, Perez-Carrion R, Becquart D et al. Letrozole (Femara) vs. tamoxifen: preliminary data of a first-line clinical trial in postmenopausal women with locally advanced or metastatic breast cancer. Eur J Cancer 2000; 36(suppl 5): S88.

93. Thürlimann B, Beretta K, Bacchi M et al. First-line fadrozole HCL (CGS-16949A) vs. tamoxifen in postmenopausal women with advanced breast cancer. Prospective randomized trial of the Swiss Group for Clinical Cancer Research SAKK 20/88. Ann Oncol 1996; 7: 471.

94. Buzdar KA, Smith R, Vogel C et al. Fadrozole HCL (CGS-16949A) vs. megestrol acetate treatment of postmenopausal patients with advanced breast carcinoma: results of two randomized double blind controlled multi-institutional trials. Cancer 1996; 77: 2503.

95. Muss HB. Endocrine treatment for advanced breast cancer: a review. Breast Cancer Res Treat 1992; 21: 15.

96. Ingle J, Ahman D, Green S et al. Randomized clinical trial of diethylstilbestrol vs. tamoxifen in postmenopausal women with advanced breast cancer. N Engl J Med 1981; 304: 16.

97. Beex L, Pieters G, Smals A et al. Tamoxifen vs. ethinyl estradiol in the treatment of postmenopausal women with advanced breast cancer. Cancer Treat Rep 1981; 65: 179.

98. Westerberg H. Tamoxifen and fluoxymesterone in advanced breast cancer: a controlled clinical trial. Cancer Treat Rep 1980; 64: 117.

99. Kaufmann M, Jonat W, Kleeberg U et al. Goreselin, a depot gonadotropin-releasing hormone agonist in the treatment of premenopausal patients with metastatic breast cancer. J Clin Oncol 1989; 7: 1113.

100. Saphner T, Troxel AB, Tormey DC et al. Phase II study of goreselin for postmenopausal patients with metastatic breast cancer. J Clin Oncol 1993; 11: 1529.

101. Ingle JN, Twito DI, Schaid DJ et al. Combination hormonal therapy with tamoxifen plus fluoxymesterone vs. tamoxifen alone in postmenopausal women with metastatic breast cancer. An updated analysis. Cancer 1991; 67: 886.

102. Tormey DC, Lippman ME, Edwards BK et al. Evaluation of tamoxifen doses with and without fluoxymesterone in advanced breast cancer. Ann Intern Med 1983; 98: 139.

103. Powles TJ, Ford HT, Nash AG et al. Treatment of disseminated breast cancer with tamoxifen, aminoglutethimide, hydrocortisone, and danazol, used in combination or sequentially. Lancet 1984; June: 1369.

104. Smith IE, Harris AL, Morgan M et al. Tamoxifen vs. aminoglutethimide vs. combined tamoxifen and aminoglutethimide in the treatment of advanced breast cancer. Cancer Res 1982; 42(suppl): 3430S.

105. Corkery J, Leonard RCF, Henderson IC et al. Tamoxifen and aminoglutethimide in advanced breast cancer. Cancer Res 1982; 42(suppl): 3409S.

106. Ingle JN, Green SJ, Ahmann DL et al. Randomized trial of tamoxifen alone or combined with aminoglutethimide and hydrocortisone in women with metastatic breast cancer. J Clin Oncol 1986; 4: 958.

107. Gill PG, Gebski V, Snyder R et al. Randomized comparison of the effects of tamoxifen, megestrol acetate, or tamoxifen plus megestrol acetate on treatment response and survival in patients with metastatic breast cancer. Ann Oncol 1993; 4: 741.

108. Scott WW, Menon M, Walsh PC. Hormonal therapy of prostate cancer. Cancer 1980; 45: 1929.

109. Smith JA. New methods of endocrine management of prostate cancer. J Urol 1987; 137: 1.

110. Scher HI, Shung LWK. Bone metastases: improving the therapeutic index. Semin Oncol 1994; 21: 630.

111. Macaluso MP, De Voogt HJ, Viggiano G et al. Comparison of diethylstilbestrol, cyproterone acetate and medroxyprogesterone acetate in the treatment of advanced prostatic cancer: final analysis of a randomized phase III trial of the European Organization for Research on Treatment of Cancer Urological Group. J Urol 1986; 136: 624.

112. Smith PH, Suciu S, Robinson MRG et al. A comparison of diethylstilbestrol with low dose estramustine phosphate in the treatment of advanced prostatic cancer: final analysis of a phase III trial of the European Organization for Research on Treatment of Cancer. J Urol 1986; 136: 619.

113. Leuprolide vs. diethylstilbestrol for metastatic prostate cancer. The leuprolide study group. N Engl J Med 1984; 311: 1281.

114. Goldenberg SL, Bruchovsky N. Use of cyproterone acetate in prostate cancer. Urol Clin N Am 1991; 18: 111.

115. Neuman F, Jacobo GE. Anti-androgens in tumor therapy. Clin Oncol 1982; 1: 41.

116. Vogelzang NJ, Chodak G, Soloway MS et al. Goreselin vs. orchiectomy in the treatment of advanced prostate cancer: final results of a randomized trial. Urology 1995; 46: 220.

117. Kaisary AV, Tyrell CJ, Peeling WB, Griffiths K. Comparison of LHRH analogue (Zoladex) with orchiectomy in patients with metastatic prostatic carcinoma. Br J Urol 1991; 67: 502.

118. Citrin DL, Resnick MI, Guinan P et al. Comparison of Zoladex R and DES in the treatment of advanced prostate cancer: results of a randomized multicenter trial. Prostate 1991; 18: 139.

119. Kuhn JM, Billebaud T, Navratil H et al. Prevention of the transient adverse events of gonadotropin-releasing hormone analogue (bureselin) in metastatic prostatic carcinoma by administration of an antiandrogen (nilutamide). N Engl J Med 1989; 321: 413.

120. Sogani PC, Vagaiwala MR, Whitmore WF. Experience with flutamide in patients with advanced prostate cancer without prior endocrine therapy. Cancer 1983; 54: 744.

121. Schellhammer P, Scharifi R, Block N et al. A controlled trial of bicalutamide vs. flutamide, each in combination with lutenizing hormone-releasing hormone analogue therapy in patients with advanced prostate cancer. Urology 1995; 45: 745.

122. Crawford ED, Eisenberger MA, McLoed DG et al. A controlled trial of leuprolide with and without flutamide in prostatic carcinoma. N Engl J Med 1989; 321: 419.

123. Janknegt RA, Abbou CC, Bartoleti R et al. Orchiectomy and nilutamide or placebo as treatment of metastatic prostate cancer in a multinational double-blind randomized trial. J Urol 1993; 149: 77.

124. Beland G, Elhiali M, Fradet Y et al. A controlled trial of castration with and without nilutamide in metastatic prostatic carcinoma. Cancer 1990; 66(suppl): 1074.

125. Iversen P, Rasmussen F, Klarskov P et al. Long-term results of Danish Prostatic Cancer Group Trial 86. Goreselin acetate plus flutamide vs. orchiectomy in advanced prostate cancer. Cancer 1993; 72: 3851.

126. Bertagna C, De Gery M, Hucher JP et al. Efficacy of the combination of nilutamide plus orchidectomy in patients with metastatic prostatic cancer. A meta-analysis of seven randomized double-blind trials (1056 patients). Br J Urol 1994; 73: 396.

127. Prostate Cancer Trialists' Collaborative Group. Maximum androgen blockade in advanced prostate cancer: an overview of 22 randomized trials with 3283 deaths in 5710 patients. Lancet 1995; 346: 265.

128. Eisenberger MA, Blumenstein BA, Crawford ED et al. Bilateral orchiectomy with or without flutamide for metastatic prostate cancer. N Engl J Med 1998; 339: 1036.

129. Wilson AJ. Response in breast cancer to a second hormonal therapy. Rev Endocr Rel Cancer 1983; 14: 5.

130. Sternberg C. Hormone refractory metastatic prostate cancer. Ann Oncol 1992; 3: 331.

131. American Society of Clinical Oncology Guideline on the role of biphosphonates in breast cancer. J Clin Oncol 2000; 18: 1378.

132. Purohit OP, Anthony C, Radstone CR et al. High dose intravenous pamidronate for metastatic bone pain. Br J Cancer 1994; 70: 554.

22

Overview of Osteoclast Inhibitors

J. J. Body

Institut Jules Bordet, Free University of Brussels, Brussels, Belgium

INTRODUCTION

The pathophysiology of tumour-induced osteolysis (TIO) explains why the introduction of osteoclast inhibitors in our therapeutic armamentarium for bone metastases has met with such success. Once cancer cells colonise the bone marrow, they are attracted to bone surfaces by products of resorbing bone and destroy bone via osteoclast stimulation. The importance of the direct osteolytic effects of metastatic cancer cells, including the effects of collagenases, remains unknown but is probably more important than currently recognised. We and others have shown a marked increase in bone resorption markers in normocalcaemic women with breast cancer and bone metastases [1]. Cancer cells essentially increase osteoclast differentiation of haematopoietic stem cells. An increased osteoclast number has been demonstrated in bone biopsies in a large series of women with breast cancer and predominantly lytic bone metastases, whether in bone adjacent to tumour cells or directly in the invaded bone [2]. Osteoblasts could also be important target cells for tumour secretory products. We have thus observed that breast cancer cells secrete factors that can inhibit the proliferation of human osteoblasts and increase their second messenger response to osteolytic agents and their production of osteolytic cytokines and of enzymes degrading the collagen matrix [3,4]. On the other hand, secretory products from cancer cells can induce osteoblast apoptosis [5]. Osteoblasts could thus keep in the process of TIO the central role that they have in the physiological regulation of osteoclast resorption activity.

The propensity of breast cancer cells to metastasise and proliferate in bone could be explained by a "seed and soil" concept [6]. Breast cancer cells (the "seed") appear to secrete factors, such as PTHrP, that potentiate the development of metastases in the skeleton, which constitutes a fertile "soil" rich in cytokines and growth factors that stimulates breast cancer cell growth. Local production of PTHrP and of other osteolytic factors by cancer cells in bone would stimulate osteoclastic bone resorption, partly through the osteoblasts and the immune cells. Such factors probably induce osteoclast differentiation from haematopoietic stem cells and could activate mature osteoclasts already present in bone. PTHrP also alters the ratio between osteoprotegerin (OPG), whose production is decreased, and RANKL (receptor activator for NF-κB ligand), whose production is increased [7]. The net result of this imbalance in these newly discovered and essential regulatory factors of osteoclast-mediated bone resorption is an increase in osteoclast proliferation and activity. Increased osteoclast number and activity would then cause local foci of osteolysis, an enhanced release of growth factors and a further stimulation of cancer cell proliferation [6,8].

A similar vicious cycle probably also exists for metastatic prostate cancer [9]. Collagen cross-link metabolites are also increased in patients with bone metastases from prostate cancer, underlining an increase in bone resorption even in blastic disease. Prostate cancer cells stimulate osteoclast activity, probably also through the osteoblasts [9].

Multiple myeloma is characterised by a marked increase in osteoclast activity and proliferation. This

Textbook of Bone Metastases. Edited by C. Jasmin, R. E. Coleman, L. R. Coia, R. Capanna and G. Saillant
© 2005 John Wiley & Sons Ltd: ISBN 0 471 87742 5

excessive resorption of bone probably stimulates the growth of myeloma cells in bone through the release of growth factors from resorbed bone matrix and the secretion of interleukin-6 (IL-6) by the bone microenvironment. Using established cell lines, it has been shown that through direct cell-to-cell contact, myeloma cells can downregulate osteocalcin production but upregulate IL-6 secretion, supporting the concept of the importance of the bone microenvironment in the genesis of myeloma-induced osteolysis [10].

There are significantly fewer data for bone metastases from other cancers, but the findings summarised above indicate that bone-resorbing cells are a logical target for the treatment, and probably also the prevention, of TIO. Currently, osteoclast inhibitors essentially comprise the bisphosphonates. Other molecules will be briefly reviewed thereafter.

INDICATIONS FOR BISPHOSPHONATES

Bisphosphonates localise preferentially to sites of active bone remodelling. They can act directly on mature osteoclasts, decreasing their bone resorption activity, notably by lowering H^+ and Ca^{++} extrusion and modifying the activity of various enzymes [11]. Nitrogen-containing bisphosphonates, which are the compounds most often used in the clinic, interfere with the mevalonate pathway. This leads to an inhibition of post-translational prenylation of proteins with farnesyl or geranylgeranyl isoprenoid groups [12]. Various cellular proteins must be anchored to the cell membrane by a prenyl group to be active. Most of these proteins are GTP-binding proteins, including the protein Ras, and it is known that prenylated proteins are essential for osteoclast function, notably cell activity and attachment. This inhibition will eventually lead to osteoclast apoptosis. Moreover, at least *in vitro*, bisphosphonates can induce the death of breast cancer [13] and myeloma [14] cells. Such effects could, theoretically at least, contribute to the beneficial role of bisphosphonates in the prevention and treatment of TIO.

Table 22.1 summarises the author's opinion on the various indications of commercially available bisphosphonates in cancer patients.

Tumour-induced Hypercalcaemia (TIH)

Bisphosphonates are indicated for hypercalcaemia complicating all tumour types even though, in some instances, other compounds can be quite active, such as glucocorticoids for hypercalcaemia complicating multiple myeloma and most lymphomas. Rehydration has generally mild and transient effects on calcium levels, effecting a median decrease of only 1 mg/dl [15], but it improves the clinical status and interrupts the vicious cycle of TIH by inhibiting the increased tubular reabsorption of calcium. Rehydration should be combined with bisphosphonate therapy and administered according to the hydration status of the patient.

The superiority of pamidronate over clodronate in patients with TIH has been demonstrated in a randomised trial involving 41 patients, not significantly so in terms of success rate, but well in the duration of normocalcaemia. The median duration of action of clodronate was indeed 14 days compared with 28 days for pamidronate [16]. Large studies indicate that a dose of 90 mg achieves normocalcaemia in >90% of patients [17]. The response to lower doses of pamidronate will, however, be less in patients with humoral hypercalcaemia of malignancy compared with

Table 22.1. Indications for bisphosphonates in cancer patients—practical recommendations

1. TUMOUR-INDUCED HYPERCALCAEMIA
   (=Standard therapy) Clodronate 1500 mg over 4+ h <pamidronate 90 mg over 2+ h <ibandronate 4–6 mg over 2 h ? ?<zoledronic acid 4–8 mg over 15 min
2. METASTATIC BONE PAIN (NON-MECHANICAL)
   Analgesic effects in ≥50% of the patients with breast (and prostate?) cancer. Recommended scheme: 4 mg zoledronic acid every 3–4 weeks or 90 mg of pamidronate or 6 mg of ibandronate. ? Higher doses for patients who keep an abnormal bone resorption rate?
3. PREVENTION OF THE COMPLICATIONS OF TUMOUR BONE DISEASE
   - *Breast cancer.* At the diagnosis of symptomatic metastatic bone disease (ASCO guidelines), or when there is a lytic or a mixed metastatic lesion in weight-bearing bones, or in cases of symptomatic or multiple metastases after failure of a first-line antineoplastic therapy (4 mg zoledronic acid or 6 mg of ibandronate every 3–4 weeks or oral ibandronate 50 mg/day or oral clodronate 1600 mg/day; see text). For long-term treatment, 90 mg pamidronate is inferior to 4 mg of zoledronic acid
   - *Multiple myeloma* (stages II and III). For all patients at the time of diagnosis of lytic disease (4 mg of zoledronic acid, or 90 mg pamidronate every 3–4 weeks, or oral clodronate 1600 mg/day)
   - *Prostate cancer.* 4 mg zoledronic acid every 3–4 weeks, probably for all patients with bone metastases and hormone-refractory prostate cancer
4. PREVENTION OF BONE METASTASES
   Currently only as part of a clinical trial, although data with clodronate are extremely encouraging

patients with bone metastases, as the importance of PTHrP will become more evident [18].

Pamidronate is well tolerated, the only clinically detectable side-effect being transient fever and a flu-like syndrome in about a quarter of cases. Oral clodronate is often prescribed after successful intravenous therapy but the efficacy of this strategy has not been systematically examined.

The newer bisphosphonates, ibandronate and especially zoledronic acid, achieve better results than pamidronate for patients with severe hypercalcaemia. Two pooled, randomised, double-blind, double-dummy trials in 275 evaluable patients with moderate or severe TIH (corrected Ca $\geqslant 12\,mg/dl = 3.0\,mmol/l$) compared zoledronic acid, administered either as a 5 min 4 mg infusion or as a 5 min 8 mg infusion, to pamidronate (90 mg over 2 h). As a whole, zoledronic acid was more efficient than pamidronate. At day 10, success rates (corrected Ca $\leqslant 10.8\,mg/dl = 2.7\,mmol/l$) were 88%, 87% and 70% for the three groups, respectively [19]. The difference, however, was not impressive in patients with bone metastases (success rates of 90%, 84% and 80%, respectively) but quite marked in patients without bone metastases (success rates of 87%, 90% and 61%, respectively). There was no significant difference in the success rates between the two doses of zoledronic acid [19].

There is no consensus on the need to treat asymptomatic patients with Ca levels $< 3.0\,mmol/l$ [20]. However, symptoms of mild TIH often go unrecognised in patients with advanced cancer and serum Ca can rise quite rapidly. More importantly, TIH development is an adverse prognostic sign in patients with bone metastases and indicates that it is already quite late to start bisphosphonate therapy!

Metastatic Bone Pain

Pain is the most common symptom of bone metastases and can dramatically affect the quality of life of cancer patients. Bisphosphonates are useful for localised bone pain that can no longer be treated by radiotherapy, or in cases of widespread painful metastatic lesions. The current opinion is that the intravenous route has to be selected in such cases, and the relative inability of first-generation oral bisphosphonates to reduce metastatic bone pain has recently been confirmed in a placebo controlled study of oral clodronate after a median study time of almost 2 months in patients with progressing bone metastases [21]. To obtain optimal analgesic effects, the intravenous route is the route of choice, at least until more potent and well-tolerated oral bisphosphonates, such as ibandronate are widely available [22].

Short-term placebo-controlled trials have confirmed that both clodronate and pamidronate, given intravenously, can exert significant and rapid analgesic effects [23]. Bone pain relief seems to occur in about half of the patients treated with repeated pamidronate infusions [22]. In 62 evaluable patients, mostly with breast cancer or myeloma, there was no difference in the analgesic response between doses of 60 and 90 mg of pamidronate [24]. The response was essentially observed in patients with moderate or severe bone pain, and most of the effect was obtained after only two infusions, which suggests that further administrations are useless in non-responders, at least for that purpose [25]. However, other recent data suggest that such non-responding patients should perhaps be treated with higher doses. The optimal dose actually remains to be defined, especially since it is probably a function of the disease stage. Some data indicate that specific markers of bone matrix resorption, such as NTx, correlate with the analgesic effects of pamidronate and follow a similar time course [26]. However, we were not able to confirm these findings in an open "high dose" ($4 \times 4\,mg$) study of intravenous ibandronate in patients with severe metastatic bone pain [27]. A high rate of bone resorption could nevertheless be one of the factors underlying "resistance" to bisphosphonates, at least concerning their analgesic effects. A high-dose "intensive" regimen could lead to better results [27] but the efficacy of such high-dose regimens has yet to be tested in double-blind trials.

The role of bisphosphonates as an alternative or an adjunct to radiotherapy requires further study [28]. The optimal combination or sequencing of radiotherapy or radioisotopes with bisphosphonates has not been studied either.

Reduction of the Skeletal Morbidity Rate in Patients with Tumour Bone Disease

Breast Cancer

Placebo-controlled trials with oral or intravenous bisphosphonates have shown that their prolonged administration can reduce by one quarter to one half the frequency of skeletal-related events (SREs) in patients with bone metastases from breast cancer and in patients with multiple myeloma. Detailed results are reviewed in the following chapters and only a brief overview and some general considerations are given here.

Two large-scale studies in patients with breast cancer metastatic to the skeleton, one with clodronate and one with pamidronate, indicate that the administration of oral bisphosphonates until death can reduce the frequency of SREs. The clodronate study was randomised, double-blind, placebo-controlled, and included 173 patients with breast cancer metastatic to bone. In the clodronate-treated group (1600 mg/day), there was a significant reduction in the incidence of hypercalcaemic episodes, number of vertebral fractures and rate of vertebral deformities. The combined rate of all morbid skeletal events was reduced by 28% [29]. Three randomised studies of regular pamidronate infusions are available in patients with breast cancer and bone metastases [30–32]. An open trial comparing low doses of pamidronate (infusions of 45 mg every 3 weeks) plus standard first-line chemotherapy or chemotherapy alone showed that pamidronate increased by almost 50% the median time to progression in bone [30]. Two double-blind randomised placebo-controlled trials, comparing 90 mg pamidronate infusions every 4 weeks to placebo infusions for up to 2 years, in addition to chemo- or hormonotherapy, in large series of breast cancer patients with at least one lytic bone metastasis indicate that bisphosphonates can reduce the skeletal morbidity rate by more than one-third, increase the median time to the occurrence of the first SRE by almost 50% and reduce the proportion of patients having any skeletal-related event [31,32]. There were also favourable effects on quality of life and, at the end of the evaluation, there was a significant decrease in the pain score. The results were more impressive in the chemotherapy trial than in the hormone therapy trial, probably because the skeletal disease was more aggressive at the beginning of the trial.

Results with newer, more potent bisphosphonates have recently been made available. The largest multicentre trial with zoledronic acid was randomised, double-blind and compared 4 or 8 mg zoledronic acid to 90 mg pamidronate every 3–4 weeks for up to 2 years in the treatment of osteolytic lesions in breast cancer ($n=1130$) and in multiple myeloma ($n=510$). The primary efficacy endpoint was the proportion of patients experiencing at least one SRE over 13 months [33]. Zoledronic acid was initially infused over 5 min but, because of an unacceptably high incidence of elevations in serum creatinine, the infusion time was prolonged to 15 min. Zoledronic acid 8 mg was not more effective than the 4 mg dose level but was associated with an increased frequency of renal adverse events, explaining why all patients in that treatment arm were switched to the lower dose of zoledronic acid

during the trials. The proportion of patients with at least one SRE was similar in all treatment groups (46%, 44% and 46% for zoledronic acid 8/4 mg, zoledronic acid 4 mg and pamidronate, respectively). The pre-established criterion for non-inferiority of zoledronic acid to pamidronate was thus met. Median time to first SRE was approximately 1 year in all treatment groups and SMRs were also not significantly different. There was, however, a trend for a lower skeletal morbidity rate in the zoledronic acid groups. This was confirmed in the recently presented 2 year data when, using a combined event analysis, the superiority of zoledronic acid over pamidronate was shown in breast cancer. The short infusion time (15 min as compared to 2-h for pamidronate), which offers a quite convenient therapy, nevertheless remains the most evident advantage of zoledronic acid for the patients [33,34]. Repeated 6 mg ibandronate infusions are also efficient to significantly reduce the skeletal morbidity rate of bone metastases from breast cancer ($p=0.004$ vs. placebo). Ibandronate (6 mg) also significantly reduced the number of new bone events (by 38%) and increased time to first new bone event. There was also a decrease in bone pain scores and in analgesic use. Treatment with ibandronate was well tolerated [35].

Criteria for when in the course of metastatic bone disease from breast cancer bisphosphonates should be started and stopped remain poorly determined. According to the ASCO guidelines, i.v. pamidronate 90 mg, delivered over 1–2 h every 3–4 weeks, is to be recommended in patients with metastatic breast cancer who have imaging evidence of lytic destruction of bone and who are concurrently receiving systemic therapy with hormonal therapy or chemotherapy [28]. Furthermore, the Panel considered it "reasonable" to start i.v. bisphosphonates in women with abnormal bone scan with localised pain and normal plain radiographs, but not if the abnormal bone scan is asymptomatic. The same can certainly now be said for ibandronate and zoledronic acid in place of pamidronate, especially since the treatment is more easily accepted by the patients. These recommendations are certainly valid in view of the available data and can be endorsed, but they can also be criticised by at least three arguments. First, the cost-effectiveness of an extensive and early use of bisphosphonates has not been established. A *post hoc* evaluation of the cost-effectiveness of the two double-blind pamidronate trials led to the conclusion that the costs of pamidronate therapy were higher than the cost savings from prevented SREs. However, the limitations of this evaluation are evident, since the figures were based on a model evaluating a hypothetical group of women and the costs only apply to the USA (e.g. $US 775 for each pamidronate course). Thus, for example, if the drug costs were reduced by 50%, the pamidronate strategy would then become dominant in the same evaluated model [36]. This study actually essentially underlines the need for prospective cost-effectiveness assessments [37]! Second, measures to reduce morbidity from skeletal involvement by breast cancer are evidently essential for optimising a patient's quality of life but, to take a common situation, it is not certain that monthly bisphosphonate infusions in a patient with asymptomatic osteolytic lesion(s) in non-weight-bearing bones, and who will receive a first-line endocrine therapy with at least a 50% chance of a durable response, will actually not alter her quality of life by such an intense therapeutic approach. Again, detailed prospective assessments of the quality of life are lacking. Third, the risk of an excessive anti-osteolytic therapy is often evoked. The possibility of a "frozen bone" with the prolonged use of potent bisphosphonates is still a matter of debate in the "bone community"! Mashiba et al. have recently reported that the administration for 1 year of high doses of alendronate (1 mg/kg/day orally) or of risedronate (0.5 mg/kg/day orally) in dogs did not impair mineralisation but significantly increased microdamage accumulation (by 322% for alendronate and 155% for risedronate). Bone toughness (i.e. its ability to absorb energy or sustain deformation without breaking) declined significantly. Both microdamage accumulation and reduced toughness were significantly related to the suppression of bone turnover [38]. So far, this is only a theoretical concern but it should at least be kept in mind. For the time being, I would certainly recommend starting bisphosphonates immediately when there is lytic or mixed metastatic bone disease in weight-bearing bones, when the bone disease appears to be "aggressive", or in cases of symptomatic or multiple metastases, or after failure of a first-line antineoplastic therapy (see Table 22.1). Patients who have dominant visceral disease should probably not start bisphosphonate therapy unless they have severe uncontrolled bone pain. In any case, whatever the recommendations, clinical judgement fortunately remains essential and therapy has to be adapted to the individual patient!

Because bisphosphonates are providing supportive care, reducing the rate of skeletal morbidity but evidently not abolishing it, criteria for stopping their administration have to be different from those used for classical antineoplastic drugs and they should not be stopped when metastatic bone disease is progressing. The ASCO panel suggested that, once initiated, i.v. bisphosphonates should be continued until there is evidence of substantial decline in a patient's general performance status [28]. However, criteria are lacking to determine if and how long an individual patient benefits from their administration, and the decision to continue or stop bisphosphonate therapy, or possibly increase their dosage, remains essentially empirical. New biochemical markers of bone resorption might help to identify those patients continuing to benefit from therapy and those in whom bisphosphonate dosage may actually have to be increased as the biochemical response seems to predict for the likelihood of SREs [39]. The benefits of such an attitude have not, however, been demonstrated, but this could be relatively easily determined by a large-scale prospective trial.

The combination of occasional poor tolerance from gastrointestinal side-effects and the low absorption of oral bisphosphonates, implying the need for high doses and to swallow large capsules, at least for clodronate, remains an obstacle, especially in advanced cancer patients. As summarised above, the results obtained with the intravenous route are also more impressive than those obtained with oral clodronate but this could no longer be the case with oral ibandronate. However, the choice between the oral and the intravenous route depends on individual circumstances. For example, the oral route will be preferred for many patients on hormonal therapy, especially if the bone disease is not rapidly evolving. At the other extreme, for an aggressive osteolytic disease, the choice is often the intravenous route.

Multiple Myeloma

Multiple myeloma is typically characterised by an extensive osteolytic process with bone fractures, even when the neoplasm is responding to chemotherapy [40]. Randomised placebo-controlled trials have demonstrated that bisphosphonates are of great benefit for myeloma patients. Clodronate at 1600 mg given daily from the time of diagnosis was shown to reduce the skeletal complication rate when the effects of chemotherapy wore off. At the time of disease progression, there were fewer patients with increased back pain or deterioration in performance status and fewer new vertebral fractures after the first year [41]. The efficacy of monthly 90 mg pamidronate infusions in myeloma has also been demonstrated in a double-blind placebo-controlled trial including almost 400 patients with at least one osteolytic lesion. The proportion of patients developing a skeletal-related event was significantly smaller in the pamidronate than in the placebo group (24% vs. 41%). The mean morbidity rate was reduced by almost half. Quality of life score, performance status, pain score, incidence of pathological fractures and the need for radiotherapy were all favourably affected by bisphosphonate therapy [42]. Interestingly, vertebral fractures were significantly reduced by pamidronate therapy but the rate of non-vertebral fractures was not significantly affected, consistent with a better effect of bisphosphonates on trabecular than on cortical bone. However, I would suggest that the lack of systematic calcium supplementation could have a deleterious effect on bone turnover and repair of microfractures after such a long term suppression of bone turnover. The recently performed comparative trial between zoledronic acid and pamidronate has demonstrated the non-inferiority of the former compound [33].

These different trials clearly indicate that bisphosphonates in addition to chemotherapy are superior to chemotherapy alone for multiple myeloma. It is true that optimal therapeutic schemes remain unknown, that more cost–benefit analyses should be performed, but it can reasonably be stated that bisphosphonate treatment should now be considered for all patients with multiple myeloma at diagnosis. Bisphosphonates should probably be used very early in all patients, not only because of their beneficial skeletal effects, but also because they may slow tumour growth [43].

Other Neoplasms

Although skeletal metastases from prostate cancer are typically osteoblastic, histomorphometric and biochemical studies have shown unequivocal evidence for an increase in bone resorption. The analgesic effect of bisphosphonates has been shown in several open trials with pamidronate or newer bisphosphonates. A placebo-controlled trial has recently been conducted in 773 patients with hormone-refractory prostate cancer [44]. The therapeutic schemes of zoledronic acid used similar doses as for the breast/myeloma trial, and the primary endpoint, i.e. the proportion of patients with at least one SRE, was indeed reached (44% in the placebo group vs. 33% in the zoledronic acid group; $p=0.02$). The time to the first SRE was significantly longer for the zoledronic acid 4 mg dose group as compared to placebo. Interestingly, there were significantly fewer patients with pathological fractures in the zoledronic acid 4 mg dose group (13%) than in the placebo group (22%) and pain increased more in the placebo group. Bisphosphonates are now a new

therapeutic tool for managing prostate cancer patients with bone metastases, especially when they are hormone-refractory [45].

Lastly, in a similar placebo-controlled trial in patients with lung cancer and other solid tumours, zoledronic acid has been shown to significantly decrease the incidence of skeletal-related events [46]. Publication of full results of this important trial was not available at the time of writing.

Perspectives

Prevention of Bone Metastases in Breast Cancer

Another potentially major role for bisphosphonates is the prevention, or at least a delay in, the development of bone metastases. Several studies in animal models of bone metastases support this exciting concept [47]. In a randomised open trial involving about 300 patients with primary breast cancer and tumour cells in the bone marrow, which is an adverse risk factor for the development of metastases, it was shown that 1600 mg clodronate daily for 2 years reduced the number of bone as well as non-bone metastases by about 50% after a median follow-up of 36 months [48]. Another non-placebo-controlled trial has not confirmed these data [49]. However, a recent double-blind placebo-controlled trial involving more than 1000 breast cancer patients after surgery indicates that a 2 year treatment with 1600 mg clodronate daily can indeed reduce the incidence of bone metastases by about one-half and prolong survival [50]. Even if preventive therapy with bisphosphonates will also have the additional beneficial effect of preventing postmenopausal osteoporosis, the use of bisphosphonates in the adjuvant setting still has to be viewed as experimental, because at least one confirmatory trial appears to be mandatory. It will be equally important to determine who are the patients at high risk of developing bone metastases before recommending a general primary preventive use of bisphosphonates. Classical prognostic factors, such as tumour size, axillary node involvement and receptor status, but also expression of PTHrP or other factors by the tumour cells, could be relevant, for that matter.

Preventive therapy with bisphosphonates will also have the additional beneficial effect of preventing postmenopausal osteoporosis in a population of women for whom oestrogen replacement therapy is avoided.

Direct Antitumour Effects

It has recently been shown that bisphosphonates can directly induce cancer cell death. It was first shown that aminobisphosphonates, much more than clodronate, can induce apoptosis in human myeloma cell lines, suggesting that some bisphosphonates could have direct antitumour effects on human myeloma cells *in vivo* [51]. This induction of apoptosis in human myeloma cell lines probably occurs by inhibiting the mevalonate pathway, just as in the osteoclasts [52]. Zoledronic acid was also shown to be able to induce apoptosis in myeloma cells. The clinical relevance of these findings remains to be demonstrated, as concentrations as high as 10^{-4} M are needed, but bisphosphonate concentrations under the resorption lacunae are probably of the same order of magnitude or even higher [53]. Moreover, preliminary results suggest that pamidronate alone could induce myeloma cell apoptosis in patients [54].

Similar *in vitro* effects appear to be true for breast and prostate cancer cells. We have recently shown that several bisphosphonates can indeed inhibit the growth of both MCF-7 and T47D cell lines in a time- and dose-dependent manner (from 10^{-8} M for ibandronate and zoledronate). Cancer cell death was due to a combination of apoptosis and necrosis but apoptotic effects were preponderant for MCF-7 and PC-3 cells [13]. Again, the relevance of these *in vitro* observations to the clinical efficacy of bisphosphonates remains to be demonstrated, but a direct inhibitory effect of bisphosphonates on cancer cell growth could evidently contribute to their beneficial effects.

Prolongation of Survival

In the double-blind placebo-controlled pamidronate trials, survival was longer in patients < 50 years old in the pamidronate group, as compared to the placebo group. In the ibandronate trial mentioned above, a similar prolongation of survival has been observed in patients who had bone and non-bone metastases, as compared to the group of patients with bone metastases only. A prolongation of survival has also been reported in myeloma patients receiving pamidronate and second or subsequent lines of chemotherapy. The results of such *post-hoc* analyses have evidently to be taken with extreme caution, but they are concordant and survival prologation should now be one of the endpoints in all trials conducted with the new bisphosphonates, whether in the adjuvant or in the therapeutic setting.

OTHER OSTEOCLAST INHIBITORS

Calcitonin

Calcitonin is widely prescribed for its analgesic activity in osteoporotic crush fractures, but its efficacy in the setting of metastatic bone disease has been most often evaluated in uncontrolled trials. The results of the two main randomised double-blind trials are contradictory, even concerning the effects on bone pain [55,56].

Osteoprotegerin

Osteoprotegerin (OPG) is a potent downregulator of osteoclast formation and activity. It is a TNF receptor family member that acts as a decoy receptor for RANK ligand (RANKL; also named osteoclast differentiation factor, ODF). OPG prevents tumour-induced osteoclastogenesis and osteolytic bone destruction in animal models of bone metastases [57]. OPG acts more rapidly than pamidronate in an animal model of cancer hypercalcaemia and produces a more profound reduction in osteoclast surface [58]. A Phase I study with a recombinant OPG construct has been conducted in patients with myeloma or breast cancer metastatic to bone. A single injection caused a rapid, sustained, dose-dependent decrease in NTX levels, which was at least comparable to the profile observed after an infusion of 90 mg pamidronate. Doses of 1–3 mg/kg appeared to be appropriate for further longer-term studies [59]. Another Phase I trial with an antiserum against RANKL is being conducted with the same objective, to block the RANK–RANKL pathway.

Therapeutic Agents in Pre-clinical Development

Osteoclast attachment to bone is mediated through cell surface adhesion receptors called integrins, which can be viewed as extracellular matrix receptors. One of these is the vitronectin receptor, which is known to play a role in the attachment of osteoclasts to the resorption surface on the bone matrix. This adhesion receptor recognises arginyl-glycyl-aspartyl (RGD)-containing matrix proteins (e.g. bone sialoprotein). Antagonists of vitronectin receptors and soluble peptides containing RGD sequences which can block osteoclast attachment to bone are being developed by major pharmaceutical companies. Vitronectin receptor antagonists have already been shown to be able to inhibit bone loss in ovariectomised rats [60]. The osteoclast proton pump is another target, as well as peptidomimetic inhibitors of osteoclast proteases, such as cathepsin K. It is evident that further fundamental research and studies in animal models will be essential to develop our therapeutic armamentarium against the devastating consequences of tumour bone disease.

REFERENCES

1. Body JJ, Dumon JC, Gineyts E, Delmas PD. Comparative evaluation of markers of bone resorption in patients with breast cancer-induced osteolysis before and after bisphosphonate therapy. Br J Cancer 1997; 75: 408–12.
2. Taube T, Elomaa I, Blomqvist C et al. Histomorphometric evidence for osteoclast-mediated bone resorption in metastatic breast cancer. Bone 1994; 15: 161–6.
3. Siwek B, Lacroix M, de Pollak C et al. Secretory products of breast cancer cells affect human osteoblastic cells: partial characterization of active factors. J Bone Min Res 1997; 12: 552–60.
4. Lacroix M, Marie PJ, Body JJ. Protein production by osteoblasts: modulation by breast cancer cell-derived factors. Breast Cancer Res Treat 2000; 61: 59–67.
5. Fromigué O, Kheddoumi N, Lomri A et al. Breast cancer cells release factors that induce apoptosis in human bone marrow stromal cells. J Bone Min Res 2001; 16: 1600–10.
6. Mundy GR. Mechanisms of bone metastasis. Cancer 1997; 80: 1546–56.
7. Hofbauer LC. Osteoprotegerin ligand and osteoprotegerin: novel implications for osteoclast biology and bone metabolism. Eur J Endo 1999; 141: 195–210.
8. Lacroix M, Siwek B, Marie PJ, Body JJ. Production of interleukin-11 by breast cancer cells. Cancer Lett 1998; 127: 29–35.
9. Goltzman D, Rabbani SA. Pathogenesis of osteoblastic metastases. In Body JJ (ed.), Tumor Bone Diseases and Osteoporosis in Cancer Patients. Marcel Dekker: New York, 2000: 71–84.
10. Barillé S, Collette M, Bataille R, Amiot M. Myeloma cells upregulate interleukin-6 secretion in osteoblastic cells through cell-to-cell contact but downregulate osteocalcin. Blood 1995; 86: 3151–9.
11. Zimolo Z, Wesolowski G, Rodan GA. Acid extrusion is induced by osteoclast attachment to bone. Inhibition by alendronate and calcitonin. J Clin Invest 1995; 96: 2277–83.
12. Luckman SP, Hughes DE, Coxon FP et al. Nitrogen-containing bisphosphonates inhibit the mevalonate pathway and prevent post-translational aprenylation of GTP-binding proteins, including ras. J Bone Min Res 1998; 13: 581–9.
13. Fromigué O, Lagneaux L, Body JJ. Bisphosphonates induce breast cancer cell death *in vitro*. J Bone Min Res 2000; 15: 2211–21.
14. Derenne S, Amiot M, Barille S et al. Zoledronate is a potent inhibitor of myeloma cell growth and secretion of IL-6 and MMP-1 by the tumoral environment. J Bone Min Res 1999; 14: 2048–56.
15. Singer FR, Ritch PS, Lad TE et al. Treatment of hypercalcemia of malignancy with intravenous etidronate. A controlled, multicenter study. Arch Intern Med 1991; 151: 471–6.
16. Purohit OP, Radstone CR, Anthony C et al. A randomised double-blind comparison of intravenous pamidronate and clodronate in the hypercalcaemia of malignancy. Br J Cancer 1995; 72: 1289–93.
17. Body JJ, Dumon JC. Treatment of tumor-induced hypercalcaemia with the bisphosphonate pamidronate: dose–response relationship and influence of the tumour type. Ann Oncol 1994; 5: 359–63.
18. Walls J, Ratcliffe WA, Howell A, Bundred NJ. Response to intravenous bisphosphonate therapy in hypercalcaemic patients with and without bone metastases: the role of parathyroid hormone-related protein. Br J Cancer 1994; 70: 169–72.
19. Major P, Lortholary A, Hon J et al. Zoledronic acid is superior to pamidronate in the treatment of hypercalcemia of malignancy: a pooled analysis of two randomized, controlled clinical trials. J Clin Oncol 2001; 19: 558–67.
20. Body JJ, Bartl R, Burckhardt P et al. for the International Bone and Cancer Study Group. Current use of bisphosphonates in oncology. Journal of Clinical Oncology 1998; 16: 3890–9.
21. Robertson AG, Reed NS, Ralston SH. Effect of oral clodronate on metastatic bone pain: a double-blind, placebo-controlled study. J Clin Oncol 1995; 13: 2427–30.
22. Body JJ, Coleman RE, Piccart M. Use of bisphosphonates in cancer patients. Cancer Treat Rev 1996; 22: 265–87.
23. Ernst DS, Brasher P, Hagen N et al. E. A randomized, controlled trial of intravenous clodronate in patients with metastatic bone disease and pain. J Pain Symptom Manag 1997; 13: 319–26.
24. Koeberle D, Bacchus L, Thuerlimann B, Senn HJ. Pamidronate treatment in patients with malignant osteolytic bone disease and pain: a prospective randomized double-blind trial. Support Care Cancer 1999; 7: 21–7.
25. Body JJ. Bisphosphonates for metastatic bone pain. Support Care Cancer 1999; 7: 1–3.
26. Vinholes JJF, Purohit OP, Abbey ME et al. Relationships between biochemical and symptomatic response in a double-blind randomised trial of pamidronate for metastatic bone disease. Ann Oncol 1997; 8: 1243–50.
27. Mancini I, Dumon JC, Body JJ. Efficacy and safety of ibandronate in the treatment of opioid-resistant bone pain associated with metastatic bone disease: a pilot study. J Clin Oncol 2004; 22(17): 3582–92.
28. Hillner BE, Ingle JN, Berenson JR et al. American Society of Clinical Oncology guideline on the role of bisphosphonates in breast cancer. American Society of Clinical Oncology Bisphosphonates Expert Panel. J Clin Oncol 2000; 18: 1378–91.
29. Paterson AHG, Powles TJ, Kanis JA et al. Double-blind controlled trial of oral clodronate in patients with bone metastases from breast cancer. J Clin Oncol 1993; 11: 59–65.
30. Conte PF, Latreille J, Mauriac L et al. Delay in progression of bone metastases in breast cancer patients treated with intravenous pamidronate: results from a

multinational randomised controlled trial. J Clin Oncol 1996; 14: 2552–9.

31. Theriault RL, Lipton A, Hortobagyi GN et al. for the Protocol 18 Aredia Breast Cancer Study Group. Pamidronate reduces skeletal morbidity in women with advanced breast cancer and lytic bone lesions: a randomized, placebo-controlled trial. J Clin Oncol 1999; 17: 846–54.

32. Hortobagyi GN, Theriault RL, Lipton A et al. for the Protocol 19 Aredia Breast Cancer Study Group. Long-term prevention of skeletal complications of metastatic breast cancer with pamidronate. J Clin Oncol 1998; 16: 2038–44.

33. Rosen LS, Gordon D, Antonio BS et al. Zoledronic acid vs. pamidronate in the treatment of skeletal metastases in patients with breast cancer or osteolytic lesions of multiple myeloma: a phase III, double-blind, comparative trial. Cancer J 2001; 7: 377–87.

34. Body JJ, Lortholary A, Romieu G et al. A dose-finding study of zoledronate in hypercalcemic cancer patients. J Bone Min Res 1999; 14: 1557–61.

35. Body JJ, Diel IJ, Lichinitser MR et al. Intravenous ibandronate reduces the incidence of skeletal complications in patients with breast cancer and bone metastases. Ann Oncol 2003; 14: 1399–1405.

36. Hillner BE, Weeks JC, Desch CE, Smith TJ. Pamidronate in prevention of bone complications in metastatic breast cancer: a cost-effectiveness analysis. J Clin Oncol 2000; 18: 72–9.

37. Body JJ. Effectiveness and cost of bisphosphonate therapy in tumor bone disease. Cancer 2003; 97: 859–65.

38. Mashiba T, Hirano T, Turner CH et al. Suppressed bone turnover by bisphosphonates increases microdamage accumulation and reduces some biomechanical properties in dog rib. J Bone Min Res 2000; 15: 613–20.

39. Lipton A, Demers L, Curley E et al. Markers of bone resorption in patients treated with pamidronate. Eur J Cancer 1998; 34: 2021–6.

40. Kanis JA, McCloskey EV. Bisphosphonates in the treatment of multiple myeloma. In Body JJ (ed.), Tumor Bone Diseases and Osteoporosis in Cancer Patients. Marcel Dekker: New York, 2000: 457–81.

41. McCloskey EV, MacLennan ICM, Drayson M et al. A randomized trial of the effect of clodronate on skeletal morbidity in multiple myeloma. Br J Hematol 1998; 100: 317–25.

42. Berenson JR, Lichtenstein A, Porter L et al. for the Myeloma Aredia Study Group. Long-term pamidronate treatment of advanced multiple myeloma patients reduces skeletal events. J Clin Oncol 1998; 16: 593–602.

43. Bataille R. Management of myeloma with bisphosphonates. N Engl J Med 1996; 334: 529–30.

44. Saad F, Gleason DM, Murray R et al. A randomized, placebo-controlled trial of zoledronic acid in patients with hormone-refractory metastatic prostate carcinoma. J Natl Cancer Inst 2002; 94: 1458–68.

45. Body JJ. Rationale for the use of bisphosphonates in osteoblastic and osteolytic bone lesions. Breast 2003; 12; S37–44.

46. Rosen LS. Efficacy and safety of zoledronic acid in the treatment of bone metastases associated with lung cancer and other solid tumors. Semin Oncol 2002; 29(6, suppl 21): 28–32.

47. Yoneda T, Sasaki A, Dunstan C et al. Inhibition of osteolytic bone metastasis of breast cancer by combined treatment with the bisphosphonate ibandronate and tissue inhibitor of the matrix metalloproteinase-2. J Clin Invest 1997; 99: 2509–17.

48. Diel IJ, Solomayer EF, Costa SD et al. Reduction in new metastases in breast cancer with adjuvant clodronate treatment. N Engl J Med 1998; 339: 357–63.

49. Saarto T, Blomqvist C, Virkkunen P, Elomaa I. No reduction of bone metastases with adjuvant clodronate treatment in node-positive breast cancer patients. Proc Am Soc Clin Oncol 1999; 18(abstr 489): 128a.

50. Powles T, Paterson S, Kanis JA et al. Randomized, placebo-controlled trial of clodronate in patients with primary operable breast cancer. J Clin Oncol 2002; 20: 3219–24.

51. Shipman CM, Rogers MJ, Apperley JF et al. Bisphosphonates induce apoptosis in human myeloma cell lines: a novel anti-tumor activity. Br J Haematol 1997; 98: 665–72.

52. Shipman CM, Croucher PI, Russel RGG et al. The bisphosphonate incadronate (YM175) causes apoptosis of human myeloma cells in vitro by inhibiting the mevalonate pathway. Cancer Res 1998; 58: 5294–7.

53. Sato M, Grasser W, Endo N et al. Bisphosphonate action. Alendronate localization in rat bone and effects on osteoclast ultrastructure. J Clin Invest 1991; 88: 2095–105.

54. Gordon S, Helfrich MH, Sati HIA et al. Pamidronate and myeloma cell apoptosis: results of an in vivo study. J Bone Min Res 1999; 14(suppl 1, abstr 1121): S163.

55. Hindley AC, Hill FB, Leyland MJ, Wiles AE. A double-blind controlled trial of salmon calcitonin in pain due to malignancy. Cancer Chemother Pharmacol 1982; 9: 71–4.

56. Blomqvist C, Elomaa I, Porkka L et al. Evaluation of salmon calcitonin treatment in bone metastases from breast cancer—a controlled trial. Bone 1988; 9: 45–51.

57. Morony S, Capparelli C, Kostenuik PJ et al. Osteoprotegerin prevents osteolytic bone destruction in both athymic and syngeneic models of experimental tumor metastasis to bone. J Bone Min Res 1999; 14(suppl 1, abstr 1125): S164.

58. Capparelli C, Kostenuik PJ, Morony S et al. Comparison of osteoprotegerin and pamidronate in a murine model of humoral hypercalcemia of malignancy. J Bone Min Res 1999; 14(suppl 1, abstr 1123): S163.

59. Body JJ, Greipp P, Coleman RE et al. A phase I study of AMGN-0007, a recombinant osteoprotegerin construct, in patients with multiple myeloma or breast carcinoma related bone metastases. Cancer 2003; 97: 887–92.

60. Stroup GB, Lark MW, Miller WH et al. A potent antagonist of the osteoclast vitronectin receptor, inhibits bone resorption in an estrogen-deficient state in a non-human primate. J Bone Min Res 1999; 14(suppl 1, abstr SA406). S411.

23

Radioisotopes and Radioimmunoisotopes

Isabelle Resche, Françoise Bodéré, Caroline Rousseau
and Jean-François Chatal

Centre René Gauducheau, Saint Herblain, France

INTRODUCTION

Internal radiotherapy is a general treatment proposed at the metastatic stage of neoplastic disease, whose success depends on the uptake intensity and residence time of a radiopharmaceutical in the tumour target. Tracers can target tumour cells specifically or accumulate in normal tissue around metastases. Strontium-89 (^{89}Sr) or labelled phosphonates play a clearly defined role in antalgic treatment of painful bone metastases, providing irradiation of all metastatic sites after a single injection. However, the mechanism of this type of low-dose irradiation is still poorly understood, and most studies have evaluated the response of the entire tumour mass rather than the specific antalgic and antitumour effect of radiopharmaceuticals on bone metastases.

ANTALGIC TREATMENT
OF BONE METASTASES

The management of bone pain is a major problem in oncological practice. Two-thirds of patients with bone metastases experience incapacitating pain and in many cases marked loss of quality of life. The presence of painful bone metastases, although indicative of the progression of the disease, can be compatible with long-term survival. Internal radiotherapy can provide pain relief and improve quality of life. Three radiopharmaceuticals are currently available for this purpose: ^{89}Sr chloride (Metastron®) for metastases of prostate cancer, and phosphorus-32 (^{32}P) and samar-

ium-153 (^{153}Sm)–EDTMP (Quadramet®) for metastases of any type of primary tumour. Rhenium-186 (^{186}Re)-HEDP and tin-117m (^{117m}Sn)–DTPA are still in clinical evaluation.

Radiopharmaceuticals

The principle of metabolic radiotherapy is to administer a radiopharmaceutical that concentrates selectively in target tissue (the area of bone reaction around the metastasis) and provides direct *in situ* irradiation. Once administered, the radiopharmaceutical should leave the blood compartment very rapidly and concentrate in target tissue. Any product not taken up should be eliminated very quickly in urine. All the radiopharmaceuticals considered here (^{32}P, ^{89}Sr, ^{153}Sm–EDTMP, ^{186}Re–HEDP, ^{117m}Sn–DTPA; Table 23.1) have these properties of rapid clearance from blood and urine [1–7].

All are β-emitters, except ^{117m}Sn$^{(4+)}$, which emits conversion electrons. The electrons emitted by the radiopharmaceutical produce the therapeutic action.

The advantages and limitations of radionuclides ^{32}P, ^{89}Sr, ^{153}Sm, ^{186}Re and ^{117m}Sn$^{(4+)}$ are related to their physical half-life, maximal energy (conditioning their range in tissue), the existence or not of associated γ-irradiation, and injected activity (150 MBq for Metastron® and 37 MBq/kg for Quadramet®) (Figure 23.1).

The γ-radiation emitted by ^{186}Re and ^{153}Sm allows scintigraphic studies indicating the biodistribution of the radiopharmaceutical. Because of this γ-irradiation,

Textbook of Bone Metastases. Edited by C. Jasmin, R. E. Coleman, L. R. Coia, R. Capanna and G. Saillant
© 2005 John Wiley & Sons Ltd: ISBN 0 471 87742 5

Table 23.I. Main radionuclide characteristics

	[32]P	[89]Sr	[186]Re	[153]Sm	[117m]Sn[(4+)]
Half-life (days)	14.3	50.5	3.77	1.95	13.6
Max energy β (MeV)	1.71	1.49	1.08	0.81	0.152 (conv)
Max range (mm)	8.7	8	5	3	0.3
Energy γ (keV)	–	–	137	103	158.6
Imaging	no	no	yes	yes	yes
Tracer	Phosphate	Chloride	HEDP	EDTMP	DTPA

a short period of hospitalisation in a shielded room may be required, depending on the regulations and radiation protection standards of the country concerned.

Results of Metabolic Radiotherapy

Different studies of the antalgic effect of [89]Sr [8,9], [186]Re [10,11], [153]Sm [12–15] and [117m]Sn [7] on pain due to bone metastases have shown similar results for undesirable side-effects and therapeutic response [16].

Immediate tolerance to treatment was excellent. No side-effects (allergic reaction, nausea, heart disorders) were noted after administration of radiopharmaceuticals. Around 10% of patients complained of a diffuse increase in pain after about 48 h, which was easily controlled by temporary additional antalgic treatment. Tolerance was good with respect to the liver and kidneys. Haematological toxicity was low to moderate, although slightly greater for ^{32}P, which is taken up by bone marrow cells, than for the other radiopharmaceuticals. [117m]Sn, a low-energy radionuclide, spared bone marrow and thus produced very slight

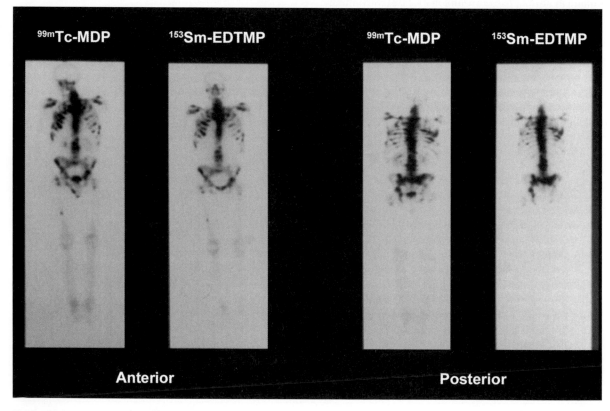

Figure 23.1. Comparison of ^{99m}Tc bone scintigraphy performed before treatment with [153]Sm scintigraphy after treatment by Quadramet: the images are superimposable

haematological toxicity. The myelosuppressive effect concerned essentially granulocytic and thrombocytic cell lines. The decrease in leukocytes and platelets was predictable and proved transient.

An antalgic effect was obtained in 70% of cases. A strong response allowing reduction or even suppression of antalgics and/or very marked improvement in quality of life was achieved in one-third of patients.

The interval before response depended on the radiopharmaceutical used, being generally long with ^{89}Sr (up to a month) and considerably shorter with ^{186}Re and ^{153}Sm (a week or more after injection). The mean response period was 6 months for ^{89}Sr and a little more than 4 months for ^{186}Re and ^{153}Sm, in accordance with the physical characteristics of the radionuclides. In fact, a rapid (but short) positive response was often observed with ^{89}Sr and a slower (but more durable) response with ^{153}Sm. The dose rate at the tumour site was probably not the only factor responsible for the effect on pain.

The recurrence of pain can justify a second course of metabolic therapy without any risk of significant haematological toxicity [17]. The long half-life of ^{89}Sr requires a minimal interval of 3 months between two injections, while the interval can be shorter for ^{186}Re and ^{153}Sm.

More recent studies have considered the concomitant use of radiosensitisers and ^{89}Sr [18,19]. Low-dose platinum compounds appear to enhance the effects of ^{89}Sr therapy without causing relevant haematological toxicity.

Role of Metabolic Radiotherapy in Therapeutic Strategy

It has been shown that treatment is effective if initiated early in the course of the disease and if the number of metastases is not too great [20]. An injection of radiopharmaceutical can be sufficient to treat initial pain at one site and prevent its occurrence at other metastatic sites. In case of failure, it is always possible to propose external radiotherapy for the refractory site. The main advantages of this procedure are the minimal risk of complications (patients are still in good health, without bone-marrow involvement) and the better overall management of pain in the oncological disease. The injections can be repeated, and other means of obtaining pain relief can also be used. The essential purpose is to delay the occurrence of pain in order to ensure adequate quality of life for as long as possible.

Some authors have suggested a choice of radiopharmaceuticals as a function of the objective sought, i.e. whether pain treatment is for patients near the end of life or for those with long life expectancy [21–23]. The cost of radiopharmaceuticals is also to be taken into account. ^{32}P administered orally, with delivery of high-energy electrons, would be preferable for patients near the end of life. For other patients whose bone pain needs to be managed over several years, radiopharmaceuticals emitting low-energy electrons would be preferable because they are less noxious for bone marrow and allow the repetition of injections and recourse to other forms of therapy without the risk of haematological toxicity.

Our knowledge of metabolic radiotherapy is still limited, particularly with regard to the mechanism of action [24]. However, it is certain that early treatment of metastatic disease offers the best chance for success [25].

Conclusion

Metabolic radiotherapy is easy to perform, not demanding on patients and well tolerated. Moreover, it provides good results, with overall pain reduction of 70% and around 30% total response, allowing discontinuation of antalgic treatment and very significant improvement in quality of life.

Internal radiotherapy is not a contraindication for external irradiation focused on a refractory or recurrent bone site, and injections can be repeated without interrupting classical antalgic treatment. Results in responders are better to the extent that therapy is begun early in the course of the disease.

The decision to apply metabolic radiotherapy should concern the entire medical staff involved (nuclear medicine specialist, radiotherapist, urologist, oncologist, pain specialist, etc.) in order to develop the best strategy for pain relief and improved quality of life.

The use of such radiopharmaceuticals concurrently with chemotherapy and/or diphosphonates is frequently debated and a few protocols are ongoing.

TREATMENT OF PRIMARY TUMOURS WITH CELL-SEEKING RADIONUCLIDES

Thyroid Carcinoma and Radioiodine-131

For nearly 50 years, iodine-131 (^{131}I) has been an integral part of the treatment of differentiated thyroid carcinoma. Radioiodine, administered as a complement to total thyroidectomy and to improve survival, constitutes the main treatment during the metastatic stage. If recurrent disease is detected, therapeutic activities of 3.7–7.4 GBq can be injected. A study performed in 394 patients with bone and/or lung metastases of differentiated thyroid cancer showed that two-thirds had ^{131}I uptake in metastases and that 46% achieved complete response [26] (Figure 23.2). Internal radiotherapy is most often associated with surgery and external irradiation for the treatment of bone metastases. In this study, bone was the only metastatic site for 108 patients,

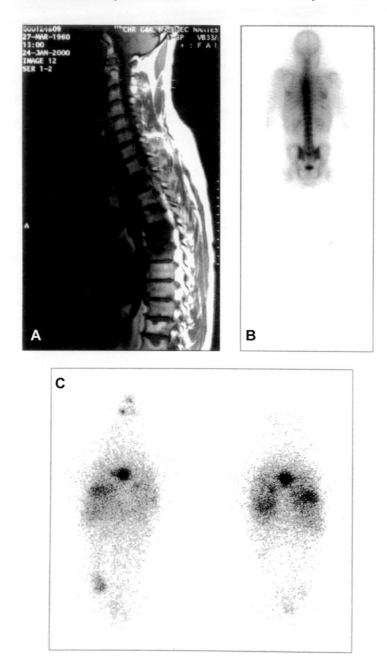

Figure 23.2. Bone metastases of differentiated thyroid carcinoma revealed by MRI (A) and bone scintigraphy (B) and treated with iodine-131 (C)

who showed a 10% remission rate and 21% survival at 10 years.

Neuroendocrine Tumours and ^{131}I-MIBG

Neuroendocrine tumours (phaeochromocytoma, para-ganglioma, carcinoid tumour, neuroblastoma and medullary thyroid cancer) develop from the diffuse neuroendocrine system (DNES) [27]. These relatively rare tumours occur in the digestive tract (56%), respiratory tract (12%) and other sites, such as the thymus and thyroid (30%) [28].

Although the frequency of bone metastases in neuroendocrine tumours is rarely reported, bone appears to be the major site of secondary localisation. The problem of detecting bone metastases is partly due to the difficulty of identifying bone lesions, which depends on the reaction of bone to the presence of tumour within it [29]: a bone metastasis may be larger than 1 cm and produce reactional osteoblastosis [30].

The diagnosis of malignant phaeochromocytoma is difficult, as it depends on the demonstration of local tissue infiltration or distant metastases, usually to the skeleton and then to regional lymph nodes, liver and lung [31]. Skeletal manifestations of malignant carci-noid tumours have rarely been reported in the literature. Bronchial and hind-gut carcinoids are less common than those of the midgut, but metastasise to bone much more frequently. Carcinoid skeletal depos-its are usually osteoblastic and most commonly affect the axial skeleton [32]. Bone metastases occur in 8–13% of patients with endocrine gastroenteropancreatic tumours and are often reported as multiple [33,34]. As indicated below, bone metastases of medullary thyroid carcinoma have not been reported, except in a clinical trial in 1999 [35] in which 21/27 patients had bone metastases or bone-marrow involvement. For neuro-blastoma, patients frequently present with haematogenous metastases, most often in bone, liver, bone marrow, lung and skin sites [36].

MIBG (meta-iodobenzyl guanidine) is a guanethi-dine analogue developed as an adrenal–medullary agent with ^{131}I radiolabelling for therapeutic purposes. More than 90% of phaeochromocytomas and para-gangliomas, 70% of carcinoids, 92% of neuroblastomas and around 35% of medullary thyroid carcinomas concentrate MIBG [37] (Figures 23.3, 23.4). It is bound at the cell membrane and transported into the cell within storage vesicles by the uptake-1 mechanism (active transport) [38]. MIBG is secreted from or diffuses out of the cell and is then recirculated by re-entering the cell by the uptake-1 mechanism [39].

Following intravenous injection, MIBG is rapidly distributed throughout the body [40] and rapidly cleared from the blood. The major elimination route for intact MIBG (84–98%) [41] is the kidney (55% of the injected dose within 24 h and up to 90% within 96 h) [42]. MIBG uptake does not normally occur in bone, and there is only vague symmetric uptake in muscle of the extremities [29]. Pregnancy is the only contraindication to ^{131}I-MIBG administration.

In view of the relative uptake of MIBG by the different neuroendocrine tumours, highly selective tumour uptake and retention of MIBG is a prerequi-site for successful treatment. When used as systemic treatment, ^{131}I-MIBG targets the primary tumour and distant metastases, which means that the decision to carry out ^{131}I-MIBG therapy should be based on a tracer study performed 24–48 h after intravenous administration of 148 MBq ^{131}I-MIBG to assess tumour uptake and retention. The dose used depends on the haematological state, especially for patients who have received other treatments previously, such as chemotherapy or interferon.

Prior to scheduling ^{131}I-MIBG therapy, it must be determined whether the patient is using any drugs known to interfere with ^{131}I-MIBG uptake and/or retention [31,37] (Table 23.2).

These medications must be stopped during four half-lives before administration of ^{131}I-MIBG. To minimise radiation to the thyroid, a stable iodine medication (5% Lugol's solution) is administered orally for 24 days (day −3 to day +21). ^{131}I-MIBG is administered by slow intravenous injection over a 90 min period. Patients need to be isolated for 4–6 days, depending on local legislation. In the case of a child, the parents or grandparents may participate in the care.

The cumulative experience of major centres was reported at the (EANM) pre-congress meeting on MIBG therapy in 1999 (Barcelona, Spain) [28]. For the 143 phaeochromocytomas treated, mean injected ^{131}I activity was 5.3 GBq for a cumulative activity of 14.8 GBq. There were 39% objective responses (4% complete and 35% partial). Symptomatic improve-ment (blood pressure and pain relief) was obtained in 52% of cases. The mean duration of response was 13 months. For the 229 carcinoids treated, mean injected activity was 6.3 GBq for a cumulative activity of 52 GBq. There were only 7.5% objective responses (no complete responses). Symptomatic improvement was observed in 23% of cases, although stability, which may be very meaningful and long-lasting, was found in 44% (Figure 23.3). For the 35 paragangliomas treated, mean injected ^{131}I activity was 7.4 GBq for a cumula-tive activity of 11.1 GBq. There were 48% objective

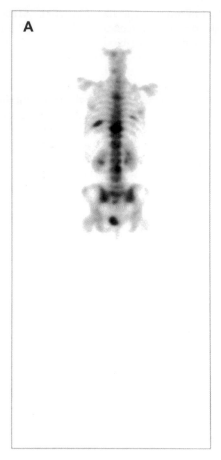
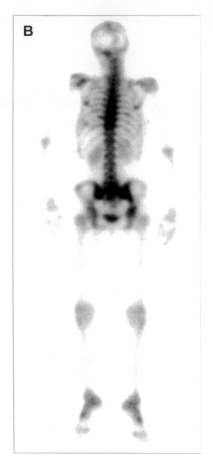

Figure 23.3. Malignant phaeochromocytoma with multiple bone metastases treated by three successive injections of ^{131}I-metaiodobenzyl guanidine (MIBG) every 4 months (5.55 GBq per injection). The bone scan (posterior view) performed after the third injection (B), as compared to the first (A), shows a reduction in uptake intensity of some tumour foci

responses (3% complete and 45% partial) relative to tumour volume. Symptomatic improvement was obtained in 70% of cases, with pain relief and a marked improvement in quality of life. The mean duration of response was 2 years. Since 1984, therapeutic doses of ^{131}I-MIBG have been given to children with metastatic or recurrent neuroblastoma not responding to conventional treatment [43]. In 1991, the pooled results from the major centres for 273 neuroblastoma patients showed an objective response rate of 35% [44]. In patients with recurrent stage IV neuroblastoma, ^{131}I-MIBG is now used in combination with hyperbaric oxygen to improve survival. In children with stage IV neuroblastoma, ^{131}I-MIBG therapy was provided early in the treatment protocol, in combination with pre-operative chemotherapy, to reduce the tumour burden and allow adequate surgical resection; 70% of the patients had complete or >95% resection of the primary tumour [45]. For the 33 medullary thyroid carcinomas treated, mean injected activity was 5.8 GBq for a cumulative activity of 47 GBq. There were 23% objective responses (no complete responses) and symptomatic improvement was observed in 73% of cases. The mean duration of response was 2 years.

Haematological effects occur most frequently, mainly as isolated thrombocytopenia [46], and may be due in part to the radiation dose to bone marrow [47] and selective uptake of ^{131}I-MIBG by thrombocytes and megakaryocytes [48]. In general, temporary myelosuppression occurs 4–6 weeks post-therapy, but is rarely of clinical significance, although cumulative. The interval between treatments may depend on the rate of platelet and leukocyte recovery. Myelosuppression is more frequent in patients with extensive bone metastases [49]. Bone-marrow harvesting is now recommended for all patients likely to undergo repeated 131I-MIBG treatments. Deterioration of renal function is occasionally observed when kidneys have been compromised by intensive chemotherapeutic pretreatment [31]. Cases of hypothyroidism are rare when the thyroid is treated with stable iodine medication. 131I-MIBG therapy is otherwise well tolerated, except for nausea 48–72 h after infusion.

The therapeutic strategy proposed for these various neuroendocrine tumours by the EANM pre-congress meeting on MIBG therapy in 1999 is to inject a high initial activity of 7.4–11 GBq (if haematological conditions are favourable) and repeat this treatment every 3–4 months with an activity of 7.4 GBq. Treatment response should be evaluated after three injections to determine whether the procedure needs to be

continued. Owing to heterogeneous uptake and the 1 mm range of iodine electrons, MIBG therapy is not likely to be effective for large tumours weighing more than a few grams. Thus, it is essential to

Table 23.2. Drugs that may interfere with MIBG uptake and/or retention

Drugs	Mechanism
Tricyclic antidepressants	Uptake-1 (active transport) inhibition
Cocaine	Uptake-1 inhibition
Labetalol	Uptake-1 inhibition
Sympathomimetics	Depletion of storage vesicle content
Antipsychotics	Uptake-1 inhibition
Calcium channel blockers	Unknown

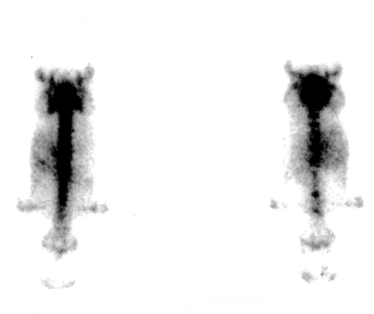

Figure 23.4. 123I-MIBG scintigraphy: diffuse bone-marrow invasion by stage IV neuroblastoma

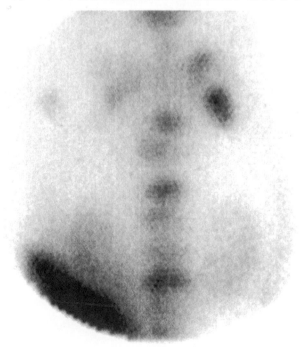

A

7 DAYS AFTER INJECTION OF 64.3 mCi

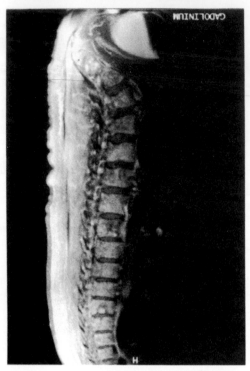

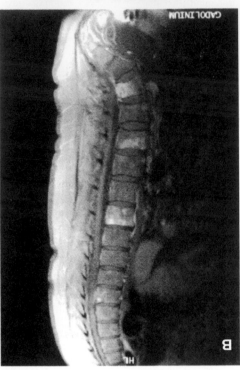

B

OCTOBER 22, 1996   FEBRUARY 11, 1997

Radioimmunotherapy (RIT)

For the last two decades, monoclonal antibodies (MAbs) have been regarded as the ideal vector for delivering high loads of radioactive isotope to tumour cells disseminated throughout the body. MAbs have the capacity to select tumour antigenic targets and, when labelled with a suitable radionuclide, can irradiate tumour cells over a distance of some fractions of a millimetre to several millimetres, corresponding to the maximum range of non-penetrating radiation. However, convincing results have been obtained only recently in RIT, using products only now in advanced stages of clinical development [50].

The efficacy of RIT depends on tumour radio-sensitivity, the biodistribution of immunoconjugates

reduce tumour volume before undertaking MIBG therapy intended to control disease progression.

and the physical properties of the radionuclide, which should take biological parameters into account, such as target size and cellular localisation of antigens [51]. The biodistribution of MAbs depends on various parameters relative to histopathology (histological type, size, tumour site), haemodynamics (blood flow, capillary permeability, tumour vascularisation), immunology (degree and homogeneity of antigen expression, MAb specificity and form, administration route) and physical aspects (choice of the radioisotope and possibly of its ligand, labelling stability). The methods developed to optimise these different parameters include the enhancement of radioactivity uptake, residence time in the tumour and reduction in non-specific uptake in normal tissues. Small subclinical or even microscopic tumours appear to be more promising targets for RIT, providing easier accessibility to antigens and containing fewer hypoxic cells. RIT doses for delivery to targets are in the range 20 150 Gy, depending on the administration route and tumour size.

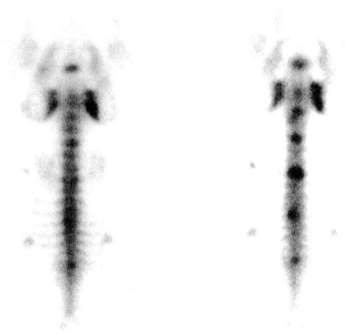

C

OCTOBER 8, 1996   FEBRUARY 11, 1997

Figure 23.5. Targeting of bone metastases of medullary thyroid carcinoma with anti-CEA × anti-DTPA bispecific antibody and di-DTPA-TL-131I hapten (A), MRI (B) and bone scan (C) performed before and 3 months after anti-CEA × anti-DTPA bispecific antibody and di-DTPA-TL-131I injections

Haematological toxicity limits the dose escalation of radiolabelled MAbs. A reduction in leukocytes and platelets usually occurs 3–5 weeks after injection, depending on the injected activity. Toxicity seems to be more frequent with bone or osteomedullary metastases, since the impoverished marrow receives a higher irradiation dose [52]. Gastrointestinal and cardiopulmonary toxicity has been reported in clinical trials involving myeloablative activities and marrow grafts [50].

Non-Hodgkin's lymphomas are favourable clinical targets for RIT, as they express well-characterised differentiation antigens and are highly radiosensitive. MAbs to B lymphocyte differentiation antigens (CD-20, CD-22, CD-37, HLA-DR) have been used with or without radioactivity [53,54]. Most of these antibodies produce significant intrinsic antitumour activity by triggering immune defence mechanisms [55]. Radioactivity appears to have a synergistic effect. The anti-CD-20 MAb provided an overall response rate of 50% (9% complete responses) in recurrences of low-grade lymphoma [53,56]. The same MAb labelled with ^{131}I and injected with non-myeloablative activities gave complete and overall response rates of 50% and 79%, respectively. These rates were further increased to 79% and 86% with myeloablative activities. RIT can be considered as a true breakthrough in the treatment of chemoresistant forms of non-Hodgkin's lymphomas. Other haematological malignancies treated by RIT include Hodgkin's disease, chronic lymphocytic leukaemia, cutaneous T cell lymphoma and acute leukaemia. The feasibility of RIT for myeloma has also been demonstrated.

Although MAbs with very high specificity for solid tumours are available [e.g. anti-carcinoembryonic antigen (CEA) for colorectal carcinomas, breast cancers or lung cancers], clinical trials to date have provided limited and controversial results. Accessibility and radiosensitivity are much lower in solid tumours than in haematological disease. Moreover, these trials have most often concerned large tumour masses inappropriate for internal radiotherapy and have used directly labelled MAbs that did not allow adequate tumour: tissue ratios for delivery of tumoricidal irradiation with acceptable toxicity. Two-step pre-targeting techniques developed to reduce the concentration of radioactivity in normal tissues [57] use bifunctional MAbs or the avidin–biotin system. In clinical studies, patients who had undergone surgery for colorectal cancer were injected with bispecific anti-CEA/anti-DTPA MAbs and then 3 days later with indium-111 (^{111}In)-labelled DTPA bivalent hapten. Tumour:tissue ratios 24h after hapten injection were four times as high as those obtained 3 days after injection of directly labelled MAb fragments [58]. A therapeutic clinical trial performed with the same bispecific MAbs and a ^{131}I-labelled hapten in patients with recurrences of medullary thyroid carcinoma (77% of patients included had bone involvement) [35] showed good targeting, especially for bone tumours (Figure 23.5). Bone pain was noted in six patients and pain relief was achieved for at least 3 months in four cases.

CONCLUSION

Radioimmunotherapy is still undergoing evaluation, but its benefit for the treatment of metastatic disease has already been demonstrated. As with other forms of internal radiotherapy, significant tumour responses are more frequent for small (more radiosensitive) lesions. In the case of larger lesions, the response is generally only antalgic or biological. For treatment of bone metastases, internal radiotherapy should be used at an early stage of metastatic disease. For example, a new therapeutic strategy seems appropriate for bone metastases of prostatic carcinoma. A bone scan may be performed once pain occurs after the hormonal dependence phase. Internal radiotherapy can be started immediately when several metastatic sites exist, even though only one is painful, whereas external radiotherapy is reserved for cases in which a single focus is visualised. Thus, the transition to opiates can be delayed and the quality of life improved. Moreover, earlier introduction of internal radiotherapy can provide a greater oncolytic effect and improve survival. In the future, in the context of treating primary tumours by cell-seeking radionuclides, internal radiotherapy will probably be used in therapeutic strategies combining different treatments to produce a potentiation effect.

REFERENCES

1. Blake GM, Wood JF, Wood PJ et al. ^{89}Sr therapy: strontium plasma clearance in disseminated prostatic carcinoma. Eur J Nucl Med 1989; 15: 49–54.
2. Maxon HR, Deutsch EA, Thomas SR et al. Re-186(Sn) HEDP for treatment of multiple metastatic foci in bone: human distribution and dosimetric studies. Radiology 1988; 166: 501–7.
3. de Klerk JMH, van Dijk A, van het Schip AD et al. Pharmacokinetics of rhenium-186 after administration of rhenium-186-HEDP to patients with bone metastases. J Nucl Med 1992; 33: 646–51.

4. Eary JF, Collins C, Stabin M et al. Samarium-153-EDTMP biodistribution and dosimetry estimation. J Nucl Med 1993; 34: 1031–6.

5. Bayouth JE, Macey DJ, Kasi LP, Fossella FV. Dosimetry and toxicity of samarium-153-EDTMP administered for bone pain due to skeletal metastases. J Nucl Med 1994; 35: 63–9.

6. Goeckeler WF, Stoneburger LK, Kasi LP et al. Analysis of urine samples from metastatic bone cancer patients administered [153]Sm–EDTMP. Nucl Med Biol 1993; 20: 657–61.

7. Srivastava SC, Atkins HL, Krishnamurthy GT et al. Treatment of metastatic bone pain with tin-117m stannic diethylenetriamine pentaacetic acid: a Phase I/II clinical study. Clin Cancer Res 1998; 4: 61–8.

8. Lewington VJ, McEwan AJ, Ackery DM et al. A prospective, randomised double-blind cross-over study to examine the efficacy of strontium-89 in pain palliation in patients with advanced prostate cancer metastatic to bone. Eur J Cancer 1991; 27: 954–8.

9. Porter AT, McEwan AJB, Powe JE et al. Results of a randomized Phase III trial to evaluate the efficacy of strontium-89 adjuvant to local field external beam irradiation in the management of endocrine-resistant metastatic prostate cancer. Int J Rad Oncol Biol Phys 1993; 25: 805–13.

10. de Klerk JMH, Zonnenberg BA, van het Schip AD et al. Dose escalation study of rhenium-186 hydroxyethylidene diphosphonate in patients with metastatic prostate cancer. Eur J Nucl Med 1994; 21: 1114–20.

11. de Klerk JMH, van het Schip AD, Zonnenberg BA et al. Phase 1 study of rhenium-186–HEDP in patients with bone metastases originating from breast cancer. J Nucl Med 1996; 37: 244–9.

12. Collins C, Eary JF, Donaldson G et al. Samarium-153–EDTMP in bone metastases of hormone-refractory prostate carcinoma: a Phase-I/II trial. J Nucl Med 1993; 34: 1839–44.

13. Resche I, Chatal JF, Pecking A et al. A dose-controlled study of 153-Sm–ethylenediamine tetramethylenephosphonate (EDTMP) in the treatment of patients with painful bone metastases. Eur J Cancer 1997; 10: 1583–91.

14. Tian J, Zhang J, Hou Q et al. Multicentre trial on the efficacy and toxicity of single-dose samarium-153–ethylene diamine tetramethylene phosphonate as a palliative treatment for painful skeletal metastases in China. Eur J Nucl Med 1999; 26: 2–7.

15. Serafini AN, Houston SJ, Resche I et al. Palliation of pain associated with metastatic bone cancer using samarium-153 lexidronam: a double-blind placebo-controlled clinical trial. J Clin Oncol 1998; 16/4: 1574–81.

16. McEwan AJ. Palliation of bone pain. In Murray IPC, Ell PJ (eds), Nuclear Medicine in Clinical Diagnosis and Treatment, vol 2. Churchill Livingstone, Edinburgh, 1994; 877–92.

17. Kasalicky J, Krajska V. The effect of repeated strontium-89 chloride therapy on bone pain palliation in patients with skeletal cancer metastases. Eur J Nucl Med 1998; 25/10: 1362–7.

18. Geldof AA, de Rooij L, Versteegh RT et al. Combination 186Re–HEDP and cisplatin supra-additive treatment effects in prostate cancer cells. J Nucl Med 1999; 40/4: 667–1.

19. Scioto R, Festa A, Tofani A et al. Platinum compounds as radiosensitizers in strontium-89 metabolic radiotherapy. Clin Therap 1998; 149/1: 43–7.

20. Kraeber-Bodéré F, Campion L, Rousseau C et al. Traitement des métastases d'origine osseuse par le chlorure de strontium-89: efficacité en fonction du degré d'envahissement osseux. Méd Nucl Imag Fonct Métab 2000; 24/2: 153–62.

21. Bouchet LG, Bolch WE, Goddu SM et al. Considerations in the selection of radiopharmaceuticals for palliation of bone pain from metastatic osseous lesions. J Nucl Med 2000; 41/4: 682–7.

22. Nair N. Relative efficacy of ^{32}P and ^{89}Sr in palliation in skeletal metastases. J Nucl Med 1999; 40/2: 256–61.

23. Krishnamurthy GT, Krishnamurthy S. Radionuclides for metastatic bone pain palliation: a need for rational re-evaluation in the new millennium. J Nucl Med 2000; 41/4: 688–91.

24. Silberstein EB. Advances in our understanding of the treatment of painful bone metastases. J Nucl Med 2000; 41/4: 655–7.

25. Papatheofanis FJ. Variation in oncologic opinion regarding management of metastatic bone pain with systemic radionuclide therapy. J Nucl Med 1999; 40/9: 1420–3.

26. Schlumberger M, Challeton C, De Vathaire F et al. Radioactive iodine treatment and external radiotherapy for lung and bone metastases from thyroid carcinoma. J Nucl Med 1996; 37: 598–605.

27. Capella C, Heitz PH, Höfler H et al. Revised classification of neuroendocrine tumours of the lung, pancreas and gut. Virchows Arch 1995; 425: 547.

28. Chatal JF, Le Bodic MF, Kraeber-Bodéré F et al. Nuclear medicine applications for neuroendocrine tumors. J Surg 2000 (in press).

29. Shapiro B, Fig LM, Gross MD et al. Neuroendocrine tumors. In Aktolun C, Tauxe WN (eds), Nuclear Oncology. Springer-Verlag: Berlin, 1999: 3–31.

30. De Kerviler E et al. Diagnostic, bilan d'extension et évaluation de l'évolutivité des métastases osseuses. John Libbey Eurotext: Euro Cancer 2000, Paris, 2000: 357–8.

31. Hoefnagel CA, Lewington VJ et al. MIBG therapy. In Murray IPC, Ell P (eds), Nuclear Medicine in Clinical Diagnosis and Treatment, 2nd edn. Churchill Livingstone: Edinburgh, 1998: 851–64.

32. Powell JM et al. Metastatic carcinoid of bone. Report of two cases and review of the literature. Clin Orthop 1998; 230: 266–72.

33. Gibril F, Doppman JL, Reynolds JC et al. Bone metastases in patients with gastronomas: a prospective study of bone scanning, somatostatin receptor scanning, and magnetic resonance image in their detection, frequency, location, and effect of their detection on management. J Clin Oncol 1998; 16(3): 1040–53.

34. Lebtahi R, Cadiot G, Delahaye N et al. Detection of bone metastases in patients with endocrine gastroentero-pancreatic tumors: bone scintigraphy compared with somatostatin receptor scintigraphy. J Nucl Med 1999; 40: 1602 8.

35. Kraeber-Bodéré F, Bardet S, Hoefnagel CA et al. Radioimmunotherapy in medullary thyroid cancer using bispecific antibody and iodine 131-labeled bivalent hapten: preliminary results of a Phase I/II clinical trial. Clin Cancer Res 1999; 5(10, suppl): 3190–8S.

36. Green DM et al. Diagnosis and Management of Solid Tumors in Infants and Children. Martinus Nijhoff: Boston, MA, 1985.

37. Hoefnagel CA et al. *Meta*-Iodobenzylguanidine and somatostatin in oncology: role in the management of neural crest tumours. Eur J Nucl Med 1994; 21: 561–81.

38. Smets LA, Loesberg L, Janssen M et al. Active uptake and extravesicular storage of *meta*-iodobenzyl guanidine in human SK-N-SH cells. Cancer Res 1995; 49: 2941–9.

39. Sisson JC, Bolgos G, Johnson J et al. Measuring acute changes in adrenergic nerve activity of the heart in the living animal. Am Heart J 1991; 121: 1119–23.

40. Guilloteau D, Baulieu JL, Huguet F et al. *Meta*-iodobenzyl guanidine adrenal medulla localization: autoradiographic and pharmaceutical studies. Eur J Nucl Med 1984; 9: 278–81.

41. Mangner TJ, Tobes MC, Wieland DM et al. Metabolism of *meta*-^{131}I-iodobenzyl guanidine in patients with metastatic phaeochromocytoma: concise communication. J Nucl Med 1986; 27: 37–44.

42. McEvan AJ, Shapiro B, Sisson JC et al. Radio-iodobenzyl guanidine from the scintigraphic location and therapy of adrenergic tumors. Semin Nucl Med 1985; 15: 132–53.

43. Chatal JF, Hoefnagel CA et al. Radionuclide therapy, Lancet 1999; 354: 931–5.

44. Troncone L, Galli G et al. Proceedings of international workshop on the role of ^{131}I]*meta*-iodobenzyl guanidine in the treatment of neural crest tumours, J Nucl Biol Med 1991; 35: 177–362.

45. De Kraker J, Hoefnagel CA et al. First-line targeted radiotherapy, a new concept in the treatment of advanced stage neuroblastoma. Eur J Cancer 1995; 31A: 600–2.

46. Hoefnagel CA, Voûte PA, De Kraker J et al. [131]I-*Meta*-iodobenzylguanidine therapy after conventional therapy for neuroblastoma. J Nucl Biol Med 1991; 35: 202–6.

47. Sisson JC, Hutchinson RJ, Carey JE et al. Toxicity from treatment of neuroblastoma with ^{131}I-iodobenzyl guanidine. Eur J Nucl Med 1988; 14: 337–40.

48. Rutgers M, Tutgat GAM et al. Uptake of the neuroblocking agent *meta*-iodobenzylguanidine and serotonin by human platelets and neuroadrenergic tumour cells. Int J Cancer 1993; 54: 290–5.

49. Ackery DM, Troncone L et al. Chairman's report: the role of [131]I-*meta*-iodobenzyl guanidine in the treatment of malignant pheochromocytoma. J Nucl Biol Med 1991; 34: 318–20.

50. Chatal JF, Mahé M. Therapeutic use of radiolabelled antibodies. In Murray IPC, Ell PJ (eds), Nuclear Medicine in Clinical Diagnosis and Treatment, 2nd edn. Churchill Livingstone: Edinburgh, 1998; 1101–14.

51. Devys A, Kraeber-Bodéré F, Chatal JF. Biodistribution and pharmacokinetics of radiolabeled antibodies. In Riva P (ed.), Cancer Radioimmunotherapy. Harwood Academic, 1998; 51–72.

52. Juweid M, Sharkey RM, Behr T et al. Radioimmunotherapy of medullary thyroid cancer with ^{131}I-labeled anti-CEA antibodies. J Nucl Med 1996; 37: 905–11.

53. Kaminski MS, Zasadny KR, Francis IR et al. Iodine-131-anti-B1 radioimmunotherapy for B-cell lymphoma. J Clin Oncol 1996; 14: 1974–81.

54. Press OW, Eary JF, Appelbaum FR et al. Radiolabeled-antibody therapy of B-cell lymphoma with autologous bone marrow support. N Engl J Med 1993; 329: 1219–24.

55. Maloney DG, Grillo-Lopez AJ, White CA et al. IDEC-C2B8 (Rituximab) anti-CD20 monoclonal antibody therapy in patients with relapsed low-grade non-Hodgkin's lymphoma. Blood 1997; 90: 2188–95.

56. Wahl RL, Zasadny KR, MacFarlane D et al. Iodine-131 anti-B1 antibody for B-cell lymphoma: an update on the Michigan Phase I experience. J Nucl Med 1998; 39: 21S–7S.

57. Barbet J, Kraeber-Bodéré F, Vuillez JP et al. Pretargeting with the affinity enhancement system for radioimmunotherapy. Cancer Biother Rad 1999; 14: 153–66.

58. Le Doussal JM, Barbet J, Delaage M. Bispecific-antibody-mediated targeting of radiolabeled bivalent hapten: theoretical, experimental and clinical results. Int J Cancer 1992; 7: 58–62.

24

Immunotherapy

T. A. Plunkett and D. W. Miles

Guy's Hospital, London, UK

INTRODUCTION

As our understanding of the immune system, carcinogenesis and the metastatic process have increased, so too have opportunities for tumour immunotherapy. The concept of tumour immunotherapy is not new. It is more than 100 years since William Coley observed that tumour regression could be induced by stimulating the immune system with bacterial toxins [1]. Interest has waxed and waned in the intervening years, but immunotherapy is now entering mainstream clinical practice.

In general, immunotherapies can be considered as non-specific (e.g. general immunomodulators, such as cytokines) or antigen-specific (e.g. tumour vaccines). This chapter will consider both forms of immunotherapy. There are no clinical trials examining the role of immunotherapy specifically for skeletal metastases. However, pre-clinical data and results from recent studies suggest that immunotherapy may be effective for bone metastases from some tumour types.

CYTOKINE THERAPY

Cytokines regulate cell behaviour via autocrine and/or paracrine pathways. They bind to specific cell surface receptors and have overlapping or pleiotrophic regulatory activities. The observations that they are direct regulators of cell division and differentiation, and that some are toxic, either directly to tumours or indirectly via the host immune system, have led to their use in immunotherapy. The majority of work in tumour immunotherapy has involved the interferons and the interleukins (Table 24.1).

Interferons

Interferons are naturally occurring glycoproteins. Three types of interferon have been identified in man: interferon-α (IFNα), which is principally produced by leukocytes, interferon-β (IFNβ), which is mainly derived from fibroblasts and interferon-γ (IFNγ), which is mainly produced by T lymphocytes.

The interferons have potent immunomodulatory effects on the expression of MHC class I and class II as well as tumour-associated antigens, resulting in increased natural killer (NK) cell and T cell cytotoxicity [2]. These and other actions have led to their use in oncology (Table 24.1). It was not until the early 1980s that sufficient amounts of interferons were available for clinical trials. They were originally produced from cell cultures, but recombinant DNA technology soon superseded this method.

Malignant Melanoma

Melanoma has been a target for tumour immunotherapy, as immunological factors may modify the course of the disease. Evidence for this includes the profuse lymphocytic infiltrate sometimes seen in primary and secondary lesions and the instances of spontaneous remission or stabilisation of disease. There are little clinical data on the effectiveness of IFNβ in patients with melanoma. A randomised trial

Textbook of Bone Metastases. Edited by C. Jasmin, R. E. Coleman, L. R. Coia, R. Capanna and G. Saillant
© 2005 John Wiley & Sons Ltd: ISBN 0 471 87742 5

Table 24.1.   Activity of selected interferons and interleukins

Cytokine	Molecular weight (kDa)	Effects
Interferons		
Type 1: IFNα	17–23	Antiviral
		Cytostatic
		Immunoregulatory (increased MHC class I expression, enhanced NK activity)
Type 2: IFNγ	20	Immunoregulatory (increased MHC class I and II expression, T cell proliferation, enhanced NK activity, activate macrophages, increased B cell differentiation), inhibitory to CD4 Th2 cells
		Antiviral
		Growth-inhibitory for tumour and endothelial cells
TNF	17	Cytotoxic for tumour/endothelial cells
		Increased cytotoxicity of LAK, TIL and macrophages, increased MHC class I expression
		Increased osteoclastic resorption of bone
IL-1	17	Macrophage activation, increased T and B cell proliferation and differentiation, chemotactic, LAK induction (with IL-2), increased NK activity (with IFN), secretion of acute phase proteins, increased IL-6 and TNF secretion, proliferation and differentiation of stem cells. Increased osteoclastic resorption of bone
IL-2	15.5	Increased T and B cell proliferation and differentiation
		Increased NK, LAK, TIL and CTL activity, macrophage activation
IL-3	28	Growth factor for multipotential progenitor cells, megakaryocytes, erythrocyte precursors, NK cells, T cells (with IL-2)
IL-4	20	Increased proliferation and immunoglobulin secretion of B lymphocytes, differentiation of Th2 cells, activation of LAK cells and dendritic cells
IL-5	12–18	Increased growth and differentiation of eosinophils, growth and Ig secretion of B cells, differentiation of T cells (with IL-2), activation of LAK and NK cells (with IL-2)
IL-6	25	Differentiation and Ig secretion of B cells, differentiation and activation of T cells (with IL-2), secretion of acute phase proteins
IL-7	25	Growth and differentiation of precursor T and B cells. Growth and activation of monocytes, macrophages. Activation of NK, LAK and TIL, growth and antigen presentation by dendritic cells
IL-8	8	Chemotactic for T cells, neutrophils, mast cells, endothelial cells, eosinophils, NK cells
IL-9	32–39	Co-stimulatory factor for erythroid precursors (with erythropoietin), T cells (with IL-2)
IL-10	17	Impaired cellular immunity, decreased Ag presentation, macrophage activation, IL-12 production and T cell stimulation
IL-12	70	Increased growth and cytotoxicity of NK cells. Increased cytotoxicity of CD8 T cells and proliferation of CD4 Th1 cells

of IFNγ as adjuvant therapy reported unacceptable toxicity [3]. The majority of published studies have examined the role of IFNα.

Early reports showed evidence of activity for IFNα in the treatment of metastatic disease. However, the overall response rates were no better than the most active standard cytotoxic agents [4]. The reported clinical responses to single-agent IFNα have generally been in soft tissue, lymph nodes or lung. Few responses have been reported in bone. Some studies have suggested a benefit for combination therapy, using standard chemotherapy and cytokines in the treatment of metastatic disease, but a lack of well-designed, prospective randomised trials precludes definite conclusions. Such trials are now under way.

There have been many studies of IFNα as adjuvant therapy for malignant melanoma. Recent evidence suggests a possible benefit for high-dose IFNα as an adjuvant therapy in patients with high-risk malignant melanoma. In a randomised controlled trial, compared to observation alone, adjuvant therapy with IFNα significantly increased 5 year disease-free (26% vs.

37%) and overall survival (2.8 vs. 3.8 years) in patients with high-risk resected cutaneous malignant melanoma [5].

The toxicity from the high-dose IFNα was probably excessive; more than two-thirds of patients overall required a dose reduction or delay and two patients died from liver failure. Notably, when the original study data were re-analysed taking into account toxicity, overall survival adjusted for quality of life was no longer statistically significant using a two-tailed *t*-test [6]. The results of a confirmatory study of high-dose IFNα are awaited; preliminary results suggest that there is a benefit in relapse-free survival, but not in overall survival [7]. The apparent discrepancy between the two trials could result from the fact that many patients in the observation arm were treated with high-dose IFNα at relapse.

Studies of lower doses of IFNα in patients with intermediate-risk melanoma demonstrated a prolongation of relapse-free survival, but this effect was gradually lost following discontinuation of therapy [8,9]. There was no benefit from treatment in terms of overall survival.

The published trials have varied in size and patient selection, and in dose and duration of IFNα therapy. Early results from a meta-analysis of IFNα as adjuvant therapy suggest benefits in both overall survival and, to a greater extent, disease-free survival [10]. Further studies are required before IFNα can be regarded as either a component for therapy of advanced disease or standard adjuvant therapy for patients at high risk of relapse from melanoma.

Renal Cancer

In patients with renal cancer, prolonged stabilisation of advanced disease and rare spontaneous regressions in the absence of systemic treatment suggested that host immune responses may be important in regulating tumour growth, and have led to the study of immunotherapy for this malignancy. The overall response rate to IFNα in over 1000 patients with metastatic renal cancer was 12% [11], although in patients whose predominant site of metastatic disease was pulmonary, the response rate has been reported to be as high as 30% [12]. As with melanoma, few responses have been reported in bone metastases.

A recent study compared IFNα and medroxyprogesterone acetate in 335 patients with metastatic renal cell cancer [13]. The results demonstrated a 28% reduction in the risk of death, a 12% improvement in 1 year survival and a 2.5 month improvement in median

survival for patients treated with IFNα. However, there was considerable early toxicity from IFNα treatment which, although less apparent by the end of treatment, should be set against the survival benefits.

In a recent randomised trial in patients with advanced disease, the combination of IFNα and vinblastine was superior to vinblastine alone, with significant increases in both response rate and median survival [14]. A study of patients with progressive metastatic disease suggested a benefit for combination therapy with IL-2 and IFNα [15]. However, the benefits were achieved at the cost of substantial toxicity. The use of IFNγ showed no benefit compared to placebo in a randomised controlled trial [16]. The use of IFNα in the management of early renal cell cancer, and in combination with other agents, requires further investigation.

Interleukins

Many interleukins have now been described (Table 24.1), but none has been as extensively studied in tumour immunotherapy as interleukin-2 (IL-2). IL-2 has no direct effect on tumour growth but is a critical cytokine in the activation of cellular and humoral immune responses. The activation of NK cells results in tumour antigen-independent cytotoxicity, but the activation of T cells may theoretically augment any pre-existing antigen-specific immunity.

Renal Cell Cancer

The intravenous infusion of IL-2 combined with autologous lymphokine activated killer (LAK) cells resulted in objective responses in over 30% of patients with metastatic renal cell cancer [17]. Subsequent studies showed that LAK cells could be omitted from the treatment schedule without affecting the response rate [18]. In a multicentre study, 255 patients with metastatic renal cancer were treated with high-dose IL-2 [19,20]: 14% of these patients had complete or partial responses lasting for a median of 23 months (one of the 24 partial responses was in bone). The rate and duration of the responses led the US Food and Drug Administration to approve the regimen as therapy for metastatic renal cell carcinoma. However, inpatient monitoring is required, often in an intensive care unit, and there is up to a 4% incidence of treatment-related death.

Table 24.2. Potential specific immunogens

Tumour cell-based	Autologous tumour cells ± adjuvant
	Allogeneic cell lines ± adjuvant
	Genetically modified tumour cells
Dendritic cell-based vaccines	Fused with tumour cell lines
	Pulsed with defined antigens/tumour cell lysates
	Transfected with tumour antigens
Defined antigens	Peptide, e.g. MAGE, gp100
	Carbohydrate, e.g. gangliosides (GM2), sialyl Tn
Antibodies	Mouse monoclonal, e.g. anti-17-1A
	Chimeric monoclonal, e.g. anti-CD20 (rhituximab)
	Humanised monoclonal, e.g. anti-*erb*B-2 (trastuzumab)

Similar response rates have been obtained with lower doses of IL-2 [21]. The toxicity was less, but response duration is not yet known. In less physically fit patients, subcutaneous IL-2 is an option for therapy. New combinations of IL-2, IFNα and fluorouracil, or IFNα and 13-*cis*-retinoic acid, have been tested, have shown promising results and are the subject of ongoing clinical trials [22].

CANCER VACCINES

Advances in the understanding of immunology have coincided with the identification of tumour-associated antigens (TAAs) [23–25]. These TAAs are potential targets for antigen-specific immunotherapy and include viral antigens, mutated proteins and oncogene products. A variety of different approaches have been taken (Table 24.2).

Tumour Cell Vaccines

Autologous or allogeneic tumour cells have been used as immunogens in the hope of inducing an immune response to putative tumour antigens (Table 24.3). Autologous vaccines have the advantage that, by definition, they are MHC-matched with the recipient.

However, they require the patient to have surgically accessible disease that will yield sufficient cells to prepare vaccine (50–100 × 10^6 cells; generally a mass of 2.5 cm diameter is required).

This criterion is most likely to be fulfilled at the primary surgical treatment of cancer. A recent trial of autologous tumour cell vaccination was reported in patients with colon cancer [26]. Two hundred and fifty-four patients were randomised to intradermal vaccination with viable, irradiated autologous tumour cells and bacille Calmette–Guérin (BCG) or no further adjuvant treatment. Patients were treated at weekly intervals for 3 weeks, with a final immunisation at 6 months. At a median follow-up of 5.3 years, overall there were no significant benefits in recurrence-free or overall survival. In a sub-group analysis of patients with node-positive disease, there was a significant increase in recurrence-free survival. However, this finding is based on a total of only 150 patients, and further investigation is required.

Allogeneic vaccines can be developed from cell lines selected to provide multiple TAAs and a broad range of MHC expression. Allogeneic vaccines may be more immunogenic than autologous vaccines, as the immune response against the foreign MHC antigens may induce a strong helper response against cross-reacting TAAs [27]. The allogeneic cell-based vaccines provide exposure to multiple known tumour antigens and as-yet unidentified tumour antigens. Therefore, allogeneic

Table 24.3. Tumour cell vaccines

Cell type	Advantages	Disadvantages
Autologous tumour cells	Identical MHC haplotype	Difficult to prepare
	May include patient-specific targets	Limited cell numbers
Allogeneic tumour cells	Unlimited cell numbers	May not be similar to patient tumour
	Easy to prepare	
	MHC-mismatch may increase immunogenicity	

vaccines have been used more widely than autologous tumour cell vaccines.

Allogeneic tumour vaccines have predominantly been used in the treatment of malignant melanoma. The most extensively studied vaccine is the so-called CancerVax. This is an allogeneic, viable, antigen-enriched melanoma cell vaccine developed from three melanoma cell lines, chosen for their high expression of immunogenic antigens [28]. The CancerVax contains an MHC haplotype match with 95% of melanoma patients [29]. Treatment with CancerVax demonstrated impressive prolongation of survival compared with historical controls [30]. These studies cannot eliminate selection bias or other unforeseen bias, and although a matched-pair analysis also demonstrated a benefit from CancerVax, the results from ongoing randomised trials are needed before definite conclusions can be drawn.

Attempts have been made to enhance the immunogenicity of tumour cell vaccines by engineering the tumour cells to secrete cytokines. A variety of cytokines have been employed to enhance the immune response, either by stimulating a local inflammatory infiltrate or by attracting or activating effector cells. These studies have shown that such modified vaccines are safe, but they have not yet demonstrated any obvious clinical benefits [31].

PEPTIDE VACCINES

Many TAAs have now been cloned. The elucidation of the structure of MHC class I and class II, and the definition of critical MHC-binding residues within peptides, has made it possible to identify putative MHC-binding peptides from the sequence of known TAAs. These peptides, with an appropriate adjuvant, have been used as vaccines.

Clinical studies of peptide vaccines have been reported in patients with melanoma. These have included an HLA-A1 restricted MAGE3 peptide [32], a combination of three melanoma-associated HLA-A2 restricted peptides [33], and an HLA-A2 restricted gp100 peptide analogue modified to increase the binding affinity to HLA-A2 [34]. In all the studies, toxicity was minimal, and immunological and clinical responses were detected.

Recently, the modified gp100 peptide was used either alone or followed by high-dose IL-2 [35]. The modified peptide induced T cell responses in 91% of patients. The administration of high-dose IL-2 reduced the frequency of T cell responses to 16%, yet in these patients a clinical response rate of 42% was observed,

with no responses seen in the patients receiving modified peptide alone. As an IL-2 treatment alone arm was not included, it is not clear whether the modified peptide contributed to the responses seen. The results demonstrate the difficulty of equating *in vitro* immunological responses with the potential for clinical responses.

HEAT SHOCK PROTEINS

Heat shock proteins (HSPs) are natural chaperones of peptides that reflect the immunological composition of the cell. They have been implicated in loading immunogenic peptides onto major histocompatibility complex molecules for presentation to T cells. When isolated from tumour cells, HSPs are complexed with a wide array of peptides, some of which serve as tumour-specific antigens. Animal studies have demonstrated that heat shock protein–peptide complexes (HSPPCs) from tumour cells can act as vaccines to prevent or treat tumours. Tumour-derived HSPs have been used as immunogens in animal models, and are being tested in human studies [36].

CARBOHYDRATE VACCINES

Carbohydrate antigens aberrantly expressed or over-expressed on tumour cells are further targets for immunotherapy. Gangliosides, particularly GM2, have been used as immunogens in patients with cancer [37]. However, a recent randomised clinical trial comparing high-dose IFNα to immunisation with a GM2 conjugate in patients with high-risk melanoma was terminated early because of lack of benefit from the GM2 conjugate.

Expression of the carbohydrate moiety sialyl-Tn (STn) is associated with a worse prognosis in colonic [38], gastric [39] and breast cancers [40]. Clinical trials using STn as a target for immunotherapy in patients with breast cancer have been reported [41]. The treatment had minimal toxicity. All patients generated an antibody response to STn, STn-positive mucin and KLH (the carrier molecule used in the vaccine). Survival was greatest in those patients who developed the highest antibody titres to STn. No association was found between survival and antibody responses to KLH. As there were no differences between the groups in terms of the natural history of their disease or the number and type of previous treatments, the results suggest a therapeutic effect for immunisation with STn. A similar association between STn antibody titres and survival has been demonstrated in patients with colorectal cancer immunised with STn [42]. A prospective, placebo-controlled, randomised trial of STn vaccine is under way in patients with advanced breast cancer.

DENDRITIC CELL VACCINES

"Cellular adjuvants" have been advocated for use with peptide vaccines. Antigen-presenting cells (APCs) include macrophages, activated B cells and dendritic cells (DCs). Although all these cells are capable of presenting antigen to T cells, DCs are: (a) the most efficient APCs in the activation of resting T cells; (b) the major APCs for the activation of naïve T cells *in vivo* [43]; and (c) the only APCs known to induce antigen-specific cytotoxic T lymphocytes (CTLs) *in vivo* [44]. DCs arise from a $CD34^+$ precursor common to granulocytes and macrophages. DCs are motile, an important attribute for their role as an APC, allowing migration from peripheral tissues to lymphoid organs.

Studies in animals and in man [45] have demonstrated that autologous DCs pulsed with antigen *in vitro* and then re-infused induced immune responses that led to inhibition of tumour growth *in vivo*. A limitation to these studies had been the generation of sufficient DCs. It is now possible to generate DCs from peripheral blood by using granulocyte/macrophage colony stimulating factor (GM-CSF) and IL-4 [46,47]. DCs are now being extensively studied for use in tumour immunotherapy [48].

A clinical trial testing peptide- and tumour cell lysate-pulsed autologous DC has been reported in patients with metastatic melanoma [49]. The pulsed DCs were administered by direct injection into lymph nodes under ultrasound guidance. Clinical responses were noted in 5/16 patients; two patients had complete responses lasting more than 1 year. All clinical responses were accompanied by antigen-specific skin test reactivity. Notably, 2/5 responding patients received tumour cell lysate-pulsed DCs in which the identity of the tumour antigens was not known. Therefore, this approach is potentially applicable to other human cancers lacking well-characterised antigens.

Peptide-pulsed DCs have also been used in patients with advanced melanoma [50]. Autologous DCs pulsed with MAGE3A1 peptide were administered to 11 patients. Significant expansions of MAGE3A1-specific CTL were demonstrated and clinical responses were observed in six patients. Three patients had bone metastases; no responses at these sites were observed.

A similar approach, particularly if a tumour antigen has not been cloned, is to fuse tumour cells with DCs [51]. The aim of fusion is to combine the TAAs from tumour cells with the antigen-processing and -presenting machinery of the DC. Theoretically, the tumour cell–DC hybrid should be able to generate antitumour immune responses. In a recent study, patients with metastatic renal cell cancer were injected subcutaneously with fusions of autologous tumour cells and allogeneic DCs [52]; 7/17 patients responded, with four complete remissions, two partial remissions and one mixed response. In several of these patients responses were noted in skeletal deposits. This strategy is now being tested in other tumour types.

DCs have also been transfected with RNA encoding defined TAAs. These cells have been demonstrated to induce primary CTL responses in human studies [53]. The optimisation of such an approach may allow the isolation of RNA from low numbers of tumour cells, and result in immune responses to shared and unique tumour antigens.

RECOMBINANT VIRAL VACCINES

Viruses transfected with cDNA encoding TAAs have also been developed. The virus acts as an adjuvant by altering the intra- and extracellular trafficking of antigen and provides an additional substrate for specific and non-specific immune recognition. In animals, vaccination with tumour cells expressing a model antigen resulted in a negligible immune response. Vaccination with recombinant viral vectors expressing the same antigen resulted in specific cell-mediated immunity and caused tumour regression [54]. It is also possible to engineer recombinant viral vaccines that express immunomodulatory molecules (such as CD80 or IL-2) together with a TAA, and this can enhance their immunogenicity [55,56].

Immunisation and repetitive boosting with the same recombinant virus can induce a strong immune response to the viral vector itself [57]. These responses limit the immunogenicity of the TAA, perhaps by rapidly eliminating the recombinant virus [58]. Alternatively, the response to immunodominant epitopes on the vector may suppress those to the weaker determinants of the TAA [59]. This problem may possibly be overcome by using different viral vectors that express the same TAA.

cDNA VACCINES

A potentially safer and easier method of vaccination is to use naked cDNA without a viral carrier system as an immunogen. The intramuscular injection of naked cDNA resulted in foreign protein expression in mice [60] and non-human primates [61]. In mice, immunisation with cDNA encoding the influenza A nucleoprotein led to the generation of specific cellular and humoral responses, and protected the mice from subsequent challenge with the virus [62]. Immunisation with cDNA encoding the carcinoembryonic antigen (CEA) showed antitumour activity [63], as have experiments using cDNA encoding for other TAAs [64]. The cDNA encoding cytokines or co-stimulatory molecules can also be used. In animal models of malaria, the use of such so-called "prime/boost vaccines" has shown considerable promise [65]. Similar combinations may be effective for tumour immunotherapy.

MONOCLONAL ANTIBODY-BASED THERAPY

Monoclonal antibodies developed against TAAs are being tested in a variety of forms in different clinical settings. Initial studies were hampered by the development of human antibody against the constant regions of xenogeneic monoclonal antibodies. The availability of human and humanised antibodies has revolutionised their use. These antibodies are produced by molecular engineering, including grafting antibody genes [66] and transgenic mice that produce human IgG in response to immunisation [67].

Antibodies can activate immune effector functions. Antibody that binds to the target antigen can mediate cell killing by complement fixation, opsonisation or antibody-dependent cell-mediated cytotoxicity. Bi-specific antibodies have been generated that bind to TAA at one antigen-binding site and to T cells at the other antigen-binding site. These antibodies can activate T cells adjacent to tumours and enhance cytotoxicity [68].

In a randomised trial, 189 colorectal cancer patients who had undergone curative resection for Dukes C cancer received either monoclonal antibody 17-1A (specific for a 34-kDa glycoprotein on the cell membrane of epithelial cells), or were assigned to observation only [69]. At a median follow-up of 5 years, the mortality and recurrence rates were reduced by 30% and 27%, respectively, in the treatment group compared to controls. The survival benefits were maintained at 7 years of follow-up [70]. Interestingly, the local recurrence rate was not affected, whilst the distant relapse rate was significantly lower in the treatment arm. This suggests that the effect of treatment may be on disseminated tumour cells rather

than local occult disease. The overall survival benefits were comparable to that of adjuvant leucovorin-primed 5-fluorouracil, but were associated with minimal toxicity. The two treatments alone or in combination are being tested in a randomised trial.

Encouraging results have also been demonstrated with antibody-based therapy in leukaemias and lymphomas. An unconjugated chimeric monoclonal antibody to CD20 was recently licensed for use in relapsed low-grade or follicular non-Hodgkins B cell lymphoma [71].

In patients with metastatic breast cancer who had received extensive prior anti-cancer therapy, treatment with monoclonal antibody to HER2/c-erbB2 (trastuzumab) produced response rates comparable to third- or fourth-line chemotherapy, but with minimal toxicity [72]. HER2/c-erbB2 is a transmembrane tyrosine kinase receptor that is overexpressed in approximately 30% of primary breast cancers. These studies have been extended and in a multicentre controlled trial, 469 women with HER2-positive metastatic breast cancer were randomised to receive doxorubicin and cyclophosphamide or paclitaxel (in those women who had received prior anthracycline therapy), with or without trastuzumab. At a median follow-up of 25 months there was a significant survival benefit for women receiving concurrent trastuzumab (25.4 months vs. 20.9 months). Since there was considerable cross-over to trastuzumab treatment from the control arm of the study, the benefits may have been underestimated.

Monoclonal antibodies directed against TAAs when conjugated with a therapeutic agent, such as a radio-isotope, can selectively deliver therapy to cancer cells. For example, in Phase II studies, radiolabelled antibodies reduced pain from skeletal metastases in patients with advanced prostate cancer [73] or advanced medullary thyroid cancer [74].

A novel means of drug delivery is by antibody-directed enzyme prodrug therapy (ADEPT), in which an antitumour antibody conjugated to an enzyme is administered intravenously. The antibody binds to tumour cells and as a result the enzyme concentration is increased around the tumour compared to normal tissues. A prodrug is then given, and is converted to an active cytotoxic agent adjacent to tumour cells by the enzyme.

The high molecular weight of antibodies (approximately 150 000 kDa) can impair their passage into cell aggregates. Single-chain Fv antibodies comprise the variable heavy and variable light regions of an IgG molecule linked by a short peptide. Studies in patients with advanced colorectal cancer demonstrated that single-chain Fv antibody specific for CEA can be more sensitive for tumour imaging than computed tomography [75]. These antibodies may have greater potential for the delivery of antitumour therapy.

CONCLUSIONS

Tumour immunotherapy has a potential role in the treatment of cancer. However, it is unlikely to be relevant to every tumour type or perhaps to every patient with a particular cancer. However, as advances in our understanding of the immune system have provided opportunities for new therapies, so too have they provided insights into the myriad ways in which tumour cells evade attack. In the future, it is likely that we will define patient or tumour characteristics that predict for potential benefit from immunotherapy. The potential role for immunotherapy in the treatment of bone metastases may have been underestimated since response assessment by conventional criteria is difficult for both immunotherapy and skeletal metastatic disease.

A better understanding of the metastatic process in bone may uncover new uses for cytokines or antigen-specific immunotherapies. For example, the expression of PTHrP in primary breast cancer has been reported to increase the risk of relapse in bone [76] and experimental studies have demonstrated that PTHrP has a causal role in the pathogenesis of human breast cancer-mediated osteolysis [77]. In animal models, neutralising antibodies to PTHrP reduced the development of bone metastases; such antibodies may have a role in the treatment of patients with skeletal metastatic disease.

REFERENCES

1. Coley W. The treatment of malignant tumors by repeated inoculations of *Erysipelas*: with a report of ten original cases. Am J Med Sci 1893; 105: 487–511.
2. Kirkwood J. Biologic therapy with interferon-α and -β: clinical applications—melanoma. In De Vita VJ, Hellman S, Rosenberg S (eds), Biologic Therapy of Cancer: Principles and Practice. Lippincott: Philadelphia, PA, 1995: 388–411.
3. Meyskens F et al. Randomized trial of adjuvant human interferon-γ vs. observation in high-risk cutaneous melanoma: a Southwest Oncology Group study. J Natl Cancer Inst 1995; 87: 1710–13.
4. Chowdury S, Vaughan M, Gore M. New approaches to the systemic treatment of melanoma. Cancer Treat Rev 1999; 25: 259–70.
5. Kirkwood J et al. Interferon α-2b adjuvant therapy of high-risk resected cutaneous melanoma: the Eastern Cooperative Oncology Group Trial EST 1684. J Clin Oncol 1996; 14(1): 7–17.
6. Cole B et al. Quality-of-life-adjusted survival analysis of interferon α-2b adjuvant treatment of high-risk resected cutaneous melanoma: an Eastern Cooperative Oncology Group study. J Clin Oncol 1996; 14(10): 2666–773.
7. Kirkwood J et al. Preliminary analysis of the E1690/S9111/C9190 intergroup post-operative adjuvant trial of high- and low-dose IFNα2b (HDI and LDI) in high-risk primary or lymph node metastatic melanoma. Proc Am Soc Clin Oncol 1999; 18: 537a.
8. Grob J et al. Randomised trial of interferon α-2a as adjuvant therapy in resected primary melanoma thicker than 1.5 mm without clinically detectable lymph node metastases. Lancet 1998; 351: 1905–10.
9. Pehamberger H et al. Adjuvant interferon α-2a treatment in resected primary stage II cutaneous melanoma. J Clin Oncol 1998; 16: 1425–9.
10. Hancock B et al. Adjuvant interferon-α in malignant melanoma: current status. Cancer Treat Rev 2000; 26: 81–90.
11. Wirth M. Immunotherapy for metastatic renal cell carcinoma. Urol Clin N Am 1993; 20: 283–95.
12. Neidhart J, Anderson S, Harris J et al. Vinblastine fails to improve response of renal cancer to interferon α-n1: high response rate in patients with pulmonary metastases. J Clin Oncol 1991; 9: 832–6.
13. MRC Collaborators. Interferon-α and survival in metastatic renal carcinoma: early results of a randomised controlled trial. Lancet 1999; 353: 14–17.
14. Pyrhonen S et al. Prospective randomized trial of interferon α-2a plus vinblastine vs. vinblastine alone in patients with advanced renal cell cancer. J Clin Oncol 1999; 17: 2859–67.
15. Negrier S et al. Recombinant human interleukin-2, recombinant human interferon α-2a, or both in metastatic renal cell cancer. N Engl J Med 1998; 338: 1272–8.
16. Gleave M et al. Interferon γ-1b compared with placebo in metastatic renal cell carcinoma. N Engl J Med 1998; 338: 1265–71.
17. Rosenberg S, Lotze M, Muul L et al. A progress report on the treatment of 157 patients with advanced cancer using lymphokine-activated killer cells and interleukin-2 or high-dose interleukin-2 alone. N Engl J Med 1987; 316: 889–97.
18. Law T, Motzer R, Mazumdar M et al. Phase III randomized trial of interleukin-2 with or without lymphokine-activated killer cells in the treatment of patients with advanced renal cell cancer. Cancer 1995; 76: 824–32.
19. Fyfe G et al. Results of treatment of 255 patients with metastatic renal cell carcinoma who received high-dose recombinant interleukin-2 therapy. J Clin Oncol 1995; 13: 688–96.
20. Fyfe G et al. Long-term response data for 255 patients with metastatic renal cell carcinoma treated with high-dose recombinant interleukin-2 therapy. J Clin Oncol 1996; 14: 2410–11.
21. Yang Y et al. Randomized comparison of high-dose and low-dose intravenous IL-2 for therapy of metastatic renal cell carcinoma: an interim report. J Clin Oncol 1994; 12: 1572–6.
22. Motzer R, Bander N, Nanus D. Renal-cell carcinoma. N Engl J Med 1996; 335: 865–75.

23. Boon T, Gajewski T, Coulie P. From defined human tumor antigens to effective immunization? Immunol Today 1995; 16: 334–6.

24. Van Pel A et al. Genes coding for tumor antigens recognized by cytolytic T lymphocytes. Immunol Rev 1995; 145: 229–50.

25. Rosenberg S. The identification of cancer antigens: impact on the development of cancer vaccines. Cancer J Sci Am 2000; 6(suppl 2): S142–9.

26. Vermoken J et al. Active specific immunotherapy for stage II and stage II human colon cancer: a randomised trial. Lancet 1999; 353: 345–50.

27. Toes R et al. Protective antitumour immunity induced by immunization with completely allogeneic tumor cells. Cancer Res 1996; 56: 3782–7.

28. Conforti A, Ollila D, Kelley M. Update on active specific immunotherapy with melanoma vaccines. J Surg Oncol 1997; 66: 55–64.

29. Hoon D et al. Is the survival of melanoma patients receiving polyvalent melanoma cell vaccine linked to the human leukocyte antigen phenotype of patients? J Clin Oncol 1998; 16: 1430–7.

30. Chan A, Morton D. Active immunotherapy with allogeneic tumour cell vaccines: present status. Semin Oncol 1998; 25: 611–22.

31. Nanni P, Forni G, Lollini P-L. Cytokine gene therapy: hopes and pitfalls. Ann Oncol 1999; 10: 261–6.

32. Marchand M et al. Tumor regression responses in melanoma patients treated with a peptide encoded by MAGE3. Int J Cancer 1995; 63: 883–5.

33. Jager E et al. GM-CSF enhances immune responses to melanoma peptides in vivo. Int J Cancer 1996; 67: 54–62.

34. Parkhurst M et al. Improved induction of melanoma-reactive CTL with peptides from the melanoma antigen gp100 modified at HLA-A*0201-binding residues. J Immunol 1996; 157: 2539–48.

35. Rosenberg S et al. Immunologic and therapeutic evaluation of a synthetic peptide vaccine for the treatment of patients with metastatic melanoma. Nature Med 1998; 4: 321–7.

36. Przepiorka D, Srivastava P. Heat shock protein–peptide complexes as immunotherapy for human cancer. Mol Med Today 1998; 4: 478–84.

37. Livingston P. Ganglioside vaccines with emphasis on GM2. Semin Oncol 1998; 25: 636–45.

38. Itzkowitz S et al. Sialosyl-Tn: a novel mucin antigen associated with prognosis in colorectal cancer patients. Br J Cancer 1990; 66: 1960–6.

39. Chun M et al. Expression of sialyl-Tn antigen is correlated with survival time of patients with gastric carcinomas. Eur J Cancer 1993; 29A: 1820–3.

40. Kinney A et al. The prognostic significance of sialyl-Tn antigen in women with breast carcinoma treated with adjuvant chemotherapy. Cancer 1997; 80: 2240–9.

41. MacLean G et al. Enhancing the effect of THERATOPE STn-KLH cancer vaccine patients with metastatic breast cancer by pre-treatment with low-dose intravenous cyclophosphamide. J Immunother 1996; 19(4): 309–16.

42. MacLean G et al. Antibodies against mucin-associated sialyl-Tn epitopes correlate with survival of metastatic adenocarcinoma patients undergoing active specific immunotherapy with synthetic STn vaccine. J Immunother Emphasis Tumor Immunol 1996; 19: 59–68.

43. Steinman R. The dendritic cell and its role in immunogenicity. Ann Rev Immunol 1991; 9: 271–96.

44. Porgador A, Gilboa E. Bone marrow-generated dendritic cells pulsed with a class I-restricted peptide are potent inducers of cytotoxic T lymphocytes. J Exp Med 1995; 182: 255–60.

45. Hsu F, Benike C, Fagnoni F et al. Vaccination of patients with B cell lymphoma using autologous antigen-pulsed dendritic cells. Nature Med 1996; 2: 52–8.

46. Romani N, Lanzavecchia A. Proliferating dendritic cell progenitors in human blood. J Exp Med 1994; 180: 83–93.

47. Sallusto F, Lanzavecchia A. Efficient presentation of soluble antigen by cultured human dendritic cells is maintained by granulocyte/macrophage colony stimulating factor plus interleukin-4 and downregulated by tumour necrosis factor α. J Exp Med 1994; 179: 1109–18.

48. Fong L, Engelman E. Dendritic cells in cancer immunotherapy. Ann Rev Immunol 2000; 18: 245–73.

49. Nestle F et al. Vaccination of melanoma patients with peptide or tumor lysate-pulsed dendritic cells. Nature Med 1998; 4: 328–32.

50. Thurner B et al. Vaccination with Mage-3-A1 peptide-pulsed mature, monocyte-derived dendritic cells expands specific cytotoxic T cells and induces regression of some metastases in advanced stage IV melanoma. J Exp Med 1999; 190: 1669–78.

51. Gong J et al. Induction of antitumour activity by immunization with fusions of dendritic and carcinoma cells. Nature Med 1997; 3: 558–61.

52. Kugler A et al. Regression of human metastatic renal cell carcinoma after vaccination with tumour cell–dendritic cell hybrids. Nature Med 2000; 6: 332–6.

53. Nair S et al. Induction of primary carcinoembryonic antigen (CEA)-specific cytotoxic T lymphocytes in vitro using human dendritic cells transfected with RNA. Nature Biotechnol 1998; 16: 364–9.

54. Wang M et al. Active immunotherapy of cancer with a non-replicating recombinant fowlpox virus encoding a model tumor-associated antigen. J Immunol 1995; 154: 4685–92.

55. Bronte V et al. IL-2 enhances the function of recombinant poxvirus-based vaccines in the treatment of established pulmonary metastases. J Immunol 1995; 154: 5482–92.

56. Chamberlain R et al. Co-stimulation enhances the active immunotherapy effect of recombinant anti-cancer vaccines. Cancer Res 1996; 56: 2832–6.

57. Murata K et al. Characterization of in vitro primary and secondary CD8+ T cell responses induced by recombinant influenza and vaccinia viruses. Cell Immunol 1996; 173: 96–107.

58. Battegay M et al. Impairment and delay of neutralizing antiviral antibody responses by virus-specific cytotoxic T cells [published erratum appears in J Immunol 1994; 152: 1635]. J Immunol 1993; 151: 5408–15.

59. Deng Y et al. MHC affinity, peptide liberation, T cell repertoire, and immunodominance all contribute to the paucity of MHC class I restricted peptides recognized by anti-viral CTL. J Immunol 1997; 158: 1507–15.

60. Wolff J et al. Direct gene transfer into muscle in vivo. Science 1990; 247: 1465–8.

61. Jioa S et al. Direct gene-transfer in non-human primate myofibres in vivo. Hum Gene Ther 1992; 3: 21–33.

62. Ulmer J et al. Protective immunity by intramuscular injection of low doses of influenza virus DNA vaccines. Vaccine 1994; 12: 1541–4.

63. Conry R et al. A carcinoembryonic antigen polynucleotide vaccine has *in vivo* antitumour activity. Gene Ther 1995; 2: 59–65.

64. Graham R et al. MUC1-based immunogens for tumour therapy: development of murine model systems. Tumour Targeting 1995; 1: 211–21.

65. Schneider J et al. Enhanced immunogenicity for CD8[+] T cell induction and complete protective efficacy of malaria DNA vaccination by boosting with modified vaccinia virus Ankara. Nature Med 1998; 4: 397–402.

66. Winter G, Milstein C. Man-made antibodies. Nature 1991; 349: 293–9.

67. Jakobovits A, Grenn L, Hardy M et al. Production of antigen-specific human antibodies from mice engineered with human heavy and light chain YACs. Ann NY Acad Sci 1995; 764: 525–35.

68. Renner C, Jung W, Sahin U et al. Cure of xenografted human tumors by bispecific monoclonal antibodies and human T cells. Science 1994; 264: 833–5.

69. Riethmuller G, Schneider-Gadicke E, Schlimok G et al. Randomised trial of monoclonal antibody for adjuvant therapy of resected Dukes' C colorectal carcinoma. Lancet 1994; 343: 1177–83.

70. Riethmuller G et al. Monoclonal antibody therapy for resected Dukes C colorectal cancer: seven year outcome of a multicentre randomized trial. J Clin Oncol 1998; 16: 1788–94.

71. Maloney D, Press O. New treatments for non-Hodgkins lymphoma: monoclonal antibodies. Oncology 1998; 12: 63–76.

72. Baselga J et al. Phase II study of weekly intravenous recombinant humanized anti-p185HER2 monoclonal antibody in patients with HER2/neu-overexpressing metastatic breast cancer. J Clin Oncol 1996; 14(3): 737–44.

73. Meredith R et al. Phase II study of interferon-enhanced ^{131}I-labelled high-affinity CC49 monoclonal antibody therapy in patients with metastatic prostate cancer. Clin Cancer Res 1999; 5: 3524–8S.

74. Kraeber-Bodere F et al. Radioimmunotherapy in medullary thyroid cancer using bispecific antibody and iodine 131-labelled bivalent hapten: preliminary results of a Phase I/II clinical trial. Clin Cancer Res 1999; 5: 3190–8S.

75. Begent R, Verhaar M, Chester K et al. Clinical evidence of efficient tumour targeting based on single-chain Fv antibody selected from a combinatorial library. Nature Med 1996; 2: 979–83.

76. Bouizar Z et al. Polymerase chain reaction analysis of parathyroid hormone-related protein gene expression in breast cancer patients and occurrence of bone metastases. Cancer Res 1993; 53: 5076–8.

77. Guise T et al. Evidence for a causal role of parathyroid hormone-related protein in the pathogenesis of human breast cancer-mediated osteolysis. J Clin Invest 1996; 98: 1544–9.

6

Bisphosphonates

Editor: Robert E. Coleman

25

Mechanisms of Action of Bisphosphonates

Michael J. Rogers

University of Aberdeen, Scotland, UK

INTRODUCTION

Despite becoming accepted as an effective treatment for osteolytic lesions and hypercalcaemia in patients with metastatic bone disease, the exact molecular mechanisms by which bisphosphonate drugs inhibit bone resorption have remained unclear for more than 30 years. A major reason for this lack of understanding has been the difficulty in isolating large numbers of pure osteoclast cells for performing biochemical and molecular studies, together with the fact that bisphosphonates have diverse effects on osteoclasts as well as on many other cell types *in vitro*. However, several major advances have recently been made that have clarified the molecular pharmacology of these drugs. Most notable has been the discovery that nitrogen-containing bisphosphonates (including pamidronate, alendronate, minodronate and zoledronate) are potent inhibitors of farnesyl diphosphate (FPP) synthase. Inhibition of this enzyme prevents lipid modification of signalling proteins, accounting for the effects of these drugs on osteoclasts *in vivo* and on other cell types *in vitro*. The exact mechanism of action of the less potent bisphosphonates that lack a nitrogen group (such as etidronate and clodronate) is somewhat less certain, but most likely involves the formation of cytotoxic metabolites or inhibition of protein tyrosine phosphatases in osteoclasts.

STRUCTURE OF BISPHOSPHONATES AND TARGETING TO BONE

Bisphosphonates are synthetic, non-hydrolysable analogues of pyrophosphate. All bisphosphonates have a P–C–P backbone, with two side chains (R^1 and R^2) attached to the central, geminal carbon atom (Figure 25.1). *In vivo*, the least potent anti-resorptive bisphosphonates are those that most closely resemble PPi. These include bisphosphonates with R^1 and R^2 side chains of a simple chemical structure, such as clodronate (dichloromethylenebisphosphonate, where R^1 and R^2=chlorine) and etidronate (hydroxyethylidenebisphosphonate, where R^2=CH_3, R^1=OH). Tiludronate differs somewhat from the bisphosphonates that closely resemble PPi, since it contains a larger R^2 side-chain consisting of a chlorophenyl group attached to the geminal carbon by a thiomethylene bond [1–3]. However, recent studies suggest that it has a similar molecular mechanism of action to that of clodronate and etidronate [4], and is of similar anti-resorptive potency to clodronate *in vivo*.

Bisphosphonates with an R^2 side chain containing a primary amino (–NH_2) group at the terminus of an alkyl chain (as in pamidronate, alendronate and neridronate, respectively) are up to 1000-fold more potent than etidronate *in vivo*. The optimum length of the amino-alkyl chain appears to be C_4 (including the geminal carbon atom), as in alendronate [5]. The potency can be further increased by modification of the primary amine in the R^2 side chain to form a tertiary amine. The addition of two methyl (CH_3) groups to the primary amine of pamidronate (to form olpadronate) [6,7], or the inclusion of the nitrogen within a heterocyclic ring (as in EB1053) [8], gives rise to a 3–10-fold increase in anti-resorptive potency. However, the addition of a methyl (CH_3) and pentyl (C_5H_{11}) group to the primary amine of pamidronate (to form ibandronate) increases potency *in vivo*

Textbook of Bone Metastases. Edited by C. Jasmin, R. E. Coleman, L. R. Coia, R. Capanna and G. Saillant
© 2005 John Wiley & Sons Ltd: ISBN 0 471 87742 5

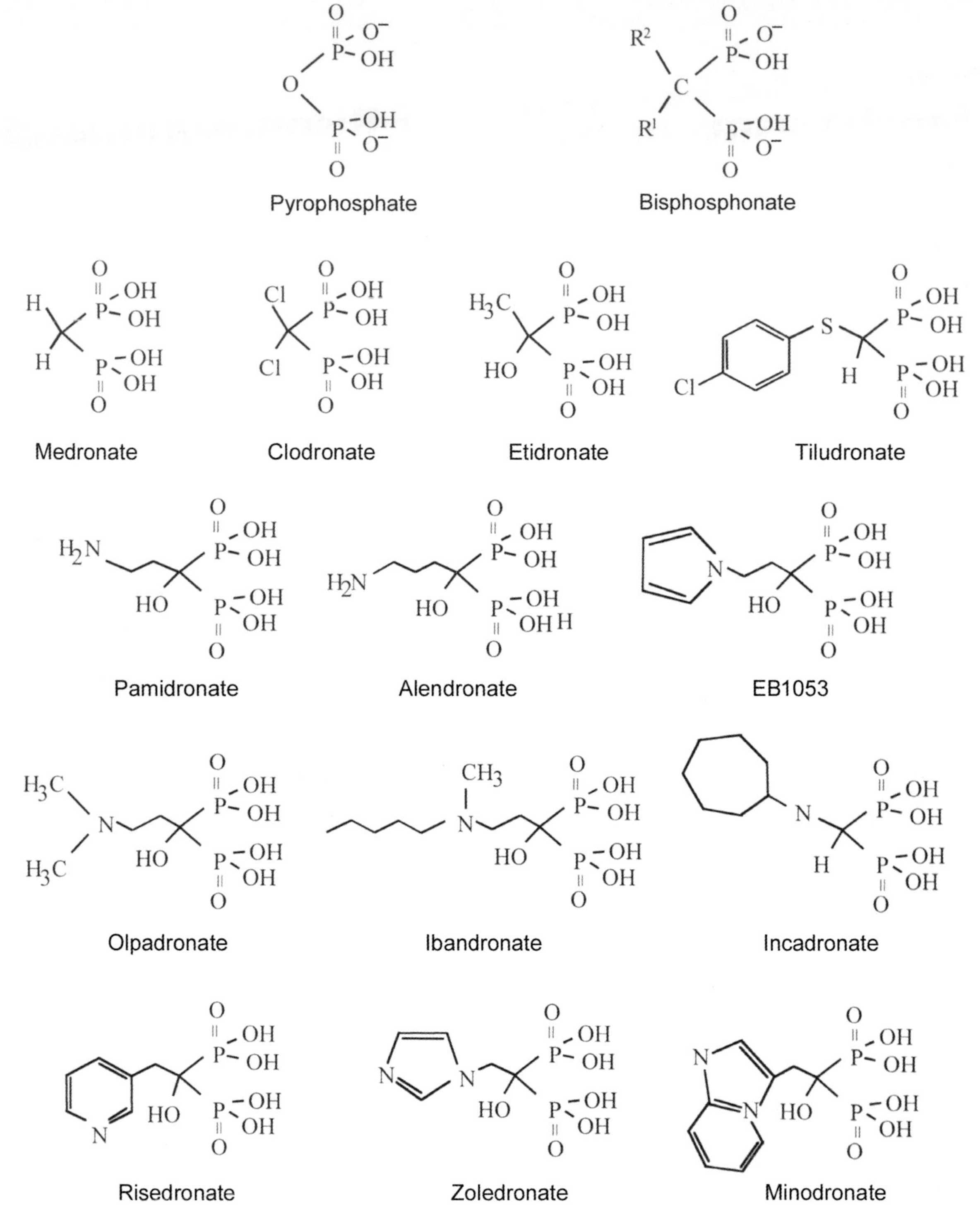

Figure 25.1. A comparison between the general structure of a bisphosphonate and pyrophosphate. The structures of bisphosphonates (shown as the protonated, bisphosphonic acid forms) studied extensively *in vitro* and *in vivo* are also illustrated

300-fold [9]. Several bisphosphonates containing a secondary amine group in the R^2 side-chain have also been found to be more potent than those containing a primary amine. YM175 (incadronate), containing a seven-membered cycloheptyl ring in the R^2 side-chain covalently attached to the geminal carbon by a secondary amine –NH– group, is 30-fold more potent than pamidronate in vivo [10].

Bisphosphonates containing a tertiary nitrogen within a ring structure in the R^2 side-chain appear to be the most potent anti-resorptive bisphosphonates discovered to date. These heterocycle-containing bisphosphonates include risedronate (containing a 3-pyridyl ring) [11], zoledronate and minodronate (both containing an imidazole ring) [12–14], which are up to 10 000-fold more potent than etidronate in vivo in rodent models to assess anti-resorptive potency.

The P–C–P backbone of bisphosphonates forms a three-dimensional structure capable of binding divalent metal ions such as Ca^{2+}, Mg^{2+} and Fe^{2+} in a bidentate manner, by coordination of one oxygen from each phosphonate group with the divalent cation. Ca^{2+} binds more effectively if one side-chain (R^1) is a hydroxyl (–OH) or a primary amino (–NH_2) group, allowing the formation of a tridentate conformation [15]. The high affinity of bisphosphonates for Ca^{2+} causes selective targeting to bone mineral in vivo, especially to sites of active bone remodelling. This avidity for bone mineral in vivo leads to rapid clearance of the drugs from the circulation and localisation to hydroxyapatite bone mineral surfaces [16], especially at sites of osteoclastic bone resorption [17–19]. The specific targeting of bisphosphonates to bone mineral, especially to sites of osteoclast activity, suggests that bisphosphonates inhibit bone resorption by direct effects on osteoclasts or other bone cells in the immediate microenvironment.

EFFECTS OF BISPHOSPHONATES ON BONE CELLS

Since bisphosphonates target bone mineral, the inhibitory effects on resorption are likely to be due to effects on cells in the immediate bone microenvironment, such as direct effects on resorbing osteoclasts or indirect effects by acting on osteoclast precursors or osteoblasts (Figure 25.2). Bisphosphonates bound to bone mineral are released from the bone surface in the acidic environment of the resorption lacuna beneath the osteoclast, since the ability to chelate Ca^{2+}, and hence bind to hydroxyapatite, is reduced at low pH [20]. This release of bisphosphonate from bone mineral

appears to be essential for their mechanism of action, since osteoclasts derived from oc/oc mice, which are unable to form ruffled borders and cannot resorb bone mineral, were not affected when cultured on bisphosphonate-coated bone [21]. Furthermore, inhibition of osteoclastic resorption by calcitonin (and hence inhibition of the release of bisphosphonates) may protect osteoclasts from the anti-resorptive action of clodronate or pamidronate bound to bone mineral [22–24].

Although bisphosphonates are not readily membrane-permeable due to their high negative charge, they can still be internalised by cells. Using radiolabelled etidronate and clodronate, Felix et al. demonstrated that bisphosphonates were taken up by calvarial cells in vitro and confirmed that the bisphosphonates could enter the cytoplasm as well as mitochondria and other organelles [25]. Furthermore, radiolabelled bisphosphonates could be visualised within endocytic vacuoles and other organelles in osteoclasts following in vivo administration [17,18]. Studies with slime mould amoebae, the growth of which is inhibited by bisphosphonates [26], have also demonstrated that cellular uptake occurs initially by fluid-phase endocytosis and that the mechanism of growth inhibition is intracellular rather than extracellular [27]. Since bisphosphonates appear to inhibit proliferation of Dictyostelium slime mould amoebae and inhibit osteoclastic bone resorption by the same molecular mechanism [28] (involving inhibition of FPP synthase or the formation of cytotoxic metabolites; see below), this strengthens the view that bisphosphonates inhibit bone resorption through an intracellular mechanism in osteoclasts.

DIRECT EFFECTS ON OSTEOCLASTS

As a result of the high affinity of bisphosphonates for hydroxyapatite bone mineral, these drugs target areas of bone turnover and are especially concentrated to sites of osteoclastic bone resorption [17–19]. This, together with the fact that osteoclasts can internalise negatively-charged compounds by endocytosis [29], indicates that osteoclasts are the cells most likely to be exposed to bisphosphonates and therefore the most likely route by which these drugs inhibit bone resorption is by a direct effect on resorbing osteoclasts (Figure 25.3)

There have been many reports supporting the view that bisphosphonates have direct effects on osteoclasts derived from a number of species [17,30,31]. Rowe et al. and others [22,23,32–34] observed that several bisphosphonates, including clodronate, etidronate

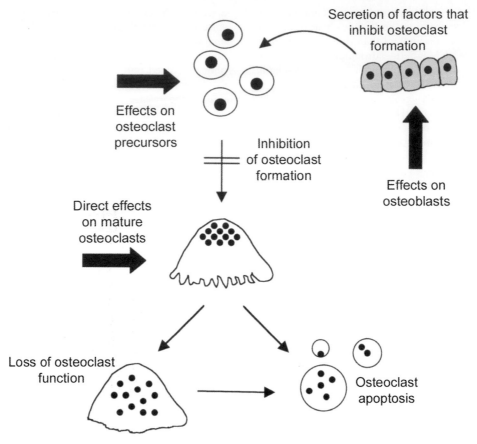

Figure 25.2.   Possible routes by which biphosphonates could inhibit osteoclast-medicated bone resorption

and pamidronate, caused degenerative changes suggestive of a toxic effect on rat and mouse osteoclasts *in vitro* and *in vivo*, including osteoclast retraction, condensation and cellular fragmentation. More recently, several studies have demonstrated that bisphosphonates, at concentrations of 10^{-7} M and above, can cause apoptotic cell death of mouse, rat and rabbit osteoclasts both *in vitro* [35–38] and *in vivo* [35,39]. Bisphosphonate-induced apoptosis of osteoclasts involves loss of mitochondrial membrane potential and the activation of caspase-3 [38], with subsequent caspase-mediated cleavage of Mst-1, an apoptosis-promoting kinase [40]. Cells undergoing apoptosis often lose adherence, whilst loss of cell adhesion to substrate can also induce osteoclast apoptosis [41], raising the possibility that bisphosphonates could induce apoptosis by inhibiting osteoclast attachment. Although several studies have concluded that bisphosphonates do not prevent the

attachment of osteoclasts to bone [17,19,30], Colucci et al. have suggested that alendronate may interfere with the attachment of osteoclasts to certain bone matrix proteins via cell-surface integrins [42]. This is in agreement with the observation that bisphosphonates can prevent the attachment of tumour cells to bone surfaces [43,44].

Induction of osteoclast apoptosis does not account totally for the inhibition of bone resorption caused by bisphosphonates, since studies with human osteoclast-like cells and rat osteoclasts *in vitro* showed that inhibition of bone resorption by alendronate, pamidronate and etidronate was not associated with signs of toxicity or a decrease in osteoclast number, except at high concentrations (10^{-5} M or above) [31,45]. Furthermore, Halasy-Nagy and colleagues found that preventing osteoclast apoptosis *in vitro* using a caspase inhibitor did not prevent alendronate or risedronate from inhibiting bone resorption, although the ability

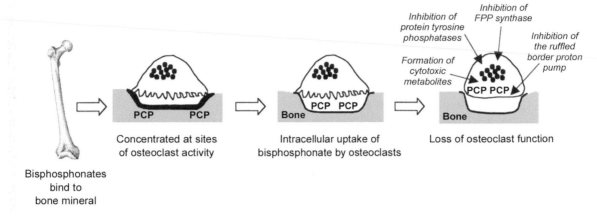

Figure 25.3. The likely mode of action of bisphosphonates on mature osteoclasts

of clodronate and etidronate to inhibit bone resorption was overcome when apoptosis was prevented [46]. Hence, it appears that certain bisphosphonates, i.e. clodronate and etidronate, inhibit bone resorption primarily by inducing osteoclast cell death by apoptosis, whereas nitrogen-containing bisphosphonates (such as alendronate, risedronate and zoledronate) inhibit bone resorption primarily by mechanisms that inhibit the resorptive activity of osteoclasts, although osteoclast apoptosis may occur as a secondary effect.

The ruffled border, a convoluted region of plasma membrane adjacent to the bone surface and essential for the resorption process, is absent in osteoclasts treated with bisphosphonates *in vitro* or *in vivo* [21,32,33,45,47,48]. In addition, bisphosphonates can also disrupt the osteoclast cytoskeleton, resulting in the loss of actin rings [17,21,34,37]. These adhesion structures, unique to osteoclasts, are comprised of actin-rich podosomes associated with other cytoskeletal proteins, and are essential for the bone resorption process [34]. As would be expected, loss of the osteoclast ruffled border and disruption of actin rings caused by bisphosphonates appears to be sufficient to prevent bone resorption [45]. In addition, bisphosphonates have been shown to inhibit the release of lysosomal enzymes in mouse calvariae [49], which would prevent resorption, since these enzymes are required for degradation of the bone matrix. This effect could be due to altered vesicular trafficking in osteoclasts, since the regulated transport of vesicles to and from the ruffled border is essential for bone resorption and appears to be disrupted in osteoclasts following bisphosphonate treatment [50]. Bisphosphonates could also inhibit resorption by indirectly preventing acidification of the resorption lacuna, since

clodronate, etidronate, pamidronate and alendronate inhibited vacuolar acidification in intact osteoclasts [51].

Although bisphosphonates clearly have diverse, detrimental effects on osteoclasts, recent studies strongly suggest that (for the nitrogen-containing bisphosphonates) most, if not all, of these effects can be accounted for as a result of inhibition of FPP synthase and subsequent loss of prenylated signalling proteins in osteoclasts (see below).

EFFECTS ON OSTEOCLAST PRECURSORS

Bisphosphonates may indirectly inhibit bone resorption by acting on osteoclast precursors and preventing osteoclast formation. Using 17 day-old fetal mouse metacarpals (which lack mature osteoclasts), low concentrations ($< 1 \mu M$) of pamidronate were found to prevent the recruitment, differentiation or fusion of osteoclast precursors [52]. This inhibitory effect on osteoclast formation is probably dependent on bisphosphonate bound to bone mineral, since pamidronate (and, in later studies, other nitrogen-containing bisphosphonates [7,53]) did not prevent the proliferation or migration of osteoclast precursors to the site of cell fusion at the bone surface, and since direct treatment of osteoclast precursors in the absence of bone mineral did not inhibit osteoclast formation [6]. The requirement of bone mineral-bound bisphosphonate for the anti-osteoclastogenic effect was further emphasised by the study of van Beek et al., who showed that bone marrow isolated from the long bones of mice treated with alendronate *in vivo* could still form osteoclasts when cultured with osteoclast-free bone explants *ex vivo* [54].

In addition to the above studies, Hughes et al. found that the potency of several bisphosphonates for preventing the formation of osteoclast-like cells in cultures of human bone marrow matched the order of anti-resorptive potency [55]. By contrast, low concentrations of the nitrogen-containing bisphosphonates pamidronate and olpadronate can actually enhance osteoclastic resorption [45,56], whilst the number of osteoclasts (although inactive at resorbing bone) may transiently increase *in vivo* immediately following bisphosphonate administration [22,57–59]. The paradoxical increase in osteoclast number observed with some nitrogen-containing bisphosphonates may be due to a transient increase in PTH (and hence osteoclast recruitment) in response to inhibition of resorption, or to stimulation of histidine decarboxylase and release of histidine by bone marrow cells [60], which could also enhance osteoclast recruitment.

Finally, several studies have concluded that bisphosphonates inhibit resorption at concentrations that do not affect osteoclast formation *in vitro*, suggesting that bisphosphonates act on mature osteoclasts rather than on osteoclast precursors [31,61,62]. Whether decreased osteoclast formation contributes to the inhibitory effect of bisphosphonates on bone resorption *in vivo* therefore remains uncertain.

EFFECTS ON OSTEOBLASTS AND OSTEOCYTES

A number of effects of bisphosphonates on bone-forming osteoblasts have been described. *In vitro*, bisphosphonates can both inhibit and stimulate the proliferation of osteoblast-like cells and other connective tissue cells [63–65]. Alendronate has been shown to stimulate the expression of collagenase 3 by rat calvarial osteoblasts *in vitro* [66], whilst pamidronate and zoledronate can stimulate the differentiation and bone mineral-forming ability of osteoblasts *in vitro* [65].

Low concentrations of bisphosphonates appear to stimulate osteoblasts to release a factor that subsequently inhibits osteoclast formation. Sahni et al. discovered that treatment of osteoblast-like CRP10/30 cells *in vitro* with 0.1 μM ibandronate or 1 μM clodronate inhibited bone resorption when these cells were subsequently cultured for 24 h with osteoclasts [67]. Similar effects were obtained when osteoclasts were cultured with conditioned medium taken from the bisphosphonate-treated osteoblast-like cells,

suggesting that the osteoblasts released a soluble factor that inhibited bone resorption. Subsequent studies concluded that this factor was of low molecular weight (<10 kDa) and acted on osteoclast precursors, thereby preventing osteoclast formation [68]. Given that bisphosphonates appear to act intracellularly, it is remarkable that concentrations of bisphosphonates as low as 10 pM had an effect on osteoblasts. Furthermore, treatment of osteoblasts for just 5 min appeared to be sufficient to cause release of this factor, although this may be an artefact, since negatively charged bisphosphonates may be sequestered and retained in culture by binding electrostatically to cell membranes or extracellular matrix proteins during the 5 min treatment. Other studies have shown that UMR106 osteoblast-like cells [69] and calvarial osteoblasts [70] treated with bisphosphonates *in vitro* are also capable of releasing some factor(s) that inhibit bone resorption by osteoclasts. However, as with many of the above effects on osteoblasts observed *in vitro*, the significance of these observations *in vivo* is not clear.

The effects of bisphosphonates on osteocytes have only recently been studied. Plotkin et al. found that a range of bisphosphonates, at concentrations of 1 μM–1 nM, prevented apoptosis of calvarial osteoblasts and the osteocyte-like cell line MLO-Y4 induced by etoposide, TNFα or dexamethasone *in vitro* [71]. The anti-apoptotic effect of bisphosphonates appears to be due to the rapid activation of extracellular signal-regulated kinases (ERKs), and involves hexameric connexin-43 hemichannels and calcium influx [72,73]. Treatment of mice with alendronate *in vivo* also prevented the increase in apoptosis of osteocytes and osteoblasts following prednisolone administration to mice, suggesting that this effect could contribute to the anti-fracture efficacy of bisphosphonates [71]. However, since it is not known whether bisphosphonates can directly affect osteocytes *in vivo*, the importance of these effects in humans *in vivo* remain unclear.

INHIBITION OF FPP SYNTHASE BY NITROGEN-CONTAINING BISPHOSPHONATES

It is now clear that the major molecular mechanism of action of nitrogen-containing bisphosphonates, accounting for most if not all of the cellular effects on osteoclasts described above, involves inhibition of the intracellular mevalonate pathway. More specifically, these bisphosphonates (zoledronate, minodronate, risedronate, ibandronate, incadronate,

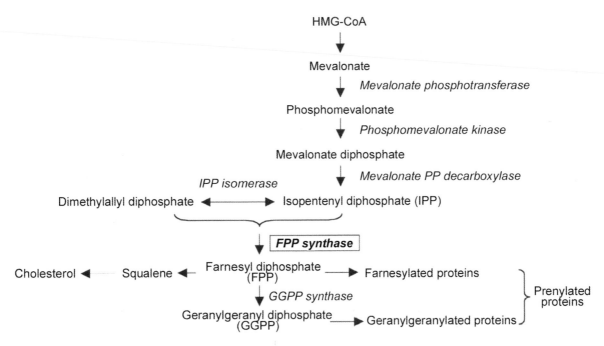

HMG-CoA

↓

Mevalonate

↓ *Mevalonate phosphotransferase*

Phosphomevalonate

↓ *Phosphomevalonate kinase*

Mevalonate diphosphate

IPP isomerase   ↓ *Mevalonate PP decarboxylase*

Dimethylallyl diphosphate ◄————► Isopentenyl diphosphate (IPP)

↓ **FPP synthase**

Cholesterol ◄——— Squalene ◄—— Farnesyl diphosphate ————► Farnesylated proteins
(FPP)   ⎫
                                ↓ *GGPP synthase*   ⎬ Prenylated
Geranylgeranyl diphosphate ————► Geranylgeranylated proteins ⎭ proteins
(GGPP)

Figure 25.4. Schematic diagram of the mevalonate pathway. Nitrogen-containing bisphosphonates inhibit FPP synthase, thereby preventing the synthesis of FPP and GGPP required for protein prenylation

alendronate, pamidronate) are all inhibitors of farnesyl diphosphate synthase (FPP synthase), an enzyme at a branch point of the mevalonate pathway (Figure 25.4). This multi-step, biochemical pathway is required for the synthesis of cholesterol via farnesyl diphosphate (FPP), a 15-carbon isoprenoid lipid. FPP can be also metabolised to dolichol and ubiquinone, as well as to geranylgeranyl diphosphate (GGPP), a 20-carbon isoprenoid lipid. Both FPP and GGPP are substrates for post-translational protein prenylation, a process involving the transfer of the farnesyl or geranylgeranyl lipid groups (of FPP or GGPP, respectively) onto a cysteine residue in characteristic, carboxy-terminal motifs of specific target proteins [74], giving rise to farnesylated and geranylgeranylated proteins, respectively (Figure 25.5). Prenylation is required for the

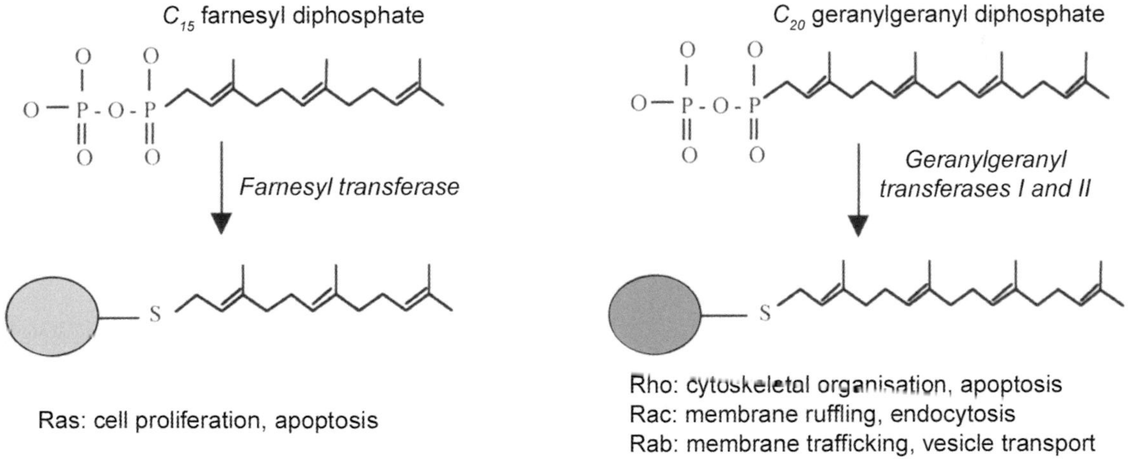

C_{15} farnesyl diphosphate

Farnesyl transferase

Ras: cell proliferation, apoptosis

C_{20} geranylgeranyl diphosphate

Geranylgeranyl transferases I and II

Rho: cytoskeletal organisation, apoptosis
Rac: membrane ruffling, endocytosis
Rab: membrane trafficking, vesicle transport

Figure 25.5. The process of protein prenylation, involving the transfer of a farnesyl or geranylgeranyl isoprenoid lipid group onto small GTP-binding proteins.

correct function of these proteins, since the lipid group serves to anchor the proteins in cell membranes and also participates in protein–protein interactions [74].

Amin et al. were the first to demonstrate that bisphosphonates could interfere with the mevalonate pathway, after finding that the nitrogen-containing bisphosphonates ibandronate and incadronate could inhibit cholesterol biosynthesis in mouse J774 macrophages by inhibiting squalene synthase and possibly other enzymes of the pathway [75,76]. By contrast, pamidronate and alendronate inhibited cholesterol synthesis but did not inhibit squalene synthase, indicating that these bisphosphonates inhibit enzymes further up the pathway, whilst clodronate and etidronate did not affect cholesterol synthesis [75]. These findings were confirmed recently when FPP synthase was shown to be inhibited by nanomolar concentrations of nitrogen-containing bisphosphonates (Table 25.1) [77–81]. Furthermore, there is a highly significant correlation between the order of potency for inhibiting FPP synthase *in vitro* and anti-resorptive potency *in vivo* (Figure 25.6), with zoledronate and minodronate being extremely potent inhibitors of FPP synthase (IC_{50} 3 nM with recombinant human FPP synthase) [80]. Minor modifications to the structure and conformation of the R^2 side-chain that were known to affect anti-resorptive potency have also now been shown to affect the ability to inhibit FPP synthase. For example, increasing the length of the chain between the geminal carbon of the P–C–P group and the heterocyclic group of risedronate dramatically decreases the potency for inhibiting FPP synthase and the *in vivo* anti-resorptive potency (Figure 25.7). Similarly, methylation of the heterocyclic group of NE11808 also dramatically decreases the potency for inhibiting FPP synthase and the *in vivo* anti-resorptive potency [80]. These observations have helped explain the relationship between bisphosphonate structure and anti-resorptive potency, strongly suggesting that FPP synthase is the major pharmaco-

logical target of nitrogen-containing bisphosphonates *in vivo*. Studies with amoebae of the slime mould *Dictyostelium discoideum* have provided further evidence that FPP synthase is the major target of nitrogen-containing bisphosphonates, since the growth-inhibitory potency toward the amoebae [26,28] is reduced in spontaneous mutant strains overexpressing FPP synthase [81].

To date, only one bisphosphonate (NE21650) has been found to inhibit protein prenylation by affecting an additional enzyme of the mevalonate pathway. NE21650, in addition to inhibiting FPP synthase, is a weak inhibitor of IPP isomerase [82]. Inhibition of both FPP synthase and IPP isomerase appears to confer only a slight increase in anti-resorptive potency compared to a corresponding bisphosphonate that inhibits FPP synthase alone. These data also strongly suggest that FPP synthase is the major molecular target of nitrogen-containing bisphosphonates.

The exact mechanism by which nitrogen-containing bisphosphonates inhibit FPP synthase has not yet been determined. Martin et al. used molecular modelling to suggest that nitrogen-containing bisphosphonates could inhibit FPP synthase by acting as isoprenoid transition state analogues [83]. The phosphonate groups of bisphosphonates may fit into the diphosphate binding site of the enzyme, thus explaining why modifications to either or both of the phosphonate groups (such as methylation) prevents these compounds from inhibiting the mevalonate pathway and reduces anti-resorptive potency [84,85]. Importantly, this confirms the proposal that the two phosphonate groups have a dual purpose [28,84], being required for

Table 25.1. Values of IC_{50} for inhibition of recombinant human FPP synthase *in vitro* by nitrogen-containing bisphosphonates. Data from Dunford et al. [80]

Bisphosphonate	IC_{50} (nM)
Pamidronate	200
Alendronate	50
Incadronate	30
Ibandronate	20
Risedronate	10
Zoledronate	3
Minodronate	3

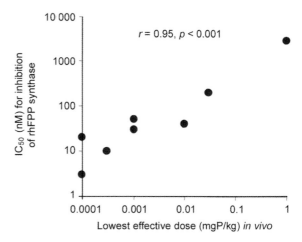

Figure 25.6. Correlation between inhibition of recombinant human FPP synthase *in vitro* and anti-resorptive potency *in vivo* for eight nitrogen-containing bisphosphonates. Data from [80]

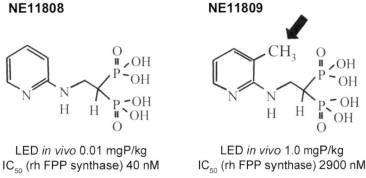

Risedronate

LED *in vivo* 0.0003 mgP/kg
IC_{50} (rh FPP synthase) 10 nM

NE58051

LED *in vivo* 1.0 mgP/kg
IC_{50} (rh FPP synthase) 2930 nM

NE11808

LED *in vivo* 0.01 mgP/kg
IC_{50} (rh FPP synthase) 40 nM

NE11809

LED *in vivo* 1.0 mgP/kg
IC_{50} (rh FPP synthase) 2900 nM

Figure 25.7. Modifications to the structure of the R^2 side-chain of bisphosphonates (arrows) affects the ability to inhibit recombinant human FPP synthase and hence affects anti-resorptive potency. Values of LED (lowest effective dose to inhibit bone resorption *in vivo* in rats) and IC_{50} for inhibition of recombinant human FPP synthase are from [80]

the molecular mechanism of action as well as for targeting to bone mineral. Martin et al. also suggested that the nitrogen in the R^2 side-chain may act as a carbocation transition state analogue, which could be stabilised by oxygen atoms in the active site cleft of FPP synthase. The length and orientation of the bisphosphonate R^2 side-chain appears to affect the interaction of the nitrogen in the side-chain with amino acid residues in the active site cleft, hence explaining why minor changes to the structure or conformation of the side-chain also affect the ability to inhibit FPP synthase [80,84] and markedly influence anti-resorptive potency [5,11,28,86,87].

INHIBITION OF FPP SYNTHASE CAUSES LOSS OF PRENYLATED PROTEINS IN OSTEOCLASTS

Inhibition of FPP synthase prevents the synthesis of FPP and its downstream metabolite, GGPP, both of which are required for post-translational protein prenylation (Figures 25.4, 25.5). The majority of prenylated proteins are geranylgeranylated small

GTPases [74], important signalling proteins that regulate a variety of cell processes important for osteoclast function, including cytoskeletal arrangement, membrane ruffling, trafficking of endosomes and apoptosis [88–92]. We therefore hypothesised that inhibition of the mevalonate pathway by nitrogen-containing bisphosphonates and loss of prenylated proteins could account for most, if not all, of the various effects on osteoclast function, including loss of the ruffled border, disruption of membrane trafficking and lysosomal enzyme secretion, disruption of the actin ring and induction of osteoclast apoptosis [93] (Figure 25.8). This hypothesis was strengthened by the observations that statins such as lovastatin and mevastatin, which inhibit the mevalonate pathway and prevent protein prenylation by inhibiting HMG-CoA reductase (an enzyme upstream of FPP synthase in the mevalonate pathway that catalyses the synthesis of mevalonate), are even more effective than alendronate or risedronate at inhibiting bone resorption by rabbit osteoclasts and in mouse calvarial cultures [93–95], at preventing osteoclast formation in bone marrow cultures [94,95] and at inducing apoptosis of mouse

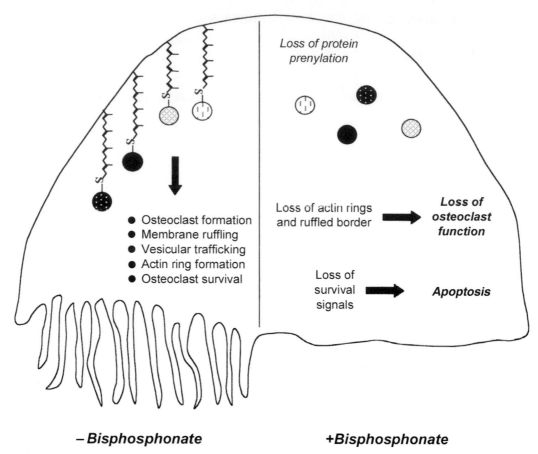

Figure 25.8.   The likely role of prenylated, small GTP-binding proteins in osteoclasts and the effect of loss of protein prenylation following bisphosphonate treatment

osteoclasts *in vitro* [93]. The similarity between the mechanism by which statins and bisphosphonates cause apoptosis has also been highlighted in macrophages. In both cases, apoptosis is dependent on protein synthesis and occurs after a lag period of 15–24 h, which may represent the time required for the levels of prenylated proteins already present in the cells to subside [96]. This may help to explain why bisphosphonates do not cause immediate cessation of osteoclast activity [30] and why some studies (utilising short exposures of cells to bisphosphonates) have not detected effects of some bisphosphonates on cell viability [97].

Studies with J774 macrophages provided direct evidence that nitrogen-containing bisphosphonates inhibit protein prenylation, since these compounds prevent the incorporation of [14C]mevalonate into both farnesylated and geranylgeranylated proteins in intact cells, whereas the bisphosphonates that lack a nitrogen

in the R^2 side (clodronate and etidronate) have no effect [4,93]. Risedronate almost completely inhibits protein prenylation in J774 cells at a concentration of 10^{-5} M, which is similar to the concentration that affects osteoclast viability *in vitro* [30,31,45] and could be achieved within the osteoclast resorption lacuna [17]. Moreover, we and others have recently confirmed that nitrogen-containing bisphosphonates inhibit the incorporation of [14C]mevalonate into prenylated proteins in purified osteoclasts *in vitro* (Figure 25.9). Zoledronate prevents protein prenylation in purified rabbit osteoclasts *in vitro* at concentrations $\geqslant 10^{-5}$ M [98]; similar effects have been reported with alendronate in murine osteoclast-like cells *in vitro* [78].

Two lines of evidence have now been provided that nitrogen-containing bisphosphonates also act *in vivo* by inhibiting the mevalonate pathway in osteoclasts. First, alendronate, ibandronate and risedronate were found to suppress the level of HMG-CoA reductase

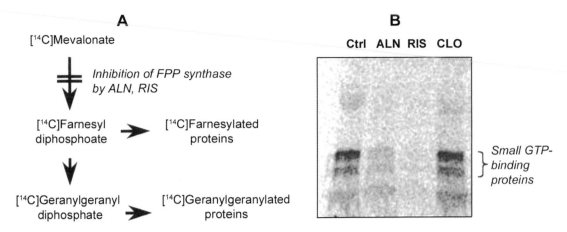

Figure 25.9. Demonstration that nitrogen-containing bisphosphonates inhibit protein prenylation in osteoclasts *in vitro*. Purified rabbit osteoclasts were incubated with [14C]mevalonate, which becomes incorporated through the mevalonate pathway into radiolabelled, prenylated proteins (A). Osteoclast lysates were then separated by electrophoresis and the radiolabelled, prenylated protein bands were detected by autoradiography (B). Both alendronate (ALN) and risedronate (RIS) prevent the incorporation of [14C]mevalonate into prenylated proteins, whereas clodronate (CLO) has no effect. Reproduced from [98] with permission of the American Society for Bone and Mineral Research

(the proximal enzyme in the pathway) in osteoclasts *in vivo*, detected by immunostaining sections of rat tibia [99]. Etidronate and clodronate, which do not inhibit FPP synthase, had no effect. This is consistent with the fact that expression of HMG-CoA reductase is modulated by feedback inhibition from downstream metabolites, which accumulate due to inhibition of FPP synthase. Second, we have demonstrated directly that protein prenylation is inhibited in osteoclasts from alendronate-treated rabbits, using immunomagnetic beads to purify osteoclasts from the long bones *ex vivo* [100]. Together, these observations confirm that nitrogen-containing bisphosphonates can inhibit FPP synthase and prevent protein prenylation in osteoclasts *in vivo*.

Compelling evidence has now accumulated that loss of protein prenylation is the major cause of the anti-resorptive effects of nitrogen-containing bisphosphonates. Addition of certain components of the mevalonate pathway can overcome the anti-resorptive effects of alendronate and statins *in vitro*, by bypassing inhibition of FPP synthase and replenishing cells with substrates for protein prenylation. In particular, addition of geranylgeraniol (a cell-permeable form of GGPP) prevents inhibition of osteoclast formation and bone resorption by alendronate [94], prevents the decrease in osteoclast number in ibandronate-treated mouse metacarpal bones *in vitro* [101] and prevents osteoclast apoptosis and caspase-mediated cleavage of Mst 1 [40]. Since geranylgeraniol can be used as a substrate for protein geranylgeranylation only, and

since farnesol has little protective effect [94,101], this strongly suggests that the inhibitory effect of nitrogen-containing bisphosphonates on both osteoclast formation and function is due to loss of geranylgeranylated proteins, rather than loss of farnesylated proteins. Studies with macrophages and myeloma cells have also concluded that apoptosis and activation of proteolytic caspases by nitrogen-containing bisphosphonates is due to loss of geranylgeranylated proteins, since these effects can be prevented by the addition of geranylgeraniol rather than farnesol [38,102].

Two studies have directly confirmed the importance of geranylgeranylated proteins in osteoclasts, since GGTI-298 (a specific inhibitor of protein geranylgeranylation) prevents osteoclast formation, disrupts the osteoclast actin ring, inhibits bone resorption and causes osteoclast apoptosis *in vitro*, whereas FTI-277 (a specific inhibitor of protein farnesylation) has little effect [38,98]. The signalling pathways involving geranylgeranylated small GTPases that regulate osteoclast morphology, function and apoptosis remain to be determined [88].

METABOLISM OF NON-NITROGEN-CONTAINING BISPHOSPHONATES TO ATP ANALOGUES

Since the non-nitrogen-containing bisphosphonates (such as clodronate and etidronate) are not inhibitors of FPP synthase [77,78,80,103], do not affect the mevalonate pathway or inhibit protein prenylation [4,75,93,94,101,103], these bisphosphonates must have a different molecular mechanism of action to that of the nitrogen-containing bisphosphonates. Early studies suggested that clodronate and etidronate could affect a variety of metabolic processes, including glycolysis, lactate production, fatty acid oxidation, adenylate cyclase and phosphohydrolases, which could all contribute to the inhibitory effect on osteoclastic bone resorption [63,104,105]. These effects are probably a result of the close structural similarity of these bisphosphonates with pyrophosphate (PPi). Hence, it is not surprising that the bisphosphonates may affect a wide variety of enzymes and metabolic pathways that utilise pyrophosphate-containing or phosphate-containing compounds. However, none of these effects satisfactorily explain the ability of clodronate and etidronate to inhibit osteoclast function and cause osteoclast apoptosis.

Although bisphosphonates have long been considered metabolically inert, Klein et al. found that methylenebisphosphonate (medronate) could be metabolically incorporated into non-hydrolysable, methylene-containing analogues of adenosine triphosphate (ATP) and diadenosine tetraphosphate (Ap$_4$A) in *Dictyostelium* slime mould ameobae [106]. The metabolites, AppCH$_2$p and AppCH$_2$ppA, contained the P–C–P moiety of medronate in place of a P–O–P moiety, and are thus resistant to hydrolysis. Rogers et al. [107,108] and others [109] then found that clodronate and other bisphosphonates that closely resemble PPi, such as etidronate, could also be metabolised to methylene-containing (AppCp-type) analogues of ATP, but not to analogues of Ap$_4$A. However, the nitrogen-containing bisphosphonates, with larger, bulkier R^2 side-chains, were not metabolised. Similar results were obtained using cell-free extracts of human cells as well as human cell lines, in particular highly endocytic macrophages [4,110,111]. The identity of the bisphosphonate metabolites of clodronate, etidronate and tiludronate (Figure 25.10) has recently been confirmed using electrospray mass spectrometry [4,112].

The incorporation of bisphosphonates into nucleotide analogues appears to be brought about by members of the family of Type II aminoacyl-tRNA synthetases [108,110], which play an essential role in protein synthesis. Tiludronate and bisphosphonates with short side-chains can probably replace PPi and be accommodated into the enzymes' active site. The inability of the bulkier bisphosphonates, such as alendronate, pamidronate and ibandronate, to be metabolised by macrophages has recently been confirmed using electrospray mass spectrometry, which

failed to detect AppCp-type metabolites of the predicted molecular mass in cell lysates [4].

Importantly, recent studies have confirmed that osteoclasts *in vitro* can metabolise clodronate and etidronate to AppCp-type nucleotides, whilst osteoclasts *in vivo* have been shown to metabolise clodronate [100]. Using immunomagnetic beads to isolate osteoclasts *ex vivo* from clodronate-treated rabbits, we could detect the AppCp-type metabolite of clodronate (AppCCl$_2$p) in osteoclast lysates using electrospray mass spectrometry. Owing to the non-hydrolysable nature of the ATP analogues, their accumulation is likely to inhibit numerous intracellular metabolic enzymes, thus having detrimental effects on cell function and survival. In accord, we found that treatment of osteoclasts with AppCCl$_2$p *in vitro* inhibits bone resorption and causes osteoclast apoptosis to the same extent as treatment with clodronate [100]. Similarly, AppCCl$_2$p contained within liposomes was of similar potency at reducing cell viability as clodronate itself and mimicked the morphological features of clodronate-treated macrophages [100,111]. The molecular pathway by which AppCp-type metabolites of bisphosphonates cause caspase activation and apoptosis of osteoclasts remains to be clarified, although Lehenkari et al. have reported that AppCCl$_2$p inhibits adenine nucleotide translocase, a component of the mitochondrial permeability transition pore [113]. Apoptosis could therefore result from inhibition of the adenine nucleotide translocase and disruption of mitochondrial membrane potential, resulting in the mitochondrial permeability transition [114], release of cytochrome *c* and subsequent activation of caspase-3 [38].

Taken together, the above observations strongly suggest that clodronate, etidronate and tiludronate probably act as pro-drugs, being converted to AppCp-type metabolites following intracellular uptake by osteoclasts *in vivo*. The accumulation of these metabolites has a cytotoxic effect on osteoclasts (Figures 25.11, 25.12), thus inhibiting bone resorption by causing osteoclast apoptosis [35,36,38,113]. The targeting of bisphosphonates to bone and their selective uptake by osteoclasts presumably accounts for the ability of these bisphosphonates to selectively cause apoptosis of osteoclasts but not other bone cells.

OTHER POTENTIAL MOLECULAR MECHANISMS OF ACTION

Since bisphosphonates inhibit acidification by osteoclasts, a potential molecular target (Figure 25.3) is the vacuolar-type, ATP-dependent proton pump in the ruffled border, which is required for acidification of the resorption lacuna and dissolution of bone mineral [115–117]. Moreover, this enzyme can be inhibited by phosphate and PPi [118], supporting the possibility that it could be a target for bisphosphonates. David et al. found that alendronate, incadronate (YM175) and etidronate can inhibit the proton-pumping activity of inside-out vesicles derived from osteoclast plasma membranes [119] with potencies similar to or less than that of PPi or phosphate (IC_{50} approximately 5 mM). Tiludronate is much more potent, with an IC_{50} of about 0.5 µM. Although inhibition of the proton pump by tiludronate is reversible and pH-dependent, it

appears to act at a site other than the catalytic, ATP-binding site [119]. Since the concentration of tiludronate required to inhibit the osteoclast proton-ATPase *in vitro* is likely to be in the range that could be achieved intracellularly in osteoclasts, this may contribute to the ability of tiludronate to inhibit bone resorption *in vivo*. However, others have found that although bisphosphonates inhibited vacuolar acidification in intact osteoclasts, this effect did not appear to be due to direct inhibition of the proton-ATPase [30,51], but may be the result of some form of metabolic inhibition [30]. Bisphosphonates have also been shown to inhibit directly the activity of certain hydrolytic enzymes, e.g. metalloproteases [120], phos-

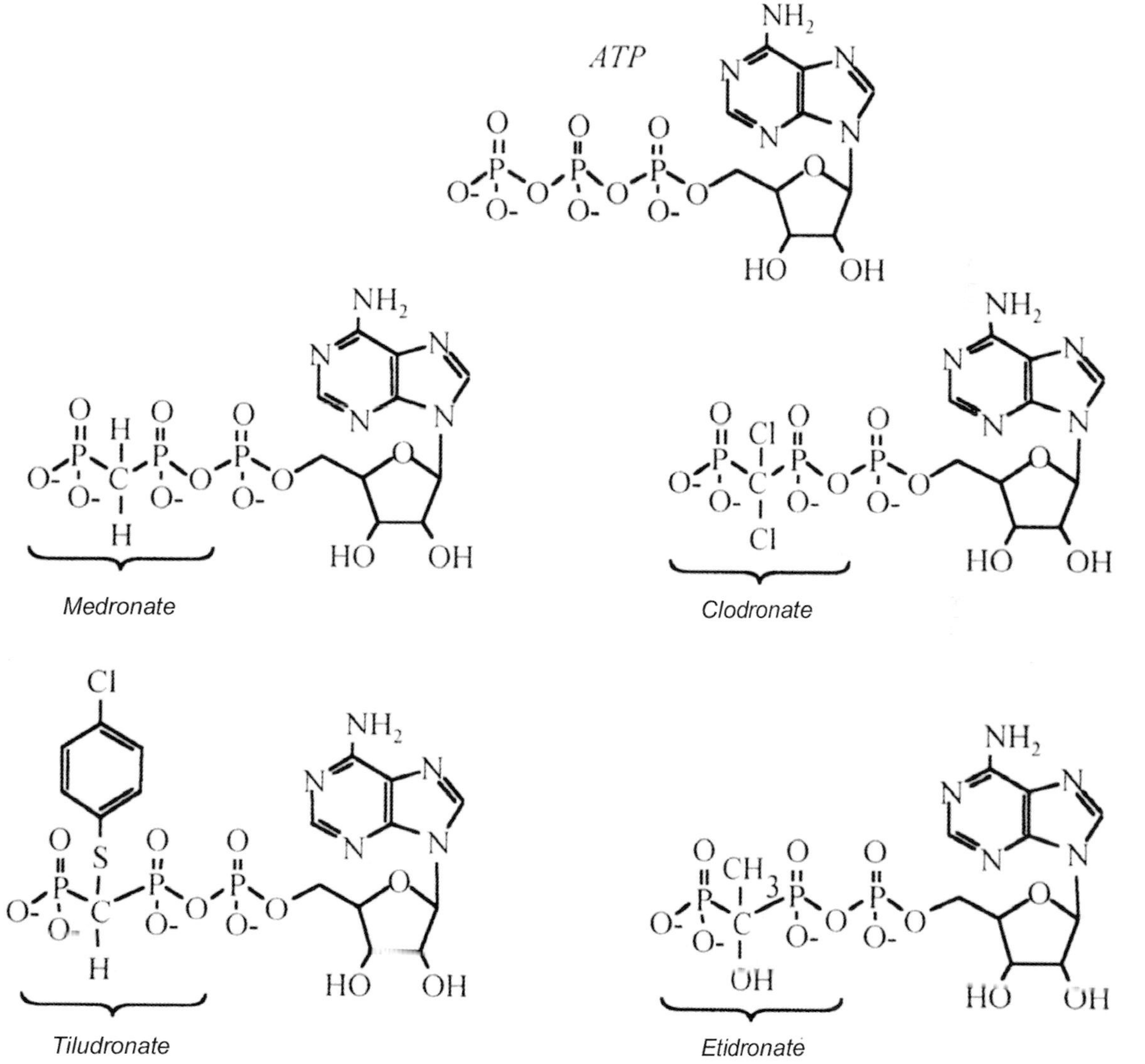

Figure 25.10. The structure of ATP in comparison to the AppCp-type metabolites of bisphosphonates.

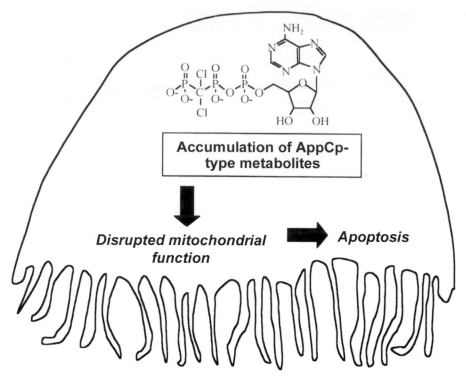

Figure 25.11. The likely major mechanism by which non-nitrogen-containing bisphosphonates such as clodronate, affect osteoclasts

phatases and acid phosphohydrolases [105]. Since bone resorption requires hydrolytic degradation of bone matrix proteins, these effects may also contribute to the overall inhibition of bone resorption. However, effects on hydrolytic enzyme activity and acidification are unlikely to account for the morphological changes of bisphosphonate-treated osteoclasts.

More recently, it has been demonstrated that bisphosphonates can inhibit protein tyrosine phosphatases (PTPs) [121], enzymes that are essential for both osteoclast formation and osteoclast resorptive activity, since inhibition of PTPs by orthovanadate or phenylarsine oxide prevents osteoclast formation in mouse marrow cultures and inhibits resorption by rat

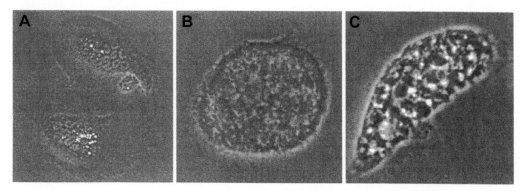

Figure 25.12. The morphology of multinucleated rabbit osteoclasts (A) and osteoclasts undergoing apoptotic cell death *in vitro*, showing cytoplasmic and nuclear condensation (B,C). Bisphosphonates that lack a nitrogen group (e.g. clodronate and etidronate) appear to act primarily by inducing osteoclast apoptosis owing to the accumulation of cytotoxic AppCp-type metabolites (see Figure 25.10). Photographs reproduced from [38], with permission of Elsevier Science © 2001

osteoclasts *in vitro* [122]. Schmidt et al. and others recently found that alendronate and other bisphosphonates can inhibit several PTPs, such as PTPmeg1, PTPσ, PTP1B and PTPε, without affecting serine or threonine phosphatases [64,121–123]. PTPε, which is highly expressed in osteoclasts, is inhibited by both alendronate and etidronate with IC_{50}s of $3\,\mu M$ and $2\,\mu M$, respectively [122], whilst recombinant PTPσ is inhibited with IC_{50}s of $0.5\,\mu M$ and $0.2\,\mu M$, respectively [64]. Inhibition appears to be due to oxidation of the conserved cysteine residue in the active site of PTPs. Murakami et al. have shown that tiludronate inhibits PTPase activity when added to lysates of osteoclast-like cells, and that a concentration ($100\,\mu M$), which disrupts actin ring formation in osteoclast-like cells *in vitro*, modestly increases the level of tyrosine phosphorylation of some intracellular proteins [124]. However, the lack of correlation between the ability of bisphosphonates to inhibit the PTPases examined to date and their anti-resorptive potency indicates that inhibition of PTPs is not the major mechanism by which bisphosphonates inhibit bone resorption. Nevertheless, disruption of PTPase-dependent signalling pathways in osteoclasts (such as c-src, which is required for organisation of the osteoclast cytoskeleton and ruffled border formation) may contribute to the decreased ability of osteoclasts to resorb bone.

SUMMARY

Bisphosphonates may inhibit osteoclast-mediated bone resorption *in vivo* by several routes, depending on the chemical structure of the bisphosphonate and the concentration that is achieved in the bone microenvironment. Due to the targeting of bisphosphonates to hydroxyapatite and the ability of osteoclasts to release the drugs in the acidic local microenvironment, a direct effect of bisphosphonates on mature osteoclasts is probably the most important route of action. As a result of recent discoveries concerning their mechanism of action, bisphosphonates can be categorised into two groups, according to the molecular mechanisms by which they affect osteoclasts. The simpler bisphosphonates that closely resemble PPi (such as clodronate, etidronate and tiludronate) can be metabolically incorporated into non-hydrolysable analogues of ATP that accumulate intracellularly in osteoclasts, resulting in induction of osteoclast cell death by apoptosis. By contrast, the more potent, nitrogen-containing bisphosphonates (such as pamidronate, alendronate, ibandronate, risedronate, zoledronate and minodronate) inhibit the intracellular enzyme

FPP synthase in osteoclasts, thereby preventing the biosynthesis of isoprenoid lipids (FPP and GGPP) that are essential for the post-translational farnesylation and geranylgeranylation of small GTPases. Loss of osteoclast activity and apoptosis is the consequence of loss of geranylgeranylation of small GTPases and hence loss of function of one or more of these important signalling proteins. Furthermore, it is possible that individual bisphosphonates also have additional effects, such as inhibition of the osteoclast proton-ATPase or protein tyrosine phosphatases, which may contribute to the overall ability to inhibit osteoclastic bone resorption.

REFERENCES

1. Reginster JY, Jeugmans-Huynen AM, Albert A et al. Biological and clinical assessment of a new bisphosphonate, (chloro-4 phenyl)-thiomethylene bisphosphonate, in the treatment of Paget's disease of bone. Bone 1988; 9: 349–54.
2. Reginster JY. Oral tiludronate: pharmacological properties and potential usefulness in Paget's disease of bone and osteoporosis. Bone 1992; 13: 351–4.
3. Bonjour JP, Ammann P, Barbier A et al. Tiludronate: bone pharmacology and safety. Bone 1995; 17: 473–7S.
4. Benford HL, Frith JC, Auriola S et al. Farnesol and geranylgeraniol prevent activation of caspases by amino-bisphosphonates: biochemical evidence for two distinct pharmacological classes of bisphosphonate drugs. Mol Pharmacol 1999; 56: 131–40.
5. Schenk R, Eggli P, Fleisch H, Rosini S. Quantitative morphometric evaluation of the inhibitory activity of new aminobisphosphonates on bone resorption in the rat. Calcif Tissue Int 1986; 38: 342–9.
6. Lowik CW, Van der Pluijm G, van der Wee-Pals LJ et al. Migration and phenotypic transformation of osteoclast precursors into mature osteoclasts: the effect of a bisphosphonate. J Bone Min Res 1988; 3: 185–92.
7. Papapoulos SE, Hoekman K, Lowik CW et al. Application of an *in vitro* model and a clinical protocol in the assessment of the potency of a new bisphosphonate. J Bone Min Res 1989; 4: 775–81.
8. Van der Pluijm G, Binderup L, Bramm E et al. Disodium 1-hydroxy-3-(1-pyrrolidinyl)-propylidene-1,1-bisphosphonate (EB-1053) is a potent inhibitor of bone resorption *in vitro* and *in vivo*. J Bone Min Res 1992; 7: 981–6.
9. Muhlbauer RC, Bauss F, Schenk R et al. BM 21.0955, a potent new bisphosphonate to inhibit bone resorption. J Bone Min Res 1991; 6: 1003–11.
10. Takeuchi M, Sakamoto S, Yoshida M et al. Studies on novel bone resorption inhibitors. I. Synthesis and pharmacological activities of aminomethylenebisphosphonate derivatives. Chem Pharm Bull 1993; 41: 688–93.
11. Sietsema WK, Ebetino FH, Salvagno AM, Bevan JA. Antiresorptive dose–response relationships across three generations of bisphosphonates. Drugs Exp Clin Res 1989; 15: 389–96.

12. Green JR, Muller K, Jaeggi KA. Preclinical pharmacology of CGP 42'446, a new, potent, heterocyclic bisphosphonate compound. J Bone Min Res 1994; 9: 745–51.

13. Green JR, Rogers MJ. Pharmacologic profile of zoledronic acid: a highly potent inhibitor of bone resorption. Drug Dev Res 2002; 55: 210–24.

14. Sasaki A, Kitamura K, Alcalde RE et al. Effect of a newly developed bisphosphonate, YH529, on osteolytic bone metastases in nude mice. Int J Cancer 1998; 77: 279–85.

15. Jung A, Bisaz S, Fleisch H. The binding of pyrophosphate and two diphosphonates by hydroxyapatite crystals. Calcif Tissue Res 1973; 11: 269–80.

16. Lin JH. Bisphosphonates: a review of their pharmacokinetic properties. Bone 1996; 18: 75–85.

17. Sato M, Grasser W, Endo N et al. Bisphosphonate action. Alendronate localization in rat bone and effects on osteoclast ultrastructure. J Clin Invest 1991; 88: 2095–105.

18. Masarachia P, Weinreb M, Balena R, Rodan GA. Comparison of the distribution of 3H-alendronate and 3H-etidronate in rat and mouse bones. Bone 1996; 19: 281–90.

19. Azuma Y, Sato H, Oue Y et al. Alendronate distributed on bone surfaces inhibits osteoclastic bone resorption in vitro and in experimental hypercalcemia models. Bone 1995; 16: 235–45.

20. Ebetino FH, Francis MD, Rogers MJ, Russell RGG. Mechanisms of action of etidronate and other bisphosphonates. Rev Contemp Pharmacother 1998; 9: 233–43.

21. Murakami H, Takahashi N, Sasaki T et al. A possible mechanism of the specific action of bisphosphonates on osteoclasts: tiludronate preferentially affects polarized osteoclasts having ruffled borders. Bone 1995; 17: 137–44.

22. Marshall MJ, Wilson AS, Davie MW. Effects of (3-amino-1-hydroxypropylidene)-1,1-bisphosphonate on mouse osteoclasts. J Bone Min Res 1990; 5: 955–62.

23. Flanagan AM, Chambers TJ. Dichloromethylenebisphosphonate (Cl2MBP) inhibits bone resorption through injury to osteoclasts that resorb Cl2MBP-coated bone. Bone Min 1989; 6: 33–43.

24. Rowe DJ, Hausmann E. The effects of calcitonin and colchicine on the cellular response to diphosphonate. Br J Exp Pathol 1980; 61: 303–9.

25. Felix R, Guenther HL, Fleisch H. The subcellular distribution of [^{14}C]dichloromethylenebisphosphonate and [^{14}C]1-hydroxyethylidene-1,1-bisphosphonate in cultured calvaria cells. Calcif Tiss Int 1984; 36: 108–13.

26. Rogers MJ, Watts DJ, Russell RG et al. Inhibitory effects of bisphosphonates on growth of amoebae of the cellular slime mold Dictyostelium discoideum. J Bone Min Res 1994; 9: 1029–39.

27. Rogers MJ, Xiong X, Ji X et al. Inhibition of growth of Dictyostelium discoideum amoebae by bisphosphonate drugs is dependent on cellular uptake. Pharm Res 1997; 14: 625–30.

28. Rogers MJ, Xiong X, Brown RJ et al. Structure–activity relationships of new heterocycle-containing bisphosphonates as inhibitors of bone resorption and as inhibitors of growth of Dictyostelium discoideum amoebae. Mol Pharmacol 1995; 47: 398–402.

29. Stenbeck G, Horton MA. A new specialized cell–matrix interaction in actively resorbing osteoclasts. J Cell Sci 2000; 113: 1577–87.

30. Carano A, Teitelbaum SL, Konsek JD et al. Bisphosphonates directly inhibit the bone resorption activity of isolated avian osteoclasts in vitro. J Clin Invest 1990; 85: 456–61.

31. Breuil V, Cosman F, Stein L et al. Human osteoclast formation and activity in vitro: effects of alendronate. J Bone Min Res 1998; 13. 1721–9.

32. Rowe EJ, Hausmann E. The alteration of osteoclast morphology by diphosphonates in bone organ culture. Calcif Tiss Res 1976; 20: 53–60.

33. Schenk R, Merz WA, Muhlbauer R et al. Effect of ethane-1-hydroxy-1,1-diphosphonate (EHDP) and dichloromethylene diphosphonate (Cl 2 MDP) on the calcification and resorption of cartilage and bone in the tibial epiphysis and metaphysis of rats. Calcif Tiss Res 1973; 11: 196–214.

34. Selander K, Lehenkari P, Vaananen HK. The effects of bisphosphonates on the resorption cycle of isolated osteoclasts. Calcif Tiss Int 1994; 55: 368–75.

35. Hughes DE, Wright KR, Uy HL et al. Bisphosphonates promote apoptosis in murine osteoclasts in vitro and in vivo. J Bone Min Res 1995; 10: 1478–87.

36. Selander KS, Monkkonen J, Karhukorpi EK et al. Characteristics of clodronate-induced apoptosis in osteoclasts and macrophages. Mol Pharmacol 1996; 50: 1127–38.

37. Hiroi-Furuya E, Kameda T, Hiura K et al. Etidronate (EHDP) inhibits osteoclastic bone resorption, promotes apoptosis and disrupts actin rings in isolate-mature osteoclasts. Calcif Tissue Int 1999; 64: 219–23.

38. Benford HL, McGowan NW, Helfrich MH et al. Visualization of bisphosphonate-induced caspase-3 activity in apoptotic osteoclasts in vitro. Bone 2001; 28: 465–73.

39. Ito M, Amizuka N, Nakajima T, Ozawa H. Ultrastructural and cytochemical studies on cell death of osteoclasts induced by bisphosphonate treatment. Bone 1999; 25: 447–52.

40. Reszka AA, Halasy-Nagy JM, Masarachia PJ, Rodan GA. Bisphosphonates act directly on the osteoclast to induce caspase cleavage of mst1 kinase during apoptosis. A link between inhibition of the mevalonate pathway and regulation of an apoptosis-promoting kinase. J Biol Chem 1999; 274: 34967–73.

41. Sakai H, Kobayashi Y, Sakai E et al. Cell adhesion is a prerequisite for osteoclast survival. Biochem Biophys Res Commun 2000; 270: 550–6.

42. Colucci S, Minielli V, Zambonin G et al. Alendronate reduces adhesion of human osteoclast-like cells to bone and bone protein-coated surfaces. Calcif Tissue Int 1998; 63: 230–5.

43. Boissier S, Magnetto S, Frappart L et al. Bisphosphonates inhibit prostate and breast carcinoma cell adhesion to unmineralized and mineralized bone extracellular matrices. Cancer Res 1977; 57: 3890–4.

44. Van der Pluijm G, Vloedgraven H, van Beek E et al. Bisphosphonates inhibit the adhesion of breast cancer cells to bone matrices in vitro. J Clin Invest 1996; 98: 698–705.

45. Sato M, Grasser W. Effects of bisphosphonates on isolated rat osteoclasts as examined by reflected light microscopy. J Bone Min Res 1990; 5: 31–40.

46. Halasy-Nagy JM, Rodan GA, Reszka AA. Inhibition of bone resorption by alendronate and risedronate does not require osteoclast apoptosis. Bone 2001; 29: 553–9.

47. Miller SC, Jee WS. The effect of dichloromethylene diphosphonate, a pyrophosphate analog, on bone and bone cell structure in the growing rat. Anat Rec 1979; 193: 439–62.

48. Plasmans CM, Jap PH, Kuijpers W, Slooff TJ. Influence of a diphosphonate on the cellular aspect of young bone tissue. Calcif Tiss Int 1980; 32: 247–66.

49. Lerner UH, Larsson A. Effects of four bisphosphonates on bone resorption, lysosomal enzyme release, protein synthesis and mitotic activities in mouse calvarial bones in vitro. Bone 1987; 8: 179–89.

50. Alakangas A, Selander K, Mulari M et al. Alendronate disturbs vesicular trafficking in osteoclasts. Calcif Tissue Int 2002; 70: 40–7.

51. Zimolo Z, Wesolowski G, Rodan GA. Acid extrusion is induced by osteoclast attachment to bone. Inhibition by alendronate and calcitonin. J Clin Invest 1995; 96: 2277–83.

52. Boonekamp PM, van der Wee-Pals LJA, van Wijk-van Lennep MLL et al. Two modes of action of bisphosphonates on osteoclastic resorption of mineralised matrix. Bone Min 1986; 1: 27–39.

53. Boonekamp PM, Lowik CWGM, van der Wee-Pals LJA et al. Enhancement of the inhibitory action of APD on the transformation of osteoclast precursors into resorbing cells after dimethylation of the amino group. Bone Min 1987; 2: 29–42.

54. van Beek ER, Lowik CW, Papapoulos SE. Effect of alendronate treatment on the osteoclastogenic potential of bone marrow cells in mice. Bone 1997; 20: 335–40.

55. Hughes DE, McDonald BR, Russell RGG, Gowen M. Inhibition of osteoclast-like cell formation by bisphosphonates in long-term cultures of human bone marrow. J Clin Invest 1989; 83: 1930–5.

56. Van der Pluijm G, Lowik CW, de Groot H et al. Modulation of PTH-stimulated osteoclastic resorption by bisphosphonates in fetal mouse bone explants. J Bone Min Res 1991; 6: 1203–10.

57. Marshall MJ, Holt I, Davie MW. Osteoclast recruitment in mice is stimulated by (3-amino-1-hydroxypropylidene)-1,1-bisphosphonate. Calcif Tiss Int 1993; 52: 21–5.

58. Holt I, Marshall MJ, Davie MW. Pamidronate stimulates recruitment and decreases longevity of osteoclast nuclei in mice. Semin Arthr Rheum 1994; 23: 263–4.

59. Endo Y, Shibazaki M, Yamaguchi K et al. Inhibition of inflammatory actions of aminobisphosphonates by dichloromethylene bisphosphonate, a non-aminobisphosphonate. Br J Pharmacol 1999; 126: 903–10.

60. Endo Y, Nakamura M, Kikuchi T et al. Aminoalkylbisphosphonates, potent inhibitors of bone resorption, induce a prolonged stimulation of histamine synthesis and increase macrophages, granulocytes, and osteoclasts in vivo. Calcif Tiss Int 1993; 52: 248–54.

61. Flanagan AM, Chambers TJ. Inhibition of bone resorption by bisphosphonates: interactions between bisphosphonates, osteoclasts, and bone. Calcif Tiss Int 1991; 49: 407–15.

62. Owens JM, Fuller K, Chambers TJ. Osteoclast activation: potent inhibition by the bisphosphonate alendronate through a non-resorptive mechanism. J Cell Physiol 1997; 172: 79–86.

63. Fast DK, Felix R, Dowse C et al. The effects of diphosphonates on the growth and glycolysis of connective tissue cells in culture. Biochem J 1978; 172: 97–107.

64. Endo N, Rutledge SJ, Opas EE et al. Human protein tyrosine phosphatase-sigma: alternative splicing and inhibition by bisphosphonates. J Bone Min Res 1996; 11: 535–43.

65. Reinholz GG, Getz B, Pederson L et al. Bisphosphonates directly regulate cell proliferation, differentiation, and gene expression in human osteoblasts. Cancer Res 2000; 60: 6001–7.

66. Varghese S, Canalis E. Alendronate stimulates collagenase 3 expression in osteoblasts by posttranscriptional mechanisms. J Bone Min Res 2000; 15: 2345–51.

67. Sahni M, Guenther HL, Fleisch H et al. Bisphosphonates act on rat bone resorption through mediation of osteoblasts. J Clin Invest 1993; 91: 2004–10.

68. Vitte C, Fleisch H, Guenther HL. Bisphosphonates induce osteoblasts to secrete an inhibitor of osteoclast-mediated resorption. Endocrinology 1996; 137: 2324–33.

69. Yu X, Scholler J, Foged NT. Interaction between effects of parathyroid hormone and bisphosphonate on regulation of osteoclast activity by the osteoblast-like cell line UMR-106. Bone 1996; 19: 339–45.

70. Nishikawa M, Akatsu T, Katayama Y et al. Bisphosphonates act on osteoblastic cells and inhibit osteoclast formation in mouse marrow cultures. Bone 1996; 18: 9–14.

71. Plotkin LI, Weinstein RS, Parfitt AM et al. Prevention of osteocyte and osteoblast apoptosis by bisphosphonates and calcitonin. J Clin Invest 1999; 104: 1363–74.

72. Plotkin LI, Manolagas SC, Bellido T. Transduction of cell survival signals by connexin-43 hemichannels. J Biol Chem 2002; 277: 8648–57.

73. Mathov I, Plotkin LI, Sgarlata CL et al. Extracellular signal-regulated kinases and calcium channels are involved in the proliferative effect of bisphosphonates on osteoblastic cells in vitro. J Bone Min Res 2001; 16: 2050–6.

74. Zhang FL, Casey PJ. Protein prenylation: molecular mechanisms and functional consequences. Ann Rev Biochem 1996; 65: 241–69.

75. Amin D, Cornell SA, Gustafson SK et al. Bisphosphonates used for the treatment of bone disorders inhibit squalene synthase and cholesterol biosynthesis. J Lipid Res 1992; 33: 1657–63.

76. Amin D, Cornell SA, Perrone MH, Bilder GE. 1-Hydroxy-3-(methylpentylamino)-propylidene-1,1-bisphosphonic acid as a potent inhibitor of squalene synthase. Arzneimittel-Forschung 1996; 46: 759–62.

77. van Beek E, Pieterman E, Cohen L et al. Farnesyl pyrophosphate synthase is the molecular target of nitrogen-containing bisphosphonates. Biochem Biophys Res Commun 1999; 264: 108–11.

78. Bergstrom JD, Bostedor RG, Masarachia PJ et al. Alendronate is a specific, nanomolar inhibitor of farnesyl diphosphate synthase. Arch Biochem Biophys 2000; 373: 231–41.

79. Keller RK, Fliesler SJ. Mechanism of aminobisphosphonate action: characterization of alendronate inhibition of the isoprenoid pathway. Biochem Biophys Res Commun 1999; 266: 560–3.

80. Dunford JE, Thompson K, Coxon FP et al. Structure–activity relationships for inhibition of farnesyl diphosphate synthase *in vitro* and inhibition of bone resorption *in vivo* by nitrogen-containing bisphosphonates. J Pharmacol Exp Ther 2001; 235–42.

81. Grove JE, Brown RJ, Watts DJ. The intracellular target for the antiresorptive aminobisphosphonate drugs in *Dictyostelium discoideum* is the enzyme farnesyl diphosphate synthase. J Bone Min Res 2000; 15: 971–81.

82. Thompson K, Dunford JE, Ebetino FH, Rogers MJ. Identification of a bisphosphonate that inhibits isopentenyl diphosphate isomerase and farnesyl diphosphate synthase. Biochem Biophys Res Commun 2002; 290: 869–73.

83. Martin MB, Arnold W, Heath HT et al. Nitrogen-containing bisphosphonates as carbocation transition state analogs for isoprenoid biosynthesis. Biochem Biophys Res Commun 1999; 263: 754–8.

84. Luckman SP, Coxon FP, Ebetino FH et al. Heterocycle-containing bisphosphonates cause apoptosis and inhibit bone resorption by preventing protein prenylation: evidence from structure–activity relationships in J774 macrophages. J Bone Min Res 1998; 13: 1668–78.

85. Ebetino FH, Jamieson LA. The design and synthesis of bone-active phosphinic acid analogues: I. The pyridyl-aminomethane phosphonoalkylphosphinates. Phosphorus, Sulfur Silicon 1990; 51/52: 23–6.

86. Shinoda H, Adamek G, Felix R et al. Structure–activity relationships of various bisphosphonates. Calcif Tiss Int 1983; 35: 87–99.

87. van Beek E, Hoekstra M, van de Ruit M et al. Structural requirements for bisphosphonate actions *in vitro*. J Bone Min Res 1994; 9: 1875–82.

88. Coxon FP, Rogers MJ. The role of prenylated small GTP-binding proteins in the regulation of osteoclast function. Calcif Tissue Int 2003; 72: 80–4.

89. Zhang D, Udagawa N, Nakamura I et al. The small GTP-binding protein, rho p21, is involved in bone resorption by regulating cytoskeletal organization in osteoclasts. J Cell Sci 1995; 108: 2285–92.

90. Razzouk S, Lieberherr M, Cournot G. Rac-GTPase, osteoclast cytoskeleton and bone resorption. Eur J Cell Biol 1999; 78: 249–255.

91. Ory S, Munari-Silem Y, Fort P, Jurdic P. Rho and Rac exert antagonistic functions on spreading of macrophage-derived multinucleated cells and are not required for actin fiber formation. J Cell Sci 2000; 113: 1177–88.

92. Chellaiah MA, Soga N, Swanson S et al. Rho-A is critical for osteoclast podosome organization, motility, and bone resorption. J Biol Chem 2000; 275: 11993–2002.

93. Luckman SP, Hughes DE, Coxon FP et al. Nitrogen-containing bisphosphonates inhibit the mevalonate pathway and prevent post-translational prenylation of GTP-binding proteins, including Ras. J Bone Min Res 1998; 13: 581–9.

94. Fisher JE, Rogers MJ, Halasy JM et al. Alendronate mechanism of action: geranylgeraniol, an intermediate in the mevalonate pathway, prevents inhibition of osteoclast formation, bone resorption and kinase activation *in vitro*. Proc Natl Acad Sci USA 1999; 96: 133–8.

95. Woo JT, Kasai S, Stern PH, Nagai K. Compactin suppresses bone resorption by inhibiting the fusion of prefusion osteoclasts and disrupting the actin ring in osteoclasts. J Bone Min Res 2000; 15: 650–62.

96. Coxon FP, Benford HL, Russell RGG, Rogers MJ. Protein synthesis is required for caspase activation and induction of apoptosis by bisphosphonate drugs. Mol Pharmacol 1998; 54: 631–8.

97. Ito M, Chokki M, Ogino Y et al. Comparison of cytotoxic effects of bisphosphonates *in vitro* and *in vivo*. Calcif Tiss Int 1998; 63: 143–7.

98. Coxon FP, Helfrich MH, van't Hof RJ et al. Protein geranylgeranylation is required for osteoclast formation, function, and survival: inhibition by bisphosphonates and GGTI-298. J Bone Min Res 2000; 15: 1467–76.

99. Fisher JE, Rodan GA, Reszka AA. *In vivo* effects of bisphosphonates on the osteoclast mevalonate pathway. Endocrinology 2000; 141: 4793–6.

100. Frith JC, Monkkonen J, Auriola S et al. The molecular mechanism of action of the anti-resorptive and anti-inflammatory drug clodronate: evidence for the formation *in vivo* of a metabolite that inhibits bone resorption and causes osteoclast and macrophage apoptosis. Arthr Rheum 2001; 44: 2201–10.

101. van Beek E, Lowik C, Van der Pluijm G, Papapoulos S. The role of geranylgeranylation in bone resorption and its suppression by bisphosphonates in fetal bone explants *in vitro*: a clue to the mechanism of action of nitrogen-containing bisphosphonates. J Bone Min Res 1999; 14: 722–9.

102. Shipman CM, Croucher PI, Russell RGG et al. The bisphosphonate incadronate (YM175) causes apoptosis of human myeloma cells *in vitro* by inhibiting the mevalonate pathway. Cancer Res 1998; 58: 5294–7.

103. van Beek E, Pieterman E, Cohen L et al. Nitrogen-containing bisphosphonates inhibit isopentenyl pyrophosphate isomerase/farnesyl pyrophosphate synthase activity with relative potencies corresponding to their antiresorptive potencies *in vitro* and *in vivo*. Biochem Biophys Res Commun 1999; 255: 491–4.

104. Felix R, Fleisch H. Increase in fatty acid oxidation in calvaria cells cultured with diphosphonates. Biochem J 1981; 196: 237–45.

105. Felix R, Graham R, Russell G, Fleisch H. The effect of several diphosphonates on acid phosphohydrolases and other lysosomal enzymes. Biochim Biophys Acta 1976; 429: 429–38.

106. Klein G, Martin J-B, Satre M. Methylenediphosphonate, a metabolic poison in *Dictyostelium discoideum*. ^{31}P NMR evidence for accumulation of adenosine $5'$-(β,γ-methylenetriphosphate) and diadenosine $5',5'''$-P1, P4-(P2,P3-methylenetetraphosphate). Biochemistry 1999; 27: 1897–901.

107. Rogers MJ, Russell RGG, Blackburn GM et al. Metabolism of halogenated bisphosphonates by the cellular slime mould *Dictyostelium discoideum*. Biochem Biophys Res Commun 1992; 189: 414–23.

108. Rogers MJ, Ji X, Russell RG et al. Incorporation of bisphosphonates into adenine nucleotides by amoebae of the cellular slime mould *Dictyostelium discoideum*. Biochem J 1994; 303: 303–11.

109. Pelorgeas S, Martin JB, Satre M. Cytotoxicity of dichloromethane diphosphonate and of 1-hydroxy-ethane-1,1-diphosphonate in the amoebae of the slime mould *Dictyostelium discoideum*. A ^{31}P NMR study. Biochem Pharmacol 1992; 44: 2157–63.

110. Rogers MJ, Brown RJ, Hodkin V et al. Bisphosphonates are incorporated into adenine nucleotides by

human aminoacyl-tRNA synthetase enzymes. Biochem Biophys Res Commun 1996; 224: 863–9.

111. Frith JC, Monkkonen J, Blackburn GM et al. Clodronate and liposome-encapsulated clodronate are metabolized to a toxic ATP analog, adenosine 5′-(β,γ-dichloromethylene) triphosphate, by mammalian cells *in vitro*. J Bone Miner Res 1997; 12: 1358–67.

112. Auriola S, Frith J, Rogers MJ et al. Identification of adenine nucleotide-containing metabolites of bisphosphonate drugs using ion-pair liquid chromatography–electrospray mass spectrometry. J Chrom B 1997; 704: 187–95.

113. Lehenkari PP, Kellinsalmi M, Napankangas JP et al. Further insight into mechanism of action of clodronate: inhibition of mitochondrial ADP/ATP translocase by a non-hydrolyzable, adenine-containing metabolite. Mol Pharmacol 2002; 61: 1255–62.

114. Kroemer G, Reed JC. Mitochondrial control of cell death. Nature Med 2000; 6: 513–19.

115. Chatterjee D, Chakraborty M, Leit M et al. Sensitivity to vanadate and isoforms of subunits A and B distinguish the osteoclast proton pump from other vacuolar H⁺ ATPases. Proc Natl Acad Sci USA 1992; 89: 6257–61.

116. Blair HC, Teitelbaum SL, Ghiselli R, Gluck S. Osteoclastic bone resorption by a polarized vacuolar proton pump. Science 1989; 245: 855–7.

117. David P, Baron R. The vacuolar H⁺-ATPase: a potential target for drug development in bone diseases. Exp Opin Invest Drugs 1995; 4: 725–39.

118. David P, Baron R. The catalytic cycle of the vacuolar H(+)-ATPase. Comparison of proton transport in kidney- and osteoclast-derived vesicles. J Biol Chem 1994; 269: 30158–63.

119. David P, Nguyen H, Barbier A, Baron R. The bisphosphonate tiludronate is a potent inhibitor of the osteoclast vacuolar H(+)-ATPase. J Bone Min Res 1996; 11: 1498–507.

120. Teronen O, Heikkila P, Konttinen YT et al. MMP inhibition and downregulation by bisphosphonates. Ann NY Acad Sci 1999; 878: 453–65.

121. Skorey K, Ly HD, Kelly J et al. How does alendronate inhibit protein–tyrosine phosphatases? J Biol Chem 1997; 272: 22472–80.

122. Schmidt A, Rutledge SJ, Endo N et al. Protein–tyrosine phosphatase activity regulates osteoclast formation and function: inhibition by alendronate. Proc Natl Acad Sci USA 1996; 93: 3068–73.

123. Opas EE, Rutledge SJ, Golub E et al. Alendronate inhibition of protein–tyrosine-phosphatase-meg1. Biochem Pharmacol 1997; 54: 721–7.

124. Murakami H, Takahashi N, Tanaka S et al. Tiludronate inhibits protein tyrosine phosphatase activity in osteoclasts. Bone 1997; 20: 399–404.

26

Antitumour Effects of Bisphosphonates

Philippe Clézardin

Faculty of Medicine Laënnec, Lyon, France

INTRODUCTION

A very common metastatic site for multiple myeloma, prostate and breast carcinomas is bone (reviewed in [1]). In bone metastases, tumour cells stimulate osteoclast-mediated bone resorption, leading to osteolysis. Osteolysis in patients is reflected by the occurrence of pathological fractures, hypercalcaemia and intractable bone pain. Thus, any agent that could interfere with osteolysis would be a major therapeutic advance in the treatment of bone metastases.

Bisphosphonates are potent inhibitors of osteoclast-mediated bone resorption and have demonstrated clinical utility in the palliative treament of bone metastases (reviewed in [2]). Bisphosphonates are analogues of the naturally occurring compound pyrophosphate (reviewed in [3]). They contain two phosphonate groups attached to a single carbon atom, forming a P–C–P structure. Two chains (usually referred to as R_1 and R_2) are covalently bound to the carbon atom. The P–C–P backbone and the R_1 chain allow the binding of bisphosphonates to bone mineral, whereas the R_2 chain is mediating the antiosteoclastic activity of bisphosphonates [3]. The molecular mechanisms by which bisphosphonates inhibit osteoclast activity can be classified into two groups. Bisphosphonates that lack a nitrogen in the chemical structure of the R_2 chain (such as etidronate, clodronate and tiludronate) are metabolically incorporated into non-hydrolysable analogues of ATP that inhibit ATP-dependent intracellular enzymes [3]. In contrast, nitrogen-containing bisphosphonates (e.g. pamidronate, risedronate, alendronate, ibandronate and zoledronic acid) inhibit enzymes of the mevalonate pathway, thereby preventing the prenylation of GTPases that are essential for osteoclast function [3]. However, bisphosphonates not only act on osteoclasts but also on other cell types including tumour cells. We review the preclinical evidence here and discuss the possible mechanisms by which bisphosphonates act on tumour cells *in vitro* and *in vivo*.

MECHANISMS OF ACTION OF BISPHOSPHONATES ON TUMOUR CELLS *IN VITRO*

Bone metastasis formation is a multiple-step process involving tumour cell adhesion to bone, invasion and proliferation at the bone metastatic site. The potential inhibitory effect of bisphosphonates has been studied on each of these steps.

Effect of Bisphosphonates on Tumour Cell Adhesion to Bone

Breast and prostate carcinoma cells strongly adhere to bone mineral [4,5]. Pretreatment of cortical bone slices with different bisphosphonates (pamidronate, alendronate, ibandronate) inhibit adhesion of MDA-MB-231 breast carcinoma cells to bone [4]. However, bisphosphonate concentrations used in this study were rather high (10^{-5}–10^{-4}M), suggesting that such concentrations could not be achieved *in vivo*. We have therefore conducted a similar study in which breast and prostate carcinoma cells, instead of bone, were treated with increasing concentrations of bisphosphonates [5] We

Textbook of Bone Metastases. Edited by C. Jasmin, R. E. Coleman, L. R. Coia, R. Capanna and G. Saillant
© 2005 John Wiley & Sons Ltd: ISBN 0 471 87742 5

have found that bisphosphonates (clodronate, pamidronate, risedronate, ibandronate) dose-dependently inhibit tumour cell adhesion to bone. The relative order of potency of these bisphosphonates in inhibiting tumor cell adhesion to bone *in vitro* corresponds to their relative anti-resorptive potencies *in vivo* (i.e. ibandronate > risedronate > pamidronate > clodronate). More importantly, maximal inhibitory activity of bisphosphonates is achieved at concentrations of 10^{-8}–10^{-6} M, which are similar to the peak plasma concentration of each of these bisphosphonates. Thus, soluble bisphosphonates have a higher potency than matrix-bound bisphosphonates in inhibiting tumour cell adhesion. To demonstrate that bisphosphonates directly act on tumour cells to inhibit adhesion, we have compared the potency of pairs of analogues of risedronate (NE-10244 and NE-58051) that have slightly different structures but markedly different anti-resorptive potencies [5]. The bisphosphonate NE-58051 is 10 000-fold less potent than NE-10244 as an anti-resorptive agent *in vivo*. Similarly, NE-58051 is totally inactive at inhibiting breast and prostate tumour cell adhesion to bone when compared to that observed with NE-10244. Such markedly different potencies result in the increase in the R_2 chain length of NE-58051 by only one –$CH2$ group when compared to the R_2 chain of NE-10244. This increase in the chain length confers a planar conformation to the bisphosphonate NE-58051, whereas the NE-10244 adopts a chair conformation. Thus, our results are strongly suggestive of a stereospecific recognition of the bisphosphonates by breast and prostate carcinoma cells. The mechanisms of action of bisphosphonates as inhibitors of tumour cell adhesion are presently unknown. Although integrins mediate cell attachment to extracellular matrix, we do not observe any inhibition of the cell surface expression of integrins upon treatment of breast and prostate carcinoma cells with bisphosphonates [5]. However, it has been proposed that nitrogen-containing bisphosphonates, by affecting enzymes of the mevalonate pathway, interfere with the prenylation of the small GTPases [3]. Members of the small GTP-binding protein family such as Ras and Rho, play a key role during cell adhesion upon integrin ligation (reviewed in [6]). In addition, integrins must switch from an inactive to an active state to interact with extracellular matrix proteins [6]. It is therefore possible that bisphosphonates inhibit tumour cell adhesion by modulating the integrin affinity state and/or the subsequent activation of some prenylated GTPases. These questions are currently being investigated in our laboratory because we have previously shown that integrin $\alpha v \beta 3$ expression confers on tumour cells a greater propensity to metastasise to bone [7].

Effect of Bisphosphonates on Tumour Cell Invasion

Tumour cell invasion is an important process during bone metastasis formation [1]. It requires both cell migration and a localised cell surface proteolytic activity, which favours cell detachment from matrix proteins. Among proteases produced by tumour cells, matrix metalloproteinases (MMPs) play a key role in promoting tumour cell invasion [1]. We have therefore investigated the effect of bisphosphonates on breast and prostate carcinoma cell invasion *in vitro* [8]. Pretreatment of MDA-MB-231 and PmPC3 cancer cells with bisphosphonates (clodronate, risedronate, ibandronate, zoledronic acid) inhibits tumour cell invasion and their relative order of anti-invasive potency *in vitro* corresponds to their relative anti-resorptive potencies *in vivo* (i.e. zoledronic acid > ibandronate ≥ risedronate > clodronate) [8]. Maximal inhibitory activity of bisphosphonates is achieved at concentrations of 10^{-8}–10^{-6} M. Similarly, a substantial inhibition of tumour cell invasion is observed when PC-3 and DU-145 prostate carcinoma cells are treated with the bisphosphonate alendronate at concentrations of 10^{-12}–10^{-6} M [9]. As previously observed for tumour cell adhesion [5], the inactive analogue of risedronate, NE-58051, does not inhibit tumour cell invasion [8]. Moreover, NE-10790 (a phosphonocarboxylate analogue of risedronate, in which one of the phosphonate groups is substituted by a carboxyl group) inhibits tumour cell invasion to an extent similar to that observed with NE-10244, the active analogue of risedronate [8].

Taken together, our results [5,8] strongly suggest that the antitumour activity of bisphosphonates against invasion (and adhesion to bone) involves the R_2 side-chain (but not the P–C–P structure) of the molecule. Mechanisms of inhibition of tumour cell invasion by nitrogen-containing bisphosphonates are likely to involve the mevalonate pathway, because geranylgeraniol reverses the inhibitory effect of alendronate on PC-3 cell invasion [9]. Besides the fact that bisphosphonates inhibit tumour cell invasion, we and others [8,10] have shown that they also inhibit MMP activity. Surprisingly, bisphosphonates are about 1000-fold less potent at reducing MMP activity than they are at inhibiting tumour cell invasion [8,10]. Moreover, despite structural differences in their bioactive moiety, all of the bisphosphonates (including the inactive bisphosphonate NE-58051) are equipotent in inhibiting the proteolytic activity of MMPs [8]. In contrast, the phosphonocarboxylate NE-10790 (in which one of the phosphonate groups is substituted by a carboxyl group) does not inhibit the proteolytic activity of MMPs [8]. MMPs are zinc-dependent endopeptidases and we have shown that an excess of zinc ($50 \, \mu M$) completely abrogates the inhibitory effect of bisphosphonates on MMP activity [8]. Overall, our findings indicate that the phosphonate groups of bisphosphonates inhibit the proteolytic activity of MMPs through zinc chelation [8]. Therefore, inhibition of tumour cell invasion by bisphosphonates occurs through two distinct mechanisms: at low concentrations (10^{-8}–$10^{-6} M$), bisphosphonates inhibit the mevalonate pathway, whereas at higher concentrations ($10^{-4} M$), they inhibit MMP activity.

Effect of Bisphosphonates on Tumour Cell Proliferation and Survival

Bisphosphonates inhibit *in vitro* growth of human myeloma, breast and prostate carcinoma cell lines [11–17]. Although tumour cell growth inhibition by bisphosphonates does not result from calcium chelation [12,14,17], concentrations of 10^{-5}–$10^{-4} M$ or more of clodronate, pamidronate, ibandronate or zoledronic acid are required to inhibit tumour cell proliferation [11–17]. This suggests that underlying mechanisms involved in the inhibition of tumour cell growth are different from those taken to inhibit tumour cell invasion and adhesion to bone. In this respect, it has been shown that the mechanisms of action of pamidronate and zoledronic acid on inhibition of MDA-MB-231 cell proliferation do not involve the mevalonate pathway [18]. However, a cautionary note must be added here, since there are other reports showing that addition of an intermediate of the mevalonate pathway (geranylgeraniol) prevents bisphosphonate-mediated growth inhibition of some breast and myeloma cell lines (MCF-7, JJN-3) [11,17]. It is possible that mechanisms of growth inhibition induced by bisphosphonates are cell-type specific. Whatever the mechanisms are, this decrease in cell proliferation has been related to an induction of cell cytostasis [12,13,16] and/or apoptosis [11–17]. In addition, bisphosphonate-mediated tumour cell apoptosis is associated with a decreased expression of Bcl-2 (antiapoptotic protein) [12,14], a release of mitochondrial cytochrome *c* [19] and caspase-3 activation [14,15,17,19].

Combined Effect of a Bisphosphonate with a Neoplastic Agent on Tumour Cells

Most clinical studies are performed using a bisphosphonate in combination with conventional chemotherapy or endocrine therapy [2]. We have therefore studied the effect of ibandronate combined with taxoids on breast cancer cell functions. We have observed that ibandronate (at a concentration as low as $10^{-6} M$) potentiates the antitumour activity of taxoids (docetaxel and paclitaxel) against invasion and adhesion of MDA-MB-231 breast carcinoma cells to bone [20]. Similarly, zoledronic acid, in combination with paclitaxel, exerts a synergistic pro-apoptotic effect on MCF-7 and MDA-MB-231 breast carcinoma cells [17]. In addition, the combination of zoledronic acid and dexamethasone synergistically induces apoptosis of different myeloma cell lines [21]. These observations [17,20,21] are clinically relevant because they suggest that low circulating doses of bisphosphonates might have a systemic antitumour effect when combined with anticancer therapies.

MECHANISMS OF ACTION OF BISPHOSPHONATES ON TUMOUR GROWTH AND METASTASIS FORMATION *IN VIVO*

Effect of Bisphosphonates on Tumour Growth

Because bisphosphonates have antitumour properties *in vitro*, their effect on growth of tumour xenografts in animals has been investigated. Bisphosphonates (risedronate, alendronate, ibandronate, zoledronic acid) do not inhibit tumour growth in immunodeficient mice when human tumour cells (MDA-MB-231, PC-3, PC3-ML) are injected subcutaneously or orthotopically (into the mammary gland) [22–25]. The lack of inhibitory effect could be related to the fact that bisphosphonates have a high affinity for bone mineral and localise to bone rapidly. Thus, tumour xenografts may be exposed to these compounds for a too short period to observe cytotoxicity. Alternatively, the use of immunodeficient animals could explain the lack of inhibitory effect of bisphosphonates on tumour growth. Nitrogen-containing bisphosphonates (pamidronate, alendronate, ibandronate) stimulate the proliferation of $\gamma\delta$ T cells and the secretion of interferon-γ which, in turn, exhibits a strong cytotoxic activity against myeloma cell lines [26]. Nitrogen-containing bisphosphonates therefore have a pronounced effect on the immune system which might contribute to the antitumour efficacy of these compounds. In the light of this finding [26], future studies using immunocompetent syngeneic animals will be required to examine the effect of bisphosphonates on tumour growth *in vivo*.

Effect of Bisphosphonates on Metastasis Formation

Several studies demonstrate that bisphosphonates (clodronate, pamidronate, risedronate, ibandronate, zoledronic acid) inhibit the formation of osteolytic lesions induced by myeloma, breast and prostate carcinoma cells [22–24,27–33]. Histomorphometric analysis of these osteolytic lesions revealed that bisphosphonates decrease osteoclast number and markedly increase apoptosis in osteoclasts, demonstrating that bisphosphonates inhibit bone metastasis formation through halted bone resorption. This contention is supported by the fact that osteoprotegerin (another inhibitor of bone resorption) also inhibits breast or prostate cancer-induced osteolysis in animals [34,35]. Interestingly, it has been shown that pamidronate and zoledronic acid dose-dependently increase osteoprotegerin production by human osteoblasts, reaching a maximum effect at 10^{-6} and 10^{-8} M, respectively [36]. These findings suggest that the upregulation of osteoprotegerin could reduce the number of osteoclasts in addition to the direct antiosteoclastic activity of bisphosphonates. Moreover, a significant reduction of breast cancer burden in bone has been reported in metastatic animals treated with risedronate, ibandronate and zoledronic acid [22,24,29,32]. Similarly, in a murine model of human multiple myeloma using myeloma cells from patients, it has been shown that treatment of animals with pamidronate or zoledronic acid not only halted osteolysis but also reduced tumour burden [33]. It has been suggested that the inhibitory effect of bisphosphonates on skeletal tumour burden might be caused by an inhibition of osteoclastic bone resorption which, in turn, decreases the release of bone-derived growth factors required for tumour growth [1,22]. Although the primary antitumour effect of bisphosphonates in bone is most probably indirect, we cannot rule out at the present time the possibility that bisphosphonates are also directly acting on tumour cells to reduce skeletal tumour burden. We have recently developed a bone metastasis model in which fluorescence imaging allows the analysis of real-time tumour cell progression in live animals [32]. This animal model should help to resolve this specific question. Besides the fact that they inhibit bone metastasis formation, the single use of bisphospho-

nates does not inhibit the formation of lung or liver metastases in animals [37]. In contrast, the combined use of a bisphosphonate with anticancer agents (doxorubicin, paclitaxel) inhibits not only bone metastases but also soft tissue metastases [23,37].

Effect of Bisphosphonates on Angiogenesis

Because angiogenesis is essential for the growth of metastases, we have examined the effects of different bisphosphonates on inhibition of endothelial cell functions *in vitro* and *in vivo* [38]. Treatment of endothelial cells with bisphosphonates (clodronate, risedronate, ibandronate, zoledronic acid) reduces proliferation, induces apoptosis, and decreases capillary-like tube formation *in vitro*. These findings have been confirmed *in vivo*. In order to develop an angiogenesis model in a non-calcified tissue where bisphosphonates could accumulate, we have first studied the tissue distribution of [14C]bisphosphonates in male rats. [14C]clodronate, [14C]ibandronate and [14C]zoledronic acid not only accumulate in bone, but also transiently and specifically accumulate in the prostate. The effects of bisphosphonates have been therefore tested in an animal model where testosterone induces the revascularisation of the prostate gland in castrated rats. We have found that treatment of castrated rats with testosterone in combination with ibandronate or zoledronic acid induces a 50% reduction of the revascularisation of the prostate compared to that observed in castrated rats treated with testosterone alone. Interestingly, the anti-angiogenic activity of bisphosphonates is not restricted to our *in vivo* model of prostate revascularisation. In another series of experiments, the systemic administration of zoledronic acid to mice results in potent inhibition of angiogenesis induced by subcutaneous implants impregnated with basic fibroblast growth factor (b-FGF) [39]. Clodronate and pamidronate also inhibit vascularisation in the chicken chorioallantoic membrane assay [40]. Finally, pamidronate decreases circulating levels of vascular endothelial growth factor (VEGF) in cancer patients with bone metastases [41] which could, in turn, inhibit angiogenesis.

CONCLUSION

There is now extensive *in vitro* and *in vivo* preclinical evidence that bisphosphonates have antitumour activity and can reduce skeletal tumour burden. These antitumour effects have been proposed to be indirect (through inhibition of bone resorption, inhibition of angiogenesis and stimulation of the immune system) and direct (through inhibition of tumour cell invasion, proliferation and adhesion to bone). Further research will be required to fully elucidate the molecular mechanisms involved. Metastasis is the most catastrophic complication of cancer, and understanding these mechanisms will provide greater insights into the most effective dose and schedule of bisphosphonates that should be given to patients to maximise their antitumour potential. Although some clinical studies suggest that bisphosphonates can reduce the occurrence of bone metastases when used in the adjuvant setting, it is not yet clear which patients are ideal candidates for prevention strategies.

REFERENCES

1. Guise TA, Mundy GR. Cancer and bone. Endocr Rev 1998; 19: 18–54.
2. Body JJ, Bartl R, Burckhardt P et al. Current use of bisphosphonates in oncology. J Clin Oncol 1998; 16: 3890–9.
3. Rogers MJ, Gordon S, Benford HL et al. Cellular and molecular mechanisms of action of bisphosphonates. Cancer 2000; 88: 2961–78.
4. van der Pluijm G, Vloedgraven H, van Beek E et al. Bisphosphonates inhibit the adhesion of breast cancer cells to bone matrices in vitro. J Clin Invest 1996; 98: 698–705.
5. Boissier S, Magnetto S, Frappart L et al. Bisphosphonates inhibit prostate and breast carcinoma cell adhesion to unmineralized and mineralized bone extracellular matrices. Cancer Res 1997; 57: 3890–4.
6. Schwartz MA. Integrin signaling revisited. Trends Cell Biol 2001; 11: 466–70.
7. Pécheur I, Peyruchaud O, Serre CM et al. Integrin $\alpha v \beta 3$ expression confers on tumor cells a greater propensity to metastasize to bone. FASEB J 2002; 16: 1266–8.
8. Boissier S, Ferreras M, Peyruchaud O et al. Bisphosphonates inhibit breast and prostate carcinoma cell invasion, an early event in the formation of bone metastases. Cancer Res 2000; 60: 2949–54.
9. Virtanen SS, Väänänen HK, Härkönen PL, Lakkakorpi PT. Alendronate inhibits invasion of PC-3 prostate cancer cells by affecting the mevalonate pathway. Cancer Res 2002; 62: 2708–14.
10. Teronen O, Konttinen YT, Lindqvist C et al. Inhibition of matrix metalloproteinase-1 by dichloromethylene bisphosphonate (clodronate). Calcif Tissue Int 1997; 61: 59–61.
11. Shipman C, Rogers MJ, Apperley JF et al. Bisphosphonates induce apoptosis in human myeloma cell lines: a novel anti-tumor activity. Br J Haematol 1997; 98: 665–72.
12. Aparicio A, Gardner A, Savage YTA et al. In vitro cytoreductive effects on multiple myeloma cells induced by bisphosphonates. Leukemia 1998; 12: 220–9.
13. Derenne S, Amiot M, Barillé S et al. Zoledronate is a potent inhibitor of myeloma cell growth and secretion of IL-6 and MMP-1 by the tumoral environment. J Bone Min Res 1999; 14: 2048–56.
14. Senaratne SG, Pirianov G, Mansi JL et al. Bisphosphonates induce apoptosis in human breast cancer cell lines. Br J Cancer 2000; 82: 1459–68.
15. Fromigue O, Lagneaux L, Body JJ. Bisphosphonates induce breast cancer cell death in vitro. J Bone Min Res 2000; 15: 2211–21.
16. Lee MV, Fong EM, Singer FR, Guenette RS. Bisphosphonate treatment inhibits the growth of prostate cancer cells. Cancer Res 2001; 61: 2602–8.
17. Jagdev SP, Coleman RE, Shipman CM et al. The bisphosphonate, zoledronic acid, induces apoptosis of breast cancer cells: evidence for synergy with paclitaxel. Br J Cancer 2001; 84: 1126–34.
18. Reinholz GR, Getz B, Sanders ES et al. Distinct mechanisms of bisphosphonate action between osteoblasts and breast cancer cells: identity of a potent new bisphosphonate analogue. Breast Cancer Res Treat 2002; 71: 257–68.
19. Senaratne SG, Mansi JL, Colston KW. The bisphosphonate zoledronic acid impairs membrane localisation and induces cytochrome c release in breast cancer cells. Br J Cancer 2002; 86: 1479–86.
20. Magnetto S, Boissier S, Delmas P, Clézardin P. Additive antitumor activities of taxoids in combination with the bisphosphonate ibandronate against invasion and adhesion of human breast carcinoma cells to bone. Int J Cancer 1999; 83: 263–9.
21. Tassone P, Forciniti S, Galea E et al. Growth inhibition and synergistic induction of apoptosis by zoledronate and dexamethasone in human myeloma cell lines. Leukemia 2000; 14: 841–4.
22. Sasaki A, Boyce BF, Story B et al. Bisphosphonate risedronate reduces metastatic human breast cancer burden in bone in nude mice. Cancer Res 1995; 55: 3551–7.
23. Stearns ME, Wang M. Effects of alendronate and taxol on PC-3ML cell bone metastases in SCID mice. Invasion Metast 1996; 16: 116–31.
24. Hiraga T, Williams PJ, Mundy GR, Yoneda T. The bisphosphonate ibandronate promotes apoptosis in MDA-MB-231 human breast cancer cells in bone metastases. Cancer Res 2001; 61: 4418–24.
25. Fournier P, Frappart L, Clézardin P. Zoledronic acid does not inhibit growth of MDA-MB-231 and PC3 tumor xenografts in animals (unpublished results).
26. Kunzmann V, Bauer E, Feurle J et al. Stimulation of $\gamma \delta T$ cells by aminobisphosphonates and induction of anti-plasma cell activity in multiple myeloma. Blood 2000; 96: 384–92.
27. Jung A, Bornand J, Mermillod B et al. Inhibition by diphosphonates of bone resorption induced by the Walker tumor of the rat. Cancer Res 1984; 44: 3007–11.
28. Nemoto R, Sato S, Nishijima Y et al. Effects of a new bisphosphonate (AHBuBP) on osteolysis induced by human prostate cancer cells in nude mice. J Urol 1990; 144: 770–4.
29. Sasaki A, Kitamura K, Alcalde RE et al. Effect of a newly developed bisphosphonate, YH529, on osteolytic bone metastases in nude mice. Int J Cancer 1998; 77: 279–85.

30. Dallas SL, Garrett IR, Oyajobi BO et al. Ibandronate reduces osteolytic lesions but not tumor burden in a murine model of myeloma bone disease. Blood 1999; 93: 1697–706.

31. Shipman CM, Vanderkerken K, Rogers MJ et al. The potent bisphosphonate ibandronate does not induce myeloma cell apoptosis in a murine model of established multiple myeloma. Br J Haematol 2000; 111: 283–6.

32. Peyruchaud O, Winding B, Pécheur I et al. Early detection of bone metastases in a murine model using fluorescent human breast cancer cells: application to the use of the bisphosphonate zoledronic acid in the treatment of osteolytic lesions. J Bone Min Res 2001; 16: 2027–34.

33. Yaccoby S, Pearse RN, Johnson CL et al. Myeloma interacts with the bone marrow microenvironment to induce osteoclastogenesis and is dependent on osteoclast activity. Br J Haematol 2002; 116: 278–90.

34. Zhang J, Dai J, Qi Y et al. Osteoprotegerin inhibits prostate cancer-induced osteoclastogenesis and prevents prostate tumor growth in the bone. J Clin Invest 2001; 107: 1235–44.

35. Morony S, Capparelli C, Sarosi I et al. Osteoprotegerin inhibits osteolysis and decreases skeletal tumor burden in syngeneic and nude mouse models of experimental bone metastasis. Cancer Res 2001; 61: 4432–6.

36. Viereck V, Emons G, Lauck V et al. Bisphosphonates pamidronate and zoledronic acid stimulate osteoprotegerin production by primary human osteoblasts. Biochem Biophys Res Commun 2002; 291: 680–6.

37. Yoneda T, Michigami T, Yi B et al. Actions of bisphosphonate on bone metastasis in animal models of breast carcinoma. Cancer 2000; 88: 2979–88.

38. Fournier P, Boissier S, Filleur S et al. Bisphosphonates inhibit angiogenesis *in vitro* and testosterone-stimulated vascular regrowth in the ventral prostate in castrated rats (submitted).

39. Wood J, Bonjean K, Ruetz S et al. Novel anti-angiogenic effects of the bisphosphonate compound zoledronic acid. J Pharm Expl Ther 2002; 302: 1055–61.

40. Steiner R, Qu BX, Laube-Gschwend E. Angiostatic activity of pamidronate and clodronate in the chicken chorioallantoic membrane assay—preliminary report. In Bijvoet OLM, Lipton A (eds), Osteoclast Inhibition in the Management of Malignancy-related Bone Disorders. Hogrefe and Huber: Lewiston, NY, 1990: 86–8.

41. Santini D, Vincenzi B, Avvisati G et al. Pamidronate induces modifications of circulating angiogenetic factors in cancer patients. Clin Cancer Res 2002; 8: 1080–4.

27

Management of Hypercalcaemia

Stuart H. Ralston

Aberdeen University Medical School, Aberdeen, UK

PRESENTATION AND DIAGNOSIS

Hypercalcaemia is a common metabolic complication of malignancy, which tends to occur at a relatively late stage in the course of most cancers. It is important to recognise and treat hypercalcaemia, however, since evidence from observational studies indicates that effective control of hypercalcaemia improves symptoms and, in some cases, prolongs survival [1]. The symptoms of hypercalcaemia in malignancy are non-specific and are easily confused with those of the underlying cancer or with the effects of anticancer treatment. In view of this, it is important to consider the possibility of hypercalcaemia in any cancer patient with suggestive symptoms (Table 27.1). The diagnosis of hypercalcaemia is made biochemically by the measurement of total serum calcium values and adjusting these for albumin concentrations. It is especially important that albumin-adjusted calcium concentrations are used in cancer patients, since hypoalbuminaemia is common in cancer [2]. Symptoms of hypercalcaemia tend to increase in proportion to severity of hypercalcaemia, but there is considerable variation between individuals, such that some patients experience severe symptoms with relatively mild hypercalcaemia, and vice versa.

TUMOURS ASSOCIATED WITH HYPERCALCAEMIA

Hypercalcaemia can occur in virtually any malignant tumour but is particularly common as a complication of multiple myeloma, breast cancer, lung cancer and genitourinary tumours [3]. These differences in incidence between tumour types reflect the ability of some but not all tumours to produce humoral factors that act locally or systemically to raise serum calcium concentrations. It is the author's clinical impression that cancer-associated hypercalcaemia is seen less commonly in hospital practice than was the case 5–10 years ago, possibly reflecting the increasing use of bisphosphonates for prevention of metastatic bone disease and general improvements in anti-cancer treatment.

PATHOPHYSIOLOGY

Under normal circumstances, serum calcium levels are held within narrow limits by homeostatic mechanisms that balance fluxes of calcium from bone, intestine and kidney into the extracellular fluid. Hypercalcaemia occurs when these mechanisms are overwhelmed and in hypercalcaemia of malignancy this generally occurs when calcium release from excessive bone resorption exceeds the rate at which calcium can be excreted by the kidney (Figure 27.1). Several tumour-produced factors have been identified that contribute to the pathogenesis of hypercalcaemia in malignancy, and these are summarised in Table 27.2. Parathyroid hormone-related protein (PTHrP) is the most important mediator of hypercalcaemia in malignancy, because it stimulates osteoclastic bone resorption and at the same time reduces urinary calcium excretion by elevating renal tubular calcium reabsorption [4]. Whilst parathyroid hormone-related protein is produced by normal cells, dysregulation of PTHrP

Textbook of Bone Metastases. Edited by C. Jasmin, R. E. Coleman, L. R. Coia, R. Capanna and G. Saillant
© 2005 John Wiley & Sons Ltd: ISBN 0 471 87742 5

Table 27.1.   Symptoms and signs of hypercalcaemia in malignancy

Kidney	Gut	CNS	CVS	Other
Polyuria	Anorexia	Confusion	Arrhythmia	Conjunctivitis
Polydipsia	Nausea	Coma	Increased sensitivity	Malaise
Thirst	Vomiting	Depression	to digoxin	Fatigue
Renal failure	Constipation	Neurological signs		
		Seizures		
		Reduced pain threshold		
		Muscle weakness		
		Hypotonia		

production occurs during tumour development, releasing excessive amounts of hormone into the systemic circulation [5]. Proinflammatory cytokines, such as interleukin-1, and tumour necrosis factors α and β (TNFα, TNFβ) are potent bone-resorbing factors which appear to play an important role in the pathogenesis of hypercalcaemia in multiple myeloma [6,7]. These factors are released locally by tumour cells and act to increase osteoclastic bone resorption in the regions surrounding tumour deposits. The active vitamin D metabolite 1,25-dihydroxyvitamin D acts as a mediator of hypercalcaemia in some lymphomas, where it is produced by the tumour cells in an unregulated fashion from its precursor 25-hydroxyvitamin D [8,9]. The resulting increase in circulating levels of 1,25-dihydroxyvitamin D contribute to

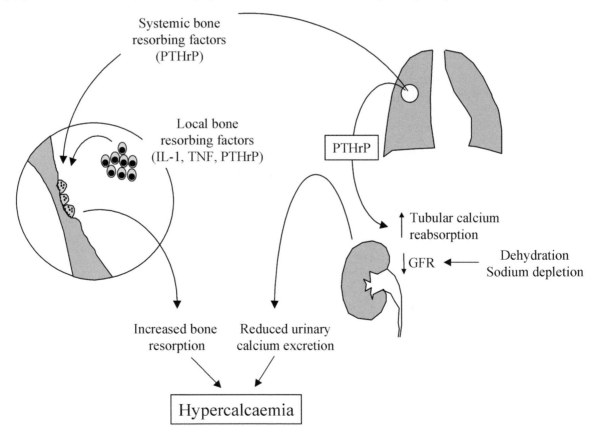

Figure 27.1.   Pathogenesis of hypercalcaemia in malignancy. PTHrP, Parathyroid hormone-related protein; IL-1, interleukin-1; TNF, tumour necrosis factors

Table 27.2. Key mediators of hypercalcaemia in malignancy

Mediator	Actions	Important in
PTHrP	Increases osteoclastic bone resorption	Lung
	Increases renal tubular calcium reabsorption	Bladder/ureter
	Increases 1,25-dihydroxyvitamin D production	Kidney
		Breast ($\sim 50\%$)
IL-1	Increases osteoclastic bone resorption	Myeloma
TNF	Increases osteoclastic bone resorption	Myeloma
1,25-Dihydroxyvitamin D	Increases osteoclastic bone resorption	Myeloma
	Increases intestinal calcium absorption	Lymphoma

hypercalcaemia by increasing bone resorption and by increasing intestinal calcium absorption. This type of hypercalcaemia can be precipitated or made worse by vitamin D administration and exposure to ultraviolet light. Rare instances of hypercalcaemia have been documented in association with overproduction of vitamin D metabolites by solid tumours. Hypercalcaemia that is responsive to treatment with cyclooxygenase inhibitors has been described and is attributed to excessive production of prostaglandins by the primary tumour or the release of factors which stimulate bone resorption through prostaglandin-mediated pathways [10]. This type of hypercalcaemia seems to be relatively rare. Several other factors with bone-resorbing effects, such as transforming growth factors alpha and beta (TNFα, TNFβ) have been isolated from tumours that cause hypercalcaemia, although the role of these factors in the pathogenesis of hypercalcaemia is poorly defined.

The kidney plays an important role in the pathogenesis of cancer-associated hypercalcaemia [11]. Dehydration and sodium depletion occur as the result of anorexia and vomiting and this reduces calcium excretion by reducing glomerular filtration rate (GFR) and increasing sodium-linked calcium reabsorption in the proximal renal tubule [12]. Once established, hypercalcaemia worsens dehydration by impairing urinary concentrating ability and promoting sodium and water excretion. Progressive renal failure may then develop, either as the result of dehydration and volume depletion, or in association with specific nephrotoxic factors, such as Bence–Jones protein. Another important factor that impairs calcium excretion is PTHrP, which acts on the distal renal tubule to enhance reabsorption of calcium, even in the absence of dehydration [13,14]. Intestinal calcium absorption seldom contributes to the pathogenesis of hypercalcaemia of malignancy, even though serum levels of 1,25-dihydroxyvitamin D can be increased in some patients

[8,9,15]. The reasons for this are not entirely clear, but possible explanations include the fact that patients with advanced malignancy have malabsorption [16], or because they are anorexic and taking little in the way of dietary calcium [17].

MANAGEMENT OF HYPERCALCAEMIA IN MALIGNANCY

Hypercalcaemia can generally be controlled by treating the underlying tumour and indeed, availability of effective antitumour therapy is the most important determinant of long-term survival [1,18]. In some cases, however, antihypercalcaemic therapy may be required to "buy time" for antitumour therapy to take effect. In others, antihypercalcaemic therapy may be indicated as a palliative manoeuvre to try to improve symptoms in those patients for whom antitumour therapy is unavailable or ineffective. Observational studies indicate that antihypercalcaemic therapy in cancer patients is associated with an improvement of symptoms (Figure 27.2).

Rehydration

Rehydration should be given to all patients with acute hypercalcaemia and should be considered in those with recurrent or persistent hypercalcaemia where there is clinical evidence of dehydration and/or serum-adjusted calcium values are > 3.0 mM. Typically, rehydration should begin with 4–6 litres of 0.9% saline daily for the first 48 h, and 2–3 litres daily thereafter until the hypercalcaemia is controlled. This regimen is sufficient to replace the sodium and water deficit in most patients and will also improve hypercalcaemia by promoting a sodium-linked calcium diuresis in the proximal renal tubule [11]. Loop diuretics should not be routinely

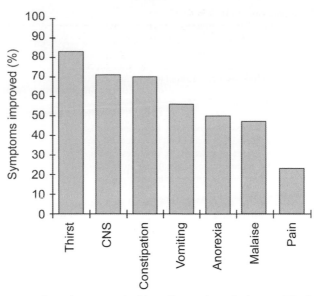

Figure 27.2. Symptomatic response in patients treated with antihypercalcaemic therapy. The figure shows percent of individual symptoms which improved after treatment in a series of patients with cancer-associated hypercalcaemia who were given various antihypercalcaemic agents. From Ralston et al. [1] Cancer-associated hypercalcemia: morbidity and mortality. Ann Intern Med 1990; 112: 499–504

used in the rehydration phase of antihypercalcaemic treatment since there is a risk that they may actually have a deleterious effect by causing extracellular volume contraction. An exception is in elderly patients with limited cardiac reserve, when it is thought that the extra fluids may provoke heart failure. The use of forced saline diuresis (combining large doses of loop diuretics with very large quantities of saline [19]) is potentially hazardous and cannot be recommended in view of the availability of safer and more effective treatments.

Bisphosphonates

Many inhibitors of bone resorption have been successfully used in the treatment of tumour-induced hypercalcaemia, but bisphosphonates are the treatment of first choice. Bisphosphonates are a group of related compounds that are potent inhibitors of osteoclastic bone resorption [20]. Many bisphosphonates have been used in the treatment of cancer-associated hypercalcaemia but most clinical experience has been gained with etidronate (ethanehydroxy bisphosphonate), clodronate (dichloromethylene bisphosphonate), pamidronate (aminohydroxypropylidene bisphosphonate), ibandronate (1-hydroxy-3-(methylpentylamino)propylidene bisphosphonate) and

zoledronate (1-hydroxy-2(1*H*-imidazol-1-yl) ethylidene bisphosphonate).

Etidronate

Etidronate was one of the first bisphosphonates to be used in the treatment of cancer-associated hypercalcaemia. In early studies, etidronate was given by intravenous (i.v.) injection in daily doses of 200–1000 mg for up to 10 days. Although this treatment was effective [21], several case reports appeared documenting an association between high-dose i.v. bisphosphonates and acute renal failure in hypercalcaemic patients [22]. Subsequently, the recommended dose of etidronate in the treatment of hypercalcaemia was reduced to 7.5 mg/kg body weight/day by slow i.v. infusion for a maximum of 3 consecutive days. At these doses etidronate is relatively ineffective in the treatment of cancer-associated hypercalcaemia and restores normocalcaemia in only 15–40% of cases [23–25]. Serum calcium values start to fall within 2–3 days of starting etidronate and the duration of action is about 10–12 days. Randomised comparative studies have shown that etidronate is significantly superior to rehydration with intravenous saline alone in the treatment of cancer-associated hypercalcaemia [26]. However, it is less effective than i.v. pamidronate

[25,27] or gallium nitrate [28] in terms of the proportion of patients achieving normocalcaemia, and in the duration of effect. Oral etidronate is relatively ineffective as a primary treatment for hypercalcaemia, but has been shown to prolong the effect of i.v. etidronate. In one study, cancer patients who became normocalcaemic following i.v. etidronate relapsed on average 30 days after treatment when also given oral etidronate (20 mg/kg/day), compared with 12 days when i.v. etidronate was given alone [23].

Adverse effects to i.v. etidronate in cancer patients are rare, although a disturbance in taste sensation has been reported [29]. Since prolonged etidronate therapy has been associated with the development of osteomalacia in Paget's disease [30], it is currently recommended that the duration of therapy be limited to 30 days in patients with tumour-induced hypercalcaemia.

Clodronate

Clodronate is an effective treatment for cancer-associated hypercalcaemia. Many dose regimens of clodronate have been used, including repeated i.v. injections of 100–300 mg [21]; slow i.v. infusions of 300–1500 mg on a single occasion; or repeated daily infusions of 300–600 mg to a total dose of 3 g or more [31,32]. Whilst some investigators have reported little or no difference between single infusions of 500–600 mg and repeated infusions of 300 mg daily for 5–10 days [33], others have reported that in certain groups of patients total doses of 1500 mg are more effective than lower doses [32,34]. The current recommended dose of clodronate for treatment of hypercalcaemia is 1500 mg, either as a single i.v. infusion over 24 h or in divided doses of 300 mg daily for 5 days [31]. Serum calcium values start to fall within 2–3 days of commencing treatment and normocalcaemia is restored in 40–80% of patients, with a maximal response at day 5–6, depending on the mix of tumour types and dose given [25,31,32,35]. The median duration of action is about 12 days. As with other bisphosphonates, patients with local osteolytic mechanisms of hypercalcaemia (e.g. myeloma) have been found to respond better to clodronate than those with humorally-mediated hypercalcaemia [33].

Two randomised studies have compared the effects of clodronate with other bisphosphonates in the treatment of hypercalcaemia. In one, a single infusion of 600 mg i.v. clodronate was slightly more effective than i.v. etidronate (7.5 mg/kg/day × 3), but significantly less effective than 30 mg i.v. pamidronate in terms of the proportion of patients achieving normocalcaemia (83% vs. 41%; $p < 0.05$) and the duration of action (12 days vs. 30 days; $p < 0.01$) [25]. In another study, higher doses of clodronate (1500 mg) and pamidronate (90 mg) were compared [35]. Clodronate restored normocalcaemia in 80% of cases when compared with 100% for pamidronate (not significant) but had a significantly shorter duration of action than pamidronate (14 days vs. 28 days; $p < 0.01$) (Figure 27.2).

Oral clodronate has been successfully used in the primary treatment of cancer-associated hypercalcaemia [36] but it is more commonly employed as an adjunct to intravenous clodronate and other bisphosphonates to prevent relapse of hypercalcaemia [37]. The recommended dose range for oral clodronate is 1600–3200 mg daily, depending on the individual response. Doses of up to 2400 mg clodronate daily are generally well-tolerated, but gastrointestinal side-effects such as diarrhoea, may occur with higher doses [38]. Intravenous clodronate is also well tolerated, but acute renal failure has been recorded in an isolated patient with severe hypercalcaemia who was given high doses (19.9 g over 30 days) by repeated i.v. infusions [22].

Pamidronate

Pamidronate is a highly effective treatment for cancer-associated hypercalcaemia. Many treatment regimens have been used in hypercalcaemia, including repeated daily infusions of 15 mg for up to 9 days and single i.v. infusions of 5–90 mg [29,39–42]. Single infusions of 30–90 mg pamidronate are generally used in routine clinical practice. There is no consistent evidence to support an increased rate of response with high-dose pamidronate (e.g. 90 mg) as compared with lower doses (e.g. 15–30 mg) [40,43]. However, there is evidence that patients with very severe hypercalcaemia (> 3.5 mM) respond more completely to higher doses [44], and escalating doses (up to 160 mg) may be required to control resistant or recurrent hypercalcaemia [45]. Reported rates of normocalcaemia in hypercalcaemic cancer patients treated with i.v. pamidronate are in the range 30–100% in different series, depending on the dose given and tumour types studied [25,29,40,41]. The onset of effect is usually seen within 1–2 days, with a nadir at day 6 and duration of effect of up to 30 days. In general terms, patients with humoral hypercalcaemia respond less well to pamidronate than those with local osteolytic hypercalcaemia. Biochemical markers of humoral hypercalcaemia, such as nephrogenous cAMP excretion, tubular phosphate threshold and PTHrP level itself, have all been shown to correlate with the calcium-lowering effect of pamidronate [46–48]. Several randomised clinical trials have been conducted comparing pamidronate with other anti-hypercalcaemic agents. An early study showed that repeated infusions of pamidronate 15 mg daily (mean dose 90 mg) were superior to mithramycin and prednisolone 40 mg plus calcitonin 100 IU t.i.d. in the treatment of cancer-associated hypercalcaemia, with respect to both the calcium-lowering effect and the duration of action [49]. In other studies, 60 mg i.v. pamidronate was found to be superior to mithramycin in terms of biochemical response and also was better tolerated [50,51].

Comparisons with other bisphosphonates have shown that 30 mg i.v. pamidronate is superior to i.v. etidronate (7.5 mg/kg/day × 3) and i.v. clodronate (600 mg) in the treatment of cancer-associated hyper-calcaemia [25] in terms of calcium-lowering response and duration of action. Another study showed that pamidronate 90 mg had a similar calcium-lowering effect to 1500 mg clodronate in the short term but had a longer duration of action (28 days vs. 14 days; $p < 0.01$) (Figure 27.3).

Intravenous pamidronate is generally well tolerated but, in common with other aminobisphosphonates, can cause a transient pyrexia and 'flu-like symptoms affecting up to 30% of patients [52]. Rare instances of allergic reactions have also been reported. Oral pamidronate has been used successfully in the treatment of hypercalcaemia associated with malignancy [53] but is not generally available for clinical use, due to problems with gastrointestinal intolerance, including dyspepsia and oesophageal ulceration.

Ibandronate

Ibandronate is a highly potent aminobisphosphonate with inhibitory effects on bone resorption approximately 50 times greater than those of pamidronate. Ibandronate has been found to be an effective treatment for hypercalcaemia at doses as low as 0.2 mg, but clinical studies have shown that the optimal response occurs over the dose range 2–6 mg [54,55]. In one study, approximately 50% of patients achieved normocalcaemia with 2 mg ibandronate given by i.v. infusion compared with 75–77% with 4 mg and 6 mg infusions [55]. The onset of effect, time to maximal response and duration of action of ibandronate is similar to that of pamidronate. Like pamidronate, tumour type has been shown to influence response to ibandronate, such that patients with local osteolytic hypercalcaemia respond best and those with

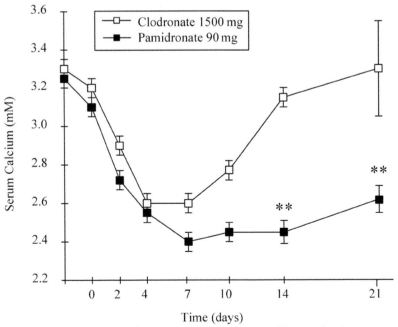

Figure 27.3. Comparison of intravenous clodronate and intravenous pamidronate in the treatment of cancer-associated hypercalcaemia. **$p < 0.01$ pamidronate compared with clodronate. From Purohit et al. A randomised double-blind comparison of intravenous pamidronate and clodronate in the hypercalcaemia of malignancy. Br J Cancer 1995; 72: 1289–93 [35]

humorally-mediated hypercalcaemia and raised PTHrP values respond less well [56]. Intravenous ibandronate is well tolerated but, like other aminobisphosphonates, has been found to cause transient pyrexia in up to 30% of cases [55].

Zoledronate

Zoledronate is an extremely potent aminobisphosphonate that is approximately 100–850 times more potent than pamidronate at inhibiting bone resorption *in vitro* and in animal models [57]. Intravenous zoledronate is a highly effective treatment for cancer-associated hypercalcaemia. In a dose-ranging study, 19/20 (93%) patients treated with i.v. zoledronate 0.02–0.04 mg/kg by single i.v. infusion over 30 min were rendered normocalcaemic and remained so for 32–39 days. The onset of effect for zoledronate appears to be more rapid than with other bisphosphonates, since a significant reduction in serum calcium occurs at day 1, with restoration of normocalcaemia in most cases by day 2 or 3. Comparative studies have shown that slow i.v. injections of zoledronate are superior to i.v. infusions of 90 mg pamidronate in the treatment of cancer-associated hypercalcaemia. Of 278 evaluable patients who took part in randomised studies of i.v. zoledronate vs. pamidronate, normocalcaemia was restored in 88.4% of those given 4 mg zoledronate and 86.7% given 8 mg zoledronate in comparison with a 69.7% rate of normocalcaemia in patients given 90 mg pamidronate ($p < 0.02$). Normalisation of serum calcium values also occurred sooner with zoledronate and the median time to relapse of hypercalcaemia was longer (30–40 days, compared with 17 days with pamidronate). Zoledronate appears to be generally well tolerated but causes fever in a proportion of treated patients. On the basis of current evidence, therefore, single i.v. doses of 4 mg or 8 mg zoledronate appear to be highly effective in the treatment of cancer-associated hypercalcaemia, with possible advantages over other bisphosphonates in terms of efficacy, onset of effect and duration of action.

Other Bisphosphonates

Alendronate has been quite extensively studied in the treatment of cancer-associated hypercalcaemia and has been found to be a highly effective agent when given intravenously and orally [37,58,59]. However, since alendronate is not marketed for this indication and is not available for i.v. use, it will not be discussed further. Experience with other bisphosphonates in the management of cancer-associated hypercalcaemia is limited. Aminohexane bisphosphonate (neridronate), administered as a single i.v. infusion of 125 mg, has been found to be an effective treatment for cancer-associated hypercalcaemia, with an overall response of 65% in terms of normocalcaemia, and kinetics of response and a duration of action similar to that of other aminobisphosphonates [60]. The heterocyclic aminobisphosphonate YM175 has been found to restore normocalcaemia in about 50% of patients when given as an i.v. infusion of 10 mg, with clear evidence of a dose–response relationship over the range 2.5–10 mg [61]. Tiludronate has been studied in the treatment of cancer-associated hypercalcaemia, with disappointing results. In the study of Dumon et al. [62], tiludronate lowered serum calcium values in most cases when given by i.v. infusion in doses of 3–6 mg/kg/day for 3 days, but the proportion of patients rendered normocalcaemic was only 20–25%. Furthermore, at these doses, one patient developed renal failure and another two increased serum creatinine levels.

Calcitonin

Calcitonin lowers serum calcium by inhibiting osteoclastic bone resorption and by promoting urinary calcium excretion [63]. Calcitonin may be given by subcutaneous (s.c.) or intramuscular (i.m.) injection in the treatment of hypercalcaemia, at doses of up to 400 IU 6–8 hourly or by slow i.v. infusion in doses of 5–10 U/kg over 6 h. Calcitonin has a rapid calcium-lowering effect, evident within 12 h of administration, but it gives less complete control of hypercalcaemia than bisphosphonates and patients tend to relapse after 2–3 days of treatment [64]. The reason for this has not been clearly established, but a suggested mechanism is the downregulation of calcitonin receptor expression on the osteoclast. There is some evidence to suggest that relapse may be prevented by co-administration of corticosteroids [65], but the combination of both agents is still less effective than 30 mg pamidronate in the treatment of cancer-associated hypercalcaemia [49]. The clearest indication for calcitonin treatment in tumour-induced hypercalcaemia is in combination with bisphosphonates during the first 1–3 days of treatment. This combination gives more rapid control of hypercalcaemia than bisphosphonates alone and may be useful in patients with severe, life-threatening hypercalcaemia where a rapid calcium-lowering effect is desired [66,67].

Mithramycin

Mithramycin reduces serum calcium by inhibiting bone resorption and by reducing renal tubular calcium reabsorption. Several randomised clinical studies have shown that mithramycin is less effective than pamidronate in the treatment of cancer-associated hypercalcaemia [49–51]. In one study, mithramycin-treated patients suffered gastrointestinal side-effects more commonly than pamidronate-treated patients [51], while in another performance status was significantly worse in mithramycin-treated patients compared with pamidronate-treated patients [50]. Because of the above, mithramycin has been superseded by the bisphosphonates and is no longer available for routine use in the UK.

Gallium Nitrate

Gallium nitrate is an effective treatment for hypercalcaemia of malignancy when given by slow continuous i.v. infusion (200 mg/m^2/day for 5–7 days) [68]. Gallium nitrate works by inhibiting osteoclastic bone resorption and starts to reduce serum calcium values within 2–3 days of administration, with a maximal effect at day 8–9 and a duration of normocalcaemia of about 6 days. Reported rates of normocalcaemia after gallium nitrate treatment have been 75–85% and randomised comparative studies have shown it to be superior to calcitonin [69] and etidronate [28] in the treatment of cancer-associated hypercalcaemia. Gallium nitrate seems to be well tolerated at the doses used for treatment of hypercalcaemia, but nephrotoxicity is a potential hazard in patients who are dehydrated or receiving other nephrotoxic agents, such as aminoglycosides. Another drawback of gallium nitrate when compared with bisphophonates is that it is slightly less convenient to administer because of the requirement for a prolonged continuous intravenous infusion.

Corticosteroids

Corticosteroids are ineffective in the treatment of cancer-associated hypercalcaemia and should not be used unless the tumour itself is corticosteroid-responsive, such as myeloma and lymphoma.

Phosphate

Intravenous neutral phosphate (40 mmol infused over 4–6 h) is an effective treatment for hypercalcaemia that works by forming insoluble calcium–phosphate complexes that are deposited in bone and soft tissues [70]. The duration of action is short, however (1–2 days), and several adverse effects, including hypotension, ectopic calcification and acute renal failure, may occur. Whilst i.v. phosphate may work when all other agents have failed [71], it has largely been superseded by other agents.

REFERENCES

1. Ralston SH, Gallacher SJ, Patel U et al. Cancer-associated hypercalcemia: morbidity and mortality. Ann Intern Med 1990; 112: 499–504.
2. Iqbal SJ, Giles M, Ledger S et al. Need for albumin adjustments of urgent total serum calcium. Lancet 1988; ii: 1477–8.
3. Fisken RA, Heath DA, Bold AM. Hypercalcaemia—a hospital survey. Qu J Med 1980; 49: 405–18.
4. Martin TJ, Suva LJ. Parathyroid hormone-related protein in hypercalcaemia of maligancy. Clin Endocrinol 1989; 31: 631–47.
5. Burtis WJ, Brady TJ, Orloff JJ et al. Immunochemical characterisation of circulating parathyroid hormone-related protein in patients with humoral hypercalcemia of malignancy. N Engl J Med 1990; 322: 1106–12.
6. Guise TA, Mundy GR. Cancer and bone [review]. Endocr Rev 1998; 19: 18–54.
7. Yamamoto I, Kawano M, Sone T et al. Production of interleukin-1β, a potent bone resorbing cytokine, by cultured human myeloma cells. Cancer Res 1989; 49: 4242–6.
8. Breslau NA, McGuire JL, Zerwekh JE et al. Hypercalcaemia associated with increased serum calcitriol levels in three patients with lymphoma. Ann Intern Med 1984; 100: 1–7.
9. Davies M, Hayes ME, Mawer EB, Lumb GA. Abnormal vitamin D metabolism in Hodgkin's lymphoma. Lancet 1985; ii: 1186–8.
10. Bringhurst FR, Bierer BE, Godeau F et al. Humoral hypercalcemia of malignancy: release of a prostaglandin-stimulating bone-resorbing factor *in vitro* by human transitional carcinoma cells. J Clin Invest 1986; 77: 456–64.
11. Heller SR, Hosking DJ. Renal handling of calcium and sodium in metastatic and non-metastatic malignancy. Br Med J 1986; 292: 583–6.
12. Wills MR, Gill JR, Barrter FC. The inter-relationships of calcium and sodium excretion. Clin Sci 1969; 37: 621–30.
13. Ralston SH, Fogelman I, Gardner MD et al. Hypercalcaemia of malignancy: evidence for a non-parathyroid humoral mediator with an effect on renal tubular calcium handling. Clin Sci 1984; 66: 187–91.
14. Yates AJP, Guttierez G, Smolens P et al. Effects of a synthetic peptide of a parathyroid hormone-related protein on calcium homeostasis, renal tubular calcium

reabsorption and bone metabolism *in vivo* and *in vitro* in rodents. J Clin Invest 1988; 81: 932–8.

15. Ralston SH, Cowan RA, Robertson AG et al. Circulating vitamin D metabolites and hypercalcaemia of malignancy. Acta Endocrinol 1984; 106: 556–63.

16. Coombes RC, Ward MK, Greenberg PB et al. Calcium metabolism in cancer: studies using calcium isotopes and immunoassays for parathyroid hormone and calcitonin. Cancer 1976; 38: 2111–20.

17. Ralston SH, Cowan RA, Gardner MD et al. Comparison of intestinal calcium absorption and 1,25-dihydroxyvitamin D3 levels in malignancy-associated hypercalcaemia and primary hyperparathyroidism. Clin Endocrinol 1987; 26: 281–91.

18. Ling PJ, A'Hern RP, Hardy JR. Analysis of survival following treatment of tumour-induced hypercalcaemia with intravenous pamidronate (APD). Br J Cancer 1995; 72: 206–9.

19. Suki WN, Yium JJ, Von Linden M et al. Acute treatment of hypercalcemia with furosemide. N Engl J Med 1970; 283: 836–40.

20. Rogers MJ, Watts DJ, Russell RGG. Overview of bisphosphonates. Cancer 1997; 80: 1652–60.

21. Jung A. Comparison of two parenteral diphosphonates in hypercalcaemia of malignancy. Am J Med 1982; 72: 221–6.

22. Bounameaux HM, Schifferli J, Montani J-P et al. Renal failure associated with intravenous diphosphonates. Lancet 1983; i: 471.

23. Ringerberg QS, Ritch PS. Efficacy of oral administration of etidronate disodium in maintaining normal serum calcium levels in previously hypercalcemic cancer patients. Clin Ther 1987; 9: 1–7.

24. Kanis JA, Urwin GH, Gray RES et al. Effects of intravenous etidronate disodium on skeletal and calcium metabolism. Am J Med 1987; 62(suppl): 55–70.

25. Ralston SH, Gallacher SJ, Patel U et al. Comparison of three intravenous bisphosphonates in cancer-associated hypercalcaemia. Lancet 1989; ii: 1180–2.

26. Hasling C, Charles P, Mosekilde L. Etidronate disodium for treating hypercalcaemia of malignancy: a double blind, placebo-controlled study. Eur J Clin Invest 1986; 16: 433–7.

27. Gucalp R, Ritch P, Wiernik PH et al. Comparative study of pamidronate disodium and etidronate disodium in the treatment of cancer-related hypercalcemia. J Clin Oncol 1992; 10: 134–42.

28. Warrell RP Jr, Murphy WK, Schulman P et al. A randomized double-blind study of gallium nitrate compared with etidronate for acute control of cancer-related hypercalcemia. J Clin Oncol 1991; 9: 1467–75.

29. Ralston SH. Medical management of hypercalcaemia [review]. Br J Clin Pharm 1992; 34: 11–20.

30. Boyce BF, Smith L, Fogelman I et al. Focal osteomalacia due to low-dose diphosphonate therapy in Paget's disease. Lancet 1984; 1: 821–4.

31. Plosker GL, Goa KL. Clodronate. A review of its pharmacological properties and therapeutic efficacy in resorptive bone disease [review]. Drugs 1994; 47: 945–82.

32. O'Rourke NP, McCloskey EV, Vasikaran S et al. Effective treatment of maligant hypercalcaemia with a single intravenous infusion of clodronate. Br J Cancer 1993; 67: 560–3.

33. Bonjour J-P, Guelpa PG, Bisetti A et al. Bone and renal components of hypercalcemia of malignancy and response to a single infusion of clodronate. Bone 1988; 9: 123–30.

34. Kanis JA, McCloskey EV, Paterson AHG. Use of diphosphonates in hypercalcaemia due to malignancy. Lancet 1990; 335: 170–1.

35. Purohit OP, Radstone CR, Anthony C et al. A randomised double-blind comparison of intravenous pamidronate and clodronate in the hypercalcaemia of malignancy. Br J Cancer 1995; 72: 1289–93.

36. Rastad J, Benson L, Johansson H et al. Clodronate treatment in patients with malignancy-associated hypercalcemia. Acta Med Scand 1987; 221: 489–94.

37. Adami S, Bolzicco GP, Rizzo A et al. The use of dichloromethylene bisphosphonate and aminobutane bisphosphonate in hypercalcemia of malignancy. Bone Min 1987; 2: 395–404.

38. Siris ES, Sherman WH, Baquiran DC et al. Effects of dichloromethylene diphosphonate on skeletal mobilisation of calcium in multiple myeloma. N Engl J Med 1980; 302: 310–15.

39. Sleeboom HP, Bijvoet OLM, Van Oosterom AT et al. Comparison of intravenous (3-amino-1-hydroxypropylidene)-1,1-bisphosphonate and volume repletion in tumour-induced hypercalcaemia. Lancet 1983; ii: 239–43.

40. Ralston SH, Alzaid AA, Gallacher SJ et al. Clinical experience with aminohydroxypropylidene bisphosphonate (APD) in the management of cancer-associated hypercalcaemia. Qu J Med 1988; 258: 825–34.

41. Nussbaum SR, Younger J, VandePol CJ et al. Single-dose intravenous therapy with pamidronate for the treatment of hypercalcemia of malignancy: comparison of 30, 60, and 90 mg dosages. Am J Med 1993; 95: 297–304.

42. Body JJ, Magritte A, Seraj F et al. Aminohydroxypropylidene bisphosphonate (APD) treatment for tumor-associated hypercalcaemia: a randomized comparison between a 3-day treatment and single 24-hour infusions. J Bone Min Res 1989; 4: 923–8.

43. Gallacher SJ, Ralston SH, Fraser WD et al. A comparison of low vs. high dose pamidronate in cancer-associated hypercalcaemia. Bone Min 1991; 15: 249–56.

44. Body JJ, Dumon JC. Treatment of tumour-induced hypercalcaemia with the bisphosphonate pamidronate: dose–response relationship and influence of tumour type. Ann Oncol 1994; 5: 359–63.

45. Judson I, Booth F, Gore M, McElwain T. Chronic high-dose pamidronate in refractory malignant hypercalcaemia. Lancet 1990; 335: 802.

46. Gallacher SJ, Fraser WD, Logue FC et al. Factors predicting the acute effect of pamidronate on serum calcium in hypercalcemia of malignancy. Calcif Tiss Int 1992; 51: 419–23.

47. Walls J, Ratcliffe WA, Howell A, Bundred NJ. Response to intravenous bisphosphonate therapy in hypercalcaemic patients with and without bone metastases: the role of parathyroid hormone-related protein. Br J Cancer 1994; 70: 169–72.

48. Body JJ, Dumon JC, Thirion M, Cleeren A. Circulating PTHrP concentrations in tumor-induced hypercalcemia: influence on the response to bisphosphonate and changes after therapy. J Bone Min Res 1993; 8: 701–6.

49. Ralston SH, Gardner MD, Dryburgh FJ et al. Comparison of aminohydroxypropylidene diphosphonate, mithramycin and corticosteroids/calcitonin in treatment of cancer-associated hypercalcaemia. Lancet 1985; ii: 907–10.

50. Ostenstad B, Andersen OK. Disodium pamidronate vs. mithramycin in the management of tumour-associated hypercalcemia. Acta Oncol 1992; 31: 861–4.

51. Thurlimann B, Waldburger R, Senn HJ, Thiebaud D. Plicamycin and pamidronate in symptomatic tumor-related hypercalcemia: a prospective randomized cross-over trial [see comments]. Ann Oncol 1992; 3: 619–23.

52. Gallacher SJ, Ralston SH, Patel U, Boyle IT. Side effects of pamidronate. Lancet 1989; ii: 42–3.

53. Thiebaud D, Portmann L, Jaegar Ph et al. Oral vs. intravenous AHPrBP (APD) in the treatment of hypercalcemia of malignancy. Bone 1986; 7: 247–53.

54. Wuster C, Schoter KH, Thiebaud D et al. Methylpentyl-aminopropylidene bisphosphonate (BM 21.0955): a new potent and safe bisphosphonate for the treatment of cancer-associated hypercalcemia. Bone Min 1993; 22: 77–85.

55. Ralston SH, Thiebaud D, Herrmann Z et al. Dose–response study of ibandronate in the treatment of cancer-associated hypercalcaemia. Br J Cancer 1997; 75: 295–300.

56. Rizzoli R, Thiebaud D, Bundred N et al. Serum parathyroid hormone-related protein levels and response to bisphosphonate treatment in hypercalcemia of malignancy. J Clin Endocrinol Metab 1999; 84: 3545–50.

57. Body JJ, Lortholary A, Romieu G et al. A dose-finding study of zoledronate in hypercalcemic cancer patients. J Bone Min Res 1999; 14: 1557–61.

58. Nussbaum SR, Warrell RP Jr, Rude R et al. Dose–response study of alendronate sodium for the treatment of cancer-associated hypercalcaemia. J Clin Oncol 1993; 11: 1618–23.

59. Rizzoli R, Buchs B, Bonjour JP. Effect of a single infusion of alendronate in malignant hypercalcaemia: dose dependency and comparison with clodranate. Int J Cancer 1992; 50: 706–12.

60. O'Rourke NP, McCloskey EV, Rosini S et al. Treatment of malignant hypercalcaemia with aminohexane bisphosphonate (neridronate). Br J Cancer 1994; 69: 914–17.

61. Fukumoto S, Matsumoto T, Takebe K et al. Treatment of malignancy-associated hypercalcemia with YM175, a new bisphosphonate: elevated threshold for parathyroid hormone secretion in hypercalcemic patients. J Clin Endocrinol Metab 1994; 79: 165–70.

62. Dumon JC, Magritte A, Body JJ. Efficacy and safety of the bisphosphonate tiludronate for the treatment of tumor-associated hypercalcemia. Bone Min 1991; 15: 257–66.

63. Hosking DJ, Gilson D. Comparison of the renal and skeletal actions of calcitonin in the treatment of severe hypercalcaemia of malignancy. Qu J Med 1984; 211: 359–68.

64. Wisneski LA, Croom WP, Silva OL, Becker KL. Salmon calcitonin in hypercalcemia. Clin Pharmacol Ther 1978, 24: 219–22.

65. Binstock ML, Mundy GR. Effect of calcitonin and glucocorticoids in combination on the hypercalcemia of malignancy. Ann Intern Med 1980; 93: 269–72.

66. Ralston SH, Alzaid AA, Gardner MD, Boyle IT. Treatment of cancer-associated hypercalcaemia with combined aminohydroxypropylidene diphosphonate and calcitonin. Br Med J 1986; 292: 1549–50.

67. Thiebaud D, Jaquet AF, Burckhardt P. Fast and effective treatment of malignant hypercalcemia: combination of suppositories of calcitonin and a single infusion of 3-amino-1-hydroxypropylidene-1-bisphosphonate. Arch Intern Med 1990; 150: 2125–8.

68. Warrell RP Jr, Bockman RS, Coonley CJ et al. Gallium nitrate inhibits calcium resorption from bone and is effective treatment for cancer-related hypercalcemia. J Clin Invest 1984; 73: 1487–90.

69. Warrell RP Jr, Israel R, Frisone M et al. Gallium nitrate for acute treatment of cancer-related hypercalcemia. A randomized, double-blind comparison to calcitonin. Ann Intern Med 1988; 108: 669–74.

70. Fulmer DH, Dimich AB, Rothschild EO, Myers WPL. Treatment of hypercalcaemia: comparison of intra-venously administered phosphate, sulphate and hydro-cortisone. Arch Intern Med 1972; 129: 923–30.

71. Rawlinson PS, Green RH, Coggins AM et al. Malignant osteopetrosis: hypercalcaemia after bone marrow transplantation. Arch Dis Child 1991; 66: 638–9.

28

Treatment of Lytic Bone Metastases

Karin Gwyn and Richard Theriault

M.D. Anderson Cancer Center, Houston, TX, USA

INTRODUCTION

Breast, prostate, lung, thyroid and kidney cancers are the most common solid tumours that result in metastatic bone disease, while multiple myeloma is the most common haematological malignancy associated with bone involvement. Those metastatic lesions that result in a net loss of bone, as seen radiographically, are osteolytic and hence termed "lytic", as is the case in multiple myeloma and metastatic renal cell carcinoma. If, however, the process involves bone formation, as seen in metastatic prostate cancer, the net increase in bone produces osteoblastic ("blastic"), sclerotic lesions. In some malignancies, including breast and lung, there are both lytic and blastic areas. In these instances, the resulting lesions are described radiographically as mixed osteolytic–osteoblastic type [1,2].

This chapter will focus on the treatment of lytic bone metastases with bisphosphonates. The use of bisphosphonates in the treatment of multiple myeloma will be discussed in Chapter 29. Thus, this chapter will focus on the use of the bisphosphonates in the treatment of those solid tumours, primarily breast, lung and renal, that produce either lytic or a combination of lytic and blastic lesions in bone. The majority of clinical data regarding the use of bisphosphonates in this group of patients has been derived from clinical trials with breast cancer patients with bone disease. Few studies have examined the use of the bisphosphonates in the treatment of bone metastases in patients with lung or renal cell carcinoma. In these patients, most of the data has focused on the use of these agents in the treatment of hypercalcaemia of malignancy. Prostate cancer

metastatic to bone will not be discussed in this chapter, as it produces lesions that are primarily blastic in nature.

BISPHOSPHONATES IN THE MANAGEMENT OF BREAST CANCER METASTATIC TO BONE

Approximately 69–73% of advanced breast cancer patients will have metastases to the skeleton [3,4]. Those who have disease metastatic to the skeleton only can survive for quite a long period of time, with 20% alive at 5 years. However, they can incur substantial morbidity from cancer-mediated bone destruction. They may develop bone pain, pathological fractures, spinal cord compression and hypercalcaemia [4]. Approximately 16% of those with bone metastases will have at least one fracture of a long bone that will require orthopaedic intervention [4]. Thus, the significant morbidity of breast cancer metastatic to bone has led to a number of clinical trials that have investigated the use of bisphosphonates as a means to improve symptoms and outcome of bone-related events.

First-generation Bisphosphonates (Etidronate and Clodronate)

Etidronate was investigated in the 1980s as a treatment for Paget's disease of bone, osteoporosis and hypercalcaemia of malignancy [5–8]. Despite its efficacy at inhibiting bone resorption, etidronate was also found to inhibit bone mineralisation [8]. The resulting

Textbook of Bone Metastases. Edited by C. Jasmin, R. E. Coleman, L. R. Coia, R. Capanna and G. Saillant
© 2005 John Wiley & Sons Ltd: ISBN 0 471 87742 5

osteomalacia made etidronate unsuitable for long-term administration. Etidronate has been combined with rhenium-186 ([186]Re), a β-emitting radionuclide. Formation of complexes between etidronate and [186]Re permits selective localisation in bone cancer lesions by bridging the hydroxyapatite crystals [9]. There are a number of small studies evaluating the safety and short- and/or long-term efficacy of [186]Re-etidronate in the management of metastatic bone disease in breast as well as other solid tumours. In a non-randomised, open-label study of 24 breast cancer patients with painful bone metastases, the effect of a single treatment with [186]Re etidronate (dosages of 1295–2960 MBq; 35–80 mCi) upon pain intensity, medication index and daily activities was examined [10]. In this study, 71% of evaluable participants reported a decrease in pain intensity of > 25% lasting more than 2 consecutive weeks. Twelve of the 14 patients with a reduction in pain also demonstrated a decrease in medication index; 58% of those treated reported an improvement in daily activities. The duration of response was in the range 2–8 weeks with the maximum follow-up period for this study of 8 weeks. Sciuto et al. [9] examined the short- and long-term effects of [186]Re-etidronate therapy in 60 patients with painful bone metastases from a number of different tumour types (45 had prostate cancer, 10 breast cancer, one leiomyosarcoma, one small cell lung cancer, one liver cancer, one colon cancer, one lung adenocarcinoma). Of the 60 patients, 55 received therapy with [186]Re etidronate once, while five patients with prostate cancer were treated twice, with the mean administered activity being 1406 MBq. Approximately 82% of patients reported prompt relief of pain with their first treatment, with clinically evident pain relief occurring within 1 week. World Health Organization grade 1–2 haematological toxicity was observed, with 32% of those treated experiencing a decrease in mean platelet count and 18% a decrease in mean leukocyte count at weeks 3 and 4, respectively. The role of this compound in the management of breast cancer metastatic to bone requires further study.

Clodronate has been reported as being 10 times more potent than etidronate in the inhibition of osteoclast activity [11]. This bisphosphonate, available in both oral and intravenous (i.v.) formulations, has been investigated as a treatment for hypercalcaemia of malignancy as well as bone metastases. In two small, randomised trials, one of which was a cross-over design, the administration of oral clodronate was associated with a decrease in markers of bone resorption and a reduction in bone pain [12,13]. One of the studies also noted a decrease in the frequency of hypercalcaemia and new bone metastases in the clodronate treatment group [12]. Of note is that the oral dose of clodronate administered in these two studies was different—one used 1600 mg/day for 3–9 months [12] while the other, the cross-over study, used 3200 mg/day for 8 weeks [13]. Of the 34 women who received oral clodronate at a dose of 1600 mg/day, no side-effects were reported, while 4/10 women who received the 3200 mg/day oral dose of clodronate experienced diarrhoea. A randomised, double-blind, placebo-controlled trial compared oral clodronate at 1600 mg/day to placebo in women with breast cancer metastatic to bone. Those who received oral clodronate ($n=85$) were found to have a significantly decreased rate of hypercalcaemic episodes (28 vs. 52, $p < 0.01$) and incidence of vertebral fractures (84 vs. 124/100 patient-years, $p < 0.025$) when compared to those who received placebo ($n=88$) [14]. The rate of vertebral deformity was also significantly decreased in the clodronate group (168 vs. 252/100 patient-years, $p < 0.001$). Non-statistically significant trends were seen with regard to improvement in non-vertebral fracture rate and radiotherapy requirements for the clodronate treatment group. However, treatment with clodronate did not improve survival. Although the oral bioavailability of clodronate is low, it appears to be efficacious in the treatment of cancer metastatic to bone [11]. Given the ease of administration of the oral formulation and the few, if any, side-effects reported with its use, oral clodronate has been used in a number of studies designed to determine its efficacy in the prevention of bone metastases in patients with a history of breast cancer or with extra-skeletal recurrent disease [15]. The use of bisphosphonates in the prevention of bone metastases will be addressed in Chapter 31. Clodronate administered intravenously has also been investigated as a treatment for hypercalcaemia as well as metastatic bone pain and has been found to be efficacious [16,17]. Untch et al. recently presented in abstract form the results of a randomised, multicentre study comparing oral clodronate at 2400 mg/day, i.v. clodronate at a dose of 900 mg every 3 weeks and i.v. pamidronate at a dose of 60 mg every 3 weeks [18]. In this study of 308 women with breast cancer metastates to bone, there were no differences seen between the three treatment arms with respect to the amount of reduction in pathological fractures. However, 89% of women who received oral clodronate achieved a reduction in their pain when compared to 80% of women treated with i.v. pamidronate and 72% of women given i.v. clodronate. Oral clodronate had the greatest frequency of gastrointestinal side-effects (6.41%), while i.v. pamidronate had the greatest amount of acute phase reactions (percentage not given). Outside the USA clodronate is approved for the treatment of metastatic bone disease.

Second-generation Bisphosphonates (Pamidronate)

Pamidronate is an aminodisodium bisphosphate analogue that inhibits bone resorption at doses that do not affect bone mineralisation. The osteoclast-inhibiting activity of pamidronate is reported to be 100 times more potent than that of etidronate [19]. The efficacy of pamidronate in the treatment of breast cancer metastatic to bone was first examined in small open-label studies by several European investigators [20–22]. In these studies, the use of i.v. pamidronate subjectively appeared to improve symptoms resulting from bone metastases as well as objectively demonstrating bone healing radiographically. An open, randomised trial of 131 breast cancer patients examined whether long-term oral pamidronate at 300 mg/day was useful in the treatment of breast cancer metastatic to bone [23]. After a median follow-up of 13 months for the 70 patients treated and a median follow-up of 14 months for the 61 controls, those who received pamidronate were significantly more likely to have fewer episodes of hypercalcaemia, fewer pathological fractures and less severe bone pain. Pamidronate therapy was also associated with a significant reduction in the need for radiotherapy for skeletal complications, as well as a decrease in the frequency of changes in systemic breast cancer therapy. The investigators concluded that oral pamidronate was a safe and effective means of decreasing skeletal morbidity for breast cancer patients with bone metastases.

A subsequent open, randomised study was then performed to determine whether oral pamidronate at 600 mg/day decreased the morbidity from bone metastases in breast cancer patients [24]. The events monitored as indicators of skeletal morbidity were the occurrence of hypercalcaemia, severe bone pain requiring radiotherapy or surgery, and/or clinically relevant symptomatic pathological or impending fractures treated by radiotherapy or surgery. Of the 81 patients who received oral pamidronate, 29 initially received 600 mg/day but this dose was subsequently reduced to 300 mg/day because of gastrointestinal toxicity, primarily nausea and vomiting; 52 patients received the lower dose, 300 mg/day, for the entire study duration. Tumour-specific treatment was unrestricted. With a median of 18 months of follow-up for the pamidronate patients and 21 months for the control patients, they found that the occurrences of

hypercalcaemia, severe bone pain and symptomatic impending fractures were decreased by 65%, 30% and 50%, respectively, for the pamidronate group when compared to controls (using an intention-to-treat analysis). In the treatment group, event-rates of systemic treatment changes and radiotherapy were significantly decreased by 35%. Pamidronate therapy did not significantly improve survival. Some differences were observed between the two treatment groups, i.e. those who received 600 mg/day pamidronate followed by 300 mg/day and those who received only 300 mg/day for the course of the study, but this may have reflected smaller numbers of a subgroup analysis. Quality of life analysis found that those individuals who received pamidronate in this study had less mobility impairment and bone pain when compared to the control group [25]. Interestingly, gastrointestinal complaints were similar over time when the treatment and control groups were compared, suggesting that other factors, such as systemic treatment, may be playing a role. Of note is that the oral absorption of pamidronate is low, with only 1.0% of the administered dose being absorbed [19].

Several multinational randomised trials have evaluated the use of i.v. pamidronate for the adjunctive treatment of skeletal metastases in breast cancer patients. In a study by Conte et al., breast cancer patients were randomised to receive chemotherapy alone (152 patients) or chemotherapy plus pamidronate (at a dose of 45 mg i.v. every 3 weeks) [26]. The chemotherapeutic regimen was not standardised among centres. Patients were maintained in the active phase of the trial until they developed progressive disease in bone on radiograph and/or bone scan. At the time of analysis, the median time to progressive disease in bone was significantly increased, by 48%, in those receiving pamidronate in combination with chemotherapy compared to those receiving chemotherapy alone. With regard to pain reduction, the other primary endpoint of the trial, 44% of pamidronate patients compared to 30% of controls experienced marked pain relief. This difference was statistically significant. The use of pamidronate did not prolong survival in this study. The investigators concluded that i.v. pamidronate was safe, well-tolerated and resulted in an increase in time to disease progression in bone, as well as an improvement in pain control.

A large, randomised double-blind placebo-controlled multinational trial investigated the efficacy of i.v. pamidronate in women with breast cancer metastatic to bone who were undergoing cytotoxic chemotherapy [27]. In this trial, reported by Hortobagyi et al., pamidronate was administered intravenously over 2 h at a dose of 90 mg every 4 weeks for a total of 12 cycles to the 185 patients randomised to the treatment arm, while the 195 controls received placebo infusions. At a median duration of follow-up of 11.9 months in the pamidronate group and 10.2 months in the placebo group, efficacy and safety were evaluated. When compared to the placebo group, the median time to the occurrence of the first skeletal complication was significantly greater in the treatment group receiving pamidronate (7 months vs. 13.1 months, $p=0.005$). The proportion of patients in whom any skeletal complication occurred was significantly lower in the pamidronate group when compared to the placebo group (43% vs. 56%, $p=0.008$). Patients receiving pamidronate also had significantly less of an increase in bone pain as well as less deterioration in their performance status. Those receiving placebo had significantly shorter times to first non-vertebral fracture, first radiation treatment to bone, first bone surgery and first episode of hypercalcaemia. There were no differences seen between the pamidronate and placebo groups with regard to proportion of patients with new vertebral pathological fractures. The infusions were well tolerated and only three patients were removed or withdrew from the study because of side-effects. Of these three patients, all from the pamidronate group, one had bone pain after each infusion and refused further pamidronate, one had symptomatic hypocalcaemia and the other was hospitalised with increased fatigue, weakness and dyspnoea. The investigators concluded that i.v. pamidronate at a dose of 90 mg every 4 weeks is useful in protecting against skeletal complications in breast cancer patients with bone metastases. Subsequent follow-up of this cohort for a total of 24 treatment cycles did not result in any substantial changes in the results seen at the end of 12 cycles, but the clinically beneficial results of pamidronate treatment persisted through 24 months [28]. At 24 cycles there was no difference in survival between the two groups.

In a parallel placebo-controlled trial, the ability of i.v. pamidronate to reduce the frequency of skeletal morbidity of breast cancer metastatic to bone was assessed in women receiving hormonal therapy for cancer [28]. One hundred and eighty two patients were randomised to receive pamidronate at a dose of 90 mg intravenously every 4 weeks for 24 cycles, while 189 received a placebo infusion. The skeletal morbidity rate was significantly decreased at 12, 18 and 24 cycles in those receiving pamidronate when compared to controls (placebo infusion). The proportion of patients receiving pamidronate having any skeletal complication at 24 cycles were 56% compared to 67% in the

placebo group ($p=0.049$). Median time to first skeletal complication was longer for those receiving pamidronate than for those receiving placebo (10.4 vs. 6.9 months, $p=0.049$). Those receiving placebo had significantly shorter times to first radiation to bone, first radiation to bone for pain relief as well as first episode of hypercalcaemia when compared to those patients receiving pamidronate. During the first year of the study, bone pain scores improved in the pamidronate group but worsened in the placebo group. This difference was statistically significant. At the final measurement, bone pain scores had increased significantly more in the placebo group than the pamidronate group. With a median estimate of survival of 23.2 months (95% CI, 19.3–25.8) for the pamidronate group and 23.5 months (95% CI, 18.7–27.4 months) for the placebo group, it could be concluded that pamidronate therapy did not improve survival ($p=0.685$). Only three serious adverse experiences were recorded: one patient in the pamidronate group was diagnosed with interstitial pulmonary infiltrates and dyspnoea several days after the first treatment; another patient on pamidronate had an allergic reaction in the left eye; while the third patient, who had received placebo, developed cellulitis within 24 h of infusion of placebo drug. The investigators concluded that treatment with 90 mg pamidronate as a 2 h i.v. infusion every 4 weeks, in addition to hormonal therapy, decreases skeletal morbidity from bone metastases.

Lipton et al. [29] recently combined and summarised the data from these two trials described by Hortobagyi et al. [27] and Theriault et al. [30]. To determine whether the two studies could be pooled, a Breslow–Day test for homogeneity was performed. It was determined that the odds ratio of having a skeleton-related event while receiving placebo to having an event while receiving pamidronate in the hormonal therapy study was not significantly different from the odds seen in the chemotherapy study. This statistical analysis justified the pooling of data from the two studies.

Of the 751 evaluable patients with breast cancer metastatic to bone in the two combined studies [30], 367 received pamidronate in conjunction with chemotherapy or hormonal therapy, while 384 patients received chemotherapy or hormonal therapy alone. Of those receiving pamidronate, 115 (31.3%) completed the trial (24 cycles of pamidronate) and 81 (22.2%) discontinued the study because of adverse events. Six members of the pamidronate group discontinued therapy due to drug-related adverse events. Of the 384 women receiving placebo, 100 (26.0%) completed the study, while 76 (19.8%) discontinued the study secondary to adverse events. The skeletal morbidity rate (the ratio of the number of skeletal complications experienced by a patient divided by the time on trial for that patient, expressed as the number of events/ year) was significantly less in the pamidronate group than the placebo group (2.4 vs. 3.7; $p < 0.001$). A smaller proportion of the pamidronate group had skeletal complications when compared to the control group (51% vs. 64%; $p < 0.001$). The median time to first skeletal complication was 7 months in the placebo group compared to 12.7 months in the pamidronate group ($p < 0.001$). Members of the placebo group had significantly worse pain and analgesic scores than the pamidronate group. The median survival in the pamidronate group was 19.8 months, while that seen in the placebo group was not significantly different at 17.8 months. As previously discussed, no significant difference in survival was seen when the data were analysed according to primary treatment, i.e. chemotherapy vs. hormonal therapy.

Although pamidronate appears to decrease skeletal morbidity, not all patients with bone metastases will respond to this therapy. Pyridinolone (PYD), deoxy-pyridinoline (DPD) and N-telopeptide (NTX) are markers of bone resorption. When compared to PYD and DPD, NTX is more often elevated in cancer patients with bone metastases. Lipton et al. [31] compared markers of bone resorption in 25 cancer patients with lytic bone disease receiving i.v. pamidronate combined with endocrine or chemotherapy, to those of 27 other cancer patients with lytic bone disease receiving placebo in addition to endocrine or chemotherapy. Although PYD, DPD and NTX levels were all measured, it was the NTX values that demonstrated the greatest change with pamidronate therapy. Of the 25 patients who received pamidronate, 21 initially had elevated NTX levels. Of these 21, 12 finished the study with normal NTX levels, while nine had NTX values that remained abnormally elevated. Although the proportion of patients with fractures between these two subgroups approached statistical significance ($p=0.07$), the proportions with bony disease progression were significantly different between these two subgroups, with progression more frequently observed in those whose NTX levels did not normalise ($p=0.03$). The investigators suggest that measurement of NTX levels may be helpful in monitoring the efficacy of bisphosphonates for the treatment of bone metastases.

The results of Lipton et al. [31] suggest that not all metastatic breast cancer patients with lytic bone disease will respond to 90 mg i.v. pamidronate each month. Costa et al. [32] recently presented the results of high-dose pamidronate in the treatment of bone metastases in 44 patients with a variety of malignancies, although most patients had breast cancer ($n=38$). In this study, cancer patients with progressive, multiple, lytic or mixed blastic/lytic bone lesions were randomised to receive one of the following treatments: treatment arm I, pamidronate 150 mg i.v daily for 3 days and then 150 mg i.v. each month; treatment arm II, pamidronate 150 mg i.v. daily for 3 days and then 90 mg i.v. each month; treatment arm III, pamidronate 90 mg i.v. each week for 6 weeks and then a 2 week rest period until bone metastases progression. The investigators concluded that high-dose pamidronate for patients with bone metastases was feasible and relatively well tolerated, with fever and flu-like symptoms the most frequent side-effects noted, particularly for treatment arms II and III (seven and six patients, respectively). Two patients had asymptomatic hypocalcaemia. Data regarding the efficacy of the different treatment arms was not presented in the published abstract. The further manipulation of pamidronate dose for those individuals who clinically, radiographically and/or biochemically do not appear to be responding to i.v. pamidronate at a dose of 90 mg every 4 weeks requires further study.

Third-generation Bisphosphonates (Zolendronate)

Zolendronate is a new, third-generation bisphosphonate that is 500–1000 times more potent than pamidronate in *in vitro* and *in vivo* model systems of bone resorption [33]. In a dose-finding study of zolendronate in the treatment of hypercalcaemia of malignancy, the two effective dose levels were 0.02 mg/kg and 0.04 mg/kg [34]. Among the 30 evaluable patients in this trial, the fall in serum calcium was rapid and normocalcaemia was often maintained for several weeks. The drug was well tolerated, with seven patients developing transient hypophosphataemia, three developing transient hypocalcaemia and 10 developing an increased body temperature. Berensen et al. reported an open-label, dose-ranging, Phase I study of zolendronate given as a single i.v. infusion in 44 cancer patients with bone metastases [35]. In this study, the majority of patients had prostate cancer ($n=16$) or non-small cell lung cancer ($n=13$). Patients were enrolled in one of five zolendronate dose-level groups (1.0, 2.0, 4.0, 8.0 or 16.0 mg) and had zolendronate administered as a single rapid (30–60 s) i.v. infusion. They were then followed for 8 weeks. Transient skeletal pain and fever were the most common adverse events reported. No grade 3 or 4 hypocalcaemia values were reported. The biochemical markers of bone resorption were suppressed throughout the 8 week observation period for all groups except the 1.0 mg dose group. The investigators concluded that zolendronate administered as a single, rapid i.v. infusion is well tolerated at doses up to 16.0 mg.

A randomised, double-blind Phase II trial comparing zolendronate and pamidronate in patients with either multiple myeloma or breast cancer has been presented in abstract form [36]. Of the 280 patients with lytic bone disease in this study, 172 had breast cancer and 108 had multiple myeloma. Participants were randomised to receive nine monthly cycles of 0.4 mg, 2.0 mg or 4.0 mg zolendronate, administered as a 5 min infusion or 90 mg pamidronate administered as a 2 h infusion. The investigators concluded that a 5 min infusion of 2–4 mg zolendronate was at least as effective as 90 mg pamidronate with regard to increasing bone mineral density and preventing skeletal complications. The safety profile of zolendronate was similar to that of pamidronate. Zolendronate is currently being studied in Phase III trials at doses of 4 and 8 mg, as there are bone marker data to suggest that higher doses may be more effective [36].

BISPHOSPHONATES IN THE MANAGEMENT OF LUNG AND RENAL CELL CARCINOMA METASTATIC TO BONE

Although bone metastases occur in approximately 30% of patients diagnosed with small cell lung cancer, no bone disease-specific therapies have been reported, neither have there been any reports of bone-specific objective response data [1]. Bone is also one of the frequent sites of metastases for non-small cell lung cancer but there are no published reports that target the use of bisphosphonates for the improvement of the morbidity from skeletal metastases in patients with this malignancy. Lung cancer patients can be found in some studies of bisphosphonates that include a number of different cancer types [35,37]. Piga et al. [37] included patients with non-small cell lung cancer in a randomised, double-blind study of oral clodronate in tumours poorly responsive to chemotherapy. Although clodronate appeared to be of some benefit in this group of patients with a variety of malignancies, the inability to follow patients for a sufficient period of time greatly impaired the ability to analyse the results of this study. A small retrospective case series

consisting of three patients with hypertrophic pulmonary osteoarthropathy secondary to bronchogenic carcinoma suggested that pamidronate may be useful therapy in this group of lung cancer patients [38].

Among those newly diagnosed with renal cell carcinoma, 30% will have distant metastases [1]. The most common sites of metastases are lung and bone, although metastases to the liver, adrenals and brain also occur. There are no published reports that specifically address the effect of bisphosphonates on skeletal morbidity from renal cell carcinoma metastatic to bone.

PUBLISHED GUIDELINES FOR THE USE OF BISPHOSPHONATES FOR THE TREATMENT OF BREAST CANCER METASTATIC TO BONE

The American Society of Clinical Oncology has published guidelines regarding the role of bisphosphonates in the management of breast cancer [39]. The expert multidisciplinary panel reviewed pertinent information from the published literature and meeting abstracts through May 1999. Intravenous pamidronate at a dose of 90 mg delivered over 1–2 hours every 3–4 weeks was recommended in patients with metastatic breast cancer who have radiographic evidence of lytic bone destruction and who are receiving concurrent hormonal therapy or chemotherapy. For those women with an abnormal bone scan but no evidence of bony destruction by imaging studies, or no localised pain, there was felt to be insufficient evidence for the initiation of bisphosphonates. The panel did not recommend starting bisphosphonates in women who do not have evidence of metastases to bone, even in the presence of other extraskeletal metastases. It was suggested that, once bisphosphonates are started for the treatment of metastatic disease to bone, they be continued until evidence of a substantial decline in the patient's performance status.

The International Bone and Cancer Study Group published guidelines for the use of bisphosphonates in the treatment of metastatic bone disease [40]. The panel recommended the prolonged administration of oral clodronate or monthly pamidronate infusions. The British Association of Surgical Oncology (BASO) has also published guidelines regarding the use of bisphosphonates in the management of breast cancer metastatic to bone. This panel recommends the use of i.v. clodronate or pamidronate for the treatment of acute and chronic bone pain, while oral clodronate could be used when the acute pain is controlled [41].

SUMMARY

The morbidity resulting from metastases to bone is a significant clinical problem in the care of cancer patients. A number of studies, including several randomised multinational trials, have demonstrated the efficacy of i.v. pamidronate in combination with either hormonal therapy or chemotherapy in the management of breast cancer metastatic to bone. The optimal schedule and duration of pamidronate therapy has yet to be elucidated. Further studies of alternative dosing or alternative bisphosphonates for those individuals who appear to "fail" pamidronate are warranted. Urinary markers of bone resorption may be useful in guiding the use of bisphosphonates in such difficult clinical situations. Ongoing studies in the treatment of breast cancer metastatic to bone with newer, more potent bisphosphonates, such as zolendronate, or bisphosphonates combined with radioactive substances, such as [186]Re-etidronate, may improve the amount and/or duration of response without a significant increase in side-effects. Further studies of these compounds are under way. Very little information exists on the use of bisphosphonates in the management of skeletal morbidity from bone metastases from either lung or renal cell carcinoma. Perhaps studies would be hampered by the aggressive biology of these tumours and the poor performance status of patients with metastatic disease, such that the follow-up required for the evaluation of response to bisphosphonates is difficult. With the lack of clinical studies on the use of bisphosphonates in patients with lung and renal cell carcinoma metastatic to bone, it would be difficult to recommend the use of bisphosphonates for the reduction of morbidity from skeletal events. Studies targeting a sufficient number of these patients are warranted to determine whether bisphosphonates are of clinical benefit in patients with either lung or renal cell carcinoma.

REFERENCES

1. Theriault RL, Hortobagyi GN. Treatment of bone metastases: chemo- and hormone therapy. In Body J-J (ed.), Tumor Bone Diseases and Osteoporosis in Cancer Patients. Marcel Dekker: New York, 2000: 227–43.
2. Kenan S, Hortobagyi GN. Skeletal complications. In Bast RC Jr, Kufe DW, Pollock RE et al. (eds), Cancer Medicine, 5th edn. BC Decker: Hamilton, 2000: Chapter 145.
3. Abrams HL, Spiro R, Goldstein N. Metastases in carcinoma: analysis of 1000 autopsied cases. Cancer 1950; 3: 74–85.
4. Coleman RE, Rubens RD. The clinical course of bone metastases from breast cancer. Br J Cancer 1987; 55: 61–6.
5. Altman RD, Johnston CC, Khairi MRA et al. Influence of disodium etidronate on clinical and laboratory manifestations of Paget's disease of the bone (osteitis deformans). N Engl J Med 1973; 289: 1379–84.
6. Storm T, Thamsborg G, Steiniche T et al. Effect of intermittent cyclical etidronate therapy on bone mass and fracture rate in women with postmenopausal osteoporosis. N Engl J Med 1990; 322: 1265–71.
7. Ryzen E, Martodam RR, Troxell M et al. Intravenous etidronate in the management of malignant hypercalcemia. Arch Intern Med 1985; 145: 449–52.
8. Kanis JA, Urwin GH, Gray RES et al. Effects of intravenous etidronate on skeletal and calcium metabolism. Am J Med 1987; 82: 55–70.
9. Sciuto R, Tofani A, Festa A et al. Short- and long-term effects of [186]Re-1, 1-hydroxyethylidene diphosphonate in the treatment of painful bone metastases. J Nucl Med 2000; 41: 647–54.
10. Han SH, Zonnenberg BA, de Klerk JMH et al. [186]Re-etidronate in breast cancer patients with metastatic bone pain. J Nucl Med 1999; 40: 639–42.
11. Plosker GL, Goa KL. Clodronate: a review of its pharmacological properties and therapeutic efficacy in resorptive bone disease. Drugs 1994; 47: 945–82.
12. Elomma I, Blomqvist C, Grohn P et al. Long-term controlled trial with diphosphonate in patients with osteolytic bone metastases. Lancet 1983: 143–8.
13. Siris ES, Hyman GA, Canfield RE. Effects of dichloromethylene diphosphonate in women with breast carcinoma metastatic to the skeleton. Am J Med 1983; 74: 401–6.
14. Paterson AHG, Powles TJ, Kanis JA et al. Double-blind controlled trial of oral clodronate in patients with bone metastases from breast cancer. J Clin Oncol 1993; 11: 59–65.
15. Theriault RL. Medical treatment of bone metastases. In Harris JR (ed.), Diseases of the Breast, 2nd edn. Lippincott Williams & Wilkins: Philadelphia, 2000: 921–9.
16. Kanis JA, McCloskey EV, Paterson AHG. Use of diphosphonates in hypercalcemia due to malignancy. Lancet 1990; 335: 170–1.
17. Ernst DS, MacDonald RN, Paterson AHG et al. A double-blind, crossover trial of intravenous clodronate in metastatic bone pain. J Pain Sympt Man 1992; 7: 4–11.
18. Untch M, Blokh E, Marschner N et al. Comparison of oral vs. parental administered bisphosphonates in breast cancer patients with bone metastases. Breast Cancer Res Treat 2000; 64(abstr 358): 90.
19. Fitton A, McTavish D. Pamidronate: a review of its pharmacologic properties and therapeutic efficacy in resorptive bone disease. Drugs 1991; 41: 289–318.
20. Coleman RE, Woll PJ, Miles M et al. Treatment of bone metastases from breast cancer with (3-amino-1-hydroxypropylidene)-1,1-bisphosphonate (APD). Br J Cancer 1988; 58: 621–5.
21. Morton AR, Cantrill JA, Pillai GV et al. Sclerosis of lytic bone metastases after disodium aminohydroxypropylidene bisphosphonate (APD) in patients with breast carcinoma. Br Med J 1988; 297: 772–3.
22. Burckhardt P, Thiebaud D, Perey L, von Fliedner V. Treatment of tumor-induced osteolysis by APD. Recent Results Cancer Res 1989; 116: 54–66.

23. van Holten-Verzantvoort ATM, Bijvoet OLM, Hermans J et al. Reduced morbidity from skeletal metastases in breast cancer patients during long-term bisphosphonate (APD) treatment. Lancet 1987: 983–5.

24. van Holten-Verzantvoort ATM, Kroon HM, Bijvoet OLM et al. Palliative pamidronate treatment in patients with bone metastases from breast cancer. J Clin Oncol 1993; 11: 491–8.

25. van Holten-Verzantvoort ATM, Zwinderman AH, Aaronson NK et al. The effect of supportive pamidronate treatment on aspects of quality of life of patients with advanced breast cancer. Eur J Cancer 1991; 27: 544–9.

26. Conte PF, Latreille J, Calabresi F et al. Delay in progression of bone metastases in breast cancer patients treated with intravenous pamidronate: results from a multinational randomized controlled trial. J Clin Oncol 1996; 14: 2552–9.

27. Hortobagyi GN, Theriault RL, Porter L et al. Efficacy of pamidronate in reducing skeletal complications in patients with breast cancer and lytic bone metastases. N Engl J Med 1996; 335: 1785–91.

28. Hortobagyi GN, Theriault RL, Lipton A et al. Long-term prevention of skeletal complications of metastatic breast cancer with pamidronate. J Clin Oncol 1998; 16: 2038–44.

29. Lipton A, Theriault RL, Hortobagyi GN et al. Pamidronate prevents skeletal complications and is effective palliative treatment in women with breast carcinoma and osteolytic bone metastases. Cancer 2000; 88: 1082–90.

30. Theriault RL, Lipton A, Hortobagyi GN et al. Pamidronate reduces skeletal morbidity in women with advanced breast cancer and lytic bone lesions: a randomized, placebo-controlled trial. J Clin Oncol 1999; 17: 846–54.

31. Lipton A, Demers L, Curley E et al. Markers of bone resorption in patients treated with pamidronate. Eur J Cancer 1998; 34: 2021–6.

32. Costa L, Coleman R, Quintela A et al. Treatment of bone metastases with high dose pamidronate. Cancer 2000; 88(abstr): 3103.

33. Lipton A. Bisphosphonates and breast carcinoma. Cancer 2000; 88: 3033–7.

34. Body JJ, Lortholary A, Romieu G et al. A dose-finding study of zolendronate in hypercalcemic cancer patients. J Bone Min Res 1999; 14: 1557–61.

35. Berenson J, Swift R, Borg T, Knight R. Phase I study of zolendronate administered as 30–60 second intravenous infusion in cancer patients. Cancer 2000; 88: 3101.

36. Berenson J, Rosen L, Knight R et al. Phase II trial of zolendronate vs. pamidronate in multiple myeloma and breast carcinoma patients with osteolytic lesions. Cancer 2000; 88: 3102.

37. Piga A, Bracci R, Ferretti B et al. A double-blind randomized study of oral clodronate in the treatment of bone metastases from tumors poorly responsive to chemotherapy. J Exp Clin Cancer Res 1998; 17: 213–17.

38. Speden D, Nicklason F, Francis H, Ward J. The use of pamidronate in hypertrophic pulmonary osteoarthropathy (HPOA). Aust NZ J Med 1997; 27: 307–10.

39. Hillner BE, Ingle JN, Berenson JR et al. American Society of Clinical Oncology guideline on the role of bisphosphonates in breast cancer. J Clin Oncol 2000; 18: 1378–91.

40. Body JJ, Bartl R, Burckhardt P et al. Current use of bisphosphonates in oncology. J Clin Oncol 1998; 16: 3890–9.

41. British Association of Surgical Oncology. The guidelines for the management of metastatic bone disease in breast cancer in the United Kingdom. Eur J Surg Oncol 1999; 25: 3–23.

29

Use in Multiple Myeloma

James R. Berenson

Institute for Myeloma and Bone Cancer Research, West Hollywood, CA, USA

INTRODUCTION

Multiple myeloma is a malignancy of B cells characterised by the accumulation of terminally differentiated plasma cells in the bone marrow. Despite sensitivity to a number of chemotherapeutic agents, the median survival of 30 months has remained unchanged over the past two decades [1]. The major clinical manifestation of this malignancy is related to osteolytic bone destruction [2]. Even patients responding to chemotherapy may have progression of skeletal disease [3,4] and recalcification of osteolytic lesions is rare. The bone disease can lead to pathological fractures, spinal cord compression, hypercalcaemia and pain, and is a major cause of morbidity and mortality in these patients [5]. These patients frequently require radiation therapy or surgery. These complications result from asynchronous bone turnover, in which increased osteoclastic bone resorption is not accompanied by a comparable increase in bone formation [6,7]. The increase in osteoclast activity in multiple myeloma is mediated by the release of osteoclast-stimulating factors [8,9]. These factors are produced locally in the bone marrow microenvironment by cells of both tumour and non-tumour origin [8–10]. Bisphosphonates are specific inhibitors of osteoclastic activity and are effective in the treatment of hypercalcaemia associated with malignancies [11]. These agents have been evaluated alone and as adjunctive therapy to primary anticancer treatment in patients with cancers involving the bone, including multiple myeloma [12–16].

Bisphosphonates have been evaluated in several large randomised trials in myeloma patients also receiving chemotherapy. Oral etidronate given daily showed no clinical benefit [3], while the use of oral clodronate daily has produced variable clinical results in three randomised trials [12,17,18]. Oral administration of pamidronate was ineffective in reducing the skeletal complications of these patients [19]. A large randomised double-blind study was conducted in which stage III multiple myeloma patients received either pamidronate (90 mg) or placebo as a 4 h intravenous (i.v.) infusion every 4 weeks for 21 cycles in addition to antimyeloma chemotherapy [20,21]. This intravenously administered bisphosphonate significantly reduced the development of skeletal complications. Although survival was not different between the pamidronate group and placebo group overall, patients receiving pamidronate who had failed first-line chemotherapy lived longer than those receiving placebo. The patients who received pamidronate also had significant decreases in bone pain, did not increase analgesic usage, unlike the placebo group, and showed a better quality of life. Recently, more potent bisphosphonates, including ibandronate and zoledronic acid, have been evaluated in large Phase III studies [23,24]. The results of these studies show that zoledronic acid (4 mg) at a much shorter infusion time (15 min) reduces skeletal complications similar to a 120 min infusion of pamidronate, whereas i.v. administered ibandronate showed no effect on skeletal morbidity compared to placebo. These findings led to the recommendation by the American Society of Clinical Oncology (ASCO) Bisphosphonates Experts Panel Guidelines of either i.v. pamidronate administered over at least 2 h or zoledronic acid given over 15 min every 3–4 weeks

Textbook of Bone Metastases. Edited by C. Jasmin, R. E. Coleman, L. R. Coia, R. Capanna and G. Saillant
© 2005 John Wiley & Sons Ltd: ISBN 0 471 87742 5

as therapy for myeloma patients showing evidence of bone loss [22].

BISPHOSPHONATES IN THE TREATMENT OF MYELOMA BONE DISEASE

These agents have been evaluated alone and as adjunctive therapy to primary anticancer treatment in patients with cancers involving the bone, including multiple myeloma [3,12,16,17,19–21,23–24]. Recent large placebo-controlled clinical trials have shown the efficacy of bisphosphonates in reducing skeletal complications in myeloma patients, and have suggested that these agents may also alter the overall course of the disease.

Although early studies involving bisphosphonates in myeloma patients suggested a reduction in bone pain and healing of lytic lesions, the trials involved relatively few patients. Large randomised trials of long-term bisphosphonate use have now been published, and involved evaluation of oral administration of daily etidronate, clodronate, or pamidronate or i.v. pamidronate, ibandronate or zoledronic acid.

Etidronate

In the Canadian study involving etidronate [3], 173 newly diagnosed patients all received intermittent oral melphalan and prednisone as primary chemotherapy, and 166 were then randomised to receive either daily oral etidronate (5 mg/kg) or placebo until death or stopping the treatment due to side-effects. Although significant height loss occurred in both placebo- and etidronate-treated patients, no difference was found between the two arms. Similarly, the other outcome measures (new fractures, hypercalcaemic episodes, and bone pain) showed no differences between the two arms.

Clodronate

Three large randomised trials have been published using oral clodronate in myeloma patients. In the Finnish trial [12], 350 previously untreated patients were entered, and 336 randomised to receive either clodronate (2.4 g) or placebo daily for 2 years. All patients were also treated with intermittent oral melphalan and prednisolone. Only a little more than half of patients had radiographs completed at both study entry and 2 years. Given this limitation, the proportion of patients with progression of lytic lesions was less in the clodronate-treated group (12%) than in the placebo group (24%). However, the progression of overall pathological fractures, as well as both vertebral and non-vertebral fractures, was not different between the arms. In addition, the number of patients developing hypercalcaemia was similar in the two arms. Changes in pain index and use of analgesics were similar in both arms.

Clodronate has also been evaluated in an open-label randomised German trial. In this study, 170 previously untreated patients were randomised to receive either no bisphosphonate or oral clodronate (1.6 g) daily for 1 year. All patients were also treated with intermittent intravenous melphalan and oral prednisone. Unfortunately, premature termination occurred in more than half of the patients, despite the short length of the study (1 year). The results showed no difference in progression of bone disease, as assessed by plain radiographs, in the two arms. However, there was a trend toward a reduction in the number of new progressive sites in the clodronate-treated group after 6 and 12 months, although this did not reach statistical significance. Although the number of patients without pain and those not using analgesics was higher in the clodronate group, the open-label design of this trial makes it difficult to interpret these findings.

Recently, the Medical Research Council has published the results of a large trial involving 536 recently diagnosed myeloma patients randomised to receive either oral clodronate 1.6 g or placebo daily in addition to alkylator-based chemotherapy [25]. The primary endpoints of the trial were unclear. However, after combining the proportion of patients developing either non-vertebral fractures or severe hypercalcaemia, including those leaving the trial due to severe hypercalcaemia, there were fewer clodronate-treated patients experiencing these combined events than placebo patients. However, the number of patients developing hypercalcaemia was similar in the two arms. The number of patients experiencing non-vertebral fractures was lower in the clodronate group. Although vertebral fractures reportedly occurred in significantly fewer clodronate-treated patients than placebo patients, only half of patients obtained at least one post-baseline radiograph. Back pain and poor performance status were not significantly different between the two groups, except at one time point (24 months). The proportion of patients requiring radiotherapy was similar between the two arms. There was no difference in time to first skeletal event or overall survival.

Pamidronate

In multiple myeloma patients, results of small open-label trials lasting up to 24 months suggested that pamidronate disodium might be effective in reducing skeletal complications of multiple myeloma [13,14]. Thus, a large, randomised, double-blind study was conducted to determine whether monthly 90 mg infusions of pamidronate compared to placebo for 21 months reduced skeletal events in patients with multiple myeloma who were receiving chemotherapy [20,21]. This study included patients with Durie–Salmon Stage III multiple myeloma and at least one osteolytic lesion. Unlike the etidronate and clodronate trials, which involved untreated patients, patients were required to receive an unchanged chemotherapy regimen for at least 2 months before enrolment. Patients were stratified according to their antimyeloma therapy at trial entry: stratum 1, first-line chemotherapy; stratum 2, second-line or greater chemotherapy. The primary endpoint, skeletal events (pathological fractures; spinal cord compression associated with vertebral compression fracture; surgery to treat or prevent pathological fracture or spinal cord compression associated with vertebral compression fracture, or radiation to bone) and secondary endpoints (hypercalcaemia, bone pain, analgesic drug use, performance status and quality of life) were assessed monthly. Importantly, although the chemotherapeutic regimen was not uniform at study entry, the types and numbers of chemotherapeutic regimens in the two groups were similar at study entry and during the trial.

At the pre-planned primary endpoint after nine cycles of therapy, the proportions of myeloma patients having any skeletal event was 41% in patients receiving placebo but only 24% in pamidronate-treated patients. In addition, the time to first skeletal event was prolonged in the pamidronate group (Figure 29.1). In addition, the number of skeletal events/year was half in the patients treated with pamidronate. The proportion of pamidronate-treated patients with skeletal events was lower in both stratum 1 (first-line therapy) and stratum 2 ($\geqslant$ second-line therapy). The patients who received pamidronate also had significant decreases in bone pain, no increase in analgesic usage and showed no deterioration in performance status and quality of life at the end of 9 months. Similar to the results after nine cycles of therapy, the proportions of patients developing any skeletal event and the skeletal morbidity rate continued to remain significantly lower in the pamidronate group than the placebo group during the additional 12 cycles of treatment. However, there were no differences between the treatment groups in the percentage of patients with healing or progression of osteolytic lesions. Although overall survival in all patients was not significantly different between the two treatment groups, in stratum 2 the median survival time was 21

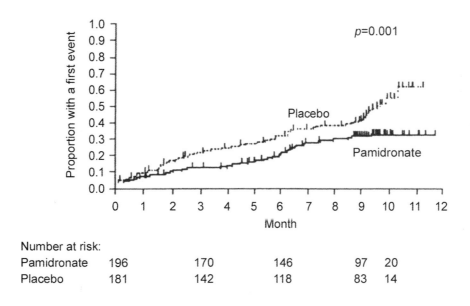

Figure 29.1. Kaplan–Meier estimates of time to first skeletal-related episode (excluding hypercalcaemia of malignancy) by treatment group (intent-to-treat patients)

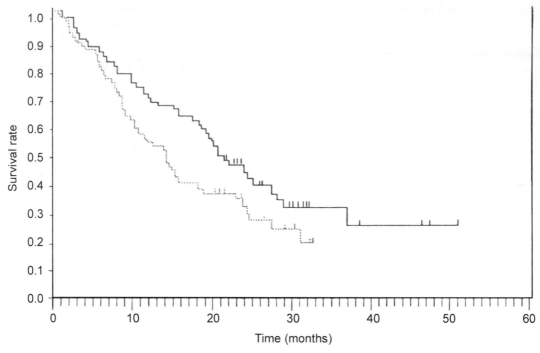

Figure 29.2. Kaplan–Meier estimates of survival in stratum 2 patients with multiple myeloma treated with pamidronate or placebo. Survival was measured from randomisation date to 1 February 1995. There was a median survival of 21 and 14 months in pamidronate (n=66) and placebo (n=65) patients, respectively. Log-rank test was adjusted for ECOG performance status and β2-microglobulin, which were the only two prognostic variables significantly influencing survival

months for pamidronate patients compared to 14 months for placebo patients (Figure 29.2).

In a double blind randomised trial, a Danish–Swedish cooperative group evaluated daily oral pamidronate (300 mg/day) compared to placebo in 300 newly diagnosed myeloma patients also receiving intermittent melphalan and prednisone [19]. After a median duration of 18 months, there was no significant reduction in the primary endpoint, defined as skeletal-related morbidity (bone fracture, surgery for impending fracture, vertebral collapse, or increase in number and/or size of lytic lesions), hypercalcaemic episodes or survival, between the arms. Fewer episodes of severe pain and less height loss were observed in the oral pamidronate-treated patients, however.

Ibandronate

Ibandronate is a nitrogen-containing bisphosphonate that in pre-clinical models shows more anti-bone-resorptive potency than pamidronate and the other non-nitrogen-containing bisphosphonates. The results of a Phase III placebo-controlled trial of 214 stage II

or III myeloma patients with osteolytic bone disease were recently published [23]. Patients either received monthly injections of 2 mg ibandronate or placebo in addition to their antineoplastic therapy. Ninety-nine patients were evaluable in each arm for efficacy. The mean number of events/patient-year on treatment was similar in both groups (ibandronate 2.13 vs. placebo 2.05). In addition, there was no difference in pain, analgesic usage or quality of life between the arms. However, among patients treated with ibandronate who showed a sustained and marked reduction in bone resorption markers, fewer skeletal complications occurred. There was no difference in overall survival. Thus, this monthly dose of intravenous ibandronate did not show significant benefits in reducing skeletal complications in myeloma patients with lytic bone disease.

Zoledronic Acid

Zoledronic acid is an imidazole-containing bisphosphonate that shows more potency in pre-clinical studies than any other bisphosphonate currently available [25]. Two small Phase I trials established the safety and marked sustained reduction in bone resorption markers for patients with myeloma and other cancers associated with metastatic bone disease, with monthly infusions of small doses given over several minutes [26,27]. A large randomised Phase II study compared this newer bisphosphonate to pamidronate in 280 patients with lytic bone metastases from either multiple myeloma ($n=108$) or breast cancer ($n=172$) [28]. Patients were randomised to nine monthly infusions of 0.4 mg, 2.0 mg, or 4.0 mg zoledronic acid, or to 90 mg pamidronate as a 2 h infusion. The primary endpoint was to determine a dose of zoledronic acid that reduced the need for radiation therapy to less than 30% of treated patients, although all skeletal events were also analysed similar to those determined in the previously reported Phase III pamidronate trials. Radiation therapy was required in a similar proportion of patients receiving pamidronate and zoledronic acid at 2.0 and 4.0 mg (18–21%), whereas more patients receiving the lowest dose of zoledronic acid underwent radiotherapy (24%). Similarly, the proportion of patients with any skeletal event was lower (30–35%) in these same groups compared to patients receiving 0.4 mg of zoledronic acid. Interestingly, significant increases in bone density (over 6% in the lumbar spine) and inhibition of bone resorption markers was observed in this latter cohort, but this failed to translate to any clinical benefit. Although the results of this study suggested that 0.4 mg was an

inadequate monthly dose of zoledronic acid to be of clinical use in the prevention of skeletal complications for patients with myeloma or breast cancer metastatic to bone, the small size of this Phase II trial did not allow for a complete assessment of the efficacy of higher doses of zoledronic acid compared to pamidronate.

Thus, a larger Phase III trial evaluated two doses of zoledronic acid (4 and 8 mg) compared to pamidronate (90 mg) infused every 3–4 weeks for treatment of myeloma or breast cancer patients with metastatic bone disease [24]. The doses and infusion time (5 min) of zoledronic acid were selected based on the safety and superiority of these doses in reversing hypercalcaemia of malignancy compared to pamidronate (90 mg) [29]. Importantly, the primary efficacy endpoint of this trial was designed to show the non-inferiority of zoledronic acid compared to pamidronate in reducing skeletal complications for patients with myeloma or breast cancer metastatic to bone. The trial involved 1643 patients who were stratified among individuals with myeloma ($n=513$) or breast cancer on either hormonal therapy or chemotherapy ($n=1130$). The proportion of patients with any skeletal event did not differ among the three treatment arms. In addition, the time to first skeletal event was similar in the three groups (12–13 months) (Figure 29.3). The effects of these treatments on pain and analgesic use were similar to those observed in prior studies. Importantly, during the clinical trial, rises in creatinine were more

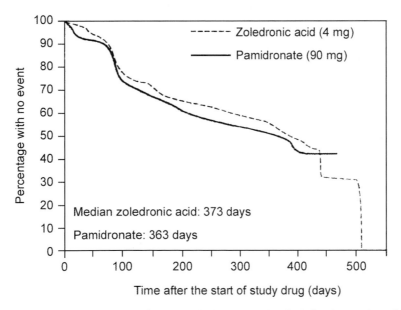

Figure 29.3. Kaplan–Meier estimates of time to first skeletal-related event (not including hypercalcaemia) by treatment group, pamidronate (90 mg) compared to zoledronic acid (4 mg)

frequently observed in the zoledronic acid arms, and the infusion time was increased to 15 min. Despite this increase in infusion time, patients receiving the 8 mg dose continued to be at a higher risk of developing rises in serum creatinine, and these patients were subsequently changed to the 4 mg dose for the remainder of the trial. Long-term follow-up data is now available and shows no difference in the renal profile between patients receiving 4 mg zoledronic acid infused over 15 min compared to 90 mg pamidronate infused over 120 min. Following the change in infusion time, zoledronic acid was well tolerated, with changes in serum creatinine observed in a similar proportion of patients receiving pamidronate 90 mg over 2 h compared to zoledronic acid 4 mg infused over 15 min.

ASCO CLINICAL PRACTICE GUIDELINES ON THE ROLE OF BISPHOSPHONATES IN MULTIPLE MYELOMA

Recently, ASCO published guidelines based on the recommendations of their Bisphosphonates Expert Panel [22]. The panel recommended that for multiple myeloma patients who have, on plain radiographs, evidence of lytic bone disease, either i.v. zoledronic acid 4 mg infused over 15 min or pamidronate 90 mg delivered over 120 min every 3–4 weeks should be given. The panel also believed it reasonable to start these agents for patients with osteopenia but without evidence of lytic bone disease. Once initiated, the panel recommended that the i.v. bisphosphonate be continued until there was a substantial decline in the patient's performance status. The panel also recommended intermittent monitoring of renal function and urinary protein evaluation to assess possible renal dysfunction from these agents. However, for patients with either solitary plasmacytoma or indolent myeloma, no data exists to suggest their efficacy. In addition, although clinical studies would be interesting to conduct for patients with monoclonal gammopathy of undetermined significance, the panel did not recommend treatment of these patients with bisphosphonates.

ANTIMYELOMA EFFECTS OF BISPHOSPHONATES

The role of bisphosphonates for myeloma patients may go beyond simply inhibiting bone resorption and the resulting skeletal complications. Some studies suggest that these drugs may have antitumour effects, both directly and indirectly [30]. Using the murine 5T2

multiple myeloma model, Radl and colleagues suggested that pamidronate might reduce tumour burden in treated mice [31]. *In vitro* studies also suggest that pamidronate may possess antimyeloma properties, as demonstrated by its ability to induce apoptosis of myeloma cells [32] and suppress the production of IL-6, an important myeloma growth factor, by bone marrow stromal cells from myeloma patients [33]. A recent *in vitro* study may help to explain the induction of apoptosis by these compounds [34]. These drugs inhibit the mevalonate pathway and, as a result, decrease the isoprenylation of proteins such as *ras* and other GTPases. The antitumour effects of these agents appear to be synergistic with glucocorticoids [35]. Several recent studies show that bisphosphonates are markedly antiangiogenic [36,37], and the recent demonstration of the marked antimyeloma clinical effects of the antiangiogenic agent thalidomide in myeloma patients [38] suggests another putative mechanism by which bisphosphonates may possess antimyeloma effects. In addition to the effects on the tumour cells and the tumoural microenvironment, recent studies suggest that nitrogen-containing bisphosphonates may stimulate $\gamma\delta$T lymphocytes and induce antiplasma cell activity in myeloma patients [39]. Several recent murine models of human myeloma show that the administration of pamidronate or zoledronic acid reduces both the development of lytic bone disease and tumour burden [40,41]. In addition to the survival advantage observed in relapsing patients in the large randomised Berenson trial [21], two recent myeloma patients treated with pamidronate alone were recently reported to show reductions in myeloma tumour cell burden [42]. Attempts to increase the dose of pamidronate to more clearly show the antimyeloma effect of this agent were accompanied by the development of albuminuria and azotemia. However, since 4 mg zoledronic acid may be administered safely over 15 min, it may be possible to increase the dose of this newer agent with longer infusion times and clearly show clinically the hoped-for antimyeloma effects that have been suggested from the pre-clinical studies mentioned above.

SUMMARY

The results of two large Phase III clinical trials show that the benefit of adjunctive use of intravenously administered monthly zoledronic acid or pamidronate in addition to chemotherapy is superior to chemotherapy alone in patients with advanced multiple myeloma, with respect to safely reducing bone complications.

Bisphosphonate treatment should now be considered for all patients with multiple myeloma and evidence of bone loss. The three large randomised studies with clodronate show inconsistent results with oral administration of this first-generation bisphosphonate. Curiously, the Finnish trial, using a larger daily dose, shows less effect than the MRC trial using a smaller amount of clodronate. In addition, in the latter trial, although the drug had some effect on reducing fractures and severe hypercalcaemia in these patients, the drug did not affect the time to first skeletal event or use of radiotherapy. Similarly, oral pamidronate has also not been effective. Given the clinical results and the poor tolerability of oral agents, this route of administration for bisphosphonates is unlikely to be of much benefit in these patients. Clearly, intravenously administered pamidronate and zoledronic acid both reduce the skeletal complications as well as improve the quality of life of these patients. Whether these drugs are effective in earlier stages of disease or for patients without bone loss is unknown. The possibility of antitumour effects of these agents, as suggested from pre-clinical studies, is now being evaluated in trials evaluating higher doses of zoledronic acid infused over several hours.

REFERENCES

1. Alexanian RH, Dimopoulos MA. Management of multiple myeloma. Semin Hematol 1995; 32: 20–30.
2. Mundy GR, Bertoline DR. Bone destruction and hypercalcemia in plasma cell myeloma. Semin Oncol 1986; 13: 291–9.
3. Belch AR, Bergsagel DE, Wilson K et al. Effect of daily etidronate on the osteolysis of multiple myeloma. J Clin Oncol 1991; 9: 1397–402.
4. Kyle RA, Jowsey J, Kelly PJ, Taves DR. Multiple myeloma bone disease. The comparative effect of sodium fluoride and calcium carbonate or placebo. N Engl J Med 1975; 293: 1334–8.
5. Kyle RA. Multiple myeloma: review of 869 cases. Mayo Clin Proc 1975; 50: 29–40.
6. Kanis JA, McCloskey EV, Taube T et al. Rationale for the use of bisphosphonates in bone metastases. Bone 1991; 12(suppl 1): S13–18.
7. Fleisch H. Bisphosphonates: a new class of drugs in diseases of bone and calcium metabolism. In Brunner KW, Fleisch H, Senn H-J (eds), Recent Results in Cancer Research, vol 116: Bisphosphonates and Tumor Osteolysis. Springer-Verlag: Berlin, 1989: 1–28.
8. Stashenko P, Dewhirst FE, Peros WJ et al. Synergistic interactions between interleukin 1, tumor necrosis factor, and lymphotoxin in bone resorption. J Immunol 1987; 138: 1464–8.
9. Mundy GR. Mechanisms of osteolytic bone destruction. Bone 1991; 12(suppl 1): S1–6.
10. Bataille R, Chappard D, Basle M. Excessive bone resorption in human plasmacytomas: direct induction by tumor cells in vivo. Br J Haematol 1995; 90: 721–4.
11. Coleman RE, Purohit OP. Osteoclast inhibition for the treatment of bone metastases. Cancer Treat Rev 1993; 19: 79–103.
12. Lahtinen R, Laakso M, Palva I et al. Randomised, placebo-controlled multicentre trial of clodronate in multiple myeloma. Lancet 1992; 340: 1049–52.
13. Man Z, Otero AB, Rendo P et al. Use of pamidronate for multiple myeloma osteolytic lesions. Lancet 1990; 335: 663.
14. Thiebaud D, Leyuraz S, Von Fliedner V et al. Treatment of bone metastases from breast cancer and myeloma with pamidronate. Eur J Cancer 1991; 27: 37–41.
15. Purohit OP, Anthony C, Radstone CR et al. High-dose intravenous pamidronate for metastatic bone pain. Br J Cancer 1994; 70: 554–78.
16. van Holten-Verzantvoort AATM, Kroon M, Bijvoet OLM et al. Palliative treatment in patients with bone metastases from breast cancer. J Clin Oncol 1993; 11: 491–8.
17. McCloskey EV, MacLennan CM, Drayson MT et al. A randomized trial of the effect of clodronate on skeletal morbidity in multiple myeloma. Br J Haematol 1998; 101: 317–25.
18. Heim ME, Clemens MR, Queisser W et al. Prospective randomized trial of dichloromethylene bisphosphonate (clodronate) in patients with multiple myeloma requiring treatment. A multicenter study. Onkologie 1995; 18: 439–48.
19. Brinker H, Westin J, Abildgaard N et al. Failure of oral pamidronate to reduce skeletal morbidity in multiple myeloma: a double-blind placebo-controlled trial. Br J Haematol 1998; 101: 280–6.
20. Berenson JR, Lichtenstein A, Porter L et al. Efficacy of pamidronate in reducing the skeletal events in patients with advanced multiple myeloma. N Engl J Med 1996; 334: 488–93.
21. Berenson J, Lichtenstein A, Porter L et al. Long-term pamidronate treatment of advanced multiple myeloma patients reduces skeletal events. J Clin Oncol 1998; 16: 593–602.
22. Berenson JR, Hillner BE, Kyle RA et al. American Society of Clinical Oncology Clinical Practice Guidelines: the role of bisphosphonates in multiple myeloma. J Clin Oncol 2002; 20: 3719–36.
23. Menssen HD, Sakalova A, Fontana A et al. Effects of long-term intravenous ibandronate therapy on skeletal-related events, survival, and bone resorption markers in patients with advanced multiple myeloma. J Clin Oncol 2002; 20: 2353–9.
24. Rosen LS, Gordon D, Kaminski M et al. Zoledronic acid vs. pamidronate in the treatment of skeletal metastases in patients with breast cancer or osteolytic lesions of multiple myeloma: a Phase III, double-blind comparative trial. Cancer J 2001; 7: 377–87.
25. Green JR, Muller K, Jaeggi KA. Preclinical pharmacology of CGP 42446, a new potent heterocyclic bisphosphonate compound. J Bone Min Res 1994; 9: 745–51.
26. Berenson JR, Vescio R, Henick K et al. A phase I open-label, dose-ranging trial of intravenous bolus zoledronic acid, a novel bisphosphonate, in cancer patients with metastatic bone disease. Cancer 2001; 91: 144–54.

27. Berenson J, Vescio R, Rosen LS et al. A phase I dose-ranging trial of monthly infusions of zoledronic acid for the treatment of metastatic bone disease. Clin Cancer Res 2001; 7: 478–85.

28. Berenson J, Rosen LS, Howell A et al. Zoledronic acid reduces skeletal-related events in patients with osteolytic metastases. Cancer 2001; 91: 1191–200.

29. Major P, Lotholary A, Hon J et al. Zoledronic acid is superior to pamidronate in the treatment of hypercalcemia of malignancy: a pooled analysis of two randomized, controlled clinical trials. J Clin Oncol 2001; 19: 558–67.

30. Mundy GR. Bisphosphonates as cancer drugs. Hospital Practice (Office edn) 1999; 34: 81–4.

31. Radl J, Croese JW, Zircher C et al. Influence of treatment with APD-bisphosphonate on the bone lesions in the mouse 5T2 multiple myeloma. Cancer 1985; 55: 1030–40.

32. Aparicio A, Gardner A, Tu Y et al. In vitro cytoreductive effects on multiple myeloma cells induced by bisphosphonates. Leukemia 1998; 12: 220–9.

33. Savage AD, Belson DJ, Vescio RA et al. Pamidronate reduces IL-6 production by bone marrow stroma from multiple myeloma patients. Blood 1996; 88: 105a.

34. Shipman CM, Croucher PI, Russell RG et al. The bisphosphonate incandronate (YM175) causes apoptosis of human myeloma cells in vitro by inhibiting the mevalonate pathway. Cancer Res 1998; 58: 5294–7.

35. Tassone P, Forciniti S, Galea E et al. Growth inhibition and synergistic induction of apoptosis by zoledronate and dexamethasone in human myeloma cell lines. Leukemia 2000; 14: 841–4.

36. Wood J, Bonjean K, Ruetsz S et al. Novel antiangiogenic effects of the bisphosphonate compound zoledronic acid. J Pharmacol Exp Ther 2002; 302: 1055–61.

37. Fournier P, Boissier S, Filleur S et al. Bisphosphonates inhibit angiogenesis in vitro and testosterone-stimulated vascular regrowth in the ventral prostate in castrated rats. Cancer Res 2002; 62: 6538–44.

38. Singhal S, Mehta J, Desikan R et al. Antitumor activity of thalidomide in refractory multiple myeloma. N Engl J Med 1999; 341: 1565–71.

39. Kunzmann V, Bauer E, Feurle J et al. Stimulation of $\gamma\delta$T cells by aminobisphosphonates and induction of anti-plasma cell activity in multiple myeloma. Blood 2000; 96: 384–92.

40. Yaccoby S, Pearse R, Epstein J et al. Reciprocal relationship between myeloma-induced changes in the bone marrow microenvironment and myeloma cell growth. Blood 2000; 96: 549a.

41. Yaccoby S, Barlogie B, Epstein J. Pamidronate inhibits growth of myeloma in vivo in the SCID-hu system. Blood 1998; 92: 106a.

42. Dhodapkar MV, Singh J, Mehta J et al. Antimyeloma activity of pamidronate in vivo. Br J Haematol 1998; 103: 530.

30

Use in Prostate Cancer

R. E. Coleman

Academic Unit of Clinical Oncology, Sheffield, UK

INTRODUCTION

Prostate cancer is a major public health problem, with a total of 265 000 men diagnosed with prostate cancer annually in the USA and Europe [1]. Prostate cancer shows a remarkable propensity for bone; around 85% of patients dying from prostate cancer display signs of malignant bone disease during the course of the disease [2,3]. Typically, bone metastases involve the spine, pelvis and rib cage. In addition to malignant bone disease, age-related and treatment-associated bone loss are common problems during hormonal therapy for prostate cancer, further compromising skeletal health in these patients [4].

Skeletal complications of bone metastases are a significant source of morbidity and mortality among men with advanced prostate cancer. The median survival is approximately 36 months after the initial diagnosis of bone metastases, and patients may experience a chronic threat of skeletal morbidity [5]. Bone metastases are the most common cause of cancer-associated pain, often requiring palliative radiotherapy. The bone destruction caused by metastatic involvement can lead to severe and debilitating complications, including pathological fractures and spinal cord compression. The degree of skeletal morbidity in patients with metastatic bone disease from hormone-resistant prostate cancer is illustrated by the control arm of a trial evaluating the bisphosphonate, zoledronic acid. In the placebo group (standard cancer treatments alone), non-vertebral and vertebral fractures developed in 16% and 8%, respectively, during the 15 month duration of the study [6]. In addition to having this high rate of pathological fractures, nearly one-third of the patients in the placebo group required palliative radiotherapy for bone pain.

Vertebral fractures may result in vertebral deformity or collapse, which can result in significant back pain, postural changes, loss of height and functional impairment. Subsequent spinal cord compression from vertebral damage may lead to severe neurological sequelae, including irreversible paraplegia. Pathological fractures of the pelvis and femur often require surgical intervention and lengthy rehabilitation. Patients with hip fractures have a particularly poor prognosis; the 30 day mortality rate for men who experience pathological or osteoporotic hip fractures is 16% [7]. The majority of long bone fractures due to cancer will never heal, and require surgical intervention to restore function. Surgical intervention to prevent an impending fracture or to restore functional mobility also requires hospitalisation and lengthy physical rehabilitation.

Effective systemic anticancer treatments may temporarily slow bone destruction. Unfortunately, although current treatment modalities are effective during the early stages of prostate cancer, they are rarely curative and, once the disease escapes from endocrine control, the disease responds poorly to any of the current antineoplastic treatments. As skeletal disease progresses, patients may be left with significant disability, loss of mobility and loss of independence.

METASTATIC BONE LESIONS IN PATIENTS WITH PROSTATE CANCER

Prostate cancer cells that metastasise to bone often trigger localised increases in bone formation by

Textbook of Bone Metastases. Edited by C. Jasmin, R. E. Coleman, L. R. Coia, R. Capanna and G. Saillant
© 2005 John Wiley & Sons Ltd: ISBN 0 471 87742 5

osteoblasts, and these osteoblastic lesions are typically associated with regions of increased osteolytic activity. Histomorphometric studies have shown that new bone formation is preceded by local osteolysis [8]. Both increased osteoblastic activity and marked osteolysis can be seen, with the osteolytic component compromising bone integrity [9]. There is also considerable biochemical evidence of increased osteoclastic activity in prostate cancer (Figure 30.1) [10,11]. Garnero et al. [12] have shown that, in addition to increases in bone formation markers, patients with prostate cancer have dramatically elevated urinary levels of bone resorption markers. These increased levels are not seen in control patients or in those with benign prostate hypertrophy.

Metastatic bone lesions from prostate cancer can appear osteoblastic, osteolytic or mixed in character on plain radiographs, and the appearance of these lesions can change during the course of the disease. However, the typical appearance is osteosclerotic. The histological and biochemical evidence of the underlying osteolytic component of osteoblastic lesions led to the hypothesis that bisphosphonates, which specifically modulate osteoclast activity, might also be successful in treating osteoblastic bone disease.

BISPHOSPHONATE THERAPY IN PATIENTS WITH PROSTATE CANCER

Although bisphosphonate therapy has primarily been evaluated in patients with osteolytic lesions associated with breast cancer and multiple myeloma, they have also been shown to reduce biochemical markers of bone resorption in patients with osteoblastic bone lesions associated with advanced prostate cancer [12–14]. However, until recently, bisphosphonates had failed to demonstrate a significant reduction in skeletal complications from bone metastases in patients with advanced prostate cancer in randomised, placebo-controlled trials (Table 30.1). Several Phase II studies have assessed bone pain and analgesic usage, with some benefit in these acute endpoints. These trials were statistically underpowered to detect significant effects on skeletal complications. Furthermore, the results were not sufficiently convincing to lead to either the regulatory approval or widespread use of bisphosphonates for metastatic bone disease in prostate cancer [12–23].

In 57 patients with hormone-refractory prostate cancer (HRPC) and bone pain at study entry, Smith concluded that intravenous etidronate (5 mg/kg) followed by oral etidronate (400 mg/day) had no significant effects on pain levels or analgesic usage over and above placebo [24]. A more recent clinical trial involving 208 patients investigated both pain and analgesic usage. In this study intravenous clodronate was added to a background treatment of mitoxantrone and prednisolone. The study also included objectively measurable skeletal complications as clinical endpoints. No significant differences between clodronate and placebo were seen [25].

The Medical Research Council in the UK has performed a moderate-sized Phase III trial of oral clodronate in 311 men with metastatic bone disease

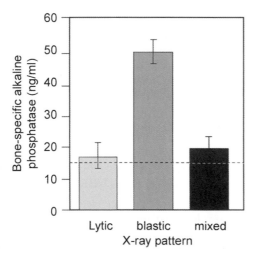
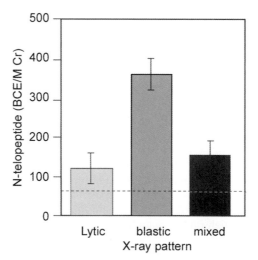

Figure 30.1. Bone formation and resorption marker measurements in metastatic bone disease classified as either "osteolytic", "ostoblastic" or "mixed" in radiographic appearance. Adapted from [11]. Upper limit of normal shown by dotted line

Table 30.1. The efficacy of bisphosphonates in randomised, placebo-controlled trials in patients with bone metastases secondary to prostate cancer

Study	Patients (n)	Drug	Dose	Efficacy results
Smith [24]	57	Etidronate	5 mg/kg (i.v., days 1–3), then 400 mg/day (oral)	No significant benefits
Elomaa et al. [21]	75	Clodronate	3200 mg/day (1st month), then 1600 mg/day (oral)	↓ Pain and analgesic use (1st month only) ↓ Serum calcium levels
Kylmala et al. [22]	57	Clodronate	300 mg/day (i.v., days 1–5) then 1600 mg/day (oral)	↓ Pain by 10% (non-significant)
Strang et al. [23]	55	Clodronate	300 mg/day (i.v., days 1–3) then 3200 mg/day (oral)	No significant benefits
Ernst et al. [25]	208	Clodronate	1500 mg (i.v.) q 3 weeks	↓ Pain (non-significant)
Lipton et al. [27]	236	Pamidronate	90 mg (i.v.) q 3 weeks	No significant benefits in pain or proportion of patients with SREs
Saad et al. [6]	643	Zoledronic acid	4 mg (i.v.) q 3 weeks	↓ Proportion of patients with ≥1 SRE (p=0.021) ↑ Time to first SRE (p=0.01) ↓ Rate of skeletal morbidity (p=0.006)
Dearnaley et al. [26]		Clodronate	1040 mg/day oral	↓ Proportion of patients with ≥1 SRE (41% vs. 49%, p=NS) Improvement in time to progression (24 vs. 19 months, p=NS)

i.v., intravenous; SRE, skeletal-related event.

from prostate cancer [26]. Quite a high dose of oral clodronate (Loron™, 1040 mg twice daily) was administered for a median duration of 43 months. A final analysis has not been published but an early analysis reported a slight reduction in the proportion of patients receiving clodronate experiencing a skeletal event (41% vs. 49%), an improvement in time to progression (24 vs. 19 months) and median survival (37 vs. 28 months). However, none of these differences were statistically significant. Further follow-up may clarify the results of this trial although, like the other studies mentioned above, the study was probably underpowered to show the likely impact of a bisphosphonate on the course of the disease.

Pamidronate has also been studied in patients with advanced prostate cancer [27]. In a multicentre, randomized, placebo-controlled trial, 236 prostate cancer patients with bone metastases were treated with intravenous (i.v.) pamidronate (90 mg) or placebo every 3 weeks for 9 months. This trial assessed bone pain as the primary endpoint and included an assessment of skeletal events (defined as pathological fracture, spinal cord compression, requirement for palliative radiotherapy or surgery to bone, or

hypercalcaemia of malignancy) as a secondary endpoint. Patients in this trial had very advanced disease (median baseline, PSA=97.8 ng/ml in the pamidronate group), very high levels of bone resorption and substantial bone pain at study entry. As in the previous trials, pamidronate did not significantly reduce the incidence of skeletal events and had only a slight effect on bone pain (Figure 30.2).

Despite the failures of other bisphosphonates, zoledronic acid was investigated in patients with advanced prostate cancer to determine whether its increased potency would translate into improved clinical benefits for this patient population. Patients (n=643) with hormone-refractory prostate cancer (HRPC) and documented bone metastases were randomised to one of three different treatment groups: 4 mg zoledronic acid (n=214); 8 mg zoledronic acid (n=221); or placebo (n=208) [6]. In the 8 mg arm, the dose was reduced by protocol amendment to 4 mg because of concerns over renal safety, and conclusions on the efficacy of this cohort are difficult to make. Zoledronic acid or placebo were administered as a 15 min, 100 ml i.v. infusion every 3 weeks for 15 months, followed by an extension phase of a further 10

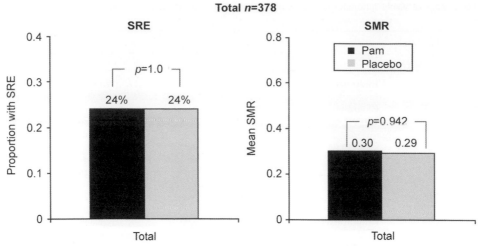

Figure 30.2. Randomised placebo-controlled trial of pamidronate in advanced prostate cancer with bone metastases. Proportion experiencing one or more skeletal-related events (SRE) and the skeletal morbidity rate (SMR) are shown. Hypercalcaemia (HCM) is excluded from this analysis of the primary endpoint. From Lipton A et al. [27] The new bisphosphonate, Zometa (zoledronic acid), decreases skeletal complications in both osteolytic and osteoblastic lesions: a comparison to pamidronate. Cancer Invest 2002; 20 (suppl 2): 45–54

months. All patients received daily oral supplements of calcium and vitamin D.

Only the results from the initial 15 months study period have been published and are presented below. However, analysis of the extension phase reveals that the effects of zoledronic acid were maintained for at least the 2 year study period (Saad, personal communication; and Novartis Data on file). The primary endpoint was the proportion of patients with a skeletal event, defined as pathological fracture, spinal cord compression, requirement for radiation therapy to treat bone pain, requirement for surgery to bone, or changes in chemotherapy resulting from bone pain. Secondary endpoints included the time to first skeletal complication, Andersen–Gill multiple-event analysis [28], levels of bone pain, and biochemical markers of bone resorption.

The disposition, demographics and prognostic factors of patients in the zoledronic acid and placebo treatment groups were well balanced (Table 30.2). At baseline, the median serum PSA levels were slightly higher in the zoledronic acid groups compared with those in the placebo group (81.7 the 4 mg zoledronic acid group vs. 61 ng/ml for the placebo patients). Similar proportions of patients reported bone pain (73% for both the zoledronic acid and placebo treatment groups), and a similar proportion of patients had experienced a prior skeletal event (31% for the zoledronic acid 4 mg group vs. 38% of the placebo group). Mean baseline pain scores were approximately two in all treatment groups.

Zoledronic acid was significantly more effective than placebo across all primary and secondary endpoints. The zoledronic acid 4 mg treatment group achieved significant reductions in the proportion of patients with any skeletal complication (33% vs. 44% with placebo; $p=0.021$) or pathological fracture (13% vs. 22% with placebo; $p=0.015$) compared with the placebo group (Figure 30.3A). Furthermore, there were consistent reductions in the proportion of patients with each type of skeletal complication, including non-vertebral fractures (Figure 30.4). Zoledronic acid 4 mg was still significantly superior to placebo when fractures were excluded, indicating that the beneficial effect was not simply as a result of the prevention of osteoporotic fractures.

Zoledronic acid also prolonged the time to first skeletal complication by more than 4 months (median not reached at 420 days vs. 321 days for placebo; $p = 0.011$). Using the Andersen–Gill multiple-event analysis, it was calculated that zoledronic acid 4 mg reduced the overall risk of skeletal complications by 36%. Zoledronic acid 8 mg appeared less effective but was not significantly different to the 4 mg dose. When the efficacy data from both dosage groups were combined, significant benefit in all analyses of efficacy is maintained (Figure 30.3B). A summary of the efficacy data is shown in Table 30.3.

Zoledronic acid reduced bone pain compared with placebo at all time points, and these differences were significant at 3 and 9 months (Figure 30.5). Significant reductions in markers of bone resorption were

Table 30.2. Prostate cancer zoledronic acid trial—demographics and prognostic factors

Demographic factor	Zoledronic acid 4 mg (n=214)	Zoledronic acid 8/4 mg (n=221)	Placebo (n=208)
Mean age (years)	71.8	71.2	72.2
Race			
Caucasian (%)	83.2	84.2	82.7
Black (%)	11.2	8.3	9.1
Performance status ECOG 0–1 (%)	92.1	91.3	91.3
Mean FACT-G score	81.0	81.4	82.2
No metastases at diagnosis (n)	115	134	116
Metastases at diagnosis (n)	99	87	92
Baseline PSA, median	82	89	61

Adapted from [6].

documented for the zoledronic acid group compared with the placebo group throughout the duration of the study (Figure 30.6). Despite the favourable effects on skeletal morbidity, there were no significant effects on disease-related endpoints, such as time to progression and survival (Figure 30.7). The results of this Phase III trial provided the first objective evidence of efficacy for a bisphosphonate in patients with bone metastases secondary to prostate cancer.

As a class, bisphosphonates are known to affect renal function. Therefore, the renal safety of zoledronic acid was monitored throughout this trial. The risk of renal function deterioration in patients treated with zoledronic acid (4 mg via a 15 min i.v. infusion) was similar to that of placebo-treated patients. The most common adverse events included bone pain, nausea, constipation, fatigue, anaemia, myalgia, vomiting, weakness, anorexia and pyrexia, but the only events that occurred at increased frequency in the zoledronic acid group compared with the placebo-treated group were fatigue, anaemia, myalgia and pyrexia. The majority of these events were manageable with simple supportive care measures and are as expected with any intravenous aminobisphosphonate therapy.

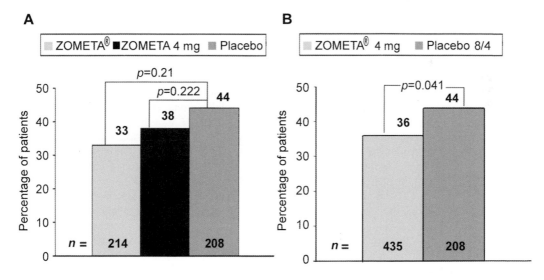

Figure 30.3. Randomised placebo-controlled trial of zoledronic acid (Zometa) in advanced endocrine prostate cancer with bone metastases. Proportion experiencing one or more skeletal-related events (SRE) is shown. Hypercalcaemia is excluded from this analysis of the primary endpoint. Based on data from [6]. Results for all three treatment arms shown in (A) and for the combined zoledronic acid groups vs. placebo in (B)

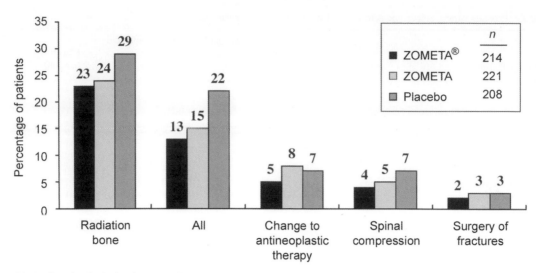

Figure 30.4. Randomised placebo-controlled trial of zoledronic acid (Zometa) in advanced endocrine prostate cancer with bone metastases. Proportion experiencing each of the skeletal-related events (SRE) comprising the primary endpoint are shown. Based on data from [6]

Table 30.3. Efficacy summary following 15 months of zoledronic acid 4 mg or placebo in hormone refractory prostate cancer

	Proportion with SRE (%)	Time to first SRE (hazard ratio)	Mean skeletal morbidity ratio	Multiple event analysis hazard ratio
Zoledronic acid, 4 mg (n=214)	33	0.669	0.80	0.643
p-value	0.021	0.011	0.006	0.004
Placebo	44		1.49	
(n=208)	—		—	

Adapted from Saad et al. [6] and Oncology Drugs Advisory Committee (ODAC) submission [34].

THE NORMAL SKELETON

Hormone deprivation therapy is associated with significant decreases in bone mineral density, even in the absence of detectable metastatic bone lesions, and the resulting osteopenia increases the risk of osteoporotic fractures in this patient population [29,30]. Approximately 5% of patients treated with luteinising hormone-releasing hormone (LHRH) agonists develop osteoporotic fractures [31]. This proportion is likely to increase because of the trend toward the earlier application of LHRH agonist therapy in patients with prostate cancer, which in turn will result in increased long-term exposure and cumulative, chronic skeletal effects.

Recently bisphosphonates have been evaluated in the prevention of bone loss secondary to androgen ablation. Smith et al. randomly assigned 47 men with advanced or recurrent prostate cancer and no bone metastases to receive either the LHRH agonist leuprolide alone, or leuprolide and pamidronate 60 mg every 3 months [32]. Bone mineral density (BMD) at the lumbar spine and hip was assessed by dual absorption X-ray absorptiometry (DEXA). In men treated with leuprolide alone, the mean ($\pm$SE) BMD decreased by $3.3 \pm 0.7\%$ in the spine and $1.8 \pm 0.4\%$ in the total hip. In contrast, the BMD did not change significantly in men treated with leuprolide and pamidronate. After 48 weeks' treatment the BMD was significantly different in each group, both at the lumbar spine ($p \leqslant 0.001$) and in the total hip ($p \leqslant 0.005$), with pamidronate preventing the bone loss associated with androgen ablation.

Subsequently a further study by Smith et al. has evaluated the more potent bisphosphonate zoledronic acid [33]. An intravenous infusion of zoledronic acid

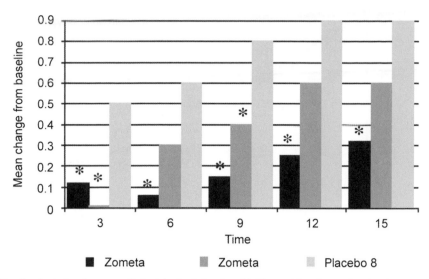

Figure 30.5. Randomised placebo-controlled trial of zoledronic acid (Zometa) in advanced endocrine prostate cancer with bone metastases. Mean change from baseline of the composite pain score by treatment shown. Higher scores indicate more pain. * $p \leqslant 0.05$ vs. placebo. Based on data from [6]

4 mg every 3 months was compared to placebo in a similar population of men with prostate cancer to those in the pamidronate study described above. Again, the men received androgen ablation with an LHRH agonist ± an antiandrogen. Zoledronic acid appeared on indirect comparison to be superior to pamidronate in that it not only prevented bone loss but also resulted in a significant gain in BMD. In the androgen ablation plus placebo patients, a 2% loss of BMD was seen at the lumbar spine. In contrast, the addition of

zoledronic acid resulted in a 5.3% increase in BMD in the lumbar spine ($p < 0.001$). A numerically smaller, but nevertheless an advantage of similar statistical significance for zoledronic acid compared with placebo was also seen in BMD changes at the hip [33].

It remains to be determined whether earlier application of bisphosphonate therapy in patients with prostate cancer would serve to further reduce skeletal morbidity. The use of zoledronic acid during hormone therapy could preserve skeletal integrity so

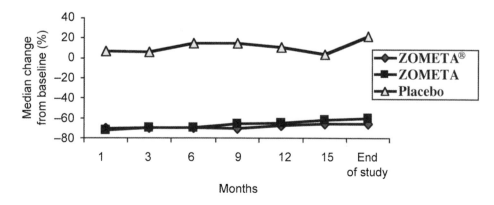

Figure 30.6. Randomised placebo-controlled trial of zoledronic acid (Zometa) in advanced endocrine prostate cancer with bone metastases. Percentage change in the bone resorption marker N-telopeptide (NTX) from baseline. Marked highly significant ($p \leqslant 0.001$) suppression with both 4 mg and 8/4 mg zoledronic acid. Based on data from [6]

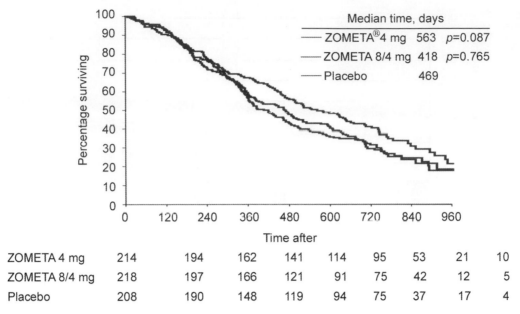

ZOMETA 4 mg	214	194	162	141	114	95	53	21	10
ZOMETA 8/4 mg	218	197	166	121	91	75	42	12	5
Placebo	208	190	148	119	94	75	37	17	4

Figure 30.7. Randomised placebo-controlled trial of zoledronic acid (Zometa) in advanced endocrine prostate cancer with bone metastases. Survival of patients on study by treatment group shown. From Saad F et al. [6] Zoledronic acid reduces skeletal complications in patients with hormone-refractory prostate carcinoma metastatic to bone: a randomized, placebo-controlled trial. J Natl Cancer Inst 2002; 94: 1458–68

that BMD would be higher before the development of bone metastases. Studies are also currently under way to determine whether the earlier application of bisphosphonate therapy can prevent the development of bone metastases.

CONCLUSIONS

It is now clear that bone resorption is also a key mechanism underlying metastatic bone disease in prostate cancer. Bisphosphonates are therefore a rational therapy to prevent skeletal morbidity. In addition to the pain relief seen with a variety of intravenous bisphosphonates, a recent large randomised trial of zoledronic acid has shown that this potent agent is able to significantly reduce the skeletal morbidity of metastatic bone disease in endocrine-resistant prostate cancer. For men earlier in the course of their disease, the bone loss associated with androgen ablation can be pevented and indeed reversed with a simple occasional intravenous bisphosphonate infusion. Further clinical trials are necessary to fully explore the optimal role of bisphosphonate therapy in patients with prostate cancer, including for the prevention of bone metastases, as well as refining their use in advanced disease.

REFERENCES

1. Jemal A, Thomas A, Murray T et al. Cancer statistics, 2002. CA Cancer J Clin 2002; 52: 23–47.
2. Koeneman KS, Yeung F, Chung LW. Osteomimetic properties of prostate cancer cells: a hypothesis supporting the predilection of prostate cancer metastasis and growth in the bone environment. Prostate 1999; 39: 246–61.
3. Carlin BI, Andriole GL. The natural history, skeletal complications, and management of bone metastases in patients with prostate carcinoma. Cancer 2000; 88: 2989–94.
4. DaniellHW. Osteoporosis after orchiectomy for prostate cancer. J Urol 1997; 157: 439–44.
5. Coleman RE. Skeletal complications of malignancy. Cancer 1997; 80(suppl): 1588–94.
6. Saad F, Gleason DM, Murray R et al. Zoledronic acid reduces skeletal complications in patients with hormone-refractory prostate carcinoma metastatic to bone: a randomized, placebo-controlled trial. J Natl Cancer Inst 2002; 94: 1458–68.
7. PoorG, Atkinson EJ, Lewallen DG et al. Age-related hip fractures in men: clinical spectrum and short-term outcomes. Osteoporosis Int 1995; 5: 419–26.
8. Urwin GH, Percival RC, Harris S et al. Generalised increase in bone resorption in carcinoma of the prostate. Br J Urol 1985; 57: 721–3.
9. Clarke NW, McClure J, George NJR. Morphometric evidence for bone resorption and replacement in prostate cancer. Br J Urol 1991; 68: 74–80.
10. Berruti A, Dogliotti L, Bitossi R et al. Incidence of skeletal complications in patients with bone metastatic

prostate cancer and hormone-refractory disease: predictive role of bone resorption and formation markers evaluated at baseline. J Urol 2000; 164: 1248–53.

11. Lipton A, Costa L, Ali S et al. Use of bone turnover for monitoring bone metastases and the response to therapy. Semin Oncol 2001; 4(suppl 11): 54–9.

12. Garnero P, Buchs N, Zekri J et al. Markers of bone turnover for the management of patients with bone metastases from prostate cancer. Br J Cancer 2000; 82: 858–64.

13. Adami S, Salvagno G, Guarrera G et al. Dichloromethylene-diphosphonate in patients with prostatic carcinoma metastatic to the skeleton. J Urol 1985; 134: 1152–4.

14. Adami S, Mian M. Clodronate therapy of metastatic bone disease in patients with prostatic carcinoma. Recent Results Cancer Res 1989; 116: 67–72.

15. Vorreuther R. Bisphosphonates as an adjunct to palliative therapy of bone metastases from prostatic carcinoma. A pilot study on clodronate. Br J Urol 1993; 72: 792–5.

16. Cresswell SM, English PJ, Hall RR et al. Pain relief and quality-of-life assessment following intravenous and oral clodronate in hormone-escaped metastatic prostate cancer. Br J Urol 1995; 76: 360–5.

17. Papapoulos SE, Hamdy NA, van der Pluijm G. Bisphosphonates in the management of prostate carcinoma metastatic to the skeleton. Cancer 2000; 88(suppl): 3047–53.

18. Coleman RE, Purohit OP, Black C et al. Double-blind, randomised, placebo-controlled, dose-finding study of oral ibandronate in patients with metastatic bone disease. Ann Oncol 1999; 10: 311–16.

19. Pelger RC, Hamdy NA, Zwinderman AH et al. Effects of the bisphosphonate olpadronate in patients with carcinoma of the prostate metastatic to the skeleton. Bone 1998; 22: 403–8.

20. Kylmala T, Tammela TL, Lindholm TS et al. The effect of combined intravenous and oral clodronate treatment on bone pain in patients with metastatic prostate cancer. Ann Chir Gynaecol 1994; 83: 316–19.

21. Elomaa I, Kylmala T, Tammela T et al. Effect of oral clodronate on bone pain. A controlled study in patients with metastatic prostate cancer. Int Urol Nephrol 1992; 24: 159–66.

22. Kylmala T, Taube T, Tammela TL et al. Concomitant i.v. and oral clodronate in the relief of bone pain—a double-blind placebo-controlled study in patients with prostate cancer. Br J Cancer 1997; 76: 939–42.

23. Strang P, Nilsson S, Brandstedt S et al. The analgesic efficacy of clodronate compared with placebo in patients with painful bone metastases from prostatic cancer. Anticancer Res 1997; 17: 4717–21.

24. Smith JA Jr. Palliation of painful bone metastases from prostate cancer using sodium etidronate: results of a randomized, prospective, double-blind, placebo-controlled study. J Urol 1989; 141: 85–7.

25. Ernst DS, Tannock IF, Venner PM et al. Randomized placebo-controlled trial of mitoxantrone/prednisone and clodronate vs. mitoxantrone/prednisone alone in patients with hormone-refractory prostate cancer (HRPC) and pain: National Cancer Institute of Canada Clinical Trials Group study. Proc Am Soc Clin Oncol 2002; 21(abstr 705): 177a.

26. Dearnaley DP, Sydes MR on behalf of the MRC PR05 collaborators. Preliminary evidence that oral clodronate delays symptomatic progression of bone metastases from prostate cancer: first results of the MRC PR05 trial. Proc Am Soc Clin Oncol 2001; 20(abs 693): 174a.

27. Lipton A, Small E, Saad F et al. The new bisphosphonate, Zometa (zoledronic acid), decreases skeletal complications in both osteolytic and osteoblastic lesions: a comparison to pamidronate. Cancer Invest 2002; 20 (suppl 2): 45–54.

28. Andersen PK, Gill RD. Cox's regression model for counting processes: a large sample study. Ann Statist 1982; 10: 1100–20.

29. Diamond T, Campbell J, Bryant C et al. The effect of combined androgen blockade on bone turnover and bone mineral densities in men treated for prostate carcinoma: longitudinal evaluation and response to intermittent cyclic etidronate therapy. Cancer 1998; 83: 1561–6.

30. Townsend MF, Sanders WH, Northway RO et al. Bone fractures associated with luteinizing hormone-releasing hormone agonists used in the treatment of prostate carcinoma. Cancer 1997; 79: 545–50.

31. Berruti A, Dogliotti L, Terrone C et al. Changes in bone mineral density, lean body mass and fat content as measured by dual energy X-ray absorptiometry in patients with prostate cancer without apparent bone metastases given androgen deprivation therapy. J Urol 2002; 167: 2361–7; discussion, 2367.

32. Smith MR, McGovern FJ, Zietman AL et al. Pamidronate to prevent bone loss during androgen deprivation therapy for prostate cancer. N Engl J Med 2001; 345: 948–55.

33. Smith MR, Shasha D, Mansour R et al. Zometa increases bone mineral density in men undergoing androgen deprivation therapy for prostate cancer. Presented at: 3rd North American Symposium: Skeletal Complications of Malignancy; Bethesda, MD, 2002. In Prostate carcinoma. Cancer 1997; 80: 1674–9.

34. Novartis submission document to Oncology Drugs Advisory Committee, February 2002.

31

Prevention of Bone Metastases

R. E. Coleman and H. L. Neville-Webbe

Academic Unit of Clinical Oncology, Sheffield, UK

INTRODUCTION

Although most patients present with a cancer that appears to be localised to the primary site, a large proportion will eventually develop metastases and die from advanced widespread disease. Micrometastatic disease represents perhaps the most important remaining challenge in breast cancer management. Adjuvant systemic therapy is now considered an integral component of the management of the vast majority of women with primary breast cancer [1] and is becoming increasingly important in the management of high-risk (Gleason grade > 6) localised prostate cancer [2], as well as a number of other solid tumours. Nevertheless, a review of the many adjuvant therapy trials for breast cancer conducted by the International Breast Cancer Study Group (IBCSG) indicated that most of the benefit of adjuvant chemotherapy and hormone therapy used in these trials was in the reduction of local, regional and distant soft tissue metastases. There had been relatively little effect on first recurrences at bone and visceral sites [3].

Bone metastases are the most common site of first metastasis from both breast and prostate cancers, and ante mortem clinical evidence of skeletal metastases is found in 70–80% of patients with these two common tumours. It has been recognised for more than 100 years that the bone microenvironment possesses special characteristics which make it a favourable site for metastasis from a number of common malignancies. The "seed and soil" hypothesis proposed by Paget suggested that the frequency of bone metastasis from breast cancer (and prostate) could not be explained by mechanical theories of embolism alone [4]. The vertebral venous plexus described by Batson links the venous drainage of many sites with the bone marrow spaces [5], and flow through this system is slow, allowing the preferential lodging of cells within the bone marrow microenvironment of the axial skeleton. Once within this environment there is a rich mixture of growth factors and cytokines, many of them derived from bone. These include insulin-like growth factor 2, (IGF2), transforming growth factor-β (TGFβ), and interleukin 6 (IL-6), among others, that can potentially facilitate and stimulate tumour cell proliferation, angiogenesis and the establishment of a metastatic focus [6].

This concept of a "vicious cycle" between bone and tumour cells makes testing of specific bone treatments a biologically rational strategy. Bisphosphonates are the most potent currently available class of pharmacological agents for the treatment of bone diseases characterised by accelerated osteoclast activity. As a result, the bisphosphonates are under evaluation for their potential benefit in preventing the development of bone metastases in the hope that this will not only preserve skeletal health but also improve survival.

All bisphosphonates are characterised by a P–C–P-containing central structure, which promotes their binding to the mineralised bone matrix, and a variable R' chain which determines the relative potency, side-effects and probably also the precise mechanism of action. Following administration, bisphosphonates bind avidly to exposed bone mineral around resorbing osteoclasts, leading to very high local concentrations

Textbook of Bone Metastases. Edited by C. Jasmin, R. E. Coleman, L. R. Coia, R. Capanna and G. Saillant
© 2005 John Wiley & Sons Ltd: ISBN 0 471 87742 5

of bisphosphonate in the resorption lacunae (up to 1000 µM). On release from the bone surface, bisphosphonates are internalised by the osteoclast, where they cause disruption of the biochemical processes involved in bone resorption [7].

Bisphosphonates also cause osteoclast apoptosis, with the appearance of distinctive changes in cell and nuclear morphology. Although the molecular targets responsible for promoting this apoptosis are unknown, the bisphosphonates have recently been shown to exert their effects via one of two molecular pathways. Bisphosphonates containing nitrogen, such as pamidronate, residronate and zoledronic acid, inhibit enzymes of the mevalonate pathway that are ultimately responsible for events that lead to the post-translational modification of GTP-binding proteins such as Ras [8]. Bisphosphonates that do not contain nitrogen, including clodronate and etidronate, exert their effects through incorporation into ATP containing non-hydrolysable analogues [9].

Bisphosphonates may have a beneficial effect on the development of bone metastases simply through their effects on osteoclast activation alone, depriving the tumour cells in the microenvironment of the stimulatory cytokines and growth factors mentioned above. However, there is increasing *in vitro* and animal evidence that bisphosphonates have direct anticancer activity, and the modern potent bisphosphonates may

have both indirect and direct effects on tumour cells in the bone microenvironment (Figure 31.1). Whether the concentrations that are required for these effects can realistically be achieved with the current pharmacological use of bisphosphonates remains to be established. There is increasing evidence that potent bisphosphonates can inhibit tumour cell adhesion and invasion [10], promote tumour cell apoptosis [11] and inhibit angiogenesis [12]. Studies of the breast cancer cell line MCF-7 have also suggested synergy between zoledronic acid and paclitaxel in the effects on both inhibition of cell proliferation and the promotion of apoptosis (Figure 31.2) [13]. These effects were also mediated via the mevalonate pathway. In add-back experiments, zoledronic acid-induced apoptosis was abolished by the addition of distal geranylgeranyl metabolites of this pathway (Figure 31.3). In addition, there are experimental data that indicate that zoledronic acid can suppress angiogenesis in a tissue chamber model implanted in the soft tissues, effects that appear to be independent of the effects of this agent on bone [12].

As a result of these experiments, the hypothesis has been proposed that potent bisphosphonates may have beneficial effects on the bone microenvironment. They may not only inhibit tumour cell proliferation by depriving them of bone-derived growth factors and cytokines, but possibly also directly exert anticancer effects on tumour cells exposed to the micromolar

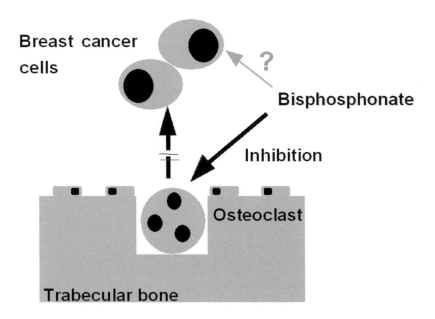

Figure 31.1. Rationale for adjuvant bisphosphonates, Bisphosphonates inhibit osteoclast function and the release of bone-derived growth factors and may have direct effects on cancer cells in the bone marrow microenvironment

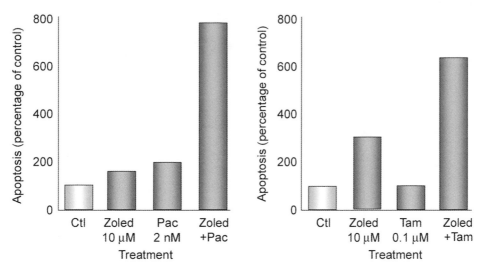

Figure 31.2.   Effect of combined treatment of MCF-7 cells with 10 μM zoledronic acid (Zoled) and 2 nM paclitaxel (Pac) or 0.1-μM tamoxifen (Tam). Cells were incubated with 10 μM zoledronic acid in the presence or absence of paclitaxel or tamoxifen for a total of 72 h. Apoptosis was assessed using the *in situ* nick translation assay. Results are expressed as percentage of control. Adapted from [13,58]

concentrations of bisphosphonate that exist around resorption cavities.

ANIMAL EXPERIMENTS INVESTIGATING ADJUVANT POTENTIAL OF BISPHOSPHONATES

There are a range of encouraging animal studies, with a variety of animal tumour models, that suggest that bisphosphonates are not only a treatment for skeletal complications but also act as a "protectant" against the development of metastases in bone [14]. Bisphosphonates have been shown to reduce skeletal tumour burden in murine tumour models and human tumour xenograft models in rats and nude mice [15–22]. Animal models generally show, as expected, that bisphosphonates inhibit tumour-induced osteolysis and preserve bone mass in animals with established bone metastases. More important, however, is the evidence that these effects are accompanied by a corresponding reduction in skeletal tumour burden compared with control animals.

In two animal models of breast cancer, zoledronic acid inhibited progression of established bone metastases, reduced tumour burden, and prevented development of new bone metastases [18,19]. In mice injected with MDA-MB-231 breast cancer cells, daily subcutaneous zoledronic acid (0.2, 1.0 or 5.0 μg/day × 10 days), administered after bone metastases were

established, reduced the bone lesion area by > 80% compared with control animals [19]. Likewise, in a murine mammary tumour model, zoledronic acid decreased the formation of new bone metastases after injection of 4T1 cells [19].

The majority of animal models suggest that bisphosphonates primarily exert antitumour effects within the bone, which is consistent with the pharmacology of bisphosphonates. However, preliminary data from a 4T1 mouse mammary tumour model have also shown an inhibitory effect of zoledronic acid (0.5 or 5.0 μg every 4 days) on bone and visceral (liver and lung) metastases [20]. Similar results were reported in a study in which mammary carcinoma cells were injected directly into the proximal tibia of rats [21]. The study showed that treatment with alendronate (8 μg/kg) reduced lung nodules by 95%. Moreover, in a 5T2 murine myeloma model, mice treated with subcutaneous zoledronic acid (120 μg/kg twice weekly) had significantly fewer osteolytic lesions and prolonged disease-free survival compared with controls [22]. These findings are certainly provocative and raise the possibility that bisphosphonates could have more systemic antitumour effects and improve survival, but based on their pharmacology, one would expect that bisphosphonates would have the greatest effect in bone.

Several potential mechanisms have been hypothesised to explain these *in vivo* antitumour effects of

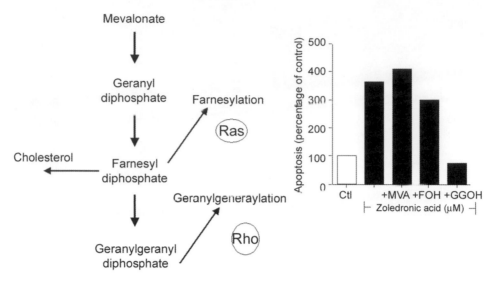

Figure 31.3. Effects of intermediates of the mevalonate pathway (left) on zoledronic acid-induced apoptosis of MCF-7 cells (right). Mevalonate (MVA) and farnesol (FOH) have little effect on zoledronic acid-induced apoptosis, whereas 50 μM geranylgeraniol (GGOH) rescues MCF-7 cells from apoptosis induced by zoledronic acid. Results are expressed as percentage of control. Adapted from [13]

bisphosphonates. Inhibition of osteoclastogenesis and tumour-induced osteolysis may make the bone a less favourable environment for tumour cells to grow in. In addition, bisphosphonates may inhibit the ability of tumour cells to invade the bone; they also have angiostatic effects, which could prevent the formation of viable tumours. Ultimately, bisphosphonates may directly cause apoptosis of tumour cells.

As early as 1996, Sterns and Wang [23] showed that the combination of paclitaxel with alendronate significantly enhanced the antitumour efficacy of paclitaxel. Human PC-3 ML subclones were injected into SCID mice. Pre-treatment of these mice with alendronate (0.04–0.1 mg/kg twice weekly or 0.1 mg/kg weekly) reduced the formation of bone metastases, but metastatic tumour grew in extra-osseous sites. However, alendronate pre-treatment (0.1 mg/kg once or twice weekly) in addition to paclitaxel (10–50 mg/kg/day once or twice weekly) not only prevented the formation of bone metastases, but also prevented the formation of non-osseous metastases, with a corresponding increase in survival rate for dual-treated mice.

When murine models metastases were treated with ibandronate and the anthracycline doxorubicin, using the heart injection model, bone and non-osseous (adrenal) metastases were more effectively suppressed by the combination than with either agent alone [24]. In an orthotopic murine model (4T1 mammary tumour cells inoculated into mammary fat pad subcutaneously), incadronate or zoledronate co-treatment with UFT (a pro-drug of fluorouracil) inhibited the formation of bone, lung and liver metastases in an additive fashion. UFT alone significantly, but only slightly, decreased the metastatic load.

Nude mice inoculated with the human breast cancer cell line MDA-231 and treated with ibandronate and the tissue inhibitor of MMP-2 (TIMP-2) did not develop osteolytic bone lesions. Mice receiving bisphosphonate (BP) alone or TIMP-2 alone developed osteolytic bone lesions, which in turn were markedly fewer than the number of lesions in control mice. Furthermore, survival was increased in mice receiving TIMP-2 alone or both BP and TIMP-2 [25]. Development of specific MMP inhibitors in the clinical setting has been beset with problems of toxicity and safety, whereas the safety and tolerability of bisphosphonates are well recognised. If the inhibition of MMPs occurs at concentrations that are achievable at the bone surface, bisphosphonates may well have a "lead" in being developed as specific MMP-inhibitors.

The data from all these animal models suggest that bisphosphonates have the potential to inhibit tumour cell growth and metastasis to bone in the clinical setting at concentrations that may be achievable in the bone at sites of active bone metabolism. For the most part, these studies used frequent subcutaneous dosing. One could argue that frequent dosing may result in more uniform incorporation of bisphosphonates into bone and optimise inhibition of tumour cell growth and metastasis. However, further clinical investigation is necessary to realise the extent of the antitumour potential of bisphosphonates *in vivo*.

CLINICAL EVIDENCE OF THE ANTITUMOUR POTENTIAL OF BISPHOSPHONATES

Bisphosphonates have demonstrated some degree of antitumour activity in a number of clinical settings. In the classic adjuvant setting, there is some evidence to suggest that oral clodronate may reduce the occurrence of bone metastases in patients with no distant metastases at study entry. Several studies have also investigated the antitumour activity of oral bisphosphonates in patients with a recurrence in extraskeletal sites but no bone metastases. Finally, studies in patients with established bone metastases suggest a reduction in tumour burden or improved survival associated with bisphosphonate therapy.

Adjuvant Studies

Two adjuvant trials have suggested that daily oral clodronate (1600 mg/day) may decrease the incidence of bone metastases and may provide a survival benefit [26,27], and one has shown an adverse outcome with clodronate [28]. In the first study, Diel et al. studied 302 breast cancer patients randomly allocated to either oral clodronate 1600 mg daily ($n=157$) for 3 years or a control group ($n=145$). These women had no overt evidence of metastatic disease, but were selected for the trial on the basis of immunocytochemical detection of tumour cells in the bone marrow, a known risk factor for the subsequent development of distant metastases [26]. Patients received appropriate adjuvant chemotherapy and endocrine treatment. There were no discernable prognostic or treatment imbalances between the two groups and the follow-up schedules were similar. The median observation period was 36 months. The incidence of osseous metastases was significantly lower in the clodronate group [11 (7%) vs. 25 (17%) patients; $p < 0.002$]. There was also an unexpected large reduction in the incidence of visceral metastases in the clodronate group [19 (13%) vs. 42 (29%) patients, $p < 0.001$]. These results have subsequently been updated [29] (Table 31.1) and show similar results, although the striking effect on extraskeletal visceral relapse seen in the earlier report is less and no longer statistically significant.

The exciting findings of the Diel study must, however, be viewed in the light of a further trial which suggested quite the reverse. Saarto et al. [28] randomised 299 women with primary node-positive breast cancer to oral clodronate 1600 mg daily ($n=149$) or a control group ($n=150$). The median follow-up was 5 years. Treatment with clodronate in this study did not lead to a reduction in the development of bone metastases [29 (19%) vs. 24 (16%) patients; $p=0.27$ for the clodronate and control groups, respectively]. Additionally in this study, the development of non-skeletal recurrence was significantly higher in the clodronate group [60 (40%) vs. 36 (24%) patients; $p=0.0007$] and, most importantly, the overall 5 year survival was significantly lower in the clodronate group (70% vs. 83%; $p=0.009$]. It is possible that there were some prognostic imbalances favouring the control group, but the safest assumption is to consider that the Diel and Saarto studies cancel each other out and probably reflect the usual heterogeneity of results seen in relatively small adjuvant studies.

Perhaps most helpful in defining the potential of adjuvant bisphosphonates are the recent results from a much larger multicentre study. 1600 mg/day oral clodronate was compared with placebo in 1069 patients with stages T_1–T_4 breast cancer [27]. Patients received treatment for 2 years and were followed for > 5 years (median follow-up, 5.5 years). Study endpoints included relapse in bone, relapse at other sites, and survival. When first reported in 1998 [30], the preliminary data showed a trend toward a reduction in the proportion of patients with bone metastases in the clodronate group (5% vs. 8% of control patients; $p=0.054$).

Powles et al. recently published the mature data from this trial [27]. These showed that during the treatment period (i.e. first 2 years) there was a significant reduction in the occurrence of bone metastases in the clodronate group (2.3% vs. 5.2% of control patients; hazard ratio, 0.44; $p=0.016$), but no survival benefit. With longer follow-up, however, the reduction in the incidence of bone metastases failed to reach statistical significance; 63 (11.9%) patients in the clodronate group vs. 80 (14.8%) patients in the placebo group developed a bone metastasis ($p=0.127$). Moreover, the incidence of extraskeletal metastases was similar for the two groups. However, in the final analysis, clodronate demonstrated a marginally significant improvement in survival (98 deaths in the clodronate group vs. 129 in the placebo group; $p=0.047$). This study, as well as the updated results of the Diel study, suggest that adjuvant clodronate may prevent bone metastases in breast cancer patients

Table 31.1.   Results of adjuvant trials with clodronate for early breast cancer

	Clodronate n (%)	Placebo n (%)	Significance
Powles et al. [27] (n=1079)			
Bone	63 (12%)	80 (15%)	p=0.127
Non-bone	112 (21%)	128 (24%)	p=0.26
Deaths	Not stated	Not stated	p=0.047
Diel et al. [29] (n=302)			
Bone	20 (14%)	34 (24%)	p=0.044
Non-bone	24 (16%)	37 (26%)	p=0.091
Deaths	13 (10%)	32 (22%)	p=0.002
Saarto et al. [28] (n=299)			
Bone	29 (21%)	24 (17%)	p=0.27
Non-bone	60 (43%)	36 (25%)	p=0.0009
Deaths	42 (30%)	24 (17%)	p=0.01

at risk, but perhaps only as long as treatment is continued. Therefore, in future trial designs, it may be necessary to continue bisphosphonate therapy indefinitely. These data also provide evidence of a potential survival benefit.

Treatment with Bisphosphonate at Recurrence (Secondary Adjuvant Trials)

Several small studies with oral clodronate or oral pamidronate have been conducted in patients who had a local or distant relapse at extraskeletal sites but did not have bone metastases at study entry. The first of these was a randomised double-blind study involving 133 breast cancer patients who received 1600 mg/day clodronate or placebo for 3 years [31]. This study demonstrated a significant reduction in the total number of bone metastases in the clodronate group (32 vs. 63; $p < 0.005$); however, the number of patients with bone metastases was not significantly reduced (15 vs. 19 patients). There was also no effect on survival. Two similar studies of oral pamidronate (150–300 mg/day) failed to show any effect on the appearance of bone metastases in breast cancer patients treated at recurrence [32,33]. This outcome may have been a result of the poor bioavailability of oral pamidronate or the fact that this patient population may not be ideal for testing the potential of bisphosphonates to prevent bone metastases.

Studies in Patients with Bone Lesions

In addition to the studies specifically designed to determine whether bisphosphonates can prevent bone metastasis, data from several studies in patients with established bone lesions provide additional support for the idea that bisphosphonates may have antitumour potential in the clinical setting (Table 31.2) [34–37]. For example, evidence of a survival benefit was reported in the long-term follow-up of a randomised, double-blind, placebo-controlled trial of oral clodronate (1600 mg/day) in conjunction with standard chemotherapy in patients with multiple myeloma [34]. Although no survival advantage was reported for the overall patient population, in patients who did not have a vertebral fracture at presentation (n=80), the median survival was extended to 59 months for the clodronate group (n=73) compared with 37 months for the placebo group.

Studies with i.v. pamidronate also provide some evidence of antitumour effects in patients with established bone metastases, based on observed bone lesion responses or a survival benefit in subsets of patients (Table 31.2) [35–37]. In the long-term follow-up of a randomised, placebo-controlled trial of pamidronate (90 mg) for the treatment of advanced multiple myeloma, subset analysis revealed a trend toward a survival advantage in a stratified subgroup of patients who were receiving second-line chemotherapy or greater [35]. Patients in the pamidronate group had a median survival of 21 months vs. 14 months for placebo (p=0.081). Adjusting for imbalances in prognostic variables between the groups actually improved the statistical significance of this survival comparison (p=0.041).

Likewise, in a pooled analysis of two randomised, placebo-controlled trials of 90 mg pamidronate in patients with breast cancer and bone metastases, a retrospective subset analysis suggested a possible survival benefit in women $\leqslant$ 50 years of age [36],

Table 31.2. Trials of bisphosphonates in patients with established bone metastases

Study	Tumour type	Bisphosphonate	Outcome
McCloskey et al. [34]	Multiple myeloma	Oral clodronate 1600 mg/day	Survival advantage in patients without a vertebral fracture at presentation
Berenson et al. [35]	Multiple myeloma	Pamidronate (90 mg every 4 weeks)	Survival advantage in stratum receiving second-line or greater chemotherapy
Lipton et al. [36]	Breast cancer	Pamidronate (90 mg every 3–4 weeks)	Survival advantage in patients $\leqslant$ 50 years of age
Hortobagyi et al. [37]	Breast cancer	Pamidronate (90 mg every 3–4 weeks)	Improved bone lesion response

although this was not a prospectively defined subgroup or stratification group. The median survival in the pamidronate group was 24.6 months compared with 15.7 months in the placebo group ($p=0.009$). Finally, in the 2 year follow-up of one of these pamidronate trials enrolling patients being treated with chemotherapy, significant treatment effects were reported for radiological bone lesion response [37]. A complete or partial response in bone was achieved by 34% of patients in the pamidronate group vs. 19% in the placebo group ($p=0.002$).

Interpreted together, the clinical data imply that bisphosphonates may prevent bone metastases in the adjuvant setting, may reduce tumour burden in bone, and may improve survival. Some clinical studies suggest that bisphosphonate therapy may alter the natural history of bone metastases in certain patient subsets, and bone lesion responses have been reported for patients with established metastases. However, further clinical trials of bisphosphonates are needed to confirm these results. Finally, given that zoledronic acid has demonstrated superior efficacy in the treatment of bone metastases, this highly potent new bisphosphonate may be useful in the adjuvant setting where other bisphosphonates have failed to yield reproducible clinical benefit.

Adjuvant Studies in Prostate Cancer

There are no published data on the role of bisphosphonates in prostate cancer for preventing metastases. Their role in preventing and treating androgen-induced bone loss has been demonstrated (see below), but the results of true adjuvant studies are awaited. The Medical Research Council (MRC) Prostate Group in the UK has completed accrual into a study of oral clodronate in prostate cancer patients at high risk of bone involvement. Results from a first analysis should be available in 2005.

A Phase III trial is examining zoledronic acid in the adjuvant setting for men with prostate cancer. The study will enrol approximately 500 men with rising levels of prostate-specific antigen and no radiological evidence of bone metastasis. Men will receive standard anticancer therapy and zoledronic acid or placebo. The dosage and schedule of zoledronic acid will be 4 mg via a 15 min infusion every 4 weeks. Men will be followed for disease-free, bone metastasis-free and overall survival endpoints.

DESIGN OF BISPHOSPHONATE TRIALS FOR THE PREVENTION OF BONE METASTASES

Identifying a definite adjuvant role for bisphosphonates will require further large randomised studies. There are many unknowns that make designing adjuvant bisphosphonate trials somewhat speculative. As with all adjuvant treatments, it is likely that any benefit of bisphosphonates will be small, even if clinically important. Relative risk reductions of around 20% are clinically worthwhile but require trials of 2000–3000 patients and sufficient follow-up for the required number of events to occur.

Which patients should be selected for these trials? Ideally, a specific prognostic factor able to predict recurrence in bone is required. However, none of the available prognostic markers are sufficiently specific. As a result, selection of patients is typically based on nodal status, although some centres have proposed the use of bone marrow immunohistochemistry to identify tumour cells in the bone marrow microenvironment. Most studies suggest that patients with positive immunocytochemistry have a higher relapse rate [38].

Having identified an appropriate population to study, what is the dose, route of administration and schedule of bisphosphonate to test (Table 31.3)? The evidence to date suggests that long-term treatment, perhaps for up to 5 years, is required for sustained

Table 31.3. Adjuvant bisphosphonate study design considerations

---

Long-term treatment probably necessary
Patient selection—node/marrow-positive
Choice of endpoint—disease-free or bone metastasis free
    survival?
"Osteoporosis" dose or "antitumour" dose?
Oral or intravenous therapy?
Class effect or drug-specific?
Large trials starting with clodronate (NSABP) and zoledronic
    acid (Novartis) (2000–3000 patients each)

---

benefit. Will potent agents, e.g. zoledronic acid, have a greater chance of success, perhaps exploiting the *in vitro* antitumour effects described earlier? Alternatively, is a weak bisphosphonate, such as clodronate, able to suppress bone resorption sufficiently and deprive the tumour cells in the microenvironment of the growth factors and cytokines necessary for tumour cell survival and proliferation?

The National Surgical Adjuvant Breast Project (NSABP) have started a 3000 patient placebo-controlled trial of oral clodronate in an attempt to resolve the value or otherwise of adjuvant clodronate. Recruitment was completed in 2003 with first results anticipated 2–3 years later. Trials are also about to start with the highly potent intravenous bisphosphonate zoledronic acid. In one study (Protocol 702), axillary lymph node positive patients will receive zoledronic acid 4 mg or placebo by i.v. infusion over 15 min every 3–4 weeks for 6 months (alongside chemotherapy where appropriate). Thereafter, zoledronic acid or placebo will be administered every 3 months for 5 years. In the second study, a broader range of stage I, II and III patients will be randomised to receive either standard adjuvant therapy plus monthly zoledronic acid for 3 years or standard adjuvant therapy and no further treatment.

PRESERVING NORMAL SKELETAL HEALTH

There are now increasing numbers of long-term survivors who have received combination chemotherapy, radiotherapy and hormonal cancer treatment. Many of these individuals are at increased risk of osteoporosis, largely because of the endocrine changes induced by treatment. However, there may also be clinically relevant, direct effects of cytotoxic drugs on bone. This is a particularly important long-term problem in women with breast cancer, for whom there are concerns about the safety of hormone replacement therapy.

Bone Loss in Women

Osteoporosis is surprisingly frequent in breast cancer patients. The occurrence of vertebral collapse with fracture is a common clinical marker of osteoporosis, and in one study [39], the annual incidence of vertebral fracture was nearly five times higher among women with breast cancer in the years after diagnosis compared with controls. Of note, 79% of the women in this study received tamoxifen and most received chemotherapy as well. Women with soft tissue relapse of their breast cancer but without known skeletal metastases had an even higher annual incidence of vertebral fracture. As the prevalence of breast cancer increases and women survive longer after treatment for breast cancer, osteoporosis is likely to become an even more important clinical problem.

Adjuvant chemotherapy commonly induces ovarian failure in premenopausal women with breast cancer. Valagussa et al. [40] found that after six cycles of cyclophosphamide, methotrexate and fluorouracil, 71% of women became amenorrhoeic compared with 16% of age-matched women with breast cancer who did not receive adjuvant chemotherapy. Women who undergo a menopause following chemotherapy have a 14% ($p \leqslant 0.05$) lower mean lumbar bone mineral density (BMD) compared with those who maintain menses [41,42]. As the indications for adjuvant chemotherapy are now extended to subgroups of patients with node-negative breast cancer, more women will be at increased risk of osteoporosis.

The effects of tamoxifen on bone are dependent on the menopausal status of the woman. In postmenopausal women, treatment with tamoxifen can increase BMD slightly [43], but tamoxifen has no effect on fracture rates and may actually increase the risk of fracture at certain sites [44]. Paradoxically, tamoxifen decreases BMD in premenopausal women [45]. In addition, tamoxifen fails to prevent the fall in BMD that occurs in women with breast cancer who become menopausal after chemotherapy [46]. Thus, tamoxifen contributes little benefit to bone and may be deleterious in some patients.

Bone Loss in Men

In men, BMD also decreases with increasing age. An increased risk of fracture (the fracture "threshold") is reached in women at approximately 65 years of age, and in men approximately 10 years later. Approximately 30% of all hip fractures in people older than 65 years occur in men, and their mortality rates from hip fracture are even higher than in women. In men, adequate oestrogen levels are also critical for bone health [47]. Oestradiol levels decrease by slightly $< 1\%$ per year and, importantly, this decrease in oestradiol has been correlated with a decrease in BMD [48]. The role of testosterone in bone health is less clear. Bioavailable testosterone levels decrease by approximately 1% per year as men age. Thus, osteoporosis is an important age-related disease in elderly men—those also at greatest risk for prostate cancer.

Orchiectomy is much less commonly performed than in previous years, but its hormonal effects are very similar to those of luteinising hormone-releasing hormone agonists (LHRH-a). Both result in a marked decrease in serum testosterone levels. Approximately one-third of men with prostate cancer receive LHRH-a as part of a neoadjuvant therapy regimen. An additional one-third receive LHRH-a if primary therapy with radiation or prostatectomy fails. Patients treated with LHRH-a or orchiectomy are at increased risk for fracture. Osteoporotic fractures are much more common in men with non-stage A prostate cancer treated with orchiectomy than in men not treated with orchiectomy (13.6% vs. 1.1%; $p < 0.001$) [49]. Approximately 6–9% of men sustain a fracture during treatment with LHRH-a [50,51] and most of these fractures are related to osteoporosis.

Not surprisingly, there is dramatic bone loss in men with prostate cancer who are androgen-depleted. Treatment with LHRH-a or orchiectomy results in a decrease in BMD. After just 6 months of treatment, men treated with an LHRH-a and an androgen antagonist experience a mean BMD loss of 6.5–7.5% at various sites [52]. Two years after orchiectomy, a mean 17% loss in BMD has been observed [53].

Bisphosphonates are probably the treatment of choice to prevent bone loss and treat osteoporosis in cancer patients. In a study by Delmas et al. [46], risedronate was administered on a cyclical basis (30 mg/day for 2 weeks, then 10 weeks off) for 2 years to women with breast cancer who had a menopause induced by chemotherapy. BMDs at the lumbar spine or hip were preserved in women treated with risedronate but decreased in patients who did not receive risedronate, even in the presence of tamoxifen. During the third year, follow-up measurements of BMD showed that bone loss occurred after stopping risedronate; as a result, continuous treatment with risedronate was recommended. Clodronate is a less potent bisphosphonate not currently available in the USA. However, several studies have reported that, at the usual dose of 1600 mg daily, clodronate also reduced bone loss induced by a chemotherapy-induced menopause [54,55].

Until recently, intravenous bisphosphonates have been avoided for the treatment of osteoporosis because of the perceived inconvenience of intravenous therapy. However, it is now recognised that the duration of intravenous potent bisphosphonates in osteoporosis is quite prolonged. In prostate cancer patients undergoing androgen ablation, a recent placebo-controlled study showed that 3 monthly infusions of pamidronate 90 mg were able to prevent the rapid bone loss associated with androgen withdrawal [56]. A subsequent study has suggested that zoledronic acid is even more effective than pamidronate, with an increase in bone mass rather than simply preservation of BMD (MJ Smith, personal communication).

Most interestingly, a recent dose- and schedule-finding study of zoledronic acid in postmenopausal women was published. This indicated that a single once-a-year 4 mg dose of intravenous zoledronic acid increased BMD by 3% at 6 months and 5% at 12 months in comparison to placebo, and was as effective as more frequent schedules of administration [57]. Further studies are awaited to ensure this strategy not only preserves BMD but also prevents fractures. If these studies are confirmatory, our prediction is that occasional intravenous zoledronic acid will replace oral therapy, at least for cancer patients with treatment-induced bone loss [58].

CONCLUSIONS

The effects of bisphosphonates on osteoclast-mediated bone resorption in metastatic bone disease have been well established. *In vitro* evidence has shown that bisphosphonates have antitumour activity against tumour cell lines and inhibit tumour cell adhesion and invasion of the extracellular matrix. Although animal models have substantiated the *in vitro* evidence, clinical studies of adjuvant bisphosphonate therapy have yielded mixed results. Adjuvant studies have suggested that oral bisphosphonates may prevent the formation of bone metastases and possibly prolong survival. However, the results of these studies have been inconsistent. Finally, evidence of a survival benefit has been suggested in subset analyses of clinical studies with intravenous pamidronate and oral clodronate in patients with advanced disease. There is also an important, but hitherto largely unrecognised, problem of treatment-induced bone loss, for which bisphosphonates, either by mouth or occasional intravenous administration, are highly effective and safe. It is hoped that the increased potency of nitrogen-containing bisphosphonates, such as zoledronic acid, along with improved prospective trial design, will translate into consistent therapeutic effects for bisphosphonates in the adjuvant setting.

REFERENCES

1. National Institutes of Health Consensus Development Conference Statement: Adjuvant therapy for breast cancer. November 1–3 2000. JNCI Monogr 2001; 30: 5–15.
2. Bolla M, Gonzalez D, Wardle P et al. Improved survival in patients with locally advanced prostate cancer treated with radiotherapy and goserelin. N Engl J Med 1997; 337: 295–300.
3. Goldhirsch A, Gelber RD, Price KN et al. Effect of systemic adjuvant treatment on first sites of breast cancer relapse. Lancet 1994; 343: 377–81.
4. Paget S. The distribution of secondary growths in cancer of the breast. Lancet 1889; i: 571–3.
5. Batson OV. The function of the vertebral veins and their role in the spread of metastases. Ann Surg 1940; 112: 138–49.
6. Mundy GR, Guise TA. Pathophysiology of bone metastases. In: Rubens RD, Mundy GR (eds), Cancer and the Skeleton. Martin Dunitz: London, 2000: 43–64.
7. Rogers MJ, Watts DJ, Russell RGG. Overview of bisphosphonates. Cancer 1997; 80/8(suppl): 1652–60.
8. Dunford JE, Thompson K, Coxon FP et al. Structure–activity relationships for inhibition of farnesyl diphosphate synthase in vitro and inhibition of bone resorption in vivo by nitrogen-containing bisphosphonates. J Pharm Exp Therap 2000; 296: 235–42.
9. Frith JC, Monkkonen J, Auriola S et al. The molecular mechanism of action of the antiresorptive and anti-inflammatory drug clodronate: evidence for the formation in vivo of a metabolite that inhibits bone resorption and causes osteoclast and macrophage apoptosis. Arthrit Rheum 2001; 44: 2201–10.
10. Boissier S, Magnetto S, Frappart L et al. Bisphosphonates inhibit prostate and breast carcinoma cell adhesion to unmineralised and mineralised bone extracellular matrices. Cancer Res 1997; 57: 3890–4.
11. Seneratne SG, Pirianov G, Mansi JL et al. Bisphosphonates induce apoptosis in human breast cancer cell lines. Br J Cancer 2000; 82: 1459–568.
12. Wood J, Bonjean K, Ruetz S et al. Novel anti-angiogenic effects of the bisphosphonate compound zoledronic acid. J Pharm Exp Therap 2002; 302: 1055–61.
13. Jagdev S, Coleman RE, Shipman CM, Croucher P. The bisphosphonate zoledronic acid induces apoptosis of breast cancer cells: evidence for synergy with paclitaxel. Br J Cancer 2001; 84: 1126–34.
14. Yoneda T, Michigami T, Yi B et al. Use of bisphosphonates for the treatment of bone metastasis in experimental animal models. Cancer Treatm Rev 1999; 25: 293–9.
15. Hiraga T, Williams PJ, Mundy GR et al. The bisphosphonate ibandronate promotes apoptosis in MDA-MB-231 human breast cancer cells in bone metastases. Cancer Res 2001; 61: 4418–24.
16. Cruz JC, Alsina M, Craig F et al. Ibandronate decreases bone disease development and osteoclast stimulatory activity in an in vivo model of human myeloma. Exp Hematol 2001; 29: 441–7
17. Yaccoby S, Pearse RN, Johnson CL et al. Myeloma interacts with the bone marrow microenvironment to induce osteoclastogenesis and is dependent on osteoclast activity. Br J Haematol 2002; 116: 278–90.
18. Peyruchaud O, Winding B, Pecheur I et al. Early detection of bone metastases in a murine model using fluorescent human breast cancer cells: application to the use of the bisphosphonate zoledronic acid in the treatment of osteolytic lesions. J Bone Min Res 2001; 16: 2027–34.
19. Green JR, Gschaidmeier H, Yoneda T et al. Zoledronic acid potently inhibits tumour–induced osteolysis in two models of breast cancer metastasis to bone. Ann Oncol 2000; 11(suppl 4, abstr 50P): 14.
20. Nobuyuki H, Hiraga T, Williams PJ et al. The bisphosphonate zoledronic acid inhibits metastases to bone and liver with suppression of osteopontin production in mouse mammary tumor. J Bone Min Res 2001; 16(suppl 1, abs F062): S191.
21. Alvarez E, Galbreath EJ, Westmore M et al. Properties of bisphosphonates in the 13762 syngeneic rat mammary carcinoma model of tumor-induced bone resorption. Proc Am Assoc Cancer Res 2002; 43(abstr 1571):316.
22. Croucher P, De Raeve H, Perry M et al. Zoledronic acid prevents the development of osteolytic bone disease and increases survival in a murine model of multiple myeloma. Bone 2002; 30(suppl): 39S.
23. Sterns ME, Wang M. Effects of alendronate and taxol on PC-3 ML cell bone metastases in SCID mice. Invasion Metast 1996; 16: 116–31.
24. Yoneda T, Michigami T, Yi B et al. Actions of bisphosphonate on bone metastasis in animal models of breast carcinoma. Cancer 2000; 88: 2979–88.
25. Yoneda T, Sasaki A, Dunstan C et al. Inhibition of osteolytic bone metastasis of breast cancer by combined treatment with the bisphosphonate ibandronate and tissue inhibitor of the matrix metalloproteinase-2. J Clin Invest 1997; 99(10): 2509–17.
26. Diel IJ, Solomayer EF, Costa SD et al. Reduction in new metastases in breast cancer with adjuvant clodronate treatment. N Engl J Med 1998; 339: 357–63.
27. Powles T, Paterson S, Kanis JA et al. Randomized, placebo–controlled trial of clodronate in patients with primary operable breast cancer. J Clin Oncol 2002; 20: 3219–24.
28. Saarto T, Blomqvist C, Virkkunen P, Elomaa I. Adjuvant clodronate treatment does not reduce the frequency of skeletal metastases in node-positive breast cancer patients: 5 year results of randomised controlled trial. J Clin Oncol 2001; 19: 10–17.
29. Diel IJ, Solomayer E, Gollan C et al. Bisphosphonates in the reduction of metastases in breast cancer—results of the extended follow-up of the first study population. Proc Am Soc Clin Oncol 2000; 82a(abstr 314).
30. Powles TJ, Paterson AHG, Nevantaus A et al. Adjuvant clodronate reduces the incidence of bone metastases in

patients with primary operable breast cancer. Proc Am Soc Clin Oncol 1998; 17(abstr 468): 123a.

31. Kanis JA, Powles T, Paterson AH et al. Clodronate decreases the frequency of skeletal metastases in women with breast cancer. Bone 1996; 19: 663–7.

32. van Holten-Verzantvoort AT, Papapoulos SE. Oral pamidronate in the prevention and treatment of skeletal metastases in patients with breast cancer. Medicina (B Aires) 1997; 57(suppl 1): 109–13.

33. Ford JM, van Oosterom A, Brincker H et al. Oral pamidronate: negative results from three double-blind, placebo-controlled trials in hypercalcaemia, myeloma, and the prevention of bone metastases. Bone 1998; 22(suppl 3, abstr B52): 58S.

34. McCloskey EV, Dunn JA, Kanis JA et al. Long-term follow-up of a prospective, double-blind, placebo-controlled randomized trial of clodronate in multiple myeloma. Br J Haematol 2001; 113: 1035–43.

35. Berenson JR, Lichtenstein A, Porter L et al. Long-term pamidronate treatment of advanced multiple myeloma patients reduces skeletal events. Myeloma Aredia Study Group. J Clin Oncol 1998; 16: 593–602.

36. Lipton A, Theriault RL, Hortobagyi GN et al. Pamidronate prevents skeletal complications and is effective palliative treatment in women with breast carcinoma and osteolytic bone metastases: long-term follow-up of two randomized, placebo-controlled trials. Cancer 2000; 88: 1082–90.

37. Hortobagyi GN, Theriault RL, Lipton A et al. Long-term prevention of skeletal complications of metastatic breast cancer with pamidronate. For the Protocol 19 Aredia Breast Cancer Study Group. J Clin Oncol 1998; 16: 2038–44.

38. Diel IJ, Cote RJ. Bone marrow and lymph node assessment for minimal residual disease in patients with breast cancer. Cancer Treatm Rev 2000; 26: 53–65.

39. Kanis JA, McCloskey EV, Powles T et al. A high incidence of vertebral fracture in women with breast cancer. Br J Cancer 1999; 79: 1179–81.

40. Valagussa P, Moliterni A, Zambetti M, Bonadonna G. Long-term sequelae from adjuvant chemotherapy. Recent Results Cancer Res 1993; 127: 247–55.

41. Bruning PF, Pit MJ, de Jong-Bakker M et al. Bone mineral density after adjuvant chemotherapy for premenopausal breast cancer. Br J Cancer 1990; 61: 308–10.

42. Headley JA, Theriault RL, LeBlanc AD et al. Pilot study of bone mineral density in breast cancer patients treated with adjuvant chemotherapy. Cancer Invest 1998; 16: 6–11.

43. Love RR, Mazess RB, Barden HS et al. Effects of tamoxifen on bone mineral density in postmenopausal women with breast cancer. N Engl J Med 1992; 326: 852–6.

44. Kristensen B, Ejlertsen B, Mouridsen HT et al. Femoral fractures in postmenopausal breast cancer patients treated with adjuvant tamoxifen. Breast Cancer Res Treat 1996; 39: 321–6.

45. Powles TJ, Hickish T, Kanis JA et al. Effect of tamoxifen on bone mineral density measured by dual-energy X-ray absorptiometry in healthy premenopausal and post-menopausal women. J Clin Oncol 1996; 14: 78–84.

46. Delmas PD, Balena R, Confravreaux E et al. Bisphosphonate risedronate prevents bone loss in women with artificial menopause due to chemotherapy of breast cancer: a double-blind, placebo-controlled study. J Clin Oncol 1997; 15: 955–62.

47. Amin S, Zhang Y, Sawin CT et al. Association of hypogonadism and estradiol levels with bone mineral density in elderly men from the Framingham study. Ann Intern Med 2000; 133: 951–63.

48. Szulc P, Munoz F, Claustrat B et al. Bioavailable estradiol may be an important determinant of osteoporosis in men: the MINOS study. J Clin Endocrinol Metab 2001; 86: 192–9.

49. Daniell HW. Osteoporosis after orchiectomy for prostate cancer. J Urol 1997; 157: 439–44.

50. Hatano T, Oishi Y, Furuta A et al. Incidence of bone fracture in patients receiving luteinizing hormone-releasing hormone agonists for prostate cancer. Br J Urol Int 2000; 86: 449–52.

51. Townsend MF, Sanders WH, Northway RO, Graham SD. Bone fractures associated with luteinizing hormone-releasing hormone agonists used in the treatment of prostate carcinoma. Cancer 1997; 79: 545–50.

52. Diamond T, Campbell J, Bryant C, Lynch W. The effect of combined androgen blockade on bone turnover and bone mineral densities in men treated for prostate carcinoma: longitudinal evaluation and response to intermittent cyclic etidronate therapy. Cancer 1998; 83: 1561–6.

53. Daniell HW, Dunn SR, Ferguson DW et al. Progressive osteoporosis during androgen deprivation therapy for prostate cancer. J Urol 2000; 163: 181–6.

54. Powles TJ, McCloskey E, Paterson AH et al. Oral clodronate and reduction in loss of bone mineral density in women with operable primary breast cancer. J Natl Cancer Inst 1998; 90: 704–8.

55. Saarto S, Blomqvist C, Valimaki M et al. Chemical castration induced by adjuvant cyclophosphamide, methotrexate, and fluorouracil chemotherapy causes rapid bone loss which is reduced by clodronate: a randomised study in premenopausal patients. J Clin Oncol 1997; 15: 1341–7.

56. Smith MR, McGovern FJ, Zietman AL et al. Pamidronate to prevent bone loss during androgen-deprivation therapy for prostate cancer. N Engl J Med 2001; 345: 948–55.

57. Reid IR, Brown JP, Burckhardt P et al. Intravenous zoledronic acid in postmenopausal women with low bone mineral density. N Engl J Med 2002; 653–61.

58. Jagdev SP, Croucher PI, Coleman RE. Zoledronate induces apoptosis of breast cancer cells *in vitro*—evidence for additive and synergistic effects with taxol and tamoxifen. Proc Am Soc Clin Oncol 2000; 19(abstr 2619).

32

Prevention of Bone Loss

Robert U. Ashford, Eugene V. McCloskey and John A. Kanis

University of Sheffield Medical School, Sheffield, UK

INTRODUCTION

Osteoporosis is defined as a systemic bone disease characterised by low bone mass and microarchitectural deterioration of bone tissue, leading to enhanced bone fragility and a consequent increase in fracture risk. While most commonly a disorder of postmenopausal women, bone loss frequently occurs in patients with malignancy. In advanced disease, rapid systemic and focal osteolysis usually reflects an interaction between tumour cells and normal bone-resorbing cells, resulting in disturbances of calcium homeostasis (hypercalcaemia) and a high incidence of skeletal complications, including pathological fracture and bone pain. It is also increasingly recognised that bone loss can occur in early stages of the disease, due to endocrine consequences of solid tumours (frequently PTHrP-mediated) and/or the effects of systemic therapy on bone cell and gonadal function. The latter is assuming increasing importance as survival times and cure rates have improved for many solid and haematological malignancies.

Irrespective of the underlying mechanisms and type of tumour, increased rates of bone loss involve disturbances of the normal bone remodelling cycle mediated by alterations to the function and proliferation of authentic bone cells. This chapter reviews the mechanisms of bone loss in patients with cancer and approaches to its prevention, primarily with bisphosphonate treatment.

BONE REMODELLING

Remodelling of the skeleton is a healthy, normal process that occurs from the age of attainment of skeletal maturity (cessation of longitudinal growth) throughout the remainder of life. The remodelling sequence consists of an ordered cycle of a resorption phase preceding a formation phase (Figure 32.1) [1]. These events occur on the surface of cancellous bone and within the Haversian canals of cortical bone, and represent a process for maintenance of skeletal integrity by permitting repair of fatigue damage in bone and accomodation of changes in mechanical forces on the skeleton. Remodelling is a bone surface event and, at any one time, 10–15% of surfaces are undergoing remodelling, with the majority occurring in cancellous bone, reflecting the larger surface area available. For this reason, disorders of bone remodelling are seen earlier and to a greater extent at sites with larger proportions of cancellous bone (e.g. the axial skeleton and the metaphyses of long bones).

MECHANISMS UNDERLYING BONE LOSS

Increased Osteoclastic Bone Resorption

The osteoclast, a multinucleated giant cell, is derived from a multipotent precursor of the monocyte–macrophage family in the bone marrow [2]. Colony stimulating factors stimulate proliferation and differentiation of the progenitor cells to form pre-osteoclasts, specialised monocytes able to proliferate and circulate in the blood stream. Pre-osteoclasts are elevated in malignant bone disease, as well as in hyperparathyroidism and Paget's disease of bone. Many factors produced in the bone microenvironment have been identified to play important roles in osteoclast development [2], and increased production of these factors

Textbook of Bone Metastases. Edited by C. Jasmin, R. E. Coleman, L. R. Coia, R. Capanna and G. Saillant
© 2005 John Wiley & Sons Ltd: ISBN 0 471 87742 5

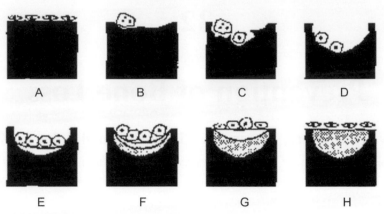

Figure 32.1. Steps in the remodelling sequence of cancellous bone. Most of the surface is quiescent (A). Surface activation is followed by the attraction of osteoclasts to the bone surface (B) and the excavation of an erosion cavity (C). When resorption is complete, osteoblasts are attracted to the erosion site (D) by the "coupling" mechanism and synthesise new osteoid (E). Subsequently mineralisation occurs (F and G) and at the completion of the cycle the bone surface is once again covered by lining cells (H)

by tumour cells or normal marrow stromal cells in response to the tumour, appears to play a significant role in osteolysis of advanced disease [2–4].

Even in early disease, bone turnover may be increased by the endocrine consequences of some solid tumours. For example, evidence suggests that products released by breast cancer cells, especially PTHrP but possibly others, such as IL-6 and IL-11, can promote RANK (receptor-activator of NF-κB) ligand formation by their actions on osteoblasts and stromal cells. These and other systemic factors may explain the observation that some patients with cancer but without skeletal metastases have increased bone turnover, as measured by biochemical markers of bone turnover. Most importantly, however, it is recognised that increased bone loss in early disease largely results from the loss of skeletal protection by gonadal hormones, either as a direct aim of the treatment in hormone-responsive tumours or as a side-effect of the systemic antitumour therapy.

Gonadal hormones, particularly oestrogen, play a vital role in the maintenance of skeletal integrity [5]. While the bone loss that results from oestrogen deficiency in women is well recognised, it now appears that oestrogen deficiency may also play a significant role in bone loss observed in hypogonadal men. Certainly, defects which decrease or prevent the peripheral conversion of androgens to oestrogen by aromatase are associated with marked reductions in bone mass, desite high circulating levels of testosterone [6]. Furthermore, defects in the oestrogen receptor are also associated with osteoporosis [7]. While the mechanisms by which oestrogen deficiency results in increased osteoclast activity are not fully elucidated,

the production and activity of a number of factors that can stimulate osteoclast differentiation, activity and survival is increased, including IL-1 and IL-6 [8,9]. A great deal of interest has recently focused on the activities of RANKL and osteoprotegerin, the relative activities of which appear to play a significant role in determining the level of osteoclast differentiation and activity [10–12].

Regardless of the mechanism underlying the increase in osteoclastic activity, resorption is usually accompanied by biochemical and histomorphometric evidence of increased bone formation as a result of coupling (Figure 32.1). However, the increase in all elements of bone turnover will still diminish skeletal mass because resorption precedes formation. It has been estimated that a five-fold increase in bone turnover will decrease bone mass by 20% at cancellous bone sites [13], but this decrease in bone mass can be exacerbated by imbalances between resorption and formation and, in later disease, by uncoupling of the two processes.

Imbalance Between Bone Resorption and Formation

Bone loss due to increased bone turnover is often exacerbated by an imbalance between osteoclast and osteoblast activity. Thus, the amount of bone deposited in a resorption cavity may be less than the volume of bone removed during resorption, accelerating skeletal losses. The imbalance is usually due to a decreased amount of new bone formed within erosion cavities, combined with an increase in resorption depth. The activity of osteoblasts may be relatively reduced in comparison to osteoclast activity, an effect that has been observed in multiple myeloma [14,15] where possible mechanisms include the production of inhibitory factors by myeloma cells [16,17]. A similar relative suppression of osteoblast function has also been described in breast cancer [18,19]. Relative suppression of bone formation also occurs in oestrogen deficiency, possibly due to decreased levels or activity of formation-stimulating cytokines such as TGFβ and IGF1 [9,20,21].

Uncoupling

The mechanisms underlying coupling are complex and poorly understood. In health, the TGFβ superfamily may play an essential role. Bone is a reservoir of inactive or latent TGFβ, which is activated and released during the process of bone resorption to inhibit osteoclast activity and stimulate osteoblast proliferation, differentiation and activity [22–24]. While suppression of bone formation in advanced or aggressive malignant disease may be severe enough to uncouple formation and resorption, this does not appear to occur in sraightforward gonadal deficiency. However, as bone loss progresses, physical uncoupling can occur as repeated waves of bone resorption result in the destruction of bone architecture and the removal of trabecular elements. At cancellous sites particularly, the increased depth of erosion transects trabecular plates and rods of bone, thus removing the surface on which new bone formation can occur.

CAUSES OF BONE LOSS

While hypogonadism has a predominant role in causing bone loss in patients with cancer, other factors also need to be considered (Table 32.1) and are discussed in more detail below.

Table 32.1. Potential causes of bone loss in patients with malignancy

Hypogonadism
  Surgical
  Post-chemotherapy
  Oestrogen or androgen antagonists
Direct toxicity of chemotherapy on bone cell function
Corticosteroids

Hypogonadism

Whether a direct aim of therapy or an unwanted consequence of systemic treatments, predominantly chemotherapy, the effects of hypogonadism on the skeleton need to be considered. This is assuming more importance as the consequences of hypogonadism in long-term survivors becomes more recognised and treatments, particularly with bisphosphonates, are known to prevent bone loss and decrease fracture risk in both hypogonadal men and women [25–32].

Women with breast cancer are particularly vulnerable to osteoporosis. At the time of first diagnosis, the prevalence of osteoporotic fractures in women with breast cancer approximates that of an age- and sex-matched control population [33,34]. Thereafter, the incidence of vertebral fractures increases to almost five times higher than in age-matched controls using morphometric criteria for the definition of vertebral fracture [34] (Figure 32.2) and more than two times higher when based on the radiologists' reports [33]. Premenopausal women are at special risk because of either the induction of an early menopause by chemotherapy [35–40] or the use of antioestrogens, most commonly tamoxifen [41].

Chemotherapy

Standard chemotherapeutic regimes for breast cancer, such as CMF (cyclophosphamide, methotrexate and 5-fluorouracil) result in ovarian failure in more than two-thirds of premenopausal women with breast cancer,

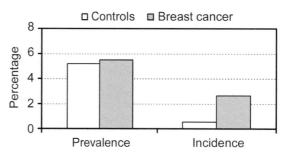

Figure 32.2. Prevalence and incidence of vertebral fracture in newly diagnosed breast cancer. The prevalence of fracture in women with newly diagnosed breast cancer is similar to that in age-matched controls. In contrast, the subsequent annual incidence of fracture is significantly higher in the breast cancer patients (Odds ratio 4.7, 95%CI 2.3–9.9) and the increased risk persisted following exclusion of patients with metastatic bone disease (OR 2.8, 95%CI 1.3–6.2). Adapted from [104]

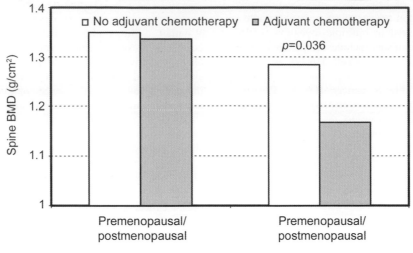

Figure 32.3. Effect of adjuvant chemotherapy on spine BMD in women with breast cancer. Subjects comprised 44 pairs of cases and controls matched for age, year of primary treatment and interval after breast surgery. In women remaining premenopausal following treatment, there was no effect of chemotherapy on spine BMD. In contrast, the induction of an early menopause by adjuvant chemotherapy was associated with a significant decrease in mean spine BMD. (Adapted from [35])

largely due to the effects of cyclophosphamide on granulosa cell function and follicle destruction in the ovary [42,43]. Ovarian failure usually occurs within 4 months of completion of the chemotherapy, with older patients at the highest risk [35,36,40]. The extent of the premature loss of bone loss was demonstrated by Bruning and colleagues, who showed a 10% lower lumbar spine bone mineral density (BMD) in women rendered amenorrhoeic by chemotherapy compared to age-matched controls [35] (Figure 32.3). Prospective studies suggest that the bone loss is rapid and detectable over the first year of treatment, with losses at the lumbar spine of 3–8% [40].

Chemotherapy, either alone or in combination with pelvic radiotherapy, can also give rise to hypogonadism in other malignancies. One- to two-thirds of premenopausal women treated with alkylating agents for lymphoma develop a premature menopause, possibly due to the use of cyclophosphamide or procarbazine. Failure to consider the use of HRT in such women is associated with significant reductions in BMD compared to healthy controls [44]. The incidence of ovarian failure increases to almost 100% in women undergoing high-dose chemotherapy and radiotherapy in preparation for bone marrow transplanation for a variety of malignancies [45].

Impairment of testicular function in men with lymphoma is not as marked as the suppression of ovarian function in women. However, reductions in BMD at several skeletal sites have been described [46] and abnormalities of LH and FSH have been described in up to two-thirds of boys after bone marrow transplantation [47,48]. Cisplatin therapy in testicular cancer is associated with low testosterone levels in up to 10% of patients, and elevated gonadotrophins are observed in the majority of patients treated with cisplatin or infra-diaphragmatic radiotherapy.

Antioestrogens and Antiandrogens

Tamoxifen is the most widely used antioestrogen in the treatment of primary and recurrent breast cancer. The effect of tamoxifen, a partial oestrogen agonist and the forerunner of the selective oestrogen receptor modulators (SERMs), on bone turnover is dependent on circulating oestrogen levels. Thus, while its weaker oestrogenic activity prevents bone loss in postmenopausal women (see later), it has been demonstrated to cause bone loss in premenopausal women [41,49] presumably by competitive agonist activity at the oestrogen receptor. In a double-blind placebo-controlled study of tamoxifen for the prevention of breast cancer, 62 premenopausal women who continued to menstruate during 3 years of tamoxifen 20 mg daily had a mean decrease in spinal BMD of approximately

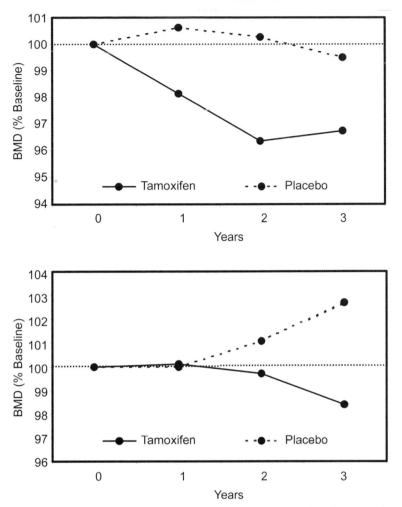

Figure 32.4. Effect of tamoxifen 20 mg daily on BMD at the spine (top) and total hip (bottom) when given over 3 years to premenopausal women at increased risk of breast cancer. Women who became postmenopausal during follow-up were excluded from this analysis. Asterisks denote the significance of differences between tamoxifen and placebo at each of the timepoints ($*p < 0.05$, $***p < 0.001$). (Based on [41])

4% compared to 63 women receiving placebo, in whom menstruation continued and spine BMD remained stable (Figure 32.4) [41]. In young women rendered postmenopausal by chemotherapy, concurrent use of tamoxifen appears to decrease but not completely prevent bone loss at the spine or hip [37].

Bone loss in premenopausal women has also been demonstrated during use of gonadotrophin-releasing hormone (GnRH) agonists in women with advanced breast cancer and those being treated for endometriosis. The resulting suppression of ovarian function is associated in premenopausal women with a steep decline in BMD, together with elevated biochemical markers of bone turnover [50–52].

Despite low circulating levels of oestrogen in postmenopausal women, the use of aromatase inhibitors can further suppress these levels by 95% and might be expected to exacerbate bone loss. Although few clinical data are available [53], endogenous oestrogen levels have been shown to relate to rates of bone loss and the future risk of fracture [54,55] as well as the future development of breast cancer [56]. It is highly likely that the use of pure antioestrogens such as faslodex will also be associated with an increased risk of osteoporosis in both pre- and postmenopausal women.

Increased rates of bone loss and fracture risk have also been observed in men undergoing orchidectomy for prostate cancer [57] and in men treated with GnRH agonists [58–60]. The simultaneous use of antiandrogens and surgical or medical castration has been shown to cause significant reductions in spine and hip BMD [61].

Direct Effects of Systemic Chemotherapy on Bone Cell Function

Perhaps surprisingly, there are few data on the direct effects of chemotherapeutic agents on bone metabolism. Cyclophosphamide has been demonstrated to have a direct effect on bone in neonatal and juvenile rats, reducing numbers of both osteoblasts and osteoclasts on the bone surface [62], but it is not clear whether these effects are of clinical significance and are largely overshadowed by the effects of cyclophosphamide on gonadal function. For example, cyclophosphamide administered in combination with methotrexate and 5-fluorouracil (CMF regimen) in premenopausal women is only associated with a small, non-significant reduction in mean spine BMD compared to breast cancer control subjects not treated by chemotherapy [35] (Figure 32.3).

Doxorubicin, an anthracycline frequently used in breast cancer, inhibits protein synthesis and hence osteoid formation with little or no effect on osteoclast number or activity. It has been demonstrated to reduce trabecular bone volume in rat vertebrae [63].

Methotrexate, an antifolate antimetabolite, also affects bone directly, leading to both decreased bone formation and increased bone resorption in rats [63,64]. It results in a marked decrease in trabecular bone volume in the tail vertebrae of rats [63] as well as an increase in osteoclast number and an increase in the percentage of the trabecular surface in contact with osteoclasts [63]. High-dose methotrexate has been reported to be associated with an increased incidence of fractures in children with acute lymphoblastic leukaemia or osteosarcoma [64,65] but low doses, such as that used in rheumatoid arthritis, appear to have little or no effect on rates of bone loss [66].

Corticosteroids

Glucocorticoids are frequently used in the management of patients with malignancy, either for the control of emesis or as part of anticancer therapy, particularly in haematological malignancy.

There is abundant evidence that corticosteroid use is associated with bone loss and increased fracture risk in non-oncological patients [67–69], mediated in part by an initial increase in osteoclastic activity and a longer-term suppression of osteoblast function. In contrast, there are relatively few data on the impact of corticosteroid use on bone loss in oncology. In some settings, e.g. multiple myeloma, the inhibitory effects on tumour cell activity and proliferation may counteract the detrimental effects on bone loss. For example, in the placebo arm of the bisphosphonate study within the MRC VIth Myelomatosis Trial [70] an unpublished analysis showed that the incidence of new vertebral fractures was similar in patients receiving the adriamycin, BCNU (carmustine), cyclophosphamide and melphalan (ABCM) regimen, with or without concurrent prednisolone (56.6% vs. 49.1%, respectively; $p=0.55$). Likewise, several reports suggest that high-dose albeit short-term use of high-dose prednisolone (up to 3 g) is not associated with acute bone loss in patients receiving treatment for lymphoma [44,71]. It is quite likely that the use of corticosteroids in patients with tumours that are not responsive to these agents will exacerbate the rates of bone loss, but this area requires further study.

PREVENTION OF BONE LOSS

Regardless of the mechanism of bone loss, its clinical sequelae, osteoporosis-related fragility fractures, are a common co-morbid event in patients with a prior history of cancer. The aims of treatment are to halt or reverse bone loss and thereby decrease the risk of fragility fractures. Many agents are available for these purposes but none are licensed specifically for use in patients with malignancy. Indeed, some agents, such as hormone replacement treatment and the anabolic steroids, may be contraindicated in the presence of tumour [72,73] and there is a need, therefore, for non-HRT alternatives. Bisphosphonates are the principal agents utilised to prevent bone loss, but other agents such as calcitonin and tamoxifen (in postmenopausal women) may also be used. In future, the use of SERMs such as raloxifene may be warranted due to the combined beneficial effects on bone mass/fracture risk and the incidence of breast cancer [28,74].

The ultimate clinical arbiter of adequate prevention of bone loss in non-malignant states, usually postmenopausal osteoporosis, is a decrease in fracture rates, and the same measure is of importance in studies of malignant skeletal disease. In advanced disease, particularly in breast cancer and multiple myeloma, bisphosphonate use has reduced the incidence of pathological vertebral and non-vertebral fractures by 30–50% [75–82]. The effects of bisphosphonate therapy to reduce these and the incidence of other skeletal-related complications is addressed elsewhere, but other studies have assessed the ability of therapies to prevent bone loss, using changes in BMD or biochemical markers of bone turnover.

Bone Mass (Bone Mineral Density)

Given the definition of osteoporosis, it can be argued that primary endpoints in studies of prevention of bone loss could be assessed by the effects of an intervention on BMD. Guidelines have recently been published for the use of bone mass measurements in clinical practice [83] and these would certainly include patients with hypogonadism, cancer-associated bone loss and exposure to drugs associated with bone loss (particularly corticosteroids). Several well-established methods are available for the measurement of bone mass, the most widely used techniques comprising either single- or dual-energy X-ray absorptiometry (SXA and DXA, respectively). DXA has the advantage of being applicable to more biologically relevant sites (e.g. the spine and proximal femur) in addition to peripheral sites of measurement (e.g. distal forearm, heel, etc.) The measurements are very reproducible (approximately 1% and 1.5% at the spine and hip, respectively) and are useful for both diagnosing and monitoring bone mass. For women, the WHO has proposed three categories of bone density (normal, osteopenia and osteoporosis), based on a comparison of the individual's value with the mean in young healthy adults of the same sex and the difference expressed as SD units (T-score) [84]. Similar thresholds may be applicable in men.

The relationship between reductions in BMD and future fracture risk appears robust and has been well documented, particularly in postmenopausal women [52,85,86,108]. While there is a somewhat weaker relationship between treatment-induced changes in BMD and the reduction in fracture risk, agents which improve or maintain BMD have been shown to reduce fracture risk in large prospective studies [25–32]. The effect of bisphosphonates and other antiresorptive therapies is in essence to prevent bone loss. The increment in bone mass that is observed in some studies, particularly at the spine, is an expected consequence of the effect on the remodelling process (i.e. a decrease in activation frequency) and should not be interpreted as an anabolic effect. Lower rates of bone turnover, documented after exposure to antiresorptive therapies, are associated with a decrease in

the resorption space within bone and a progressive increase in the mineralisation of newly formed bone.

The reduction in fracture risk is usually greater than that predicted by the magnitude of the changes in BMD, possibly reflecting the reduction in bone turnover and the progression of architectural destruction in bone. The evidence on which efficacy for bisphosphonates is based rests not only upon information on the effects on BMD, but also the effects on fracture risk and the effects on the quality of bone in clinical and in preclinical studies.

Biochemical Markers of Bone Turnover

Biochemical markers are an indirect measurement of bone turnover and can reflect either osteoblastic or osteoclastic activity. Numerous serum and urinary markers of bone turnover have been and are being developed with increasing evidence for a role in the management of patients with malignant disease. The vast majority of studies using biochemical markers in patients with malignancy are of relatively short duration ($\leqslant 6$ months) and most demonstrate a rapid reduction in markers of both bone resorption (including hydroxyproline, deoxypyridinoline, collagen telopeptides) and a slightly delayed suppression of markers of bone formation (alkaline phosphatase, bone alkaline phosphatase, osteocalcin). The clinical utility of these biochemical markers is discussed in more detail elsewhere in this textbook.

BISPHOSPHONATES

Background

While the precise mechanisms of action of the bisphosphonates in vivo remain uncertain, recent studies in vitro have suggested that the non-aminobisphosphonates (e.g. etidronate, clodronate) and the amino-bisphosphonates (e.g. pamidronate, alendronate, risedronate) inhibit osteoclast recruitment, activity and apoptosis by different intracellular mechanisms [87,88]. It is not yet certain whether these differences are of clinical relevance so that appropriate doses of the different agents (bearing in mind well-documented differences in potency) appear to confer similar clinical efficacy. A relatively small number of studies have addressed their efficacy to prevent bone loss in oncology but a large amount of data exists for their utility in postmenopausal and secondary osteoporosis.

Prevention of Bone Loss by Bisphosphonates in Patients with Cancer

Over the last 5 years, a number of controlled studies have demonstrated that the administration of bisphosphonates can prevent or decrease bone loss in women undergoing treatment for breast cancer [36–38,89,90] (Table 32.2).

In a randomised open controlled study, 67 women at first relapse of proven breast cancer were studied prospectively [90]. A total of 33 women were allocated to receive clodronate 1600 mg daily by mouth for 9 months with an entire follow-up of 24 months and the remaining women were followed as controls. Concomitant chemotherapy was used as deemed clinically necessary, largely comprising adriamycin or derivative-based regimens or cyclophosphamide-based regimens with 5-fluorouracil and methotrexate. Tamoxifen was used for the patients who were oestrogen-receptor positive. BMD of the lumbar spine, femoral neck and femoral shaft was measured by dual photon absorptiometry at baseline and, every 6 months or less, with a subgroup analysis being undertaken in patients with a normal scintigram of the lumbosacral region at baseline. An increase in the mean BMD occurred in both clodronate and control group patients. The reason for the increase in both groups of the study was the confounding effect of the presence of lumbar spinal osteoblastic metastases. When patients with lumbar metastases were excluded, control patients lost bone from the lumbar spine, whereas a marked increase occurred during treatment with clodronate [90] (Table 32.2).

Saarto and colleagues reported the use of oral clodronate 1600 mg daily in two large open randomised studies of women at the time of primary diagnosis of breast cancer (Table 32.2). These studies examined the effect of oral clodronate on spine and hip BMD in premenopausal women receiving chemotherapy, and in postmenopausal women receiving hormonal treatments [36,89]. The median age, height, weight, menopausal status and type of primary adjuvant treatment were well balanced between treatment groups. For the analysis of efficacy, data were censored if patients developed skeletal metastases, since this had been observed to impair the interpretation of changes in BMD [90]. In the study of postmenopausal women with early stage breast cancer, patients had surgery and radiotherapy followed by randomisation to either tamoxifen 20 mg daily or toremifene 60 mg daily for 3 years. All patients were also randomised to receive clodronate or act as

Table 32.2. Efficacy of bisphosphonates in premenopausal or postmenopausal women with breast cancer

Author	Population	Duration (months)	Age (mean ± SD)	Treatment	Patients assessed	LS (%)	TH/FN (%)
Rizzoli et al. [90]	Breast cancer first relapse (includes only women without skeletal metastases)	9	59	Clodronate 1600 mg daily	7	+8.1	—
				None	8	−0.9	—
Delmas et al. [37]	Premenopausal breast cancer, artificial menopause due to chemotherapy	24	46 ± 4	Risedronate 30 mg daily (2/12 weekly cycle)	27	−0.2*	−0.8*
				Placebo	26	−2.7	−3.4
Saarto et al. [36]	Premenopausal newly diagnosed breast cancer, axillary nodes involved, chemotherapy	24	44 ± 7	Clodronate 1600 mg daily	40	−2.2*	+0.9
				Control	53	−5.9	−2.0
Saarto et al. [89]	Postmenopausal newly diagnosed breast cancer, axillary nodes involved, antioestrogens	24	62 ± 7	Clodronate 1600 mg daily	44	+2.9**	+3.7**
				Control	49	−0.7	+0.5
Powles et al. [38]	Newly diagnosed breast cancer, endocrine and/or chemotherapy	24	54 ± 10	Clodronate 1600 mg daily	156	−0.16*	+1.13**
				Placebo	155	−1.88	−0.72

Data derived from published studies of double-blind, placebo-controlled studies. The two rightmost columns refer to mean changes in lumbar spine (LS) or total hip/femoral neck (TH/FN) bone mineral density from entry to the study. Asterisks refer to the statistical significance of differences between the two treatment groups (*p < 0.05, **p < 0.01).

untreated controls [89]. Spine and femoral neck BMD measurements were obtained using DXA measurements in the 49 controls and 44 women receiving clodronate. As expected from the known effects of tamoxifen on bone turnover in postmenopausal women, spine and femoral neck BMD remained stable over 2 years of treatment in the control group (Table 32.2) with no apparent differences between treatment with tamoxifen or toremifene in the study. Concomitant treatment with clodronate was associated with significant increases in BMD at both the spine and femoral neck, comprising 2.9% and 3.7% at the respective sites by the end of 2 years (Table 32.2).

In the study of premenopausal women, changes in spine and femoral neck BMD over 2 years were reported in 93 women with newly-diagnosed operable breast cancer. All of the women were treated with six cycles of CMF after initial surgery and axillary irradiation [36]. At 2 years, the severity of bone loss was less severe with clodronate (-2.0 vs. -5.9% in the vertebral spine and $+0.9\%$ vs. -2.0% in the femoral neck; $p=0.0005$ and $p=0.018$, respectively). Of the 93 women, only 16 (17.2%) continued to menstruate regularly during follow-up and a further 40 (43%) developed irregular menses, with the remainder experiencing an early menopause. In women continuing to menstruate, spine and femoral neck BMD remained stable over the 2 years, while clodronate treatment induced small increases in BMD at both sites (mean increase $+2.0\%$ and $+3.1\%$, respectively, at the spine and hip). In contrast, the induction of an early menopause was associated with dramatic bone loss at both skeletal sites over the 2 years (mean change -9.5% and -4.6% at the spine and femoral neck,

respectively). Treatment with clodronate prevented bone loss at the femoral neck ($+0.4\%$ at 2 years), while the rate of loss at the lumbar spine was approximately halved in the women receiving concomitant clodronate (mean change -5.9%) [36].

A significant prevention of bone loss in young women with breast cancer and early menopause induced by chemotherapy has also been demonstrated with the bisphosphonate risedronate [37]. Fifty-three women (aged 36–55 years) with breast cancer and an artificially induced menopause were stratified according to prior tamoxifen use ($n=36$) or non-use ($n=17$). Within each stratum, patients were randomly assigned to receive risedronate (30 mg/day, $n=27$) or placebo ($n=26$) for 2 weeks, followed by 10 weeks without treatment. The treatment cycle was repeated eight times and patients were monitored for a third year without treatment. During the 2 years of treatment, the women on placebo exhibited a significant loss of BMD at the lumbar spine and hip. In contrast, there was an increase in BMD in the risedronate group, so that at 2 years the mean difference between groups was 2.5% [95% confidence interval (CI), 0.2–4.9] at the lumbar spine ($p=0.041$) and 2.6% (95% CI, 0.3–4.8) at the femoral neck ($p=0.029$) (Table 32.2). Similar results were observed at the hip trochanteric region. Tamoxifen use alone was associated with a reduction in the rate of bone loss in young women with a chemotherapy-induced early menopause. It is important to note that when treatment with risedronate was withdrawn, there was a relatively rapid offset of action, as judged by an increase in serum osteocalcin and a parallel reduction in lumbar spine BMD in the bisphosphonate and placebo groups. This suggests that treatment needs to

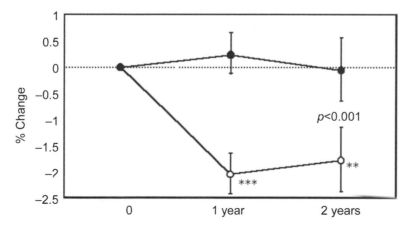

Figure 32.5. Effect of clodronate 1600 mg daily on spine BMD in women with newly diagnosed breast cancer. The open circles represent women receiving surgery and systemic treatment (chemotherapy and/or endocrine therapy) with placebo. The solid circles are mean changes in spine BMD in women receiving the same treatment plus oral clodronate given over 2 years. (Based on [38,39])

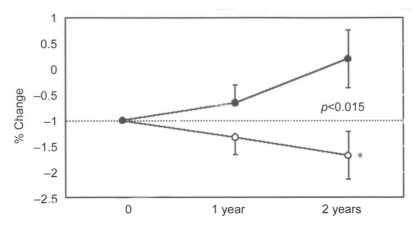

Figure 32.6. Effect of clodronate 1600 mg daily on total hip BMD in women with newly diagnosed breast cancer. The open circles represent women receiving surgery and systemic treatment (chemotherapy and/or endocrine therapy) with placebo. The solid circles are mean changes in total hip BMD in women receiving the same treatment plus oral clodronate given over 2 years. (Based on [38,39])

be continuous to maintain a protective effect on bone mass.

In a further double-blind, placebo-controlled study [38], bone mineral density (BMD) was assessed in 311 patients at first diagnosis of breast cancer allocated to oral clodronate 1600 mg daily or placebo and followed for 1 year or more. Patients allocated to the two treatment groups were well balanced with respect to age, menopause status and concomitant anti-cancer treatment [38]. After 1 year the placebo group had a mean loss in spinal BMD of 2.2%, whereas the clodronate group showed a small gain of 0.18% (treatment effect +2.38%; $p < 0.001$) (Figure 32.5); (Table 32.2). At the hip, placebo-treated patients lost less bone (0.34%) compared to a gain of 0.4% in the clodronate-treated group ($p=0.09$) (Figure 32.6). The difference in placebo and treated groups was greater at the trochanteric region of the hip (treatment effect +1.29%; $p=0.02$). After 2 years the treatment effect for clodronate in spinal BMD, total hip and trochanteric BMD remained significantly higher than in placebo-treated patients (Figures 32.1 and 32.2) [38]. As expected, the mean rate of bone loss in the first year of the study in the placebo arm of the study was greater at the lumbar spine in women receiving chemotherapy ($\pm$ tamoxifen, largely premenopausal women) than in those receiving endocrine therapy alone (largely postmenopausal women) (Figure 32.7). Treatment with clodronate reduced the rate of bone loss in all groups of systemic treatment, although this did not achieve statistical significance in women receiving chemotherapy alone [38] (Figure 32.7).

Finally, in a double-blind, randomised comparative study in patients with advanced malignant osteolytic bone disease and bone pain, intravenous pamidronate, 60 mg every 3 weeks, was noted to maintain total body bone mass over a short follow-up period (5 months), while a significant increase (mean +3.0%) was observed in patients receiving 90 mg every 3 weeks. The difference between the treatment groups was, however, not statistically significant [91].

Prevention of Bone Loss by Bisphosphonates in Postmenopausal Women and Secondary Osteoporosis

The evidence that bisphosphonates can prevent bone loss secondary to loss of gonadal function in non-malignant conditions is well established in postmenopausal women [25–27,31,32,92–94]. Several bisphosphonates are currently licensed for the prevention and/or treatment of postmenopausal bone loss, and more recently efficacy has been demonstrated for osteoporosis in men, including hypogonadal individuals [30]. The results of some of the largest trials are shown in Table 32.3. It should be borne in mind, however, that most of these studies have excluded patients with any prior history of malignancy other than basal cell carcinoma, and some doubts remain over the most appropriate dose for prevention of bone loss in malignancy. For example, clodronate 800 mg daily has been shown to reduce the incidence of vertebral fracture by approximately 50% in women

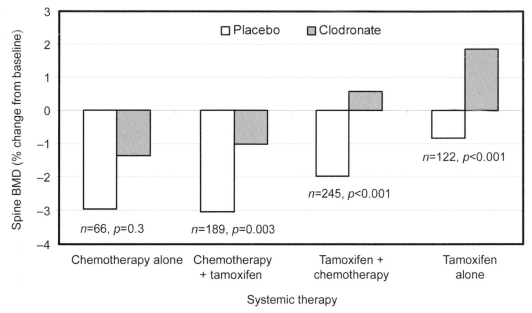

Figure 32.7. Effect of clodronate 1600 mg daily on spine BMD over the first year from diagnosis in women with newly diagnosed breast cancer treated with chemotherapy or tamoxifen alone or in combination. (Based on [38,39])

with postmenopausal or secondary osteoporosis (including women with prior non-recurrent breast cancer) [32]. The data for prevention of bone loss in women with newly diagnosed breast cancer is largely with clodronate 1600 mg daily, a dose that has also been associated with a significant reduction in the subsequent incidence of skeletal metastases [39,95]. Whether a lower dose, or indeed currently used anti-osteoporotic doses of other bisphosphonates, would be sufficient to achieve a reduction in the incidence of skeletal metastases is not known. The current data suggest that if the primary aim of treatment is to prevent skeletal metastases, then higher doses of bisphosphonates may be required.

Corticosteroid osteoporosis. In a small study addressing the effect of tamoxifen in postmenopausal women with breast cancer receiving corticosteroids, serial bone density measurements were performed at baseline and after 24 months in 46 women [96]. By 2 years, there was no significant difference between mean bone density of those receiving tamoxifen alone ($n=26$) and those receiving tamoxifen and prednisolone ($n=20$), or any significant change from baseline levels. The authors concluded that the absence of the predicted steroid-induced bone loss suggested that tamoxifen may be of more general use in prevention of

osteoporosis in patients requiring long-term steroid treatment. This conclusion should probably be interpreted cautiously, due to the absence of a treatment arm with prednisolone alone to demonstrate the expected loss of bone.

In contrast to tamoxifen, three placebo-controlled studies of bisphosphonates have demonstrated the efficacy to prevent corticosteroid-induced bone loss [97–99]. In the study of risedronate, 290 ambulatory men and women receiving high-dose oral corticosteroid therapy (prednisone $\geqslant 7.5$ mg/day or equivalent) for 6 or more months were randomised to receive placebo, risedronate 2.5 mg/day, or risedronate 5 mg/day for 12 months [99]. All patients received calcium 1 g and vitamin D 400 IU daily. Risedronate 5 mg increased BMD at 12 months by a mean (SEM) of 2.9% (0.49%) at the lumbar spine, 1.8% (0.46%) at the femoral neck, and 2.4% (0.54%) at the trochanter, whereas BMD remained unchanged in the control group. Although underpowered to examine fracture efficacy, a reduction in the incidence of vertebral fractures of 70% in the combined risedronate treatment groups, relative to placebo ($p=0.042$), was observed. Trends for reductions in vertebral fracture incidence were reported in the studies of cyclical etidronate or alendronate [97,98]. It should be borne in mind, however, that all of these studies usually excluded patients with prior histories of

Table 32.3. Efficacy of bisphosphonates in women with postmenopausal osteoporosis during bisphosphonate therapy

Author	Treatment	Duration (years)	Spine BMD [Treatment effect (%) at 1 year]	Vertebral fracture [RR (95% CI)]	Non-vertebral fracture [RR (95% CI)]
Watts et al. [92]	Cyclical etidronate 400 mg daily p.o.	2			
Storm et al. [93]	Cyclical etidronate 400 mg daily p.o.	3			
Reid et al. [94]	Pamidronate 150 mg daily p.o.	2		—	—
Black et al. [25]	Alendronate 10 mg daily p.o.	3	+3.5	0.53 (0.41–0.68)	0.72 (0.58–0.90)
Cummings et al. [54]	Alendronate 10 mg daily p.o.	4	+3.6	0.56 (0.39–0.80)	0.86 (0.73–1.01)
Pols et al. [29]	Alendronate 10 mg daily p.o.	1	+4.9	—	0.53 (0.30–0.90)
Reginster et al. [27]	Risedronate 5 mg daily p.o.	3		0.51 (0.36–0.65)	0.67 (0.44–1.04)
Harris et al. [106]	Risedronate 5 mg daily p.o.	3		0.59 (0.42–0.82)	0.61 (0.39–0.94)
McCloskey et al. [32]	Clodronate 800 mg daily p.o	1	+2.6	0.40 (0.16–1.00)	—

Data derived from published studies of double-blind, placebo-controlled studies of 1–4 years duration. In all studies, calcium supplements were also given to all the study subjects (usually 500–1000 mg daily).

malignancy, so that the use of bisphosphonates to prevent corticosteroid-induced bone loss in this setting should be monitored closely.

Additional Effects of Bisphosphonates in Postmenopausal Women Receiving Antioestrogens

In contrast to the apparently detrimental effects in premenopausal women, several studies of tamoxifen in postmenopausal women have demonstrated a positive effect on BMD at different sites [41,100–102,107]. The observed differences in BMD reflect decreases in bone turnover, with further evidence for this provided by significant decreases in biochemical markers of bone resorption and formation [100,102]. The most definitive study in postmenopausal women with a history of breast cancer is the randomised, double-blind, placebo-controlled trial [101,102] of 140 postmenopausal women with axillary node negative breast cancer. Spinal BMD increased by 0.61% per year over a 2 year period in those treated with tamoxifen compared with a 1% annual decrease in the placebo group. At the forearm there were similar reductions in the two groups (0.88% vs. 1%, NS). A later analysis of those patients continuing with or without tamoxifen for 5 years confirmed that the effect on bone density persisted throughout the duration of treatment [102].

The beneficial effect of tamoxifen on bone mass and the lowered rate of bone turnover may lower the fracture rate in postmenopausal women with breast cancer, but this remains to be confirmed by longitudinal studies. In a long-term follow-up study of over 1700 postmenopausal women randomised to receive radiotherapy with or without tamoxifen 30 mg daily for 1 year, the incidence of femoral fractures (femoral neck and trochanteric) was higher in the women who had received the tamoxifen therapy [103]. While the study design could not exclude a number of possible confounders, it was noted by the authors that the results could not be explained by a longer survival in the tamoxifen group, or by metastases with pathological fractures. It is of interest that, despite the use of tamoxifen in postmenopausal women with primary breast cancer, the incidence of vertebral fractures was noted to be higher than that in healthy age-matched controls [104]. It should be noted, however, that tamoxifen use in the primary prevention of breast cancer has been associated with a significant decrease in the incidence of hip, wrist and spine fractures [105].

It should be noted that even in postmenopausal patients receiving antioestrogens, the comcomitant use of bisphosphonate therapy is associated with a further increment in spine and hip BMD in postmenopausal women with breast cancer or in young women with an early menopause secondary to chemotherapy [37–39,89] (Figure 32.8). Whether this confers a reduction in the incidence of vertebral and other fractures remains unclear, but the incidence of skeletal metastases appears to be reduced below that observed with tamoxifen alone.

SUMMARY

The available studies indicate that bisphosphonates decrease or prevent losses of bone mineral density of

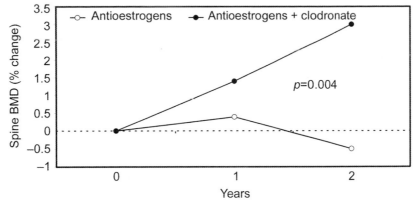

Figure 32.8. Changes in spine BMD over 2 years in postmenopausal women with breast cancer treated with antioestrogens (tamoxifen or toremifene) alone or in combination with clodronate 1600 mg daily. (Based on [89])

the spine and femur in women with early and advanced breast cancer. Data are lacking from patients with other types of malignancy but similar efficacy might be expected. For many bisphosphonates, however, the optimal dose and regimen has not been fully characterised. Most evidence exists for clodronate 1600 mg daily, with the higher dose giving comparable results to that observed with 800 mg daily in postmenopausal osteoporosis. Several bisphosphonates are of proven value in the prevention and treatment of glucocorticoid-induced osteoporosis.

The optimal duration of treatment with bisphosphonates has not been determined, but prevention of bone loss has been shown over 1–4 years in double-blind placebo-controlled studies. It is likely that long-term use of bisphosphonates will become increasingly common in survivors among patients with a number of malignancies.

REFERENCES

1. Frost HM. Bone Remodelling and Its Relationship to Metabolic Bone Disease. Thomas: Springfield, 1973.
2. Mundy GR. Bone Remodelling and Its Disorders, 2nd edn. Martin Dunitz: London, 1999.
3. Rodan GA, Martin TJ. Therapeutic approaches to bone diseases. Science 2000; 289(5484): 1508–14.
4. Croucher PI, Apperley JF. Bone disease in multiple myeloma. Br J Haematol 1998; 103: 902–10.
5. Turner RT, Riggs BL, Spelsberg TC. Skeletal effects of oestrogen. Endocr Rev 1994; 15: 275–300.
6. Carani C, Quin K, Simoni M et al. Effect of testosterone and oestradiol in a man with aromatase deficiency. N Engl J Med 1997; 337: 91–5.
7. Smith EP, Boyd J, Frank GR et al. Estrogen resistance caused by a mutation in the estrogen-receptor gene in a man. N Engl J Med 1994; 331: 1056–61.
8. Jilka RL. Cytokines, bone remodelling and estrogen deficiency: a 1998 update. Bone 1998; 23: 75–81.
9. Spelsberg TC, Subramaniam M, Riggs BL et al. The actions and interactions of sex steroids and growth factors/cytokines on the skeleton. Mol Endocrinol 1999; 13: 819–28.
10. Yasuda H, Shima N, Nakagawa N et al. Identity of osteoclastogenesis inhibitory factor (OCIF) and osteoprotegerin (OPG): a mechanism by which OPG/OCIF inhibits osteoclastogenesis in vitro. Endocrinology 1998; 139: 1329–37.
11. Simonet WS, Lacey DL, Dunstan CR et al. Osteoprotegerin: a novel secreted protein involved in the regulation of bone density. Cell 1997; 89: 309–19.
12. Tsuda H, Goto M, Mochizuki S et al. Isolation of a novel cytokine from human fibroblasts that specifically inhibits osteoclastogenesis. Biochem Biophys Res Commun 1997; 234: 137–42.
13. Kanis JA. The Pathophysiology and Treatment of Paget's Disease of Bone. Martin Dunitz: London, 1991.
14. Valentin-Opran A, Charhon S, Meunier PJ et al. Quantitative histology of myeloma-induced bone changes. Br J Haematol 1982; 52: 601–10.
15. Taube T, Beneton MNC, McCloskey EV et al. Abnormal bone remodelling in patients with myelomatosis and normal biochemical indices of bone resorption. Eur J Haematol 1993; 49: 192–8.
16. Evans CE, Galasko CSB, Ward C. Does myeloma secrete an osteoblast-inhibiting factor? J Bone Joint Surg Br 1989; 71B: 288–90.
17. Evans CE, Ward C, Rathour L, Galasko CSB. Myeloma affects both the growth and function of human osteoblast-like cells. Clin Exp Metast 1992; 10: 33–8.
18. Lacroix M, Siwek B, Body JJ. Effects of secretory products of breast cancer cells on osteoblast-like cells. Breast Cancer Res Treat 1996; 38: 209–16.
19. Siwek B, Lacroix M, dePollak C et al. Secretory products of breast cancer cells affect human osteoblastic cells: partial characterisation of active factors. J Bone Min Res 1997; 12: 552–60.
20. Ernst M, Heath JK, Rodan GA. Estradiol effects on proliferation, messenger ribonucleic acid for collagen and

insulin-like growth factor-1, and parathyroid hormone-stimulated adenylate cyclase activity in osteoblastic cells from calvariae and long bones. Endocrinology 1989; 125: 825–33.

21. Oursler MJ, Cortese C, Keeting PE et al. Modulation of transforming growth factor-β production in normal human osteoblast-like cells by 17β-estradiol and parathyroid hormone. Endocrinology 1991; 129: 3313–20.

22. Pfeilschifter J, Seyedin SM, Mundy GR. Transforming growth factor β inhibits bone resorption in fetal rat long bone cultures. J Clin Invest 1988; 82(2): 680–5.

23. Chenu C, Pfeilschifter J, Mundy GR, Roodman GD. Transforming growth factor β inhibits formation of osteoclast-like cells in long-term human marrow cultures. Proc Natl Acad Sci USA 1988; 85(15): 5683–7.

24. Noda M, Camilliere JJ. In vivo stimulation of bone formation by transforming growth factor-β. Endocrinology 1989; 124(6): 2991–4.

25. Black DM, Cummings SR, Karpf DB et al. For the Fracture Intervention Trial Research Group. Randomised trial of effect of alendronate on risk of fracture in women with existing vertebral fractures. Lancet 1996; 348: 1535–41.

26. Cummings SR, Black DM, Thompson DE et al. for the Fracture Intervention Trial Research Group. Effect of alendronate on risk of fracture in women with low bone density but without vertebral fractures. J Am Med Assoc 1998; 280: 2077–82.

27. Reginster J, Minne HW, Sorensen OH et al. Randomized trial of the effects of risedronate on vertebral fractures in women with established postmenopausal osteoporosis. Vertebral Efficacy with Risedronate Therapy (VERT) Study Group. Osteoporosis Int 2000; 11: 83–91.

28. Ettinger B, Black DM, Mitlak BH et al. for the Multiple Outcomes of Raloxifene Evaluation (MORE) Investigators. Reduction of vertebral fracture risk in postmenopausal women with osteoporosis treated with raloxifene. Results from a 3-year randomized clinical trial. J Am Med Assoc 1999; 282: 637–45.

29. Pols HAP, Felsenberg D, Hanley DA et al. for the Fosamax International Trial Study Group. Multinational, placebo-controlled, randomized trial of the effects of alendronate on bone density and fracture risk in postmenopausal women with low bone mass: results of the FOSIT study. Osteoporosis Int 1999; 9: 461–8.

30. Orwoll E, Ettinger M, Weiss S et al. Alendronate for the treatment of osteoporosis in men. N Engl J Med 2000; 343: 604–10.

31. McClung MR, Geusens P, Miller PD, Zippel H et al. Effect of risedronate on the risk of hip fracture in elderly women. N Engl J Med 2001; 344: 333–40.

32. McCloskey E, Selby P, de Takats D et al. Effects of clodronate on vertebral fracture risk in osteoporosis—a one-year interim analysis. Bone 2001; 28: 310–15.

33. Utz JP, Melton LJ, Kan SH, Riggs BL. Risk of osteoporotic fractures in women with breast cancer. A population band cohort study. J Chron Dis 1987; 40: 105–13.

34. Kanis JA, McCloskey EV, Powles T et al. A high incidence of vertebral fracture in women with breast cancer. Br J Cancer 1999; 79(7–8): 1179–81.

35. Bruning PF, Pit MJ, Jong-Bakker M et al. Bone mineral density after adjuvant chemotherapy for premenopausal breast cancer. Br J Cancer 1990; 61(2): 308–10.

36. Saarto T, Blomqvist C, Valimaki M et al. Chemical castration induced by adjuvant cyclophosphamide, methotrexate, and fluorouracil chemotherapy causes rapid bone loss that is reduced by clodronate: a randomized study in premenopausal breast cancer patients. J Clin Oncol 1997; 15: 1341–7.

37. Delmas PD, Balena R, Confravreux E et al. Bisphosphonate risedronate prevents bone loss in women with artificial menopause due to chemotherapy of breast cancer: a double-blind, placebo-controlled study. J Clin Oncol 1997; 15(3): 955–62.

38. Powles TJ, McCloskey E, Paterson AH et al. Oral clodronate and reduction in loss of bone mineral density in women with operable primary breast cancer. J Natl Cancer Inst 1998; 90(9): 704–8.

39 Powles TJ, Paterson AHG, Nevantaus A et al. Adjuvant clodronate reduces the incidence of bone metastases in patients with primary operable breast cancer. Prog Proc Am Soc Clin Oncol 1998; 17: 123a.

40. Shapiro CL, Manola J, Leboff M. Ovarian failure after adjuvant chemotherapy is associated with rapid bone loss in women with early-stage breast cancer. J Clin Oncol 2001; 19: 3306–11.

41. Powles TJ, Hickish T, Kanis JA et al. Effect of tamoxifen on bone mineral density measured by dual-energy X-ray absorptiometry in healthy premenopausal and postmenopausal women. J Clin Oncol 1996; 14(1): 78–84.

42. Mattison DR, Chang L, Thorgeirsson SS et al. The effects of cyclophosphamide, azathioprine, and 6-mercaptopurine on oocyte and follicle number in C57BL/6N mice. Res Commun Chem Pathol Pharmacol 1981; 31: 155–61.

43. Plowchalk DR, Mattison DR. Reproductive toxicity of cyclophosphamide in the C57BL/6N mouse: 1. Effects on ovarian structure and function. Reprod Toxicol 1992; 6: 411–21.

44. Ratcliffe MA, Lanham SA, Reid DM et al. Bone mineral density (BMD) in patients with lymphoma: the effects of chemotherapy, intermittent corticosteroids and premature menopause. Hematol Oncol 1992; 10: 181–7.

45. Schimmer AD, Quatermain M, Imrie K et al. Ovarian function after autologous bone marrow transplantation. J Clin Oncol 1998; 16: 2359–63.

46. Holmes SJ, Whitehouse RW, Clark ST et al. Reduced bone mineral density in men following chemotherapy for Hodgkin's disease. Br J Cancer 1994; 70: 371–5.

47. Sarafoglou K, Boulad F, Gillio A et al. Gonadal function after bone marrow transplantation for acute leukaemia during childhood. J Pediatr 1997; 130: 210–16.

48. Kauppila M, Viikari J, Irjala K et al. The hypothalamus–pituitary–gonad axis and testicular function in male patients after treatment for haematological malignancies. J Intern Med 1998; 244: 411–16.

49. Garrett TJ, Vahdat LT, Kinne DW. Systemic adjuvant therapy of breast cancer. J Surg Oncol 1997; 64: 167–72.

50. Johansen J, Riis B, Hassager C et al. The effect of gonadotrophin-releasing hormone agonist analog (nafarilin) on bone metabolism. J Clin Endocrinol Metab 1988; 67: 701–6.

51. Gambacciani M, Spinetti A, Piaggesi L et al. Ipriflavone prevents the bone mass reduction in premenopausal women treated with gonadotrophin hormone-releasing hormone agonist. Bone Min 1994; 26(1): 19–26.

52. Marshall D, Johnell O, Wedel H. Meta-analysis of how well measures of bone mineral density predict occurrence of osteoporotic fractures. Br Med J 1996; 312: 1254–9.

53. Kelloff GJ, Lubet RA, Lieberman R et al. Aromatase inhibitors as potential cancer chemopreventives. Cancer Epidemiol Biomark Prevent 1998; 7: 65–78.

54. Cummings SR, Browner WS, Bauer D et al. Endogenous hormones and the risk of hip and vertebral fractures among older women. Study of Osteoporotic Fractures Research Group [see comments]. N Engl J Med 1998; 339(11): 733–8.

55. Stone K, Bauer DC, Black DM et al. Hormonal predictors of bone loss in elderly women: a prospective study. The Study of Osteoporotic Fractures Research Group. J Bone Min Res 1998; 13(7): 1167–74.

56. Cauley JA, Lucas FL, Kuller LH et al. Bone mineral density and the risk of breast cancer in older women. J Am Med Assoc 1996; 267: 1404–8.

57. Daniell HW. Osteoporosis after orchiectomy for prostate cancer. J Urol 1997; 157(2): 439–44.

58. Collinson MP, Tyrrell CJ, Hutton C. Osteoporosis occurring in two patients receiving LHRH analogs for carcinoma of the prostate. Calcif Tissue Int 1994; 54: 327–8.

59. Maillefert JF, Sibilia J, Michel F et al. Bone mineral density in men treated with synthetic gonadotrophin-releasing hormone agonists for prostatic carcinoma. J Urol 1999; 161: 1219–22.

60. Townsend MF, Sanders WH, Northway RO et al. Bone fractures associated with luteinising hormone-releasing hormone agonists used in the treatment of prostate carcinoma. Cancer 1997; 79: 545–50.

61. Diamond T, Campbell J, Bryant C et al. The effect of combined androgen blockade on bone turnover and bone mineral densities in men treated for prostate carcinoma: longitudinal evaluation and response to intermittent cyclical etidronate therapy. Cancer 1998; 83: 1561–6.

62. Wang TM, Shih C. Study of histomorphometric changes of the mandibular condyles in neonatal and juvenile rats after administration of cyclophosphamide. Acta Anat 1986; 127: 93–9.

63. Friedlaender GE, Tross RB, Doganis AC et al. Effects of chemotherapeutic agents on bone. I. Short-term metho-trexate and doxorubicin (adriamycin) treatment in a rat model. J Bone Joint Surg Am 1984; 66(4): 602–7.

64. Schwartz AM, Leonidis JC. Methotrexate osteopathy. Skel Radiol 1984; 11: 13–16.

65. Ecklund K, Laor T, Goorin AM et al. Methotrexate osteopathy in patients with osteosarcoma. Radiology 1997; 202: 543–7.

66. Carbone LD, Kaeley G, McKown KM et al. Effects of long-term administration of methotrexate on bone mineral density in rheumatoid arthritis. Calcif Tissue Int 1999; 64: 100–1.

67. van Staa TP, Leufkens HG, Abenhaim L et al. Oral corticosteroids and fracture risk: relationship to daily and cumulative doses. Rheumatology (Oxford) 2000; 39: 1383–9.

68. van Staa TP, Leufkens HG, Abenhaim L et al. Use of oral corticosteroids and risk of fractures [review]. J Bone Min Res 2000; 15: 993–1000.

69. van Staa TP, Leufkens HG, Abenhaim L et al. Use of oral corticosteroids in the United Kingdom. Qu J Med 2000; 93: 105–11.

70. McCloskey EV, MacLennan ICM, Drayson M et al. A randomised trial of the effect of clodronate on skeletal morbidity in myelomatosis. Br J Haematol 1998; 100: 317–25.

71. Redman JR, Bajorunas DR, Wong G et al. Bone mineralization in women following successful treatment of Hodgkin's disease. Am J Med 1988; 85: 65–72.

72. Anonymous. Cautious approach warranted for ERT in breast cancer survivors. Drugs 1996; 8: 11–13.

73. Roy JA, Sawka CA, Pritchard KI. Hormone replacement therapy in women with breast cancer. Do the risks outweight the benefits? J Clin Oncol 1996; 14; 997–1006.

74. Cummings SR, Eckert S, Krueger KA et al. The effect of raloxifene on risk of breast cancer in postmenopausal women: results from the Multiple Outcomes of Raloxifene Evaluation (MORE) randomized trial. J Am Med Assoc 1999; 281(23): 2189–97.

75. Hortobagyi GN, Theriault RL, Porter L et al. Efficacy of pamidronate in reducing skeletal complications in patients with breast cancer and lytic bone metastases. Protocol 19 Aredia Breast Cancer Study Group [see comments]. N Engl J Med 1996; 335(24): 1785–91.

76. Hortobagyi GN, Theriault RL, Lipton A et al. Long-term prevention of skeletal complications of metastatic breast cancer with pamidronate. Protocol 19 Aredia Breast Cancer Study Group. J Clin Oncol 1998; 16(6): 2038–44.

77. Berenson JR, Lichtenstein A, Porter L et al. Efficacy of pamidronate in reducing skeletal events in patients with advanced multiple myeloma. Myeloma Aredia Study Group. N Engl J Med 1996; 334(8): 488–93.

78. Berenson JR, Lichtenstein A, Porter L et al. Long-term pamidronate treatment of advanced multiple myeloma patients reduces skeletal events. Myeloma Aredia Study Group. J Clin Oncol 1998; 16(2): 593–602.

79. Theriault RL, Lipton A, Hortobagyi GN et al. Pamidronate reduces skeletal morbidity in women with advanced breast cancer and lytic bone lesions: a randomized, placebo-controlled trial. Protocol 18 Aredia Breast Cancer Study Group. J Clin Oncol 1999; 17(3): 846–54.

80. Hultborn R, Gundersen S, Ryden S et al. Efficacy of pamidronate in breast cancer with bone metastases: a randomized double-blind placebo-controlled multicenter study. Acta Oncol 1996; 35(suppl 5): 73–4.

81. Paterson AH, Powles TJ, Kanis JA et al. Double-blind controlled trial of oral clodronate in patients with bone metastases from breast cancer. J Clin Oncol 1993; 11(1): 59–65.

82. Kanis JA, Powles T, Paterson AH et al. Clodronate decreases the frequency of skeletal metastases in women with breast cancer. Bone 1996; 19(6): 663–7.

83. Royal College of Physicians. Osteoporosis: Clinical Guidelines for Prevention and Management. RCOG: London, 1999.

84. World Health Organization. Assessment of fracture risk and its application to screening for postmenopausal osteoporosis. Report of the WHO Study Group. Technical Report Series 843. World Health Organization. Geneva.

85. Hui SL, Slemenda CW, Johnston CC Jr. Baseline measurement of bone mass predicts fracture in white women. Ann Intern Med 1989; 111: 355–61.

86. Cummings SR, Black DM, Nevitt MC et al. Bone density at various sites for prediction of hip fractures. The Study of Osteoporotic Fractures Research Group. Lancet 1993; 341: 72–5.

87. Frith JC, Mönkkönen J, Blackburn GM et al. Clodronate and liposome-encapsulated clodronate are metabolized to a toxic ATP analog, adenosine 5′(β,γ-dichloromethylene) triphosphate, by mammalian cells *in vitro*. J Bone Min Res 1997; 12: 1358–67.

88. Luckman SP, Coxon FP, Ebertino FH et al. Heterocycle-containing bisphosphonates cause apoptosis and inhibit bone resorption by preventing protein prenylation: evidence from structure–activity relationships in J774 macrophages. J Bone Min Res 1998; 13: 1668–78.

89. Saarto T, Blomqvist C, Valimaki M et al. Clodronate improves bone mineral density in post-menopausal breast cancer patients treated with adjuvant antioestrogens. Br J Cancer 1997; 75: 602–5.

90. Rizzoli R, Forni M, Schaad MA et al. Effects of oral clodronate on bone mineral density in patients with relapsing breast cancer. Bone 1996; 18: 531–7.

91. Koeberle D, Bacchus L, Thuerlimann B, Senn HJ. Pamidronate treatment in patients with malignant osteolytic bone disease and pain: a prospective randomized double-blind trial. Supp Care Cancer 1999; 7: 21–7.

92. Watts NB, Harris ST, Genant HK et al. Intermittent cyclical etidronate treatment of postmenopausal osteoporosis. N Engl J Med 1990; 323: 73–9.

93. Storm T, Thamsborg G, Steiniche T et al. Effect of intermittent cyclical etidronate therapy on bone mass and fracture rate in postmenopausal osteoporosis. N Engl J Med 1990; 322: 1265–71.

94. Reid IR, Wattie DJ, Evans MC et al. Continuous therapy with pamidronate, a potent bisphosphonate, in postmenopausal osteoporosis. J Clin Endocrinol Metab 1994; 79: 1595–9.

95. Diel IJ, Solomayer EF, Costa SD et al. Reduction in new metastases in breast cancer with adjuvant clodronate treatment. N Engl J Med 1998; 339(6): 357–63.

96. Fentiman IS, Saad Z, Caleffi M et al. Tamoxifen protects against steroid-induced bone loss. Eur J Cancer 1992; 28(2–3): 684–5.

97. Adachi JD, Bensen WG, Brown J et al. Intermittent etidronate therapy to prevent corticosteroid-induced osteoporosis. N Engl J Med 1997; 337: 382–7.

98. Saag KG, Emkey R, Schnitzer TJ et al. Alendronate for the prevention and treatment of glucocorticoid-induced osteoporosis. N Engl J Med 1998; 339: 292–9.

99. Reid DM, Hughes RA, Laan RF et al. Efficacy and safety of daily risedronate in the treatment of corticosteroid-induced osteoporosis in men and women: a randomized trial. European Corticosteroid-induced Osteoporosis Treatment Study J Bone Min Res 2000; 15(6): 1006–13.

100. Grey AB, Stapleton JP, Evans MC et al. The effect of the antioestrogen tamoxifen on bone mineral density in normal late postmenopausal women. Am J Med 1995; 99: 636–41.

101. Love RR, Mazess RB, Barden HS et al. Effects of tamoxifen on bone mineral density in postmenopausal women with breast cancer. N Engl J Med 1992; 326(13): 852–6.

102. Love RR, Barden HS, Mazess RB et al. Effect of tamoxifen on lumbar spine bone mineral density in postmenopausal women after 5 years. Arch Intern Med 1994; 154(22): 2585–8.

103. Kristensen B, Ejlertsen B, Mouridsen HT et al. Femoral fractures in postmenopausal breast cancer patients treated with adjuvant tamoxifen. Breast Cancer Res Treat 1996; 39(3): 321–6.

104. Kanis JA, McCloskey EV, Powles T et al. A high incidence of vertebral fracture in women with breast cancer. Br J Cancer 1999; 79(7–8): 1179–81.

105. Fisher B, Constantino JP, Wickerham DL et al. Tamoxifen for prevention of breast cancer: report of the National Surgical Adjuvant Breast and Bowel Project P-1 Study. J Natl Cancer Inst 1998; 90: 1371–88.

106. Harris ST, Watts NB, Genant HK et al. Effects of risedronate treatment on vertebral and nonvertebral fractures in women with postmenopausal osteoporosis: a randomized controlled trial. Vertebral Efficacy With Risedronate Therapy (VERT) Study Group. J Am Med Assoc 1999; 282: 1344–52.

107. Wright CD, Compston JE. Tamoxifen: oestrogen or anti-oestrogen in bone? Qu J Med 1995; 88(5): 307–10.

108. Marshall LA, Cain DF, Dmowski WP et al. Urinary N-telopeptides to monitor bone resorption while on GnRH agonist therapy. Obstet Gynecol 1996; 87(3): 350–4.

33

Cost Implications of Bisphosphonates

E. V. McCloskey,[1] **J. F. Guest,**[2] **R. U. Ashford**[1] **and J. A. Kanis**[1]

[1]*University of Sheffield Medical School, Sheffield, UK,* [2]*Catalyst Health Economics Consultants Ltd, Pinner, UK*

INTRODUCTION

Bone destruction and its clinical sequelae are a significant cause of morbidity in patients with cancer. Furthermore, despite progress in antitumour therapy and the use of more aggressive regimens, the incidence of skeletal disease remains high and, in contrast to visceral metastases, is frequently associated with prolonged survival. Bone pain is observed in both osteosclerotic and osteolytic disease, but hypercalcaemia and pathological fracture are most frequently associated with osteolysis. Regardless of the tumour type, there is compelling evidence that this bone destruction is mediated by normal osteoclasts (bone-resorbing cells) stimulated by factors produced by the tumour or by stromal cells in response to the presence of tumour [1,2]. The bisphosphonates are potent inhibitors of osteoclast-mediated bone resorption (for review, see [3,4]). These agents are now the treatment of choice for the management of hypercalcaemia due to malignancy. Several studies have examined their ability to decrease the incidence of skeletal complications in malignancies, particularly breast cancer and myelomatosis. This chapter focuses on studies addressing the long-term efficacy of bisphosphonates in breast cancer and multiple myeloma, with particular reference to controlled studies of sufficient magnitude and duration to allow confidence in the estimation of efficacy. Data from these studies have then been used to derive some estimates of the cost implications of the long-term use of bisphosphonates. Comparisons between the various bisphosphonates, and indeed between studies, are difficult due to a lack of common definitions of outcome measures. These agents have not been associated with significant improvements in overall survival in patients with malignancy, thus preventing estimates of the cost per life year gained. A number of studies have reported prolonged survival in subgroup analyses that should ideally be confirmed in appropriately designed clinical trials [5–9]. If confirmed, such effects could have a marked effect on the cost–benefit ratios of bisphosphonate therapy. Most studies have not collected or reported quality-of-life data, thus preventing the derivation of a cost–utility ratio, such as the cost per quality-adjusted life year (QALY). Finally, the use of multiple measures of clinical effectiveness that are difficult to combine into a common denominator has limited the ability to undertake analyses of cost-effectiveness.

THE BURDEN OF SKELETAL COMPLICATIONS IN MALIGNANCY

Approximately 30 000 new cases of breast cancer are diagnosed each year in the UK. Of those developing recurrent disease, 30% will develop their first metastases in bone and skeletal disease will be present in approximately 80% at death. Women with predominantly skeletal disease survive significantly longer compared to those with visceral disease (particularly liver and CNS metastases). A similar burden of disease is observed in prostate cancer in men. Multiple myeloma affects approximately 3000 new patients each year in the UK, with skeletal destruction being a prominent feature at the time of diagnosis [8].

Textbook of Bone Metastases. Edited by C. Jasmin, R. E. Coleman, L. R. Coia, R. Capanna and G. Saillant
Published 2005 by John Wiley & Sons Ltd: ISBN 0 471 87742 5. © 2001 Adis International Ltd

The most common skeletal complications of neo-plasia are hypercalcaemia, bone pain and fractures at both axial and appendicular sites. In contrast to studies documenting the prevalence of skeletal complications in malignancy, there are few data from prospective studies describing the incidence of such complications during the course of the disease. Some estimate of the incidence can be derived from the control wings of placebo-controlled studies of bisphosphonates in myeloma and breast cancer metastatic to bone (Table 33.1). There are obvious difficulties in extrapolating such data to the routine clinical setting, since selection criteria for studies can exclude patients with severe or mild disease, leading respectively to under- or over-estimation of the incidence. Further-more, the methods of reporting incidence are not uniform across the studies. Bearing these limitations in mind, the incidence of skeletal complications is high despite apparent responses to systemic therapy (Table 33.1). The incidence and event rates are particularly high in women with advanced skeletal metastases in breast cancer, where approximately 25–40% of patients will require radiotherapy for bone pain, 25–50% will sustain incident vertebral fractures and a similar proportion may sustain non-vertebral fractures. Hypercalcaemia is also common, occurring in approximately 30% of patients annually, although the incidence of severe hypercalcaemia (serum calcium adjusted for albumin $>3.00\,mmol/l$) is somewhat lower (approximately 10%). It should be noted, however, that the incidence of hypercalcaemia and pathological vertebral fracture is also substantial in women, with recurrence apparently limited to soft tissue and visceral sites. The incidence of complications in myeloma appears to be lower than in patients with skeletal disease in breast cancer, but new vertebral fractures occur in about 15–30% of patients annually and peripheral fractures occur in approximately 10%.

Multiple complications within an individual are common, so that estimates based on events per 100 patient-years (Table 33.1) exceed estimates of incidence computed as the proportion of patients with each event. The majority of studies that have reported event rates and the number of patients affected, show that the event rates are usually two- to three-fold higher (Table 33.1).

EFFECTIVENESS OF BISPHOSPHONATES IN REDUCING SKELETAL COMPLICATIONS

It is important to note that to date there have been no direct comparative studies of long-term bisphosphonates in malignancy. Differences in patient selection, concomitant therapies and the assessment of outcome complicate any attempt to draw comparisons between the various trials. These limitations need to be borne in mind when the efficacy in each of the clinical trials is expressed in a unified way, e.g. as a percentage reduction in the incidence of skeletal complications.

Although a large number of studies have examined the effects of bisphosphonates in neoplastic bone disease, many have only involved small numbers of patients or examined short-term efficacy and others have been open, uncontrolled studies. A number of relatively large (total sample sizes of more than 100 patients) randomised placebo-controlled studies of more than 6 months duration have been published that allow better estimates of the efficacy of these agents to be derived. The reduction in the incidences of skeletal complications reported in these studies are summarised in Table 33.2.

Prevention of Hypercalcaemia

The definition of hypercalcaemia has varied between studies, with thresholds ranging from $2.6\,mmol/l$ (adjusted for serum albumin) to $3.0\,mmol/l$ (usually referred to as severe hypercalcaemia). Mild hypercalcaemia is not always actively treated, however, so that some studies have utilised the higher threshold (e.g. $3.0\,mmol/l$), a level at which clinical intervention (usually rehydration, corticosteroids if appropriate and possible use of bisphosphonates) is required. All but two of the nine placebo-controlled studies have shown marked reductions in the incidence of hyper-calcaemia during treatment with bisphosphonates (Table 33.2), with estimated reductions of 63% and 37% in the number of events in breast cancer and multiple myeloma, respectively. The lower apparent efficacy in myelomatosis largely reflects the failure of pamidronate to reduce the incidence of hypercalcaemia [5,6].

Pathological Fracture

The acquisition of data on fractures differs for vertebral and non-vertebral fractures. Whilst most non-vertebral fractures are clinically obvious, vertebral fractures may be difficult to detect. Assessment of the latter can be undertaken by visual assessment of changes in shape between radiographs but vertebral fractures frequently involve subtle changes. The major limitation of purely visual assessments is that they are very subjective and lead to poor concordance between

Table 33.1. Estimated incidences of skeletal complications in multiple myeloma and advanced breast cancer

Reference	Malignancy	Number of patients	Population	Median duration (months)	Percentage of patients developing complication annually (event rate/100 patient-years)				
					Pain*	Hypercalcaemia	Fracture		
							Any	Vertebral	Non-vertebral
Belch et al. [26]	Myeloma	173	At first treatment	44	– (–)	5 (–)[b]	– (–)	– (–)	8 (–)
Lahtinen et al. [18]	Myeloma	336	At first treatment	24	– (–)	– (–)	– (–)	20 (–)[d]	12 (–)
Brincker et al. [16]	Myeloma	300	At first treatment	18	– (26)	– (13)[a]	– (59)	– (38)[d]	– (21)
Berenson et al. [5,6]	Myeloma	392	On chemotherapy	18	24 (–)	5 (–)[b]	21 (–)	15 (–)	6 (–)
McCloskey et al. [8]	Myeloma	536	At first treatment	31	–	3 (5)[b]	– (39)	31 (35)[c]	3 (4)
Paterson et al. [17]	Breast	173	Bone metastases	14	41 (89)	30 (52)	– (164)	50 (124)[c]	23 (40)
Kanis et al. [15]	Breast	133	Non-bone metastases	20	12 (19)	8 (12)	– (67)	17 (61)[c]	5 (6)
Hortobagyi et al. [14,35]	Breast	382	Bone metastases	10	23 (84)	8 (19)[b]	25 (174)	25 (74)[c]	39 (100)
Theriault et al. [7]	Breast	371	Bone metastases	16	28 (90)	6 (17)[b]	44 (210)	22 (80)[c]	31 (140)
Hultborn et al. [19]	Breast	404	Bone metastases	12	28 (40)	9 (9)[e]	–	–	16[f] (20)

Data derived from placebo arms of double-blind controlled trials. –, Not recorded. [a]Serum calcium >2.75 mmol/l; [b]serum calcium >3.00 mmol/l; [c]using vertebral morphometry (but different criteria); [d]subjective radiological reading; [e]requiring treatment (level not defined); [f]pelvis and long bones only. *Pain recorded as number of radiotherapy episodes.

Table 33.2. Reduction in skeletal complications of malignancy in double-blind placebo-controlled studies of clodronate and pamidronate

Reference	Tumour	n	Agent	Dose (mg)	Population	Estimated reduction in event rate (%)		Fracture	
						Radio-therapy	Hyper-calcaemia	Vertebral	Non-vertebral
Lahtinen et al. [18]	Myeloma	336	Clodronate	2400	At first treatment	ne (ns)	nr (ns)	−25 (ns)	0 (ns)
McCloskey et al. [8]	Myeloma	536	Clodronate	1600	At first treatment	ne (ns)	−60 (0.06)	−45 (0.001)	−45 (0.025)
Brincker et al. [16]	Myeloma	300	Pamidronate	300	At first treatment	−27 (ns)	−62 (ns)	−24 (ns)	−43 (ns)
Berenson et al. [6]	Myeloma	392	Pamidronate	90, 4-weekly	On chemotherapy	−27 (0.06)	+13 (ns)	−41 (0.005)	ne (ns)
Paterson et al. [17]	Breast	173	Clodronate	1600	Bone metastases	−6 (ns)	−46 (0.01)	−32 (0.025)	−20 (ns)
Kanis et al. [15]	Breast	133	Clodronate	1600	Soft tissue metastases	−20 (ns)	−39 (ns)	−22 (0.1)	−75 (0.1)
Hortobagyi et al. [14]	Breast	382	Pamidronate	90, 4-weekly	Bone metastases	−49 (0.001)	−67 (0.005)	−39	−34 (0.001)
Theriault et al. [7]	Breast	371	Pamidronate	90, 3/4-weekly	Bone metastases	−45 (0.011)	−65 (0.037)	−23 (0.43)	−36 (0.36)
Hultborn et al. [19]	Breast	404	Pamidronate	60, 4-weekly	Bone metastases	−10 (ns)	−71 (<0.05)	ne	−3 (ns)*
Weighted mean reduction in multiple myeloma						−27	−37	−37	−32
Weighted mean reduction in breast cancer						−31	−63	−30	−28

Values in parentheses show the *p*-values from the relevant studies.
ne, not evaluable from the data presented; nr, not reported; ns, not statistically significant; *pelvic and long bone fractures only.

classifications by different radiologists. For this reason, information on vertebral fractures is increasingly obtained using morphometric evaluations of X-rays [10]. Such approaches involve the measurement of vertebral heights on lateral spine radiographs and compare vertebral height ratios to appropriate reference data. The attraction of such approaches is that they standardise the definition of vertebral fracture and, by choosing more stringent criteria for deformity, increase the specificity of the evaluations [11,12]. The outcome of differences in detection of vertebral and non-vertebral fracture is that the effects of treatments on each type of fracture are usually reported separately.

Non-vertebral Fracture

Fractures at all sites other than the thoracic and lumbar spine are usually included in the category of non-vertebral fractures. The actual sites of fracture are rarely recorded in published reports and it is therefore not possible to comment on issues such as the method of recording simultaneous multiple fractures (e.g. do multiple rib fractures count as one event or more?) and further fracture or re-fracture within a bone. The site of fracture has a significant impact on the patient and health care resources [13]. For example, long bone fractures usually require hospitalisation and surgical fixation [13] and this has a significant bearing on the costs of therapy. It is usual practice to exclude fractures, particularly long bone fractures, which occur as the result of significant trauma (e.g. road traffic accidents).

Six of the nine studies support the conclusion that long-term treatment with a bisphosphonate reduces the incidence of non-vertebral fractures. Two studies have shown statistically significant reductions in the proportion of patients sustaining non-vertebral fractures [8,14]. A second study with clodronate in breast cancer also showed a borderline effect [15]. Non-significant decreases were observed in myeloma with pamidronate by mouth [16] and in breast cancer with oral clodronate [17]. No apparent effect was observed in two studies of myeloma [6,18] and one breast cancer study [19]. The reasons for these results are unclear. In addition to the usual possibilities of inadequate dose and poor compliance, the explanation may relate to differences in recording of non-vertebral fractures.

As stated previously, the costs of long bone fractures are greater as they require hospitalisation and surgical fixation. Three studies have reported either a reduction in long bone fractures (82% effect) [8] or in the

requirement for surgery (58% and 55%, respectively) [14,16]. Reductions in appendicular fractures have been reported with bisphosphonates in other diseases, particularly postmenopausal osteoporosis [20,21].

Vertebral Fracture

Vertebral fractures are one of the most frequent complications of malignancy (Tables 33.2 and 33.3). They may result directly from the metastatic process or alternatively reflect the effect of systemic treatment on gonadal function and bone loss [22–25]. Regardless of the mechanism, bisphosphonate therapy should be expected to decrease the incidence of vertebral fracture. Comparison between the studies in this review is complicated by the lack of uniformity in the method of defining both prevalent and incident vertebral fractures. All evaluable studies demonstrate a 20–45% reduction in vertebral fracture event rates and in three of the eight studies the reduction in risk was significant [6,8,17]. In all of the other studies, similar reductions in the incidence of vertebral fractures were observed and the lack of significance may partly relate to the type of analysis undertaken. For example, Lahtinen and colleagues observed a 25% reduction in patients sustaining vertebral fractures but did not report the total number of fractures in each group [18]. Hortobagyi and associates reported that intravenous pamidronate had no significant effect in reducing the number of patients reporting fractures, but the total number of fractures was 39% lower during pamidronate therapy [14].

It is likely that much of the discrepancy between studies lies in the lack of consensus on the definition of vertebral fracture. This lack of standardisation also raises the question of the clinical relevance of vertebral fractures recorded during clinical trials. There are obvious clinical correlates of vertebral fracture that can be examined but unfortunately these have not been reported in the majority of clinical trials. These include back pain and height loss [12]. In women with advanced metastatic breast cancer, the requirement for radiotherapy to the spine is about two-fold higher than that to the peripheral skeleton, and there is a clear association between incident vertebral fractures defined morphometrically and the requirement for spinal radiotherapy [17]. It is likely, therefore, that the reduction in radiotherapy requirements or back pain reported in most studies is at least partially mediated by a decrease in the incidence of clinically-relevant vertebral fractures.

Table 33.3. Estimates of numbers-needed-to-treat (NNT) for 1 year to prevent one skeletal complication (hypercalcaemia, vertebral or non-vertebral fracture)

Disease	Hypercalcaemia			Vertebral fracture			Non-vertebral fracture		
	Risk	RR	NNT	Risk	RR	NNT	Risk	RR	NNT
Myeloma	9	0.63	30 (20–60)	36	0.63	8 (5–15)	10	0.68	31 (21–63)
Breast cancer									
Soft tissue metastases only	12	0.61	21 (14–43)	61	0.78	7 (5–15)	6	0.25	22 (15–44)
Bone metastases	20	0.37	8 (5–16)	86	0.70	4 (3–8)	81	0.72	4 (3–8)

The risk is computed as the mean event rate per 100 patient-years, weighted by study size from Table 33.1. The relative risk (RR) during treatment with a bisphosphonate is derived from Table 33.2. Numbers in parentheses represent the NNT if the risk of event was 50% higher or 50% lower than estimated (or alternatively if the reduction in risk was 50% greater or 50% lower).

A clear relationship exists between vertebral fractures and height loss, with a progressive increase in height loss occurring with increasing numbers of prevalent and/or incident vertebral fractures [12]. Prevention of clinically relevant vertebral fractures should therefore decrease height loss and this has been demonstrated in myeloma, using clodronate 1600 mg daily over 3–4 years from initial diagnosis [8]. A reduction in height loss has also been reported during oral pamidronate therapy [16]. Despite a reported non-significant difference in the incidence of vertebral collapses, height loss was noted to be significantly less in the pamidronate group (1.5 vs. 3 cm, $p=0.02$) suggesting problems with the definition of vertebral collapses rather than the efficacy of the drug. There was no difference in reported height loss between etidronate-treated patients and placebo-treated patients in the study by the National Cancer Institute of Canada Clinical Trials Group [26]. The latter study also showed no effect of treatment to reduce deterioration in the vertebral index, a subjective grading system for vertebral deformity.

In summary, a significant reduction of pathological fracture incidence (vertebral and/or non-vertebral fractures) is reported in five of the nine studies reviewed. The estimated treatment effects are very similar for both vertebral (30–37% reduction) and non-vertebral fractures (28–32% reduction) and are also similar in breast cancer and myeloma.

Bone Pain

Like vertebral fracture, the assessment of bone pain is also fraught with difficulties, particularly in long-term studies, and has rarely been performed in an adequate manner. The relationship between reported pain, direct pain assessments and radiotherapy requirements is complex and is illustrated by the observations of Hultborn and colleagues. In their study of metastatic breast cancer, pamidronate use was associated with a highly significant reduction ($p=0.006$) in symptoms of skeletal progression, largely reflecting pain, but had no significant effect on the requirement for palliative radiotherapy and no significant reduction in bone pain assessed by visual analogue scale [19].

The effect of high dose intravenous or intramuscular bisphosphonates to treat bone pain in malignancy in the short term is well documented [27–30]. However, long-term intervention studies have demonstrated that the incidence and severity of bone pain can be reduced. In myeloma, for example, the proportion of patients who were pain-free at 24 months of follow-up in the Finnish study increased from 24% at entry to 54% during clodronate therapy ($p<0.001$) compared to an increase from 29% to 44% in the placebo group ($p<0.01$) [18]. The difference between the groups was, however, not statistically significant. Similarly, in the MRC VIth Myeloma Trial, the increased frequencies of back pain and poor performance status associated with disease relapse were significantly lower in clodronate than in placebo-treated patients (10.9 vs. 19.9%, $p<0.05$; and 18.3 vs. 30.5%, $p<0.025$, respectively) [8]. Reductions in bone pain and analgesic consumption have also been noted in small double-blind studies and open-controlled studies in myeloma [31–33]. Intermittent intravenous pamidronate has also shown reductions in pain scores, at least during the first nine cycles of treatment [5]. In a combined analysis of the Hortobagyi and Theriault studies of pamidronate in breast cancer, bone pain was assessed by a pain score that reflected both severity and frequency of pain and quality of life was measured using the Spitzer index [34]. The treatment was associated with a significant reduction in the deterioration of bone pain between the first and last visits for each patient (0.72 ± 3.49 vs. 1.65 ± 3.40 in pamidronate and placebo groups, respectively; $p<0.001$). The deterioration in quality of life was also less marked in the pamidronate group (-1.80 ± 2.81 vs. -2.13 ± 2.63), although this was not statistically significant ($p=0.088$) [34].

Many studies, particularly those in breast cancer, have utilised skeletal radiotherapy requirements as a surrogate for pain assessment (Tables 33.1 and 33.2). Decreases in radiotherapy requirements have been observed during treatment with oral and intermittent intravenous bisphosphonates [14,17,35]. In myeloma, intermittent pamidronate appears to decrease the requirements for radiotherapy in patients with more advanced disease receiving second-line chemotherapy but had no effect in patients with less advanced disease [5,6]. The latter outcome is similar to that observed in the MRC Myeloma Trial with clodronate, where the event rate for radiotherapy was low [8].

COSTS OF LONG-TERM BISPHOSPHONATE THERAPY IN MALIGNANCY

Long-term bisphosphonate therapy in malignancy is commonly regarded as relatively expensive. A total of four economic studies have been published, three of which have addressed the use of oral clodronate [13,36,37] and another the use of intravenous pamidronate [38]. Again, comparisons between studies are hindered by differences in the measurement of study outcomes and the use of multiple outcomes prevents attempts at comparative cost-effectiveness analyses. Furthermore, most studies have not collected information on quality of life to allow derivation of costs per quality-adjusted life year.

The use of clodronate in the Finnish Myeloma Study [18] was not found to significantly increase treatment costs in an analysis published by Laakso and colleagues [37]. This analysis comprised a review of the medical records of 312 patients (93%) of the study participants to document the total lengths of hospital admissions and derived costs from official national figures. They noted that the benefits of clodronate on the skeleton (a 50% reduction in patients with progressive osteolysis) were associated with a non-significant 12% reduction in hospital costs due to a lower requirement for hospitalisation (Figure 33.1). The concomitant use of clodronate was associated with a 22% increase in overall costs of treatment (278 vs. 227 FM daily) but again, the difference from placebo was not statistically significant (Figure 33.1).

A more robust analysis of the costs of treatment with clodronate in myeloma was undertaken more recently [13] using data derived from the MRC VIth Myeloma Trial [8]. Using a state-transition model for the first 4 years of the study and resource utilisation data from trial investigators, the authors estimated the mean costs of each transition state and each skeletal complication. Clodronate was found to reduce the mean costs of skeletal complications by 50% from £2860 to £1376 over the 4 years of treatment. The costs of clodronate itself increased the overall management costs by £3377 (from £19 557 to £22 934), an increase of 17% (Figure 33.2). This estimate was shown to be robust (£2605–4150) by sensitivity analysis [13]. It should be borne in mind that the additional cost does not take into account any additional benefits over and above a reduction in the costs of skeletal complications, most notably any gains in quality of life.

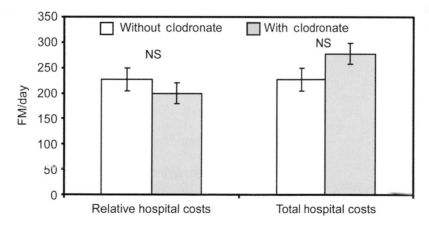

Figure 33.1. Costs of clodronate treatment derived from the Finnish multicentre trial [37]. The relative hospital costs represents the total hospital costs divided by the length of follow-up (Finnish Marks per day; 1FM £0.12). The total relative costs includes the cost of clodronate treatment

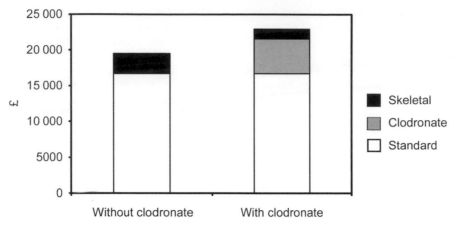

Figure 33.2. Mean costs of managing patients with multiple myeloma with and without clodronate treatment in the MRC VIth Myeloma Trial [13]. The use of clodronate was associated with a 17% increase in overall costs but achieved an approximate 50% reduction in the costs of skeletal complications

In an analysis of hospital costs associated with osteolytic metastases, Biermann and colleagues suggested that significant savings could be made if clodronate reduced the incidence of skeletal complications by at least 20% [36]. The studies included in this review suggest that such a reduction in hypercalcaemia, bone pain and pathological fractures is realistically achieved during bisphosphonate therapy. However, in a recent cost-effectiveness analysis of pamidronate usage in metastatic breast cancer, the authors concluded that the treatment is associated with high incremental costs per adverse event avoided [38]. This analysis was based on information on event rates and efficacy of pamidronate, derived from the studies of Hortobagyi and Theriault [7,14,35], with a number of well-documented assumptions being used in the model. Pamidronate use was associated with an approximate 50% reduction in the costs of treating skeletal complications but with a 28–61% increase in the total costs for management of each patient, depending on whether the analysis was conducted in patients receiving chemotherapy or hormonal therapy (Figure 33.3). The resulting cost-effectiveness ratios were $108 200 and $305 300 per quality-adjusted life year in women treated with chemotherapy or hormonal therapy, respectively. The costs of pamidronate and costs associated with pathological fractures that were asymptomatic or treated conservatively were the major cost drivers in the model. A reduction in drug costs by 38% would have resulted in a significant reduction in skeletal events at no extra cost (cost-equivalence) and the authors proposed a number of mechanisms by which this might be achieved [38]. The suggestions that a dose reduction or an increase in

treatment intervals could be beneficial are difficult to recommend, given the available data. It should be noted, however, that half of the cost reduction could be achieved if the need for an intravenous infusion could be avoided altogether. Hospitalisation is the major cost driver in the management of patients with malignancy and accounted for 32% of the total cost of managing patients over the first 4 years following diagnosis of multiple myeloma [13] (Figure 33.4). Additionally, outpatient and day-ward attendances accounted for a further 28% of the overall cost of managing patients, whereas chemotherapy accounted for only 5%. Therefore, treatment regimens that reduce the use of secondary care resources will reduce the overall cost of managing multiple myeloma, even if they do not lead to cost savings.

The achievement of cost savings, however, depends not only on the reduction by treatment but in the incidence of these complications in the population being treated. Thus, the failure of Bruce et al. to reproduce Biermann's finding of potential cost savings probably results from the lower incidence of skeletal complications in the MRC VIth Myeloma Trial [8]. It is certainly clear that the numbers-needed-to-treat (NNT) will be greater in multiple myeloma and early breast cancer than in women with established skeletal metastases in breast cancer (Table 33.3). However, even in myeloma the NNTs compare very favourably with the use of treatments as secondary prevention in other diseases, such as stroke reductions in patients with a previous stroke or transient ischaemic attacks (TIA) [39,40].

In Table 33.4, the annual additional costs for the use of bisphosphonates in multiple myeloma and breast

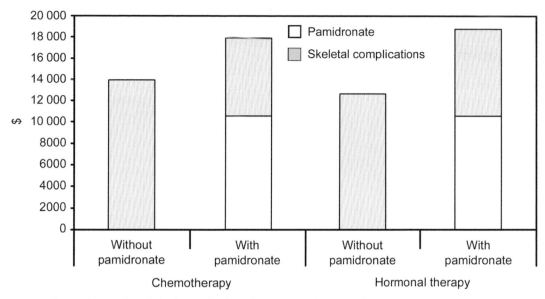

Figure 33.3. Costs of managing skeletal complications in women with metastatic breast cancer with and without the use of pamidronate [38]. Treatment reduced the cost of skeletal complications by up to 50% and increased the overall costs by 28% and 61% in patients receiving chemotherapy or hormonal therapy respectively

cancer have been computed using the NNT data from Table 33.3 and the costs of skeletal complications and drug reported from the economic analysis of the MRC VIth Myelomatosis Trial [13]. The average cost of a non-vertebral fracture was estimated to be £1902, assuming that incident non-vertebral fractures comprised fractures at long bone sites (15% and 10% of total non-vertebral fractures for lower and upper limb, respectively) and other sites (75% of the total, with costs assumed to be equivalent to rib fractures). The sites of fractures have been derived from unpublished data of a bisphosphonate intervention trial. The analysis suggests that the use of a bisphosphonate in myelomatosis is associated with an average additional

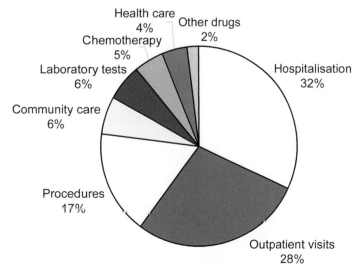

Figure 33.4. The proportion of standard management costs accounted for by different resources in the management of patients with multiple myeloma in the UK [13]

cost of £809 per patient per year, and is in keeping with the results from the economic analysis of the MRC study, in which the additional costs over 4 years were estimated to be £3377 [13]. It is of interest to note that in women with skeletal metastases in breast cancer, the average additional cost of the use of a bisphosphonate is effectively cost-neutral (Table 33.4)

OPTIONS TO REDUCE COSTS—WHEN SHOULD BISPHOSPHONATE THERAPY BE INTRODUCED AND DISCONTINUED?

None of the studies carried out to date have specifically addressed these questions. However, it is clear that long-term bisphosphonate therapy shows benefits when given early in the course of the disease [8,41,42] or at later stages in breast cancer and myeloma [5,6,14,15,17,35].

In myeloma, the progression of skeletal disease is probably at its most active at or around the time of diagnosis, as judged by biochemical markers of bone turnover and the high prevalence of baseline fractures. These observations, combined with the apparent survival benefit in patients with a lower burden of skeletal disease at diagnosis, suggest that treatment should probably be commenced as early as possible. The higher incidence of breast cancer makes the possible use of bisphosphonates in all women at the time of diagnosis problematic and perhaps undesirable. Targeting of women at high risk of skeletal metastases would seem a reasonable approach (larger

tumours, axillary node involvement, bone marrow involvement) but the optimal duration of therapy is not yet known. In women with advanced skeletal metastases, it might also be possible to target individuals at highest risk of skeletal complications but no studies have yet addressed this specific question. Guidelines have been proposed and, whilst they appear sensible, it is important to note that they have not been validated.

The decision about if and when to stop treatment is also difficult. It is important to remember that myeloma and metastatic breast cancer are presently incurable diseases and osteolysis will continue throughout their course. The speed of offset of the action of the bisphosphonates is unknown but is likely to be greater in malignancy than in other diseases associated with lower rates of bone turnover. Two double-blind controlled studies in breast cancer have suggested that the risk of skeletal disease increases within a few months after stopping bisphosphonate treatment [41,43]. A third controlled but open study suggests a more prolonged effect [42]. At present it would seem reasonable to continue treatment with bisphosphonates indefinitely.

There has been some concern about resistance developing to bisphosphonates in the later stages of malignant disease but there is little or no evidence that this is a clinically relevant problem. An increased incidence of skeletal events has been noted in only a few studies. For example, in myeloma patients receiving intermittent pamidronate, the incidence of fracture was similar or slightly higher than in those receiving placebo during the later stage of treatment and contrasted with a marked reduction during earlier cycles of treatment [5,6]. The reasons for this are not clear but are more likely to represent either an insufficient dose or frequency in patients with advancing disease, rather than resistance to treatment. The possibility that more frequent exposure may prevent this waning of effect is supported by the observation that there did not appear to be a reduction in the efficacy of oral clodronate, administered daily, in the MRC VIth Myeloma Trial [8]. A remote possibility is that long-term pamidronate, like etidronate, may impair mineralisation of bone and this might mask the benefit accruing from inhibition of bone resorption [26,44].

It is important to remember that the occurrence of complications is reduced but not totally prevented by bisphosphonates. The onset of a complication in a treated patient should therefore be regarded as an indication to consider more aggressive bisphosphonate therapy, rather than to deem it a treatment failure and

Table 33.4. Estimates of additional annual cost per treated patient for the use of bisphosphonates in preventing skeletal complications

Disease	NNT	Additional annual cost per patient (£)
Multiple myeloma	31 (21–63)	809 (622–1007)
Breast cancer with soft tissue metastases only	22 (15–44)	745 (533–973)
Breast cancer with skeletal metastases	8 (5–16)	−23 (−757–588)

NNTs, represent the numbers-needed-to-treat for 1 year to prevent at least one of each skeletal complication (hypercalcaemia, vertebral or non-vertebral fracture) derived from Table 33.3, with the numbers in parentheses representing the NNT if the risk of events were 50% higher or 50% lower than estimated. The costs used for each complication were those reported by Bruce et al. [13] (hypercalcaemia £1730, vertebral fracture £2126, peripheral fracture £1902—see text for description). The bisphosphonate costs were estimated to be £1200 per annum [13].

to discontinue therapy. The use of biochemical markers of bone resorption to monitor osteolysis and adequacy of response to bisphosphonates is undergoing evaluation and may improve clinical decision making [45–47].

SUMMARY

The rationale for the use of the bisphosphonates in tumour-induced osteolysis is well established [48]. The evidence to date supports the view that, whilst systemic chemotherapy is effective in reducing bone resorption, bone destruction continues in myeloma and breast cancer, so that supplementary bone protection should be considered. Long-term treatment with clodronate or pamidronate has been shown to modify the progression of skeletal disease. Despite the reservations of some authors, the efficacies of oral and intravenous bisphosphonates seem similar in breast cancer and myeloma [49]. The numbers-needed-to-treat, particularly in metastatic breast cancer, compare very favourably with the use of treatments as secondary prevention in other diseases. The limited economic analysis that is available currently suggests that, at least in the UK, the use of bisphosphonates in women with skeletal metastases is approximately cost-neutral. Further research is required to determine whether we can better identify sub-groups of patients who will derive particular benefit, or perhaps not benefit at all, from bisphosphonate therapy. The use of biochemical markers of bone resorption and formation to evaluate the risk of skeletal disease and its response to treatment also requires further study.

ACKNOWLEDGEMENTS

The authors wish to acknowledge that substantial parts of this chapter have been reprinted from McCloskey EV, Guest JF, Kanis JA. The clinical and cost considerations of bisphosphonates in preventing bone complications in patients with metastatic breast cancer or multiple myeloma. Drugs 2001; 61(9):1253–1274, ©Adis International Limited, 2001.

REFERENCES

1. Taube T, Elomaa I, Blomqvist C et al. Histomorphometric evidence for osteoclast-mediated bone resorption in metastatic breast cancer. Bone 1994; 15(2): 161–6.

2. Croucher PI, Apperley JF. Bone disease in multiple myeloma. Br J Haematol 1998; 103(4): 902–10.

3. Fleisch H. Bisphosphonates: mechanisms of action. Endocr Rev 1998; 19(1): 80–100.

4. Fleisch H. From polyphosphates to bisphosphonates and their role in bone and calcium metabolism. Prog Mol Subcell Biol 1999; 23: 197–216.

5. Berenson JR, Lichtenstein A, Porter L et al. Efficacy of pamidronate in reducing skeletal events in patients with advanced multiple myeloma. Myeloma Aredia Study Group [see comments]. N Engl J Med 1996; 334(8): 488–93.

6. Berenson JR, Lichtenstein A, Porter L et al. Long-term pamidronate treatment of advanced multiple myeloma patients reduces skeletal events. Myeloma Aredia Study Group [see comments]. J Clin Oncol 1998; 16(2): 593–602.

7. Theriault RL, Lipton A, Hortobagyi GN et al. Pamidronate reduces skeletal morbidity in women with advanced breast cancer and lytic bone lesions: a randomized, placebo-controlled trial. Protocol 18 Aredia Breast Cancer Study Group. J Clin Oncol 1999; 17(3): 846–54.

8. McCloskey EV, MacLennan IC, Drayson MT et al. A randomized trial of the effect of clodronate on skeletal morbidity in myeloma. MRC Working Party on Leukaemia in Adults. Br J Haematol 1998; 100(2): 317–25.

9. McCloskey EV, Dunn JA, Kanis JA. Long-term follow-up of a prospective, double-blind, placebo-controlled randomized trial of clodronate in multiple myeloma. Br J Haematol 2001; 113(4): 1035–43.

10. Cummings SR, Melton LJ III, Felsenberg D et al. Assessing vertebral fractures. J Bone Min Res 1995; 10: 518–23.

11. McCloskey EV, Spector TD, Eyres KS et al. The assessment of vertebral deformity: a method for use in population studies and clinical trials [see comments]. Osteoporosis Int 1993; 3(3): 138–47.

12. McCloskey EV, Kanis JA. The assessment of vertebral deformity. In Genant HK, Jergas M, van Kuijk C (eds), Vertebral Fractures in Osteoporosis. UCSF: San Francisco, 1996: 215–33.

13. Bruce NJ, McCloskey EV, Kanis JA, Guest JF. Economic impact of using clodronate in the management of patients with multiple myeloma. Br J Haematol 1999; 104(2), 358–64.

14. Hortobagyi GN, Theriault RL, Lipton A et al. Long-term prevention of skeletal complications of metastatic breast cancer with pamidronate. Protocol 19 Aredia Breast Cancer Study Group. J Clin Oncol 1998; 16(6): 2038–44.

15. Kanis JA, Powles T, Paterson AH et al. Clodronate decreases the frequency of skeletal metastases in women with breast cancer. Bone 1996; 19(6): 663–7.

16. Brincker H, Westin J, Abildgaard N et al. Failure of oral pamidronate to reduce skeletal morbidity in multiple myeloma: a double-blind placebo-controlled trial. Danish–Swedish Cooperative Study Group. Br J Haematol 1998; 101(2): 280–6.

17. Paterson A, Powles TJ, Kanis JA et al. Double-blind controlled trial of oral clodronate in patients with bone metastases from breast cancer. J Clin Oncol 1993; 11(1): 59–65.

18. Lahtinen R, Laakso M, Palva I et al. Randomised placebo-controlled multicentre trial of clodronate in multiple myeloma. Finnish Leukaemia Group [published erratum appears in Lancet 1992 Dec 5; 340(8832): 1420] [see comments]. Lancet 1992; 340(8827): 1049–52.

19. Hultborn R, Gundesen S, Ryden S et al. Efficacy of pamidronate in breast cancer with bone metastases: a randomized, double-blind placebo-controlled multicenter study. Anticancer Res 1999; 19(4C): 3383–92.

20. Black DM, Cummings SR, Karpf DB et al. Randomised trial of effect of alendronate on risk of fracture in women with existing vertebral fractures. Fracture Intervention Trial Research Group [see comments]. Lancet 1996; 348(9041): 1535–41.

21. Harris ST, Watts NB, Genant HK et al. Effects of risedronate treatment on vertebral and nonvertebral fractures in women with postmenopausal osteoporosis: a randomized controlled trial. Vertebral Efficacy with Risedronate Therapy (VERT) Study Group [see comments]. J Am Med Assoc 1999; 282(14): 1344–52.

22. Bruning P, Pit MJ, de Jong-Bakker M et al. Bone mineral density after adjuvant chemotherapy for premenopausal breast cancer. Br J Cancer 1990; 61(2): 308–10.

23. Kanis JA, McCloskey EV, Powles T et al. A high incidence of vertebral fracture in women with breast cancer. Br J Cancer 1999; 79(7–8): 1179–81.

24. Powles TJ, Hickish T, Kanis JA et al. Effect of tamoxifen on bone mineral density measured by dual-energy X-ray absorptiometry in healthy premenopausal and postmenopausal women. J Clin Oncol 1996; 14(1): 78–84.

25. Saarto T, Blomqvist C, Valimaki M et al. Chemical castration induced by adjuvant cyclophosphamide, methotrexate and fluorouracil chemotherapy causes rapid bone loss that is reduced by clodronate: a randomized study in premenopausal breast cancer patients. J Clin Oncol 1997; 15(4): 1341–7.

26. Belch AR, Bergsagel DE, Wilson K et al. Effect of daily etidronate on the osteolysis of multiple myeloma. J Clin Oncol 1991; 9(8): 1397–402.

27. Vinholes JJ, Purohit OP, Abbey ME et al. Relationships between biochemical and symptomatic response in a double-blind randomised trial of pamidronate for metastatic bone disease. Ann Oncol 1997; 8(12): 1243–50.

28. Adami S, Salvagno G, Guarrera G et al. Dichloromethylene diphosphonate in patients with prostatic carcinoma metastatic to the skeleton. J Urol 1985; 134: 1152–4.

29. Ernst DS, Brasher P, Hagen N et al. A randomized, controlled trial of intravenous clodronate in patients with metastatic bone disease and pain. J Pain Sympt Manag 1997; 13(6): 319–26.

30. Ernst DS, MacDonald RN, Paterson AH et al. A double-blind, cross-over trial of intravenous clodronate in metastic bone pain. J Pain Sympt Manag 1992; 7(1): 4–11.

31. Delmas PD, Charhon S, Chapuy MC et al. Long-term effects of dichloromethylene diphosphonate (Cl2MDP) on skeletal lesions in multiple myeloma. Metab Bone Dis Relat Res 1982; 4(3): 163–8.

32. Heim ME, Clemens MR, Queisser W et al. Prospective randomized trial of dichloromethylene bisphosphonate (clodronate) in patients with multiple myeloma requiring treatment. A multicentre study. Oncologie 1995; 18: 439–48.

33. Ascari E, Attardo Parrinello G, Merlini G et al. Treatment of painful bone lesions and hypercalcaemia. Eur J Haematol 1989; 51(suppl): 135–9.

34. Lipton A, Theriault RL, Hortobagyi GN et al. Pamidronate prevents skeletal complications and is effective palliative treatment in women with breast carcinoma and osteolytic bone metastases: long-term follow-up of two randomized, placebo-controlled trials. Cancer 2000; 88(5): 1082–90.

35. Hortobagyi GN, Theriault RL, Porter L et al. Efficacy of pamidronate in reducing skeletal complications in patients with breast cancer and lytic bone metastases. Protocol 19 Aredia Breast Cancer Study Group [see comments]. N Engl J Med 1996; 335(2): 1785–91.

36. Biermann WA, Cantor RI, Fellin FM et al. An evaluation of the potential cost reductions resulting from the use of clodronate in the treatment of metastatic carcinoma of the breast to bone. Bone 1991; 12(suppl 1): S37–42.

37. Laakso M, Lahtinen R, Virkkunen P, Elomaa I. Subgroup and cost–benefit analysis of the Finnish multicentre trial of clodronate in multiple myeloma. Finnish Leukaemia Group. Br J Haematol 1994; 87(4): 725–9.

38. Hillner BE, Weeks JC, Desch CE, Smith TJ. Pamidronate in prevention of bone complications in metastatic breast cancer: a cost–effectiveness analysis. J Clin Oncol 2000; 18(1): 72–9.

39. Gent M, Blakely JA, Easton JD et al. The Canadian American Ticlopidine Study (CATS) in thromboembolic stroke. Lancet 1989; 1: 1215–20.

40. Diener HC, Cunha L, Forbes C et al. European stroke prevention study 2. Dipyridamole and acetylsalicylic acid in the secondary prevention of stroke. J Neurol Sci 1996; 143: 1–13.

41. Powles TJ, Paterson AHG, Nevantaus A et al. Adjuvant clodronate reduces the incidence of bone metastases in patients with primary operable breast cancer. Prog Proc Am Soc Clin Oncol 1998; 17: 123a.

42. Diel IJ, Solomayer EF, Costa SD et al. Reduction in new metastases in breast cancer with adjuvant clodronate treatment [see comments]. N Engl J Med 1998; 339(6): 357–63.

43. Elomaa I, Blomqvist C, Porkka L et al. Treatment of skeletal disease in breast cancer: a controlled clodronate trial. Bone 1987; 8(suppl 1): 53–6.

44. Adamson BB, Gallacher SJ, Byars J et al. Mineralisation defects with pamidronate therapy for Paget's disease [see comments]. Lancet 1993; 342(8885): 1459–60.

45. Elomaa I, Risteli L, Laakso M et al. Monitoring the action of clodronate with type I collagen metabolites in multiple myeloma. Eur J Cancer 1996; 32A(7): 1166–70.

46. Vinholes J, Coleman R, Lacombe D et al. Assessment of bone response to systemic therapy in an EORTC trial: preliminary experience with the use of collagen cross-link excretion. European Organization for Research and Treatment of Cancer. Br J Cancer 1999; 80(1–2): 221–8.

47. Vinholes J, Guo CY, Purohit OP et al. Evaluation of new bone resorption markers in a randomized comparison of pamidronate or clodronate for hypercalcemia of malignancy. J Clin Oncol 1997; 15(1): 131–8.

48. Kanis JA, McCloskey EV, Taube T, O'Rourke N. Rationale for the use of bisphosphonates in bone metastases. Bone 1991; 12(suppl 1): S13–18.

49. Major PP, Lipton A, Berenson J, Hortobagyi G. Oral bisphosphonates: a review of clinical use in patients with bone metastases. Cancer 2000; 88(1): 6–14.

7

The Global Approach

Section Editor: C. Jasmin

34

Treatment of Bone Pain

D. A. Lossignol

Institut Jules Bordet, Brussels, Belgium

INTRODUCTION

Pain is one of the most distressful and most feared symptoms in cancer, which may vary from moderate to intractable, and is often associated with physical and psychological impairment [1,2]. However, in spite of the advances in physiopathology and in clinical experience and despite the interest devoted to pain control, many patients remain unrelieved during their illness and many data suggest that pain is undertreated [3,4]. Therefore, some points need to be well defined: the definition of pain syndromes and their mechanisms; the assessment and the evaluation of pain; possibilities and availability of treatment and follow-up; and the information given to the patient. These elements have been emphasised by the Ad Hoc Committee on Cancer Pain of the American Society of Clinical Oncology [5].

Bone pain secondary to cancer (metastatic or direct involvement) is a common complication in solid tumours. Some locations are life-threatening, e.g. spinal metastases with cord compression or involvement of the base of the skull with cranial nerve palsy. The incidence of bone metastases depends on the nature of the tumour. Breast, lung and prostate carcinomas are mostly associated with this complication but other types of tumour may present bone metastases, e.g. melanoma, head and neck tumours and ovarian carcinoma.

The severity of pain increases as the disease progresses, due to growth of the tumour and/or metastases, weakness of the patient, related complications (anaemia, nerve involvement, nutrition impairment, metabolic disturbances) and neuronal

sensitisation, which will contribute to reduce patients' ability to tolerate pain. This contributes to the degradation of motor function, mood and quality of life.

In this chapter, a global approach to bone pain is proposed, with a focus on pain assessment, pain management and follow-up. Expertise is necessary to achieve effective pain relief but the most important thing is to be aware that pain must be treated, away from myths and ignorance [6].

INCIDENCE AND EPIDEMIOLOGICAL ASPECTS OF BONE METASTASES

The incidence of bone metastases varies according to the origin and the histological type of the primary tumour (Table 34.1). The high prevalence of breast, lung and prostate cancer means that together they account for more than 80% of metastastic bone disease. Less frequently, bone metastases may be the first clinical manifestation of the tumour or metastases (pathological fracture), as seen in myeloma, or reveal an unknown primary. Morbidity of bone metastases is associated with a shortened life expectancy, e.g. lung carcinoma carries a poor prognosis, with a median survival of 3.5 months after diagnosis when associated with bone metastases [7]. Nevertheless, the prognosis appears to be better in breast or in prostate cancer, partly due to a higher chemotherapy and hormone therapy response rate.

Co-morbidity of bone metastases is of importance because of its impact on quality of life. Pain is the first manifestation of a bone lesion in most cases, and may

Textbook of Bone Metastases. Edited by C. Jasmin, R. E. Coleman, L. R. Coia, R. Capanna and G. Saillant
© 2005 John Wiley & Sons Ltd: ISBN 0 471 87742 5

Table 34.1. Incidence of bone metastases (%)

Breast	73
Prostate	68
Thyroid	42
Lung	36
Kidney	35

Based on Houston [23].

Table 34.2. Pain syndromes*

Due to tumour involvement
Direct compression by the tumour
Bone invasion
Nerve compression or infiltration
Visceral involvement
Other structures: vein, arteries, soft tissues
Specific peptides: endothelin I (?)

Due to cancer treatment
Post-chemotherapy
Mucositis
Neuropathy
Encephalopathy ("central pain")
Post-surgery
Post-mastectomy
Post-thoracotomy
Post-amputation pain
Post-radiation therapy
Fibrosis
Bone necrosis
Myelopathy

*Alone or in combination.

precede imaging abnormalities, sometimes for weeks. This is especially true for metastases of the spine associated with back pain [8].

CANCER PAIN SYNDROMES

The principal causes of pain in cancer are listed in Table 34.2. It is important to correlate the symptom with the underlying disease. This may indicate the possibility of a specific treatment, e.g. chemotherapy, radiation therapy or surgery, and could be of prognosis value concerning pain control. Most patients may present more than one type or cause of pain. In fact, each situation is particular and has to be assessed closely to avoid diagnostic error. Further investigations are often necessary but have to be considered according to the clinical situation and performed in view of comfort for the patient.

In the case of bone metastases, multiple sites are frequently affected [9]. The most frequent sites are the spine, femur, pelvis and skull. Those locations are directly associated with clinical complications: bone fracture, nerves and spinal cord compression.

Usually, pain is described in terms of somatic, visceral and neuropathic pain, according to the lesions responsible. Visceral and somatic pain (or nociceptive pain) are well defined by the patient. Quality (intensity, description) and location are easy to determine, although visceral pain is less specific in terms of location. Neuropathic pain (or non-nociceptive pain), although often associated with the two others, is less easy to define because of its particular presentation. It is related to the peripheral or central nerve lesion. The taxonomy of neuropathic pain is rich and describes abnormal sensitive sensations: aching, burning, squeezing or cold pain.

Bone pain is the clinical expression of somatic pain, but from a practical point of view, it must be emphasised that there is almost always a neuropathic and a visceral component to bone pain (association of muscles and peripheral nerve lesions). The identification of the pain syndrome will provide clues for adequate treatment.

ASSESSMENT AND EVALUATION OF PAIN

Guidelines for bone pain assessment are proposed in Table 34.3. A physical examination and a complete neurological testing are essential to clarify the pain complaint and to identify the pain syndrome. The characteristics of pain (onset, quality, intensity, location and temporal pattern) have to be detailed. Aggravating and relieving factors will be determined. Prior therapies will be collected (pain medications and other specific treatment).

A close neurological examination is warranted, especially when patients report a history of back pain, bladder or cranial nerve dysfunction. The need of complementary procedures [plain X-ray, computed tomography (CT) and magnetic resonance imaging (MRI)] will be considered according to clinical manifestations. Prior administration of analgesics is essential to facilitate diagnostic studies.

Numerous procedures exist to quantify and to evaluate the pain. We suggest using simple but easy and reproductive techniques, which will provide an adequate monitoring of pain (see Figure 34.1). The numeric scale (NS) is certainly the instrument of choice for quantifying the pain, and may be used in an outpatient or inpatient setting. It is a self-report tool

Table 34.3. Assessment of bone pain

Physical examination	
Neurological examination	Vital if cranial nerve palsy or back pain is present
Performance status	ECOG or Karnofsky
History of pain	Onset, progression, location(s), temporal pattern, aggravating and relieving factors, prior therapies, functional consequences, associated sleep disturbances
Evaluation of pain	Visual analogue scale Descriptive scale Numeric scale
Laboratory tests	Liver and renal function
Radiological studies	X-rays, CT, MRI
Psychological evaluation	To rule out associated depression or anxiety
Lumbar puncture	If necessary, to avoid leptomeningeal involvement

allowing the patient to give a score to his/her pain (0–10 or 0–100) and may be recorded every day. Although pain is essentially a subjective experience, NS remains the best way to assess pain and to adjust the treatment. We suggest its use to define the pain intensity at rest and during motion.

Values should be recorded four to six times a day in order to obtain a graphic representation of pain. This procedure is useful for detecting breakthrough pain and/or adapting the schedule of the drug administration. Alternatively, a visual analogue scale (VAS) without numerical graduation may help a patient to quantify his/her pain. It is important to teach the patient and family members how to use these tools to improve compliance and coping abilities.

NS and VAS may also be used to assess other subjective aspects, such as pain relief, quality of sleep, mood and sleep. The generated scales complete the pain evaluation. The introduction of a "pain-grading system" opens new horizons for pain evaluation and could offer new perspectives in terms of pain management. This system is based on objective factors (type of pain, nature of pain, tolerance to opioids, opioids intake, cognitive and psychological impairment, history of toxicomany or ethylism) and introduces the notion of prognosis regarding pain control [10]. The development of such a system is certainly a new way to evaluate cancer pain but deserves more data to be used as routine.

It must be emphasised that pain evaluation, treatments and follow-up require expertise, comprehension and availability. This is only possible in an adequate environment, in an ethos of "team spirit" and with an interdisciplinary approach.

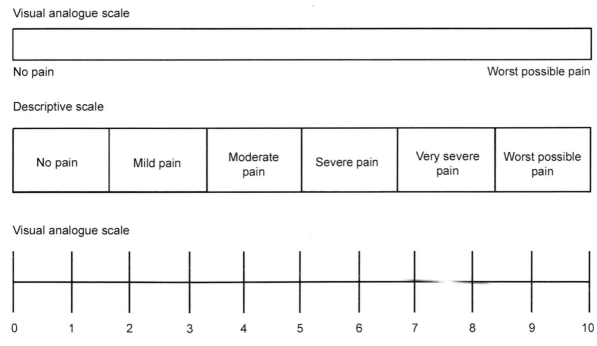

Figure 34.1. Pain assessment tools. Adapted from [25]

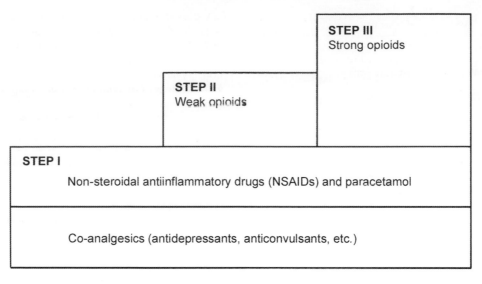

Comments:
1. Step I medications may be associated with Step II/III
2. Never associate Step II and Step III
3. Consider surgery and/or radiation therapy in each case
4. Prevent breakthrough pain with rescue medications

Figure 34.2. The WHO ladder

TREATMENT

The efficacy of pain control relies on a correct evaluation of pain, an adequate treatment and a prolonged follow-up. Beside specific treatment like biphosphonate [11], the therapeutic procedure is based on a multidisciplinary approach and includes pharmacological, radiological, anaesthetic, psychological and neurosurgical approaches. Guidelines have been developed by the Cancer Unit of the World Health Organization, who proposed an analgesic ladder to treat cancer pain [12]. According to these guidelines, anaesthetic procedures should be considered only if other approaches are ruled out. A three-step procedure for the use of oral analgesics in cancer pain, known as "the WHO ladder", has been proposed (Figure 34.2). Depending on the pain intensity, non-opioids, e.g. paracetamol or non-steroidal antiinflammatory drugs (NSAIDs), weak or strong opioids and co-analgesics may be prescribed.

NSAIDs—"Step I"

The first step entails using non-opioids such as paracetamol (or acetaminophen) and non-steroidal antiinflammatory drugs (NSAIDs). The non-opioid analgesics are effective in relieving mild-to-moderate pain. They are considered as the first-line agents in the management of cancer pain. However, their use is limited because of a ceiling effect, gastrointestinal toxicity and coagulation disturbances. They may be used in association with opioids but, in contrast, these agents do not produce tolerance and physical dependence.

Paracetamol (acetaminophen) is the most prescribed drug of this class in view of its moderate toxicity, low cost and effectiveness. Doses are in the range 2–6 g/day. Nevertheless, hepatic failure is of concern because of the risk of hepatotoxicity or hepatorenal syndrome.

NSAIDs are all antipyretic and are thought to produce their analgesic effect through the inhibition of the cyclooxygenase (COX) pathway. COX catalyses the production of prostaglandins and leukotrienes from arachidonic acid. Two COX isoforms are now recognised. COX-1 is present in the stomach and kidney and sustains the physiological function of prostaglandins, including gastric mucosal protection. COX-2 is essentially produced in response to a pathological process, including pain and inflammation. The therapeutic effect of NSAIDs may be primarily attributed to COX-2 inhibition. NSAIDs are effective in the treatment of bone metastases, soft tissue infiltration, arthritis and post-operative pain [13]. There is a wide variety of NSAIDs, exhibiting marginal differences in terms of pharmacokinetics and efficacy, but none of them is superior to any of the others [14]. NSAIDs are 1.5–2 times more effective than placebo; NSAID-induced analgesia is dose-dependent with a ceiling effect, but NSAID-induced side-effects, despite a dose–response relationship, have no ceiling and increase dramatically with multiple dosing over 7–10 days. Furthermore, it appears that NSAIDs are as effective as weak opioids (pentazocine, codeine) [15]. We therefore do not recommend one NSAID rather than another, but we suggest using only well-known molecules with respect of efficacy, safety, availability and cost. A treatment of more than 8 days, even an effective one, should be interrupted to avoid undesirable side-effects.

A new class of NSAIDs is now available, including rofecoxib and celecoxib, two COX-2 specific inhibitors. Preliminary data demonstrate their safety in terms of gastrointestinal toxicity in patients with rheumatoid arthritis [16,17]. Nevertheless, there are actually no data about their effectiveness in cancer pain and clinical experience is as yet too limited to allow their recommendation in the treatment of cancer-related bone pain. Guidelines for the use of NSAIDs are proposed in Table 34.4.

Opioids—"Step II and Step III"

The effectiveness of morphine and other narcotic analgesics is well recognised for the relief of moderate to extremely severe cancer pain. Opioids are classified according to their intrinsic activity at opioid receptors. The distinction between "weak" and "strong" opioids is arbitrary. Recommended opioids are listed in Table 34.5.

Synthetic opioids (tilidine, pentazocine, buprenorphine, etc.), although effective in acute pain syndromes, are associated with routes of administration, ceiling effects or psychomimetic side-effects that are too restricted to be used for chronic pain. Their use in the treatment of cancer pain is therefore not recommended.

In this field, some molecules deserve special attention. Tramadol hydrochloride is a central analgesic with morphine-like activity. Furthermore, it exhibits "non-opioid activity" similar to antidepressant molecules that blockade monoamine re-uptake. It has been demonstrated to be effective in cancer pain in a large

Table 34.4. NSAIDs in cancer pain

Oral route available	
No coagulation disorder	Coagulation tests required
No active peptic ulcer	
No active bleeding	
Avoid long-acting molecule	To avoid long-term side-effects
Favour short duration of treatment	6–8 days (treatment may be repeated)
Use a "well-known" molecule	Adverse events of a "new" molecule may be underestimated

variety of syndromes. The advantage of such a molecule is its good clinical tolerance and its wide availability. Although studies are still ongoing, tramadol is an alternative to strong opioids in the treatment of chronic cancer pain [18].

The introduction of the opioid rotation concept is still raising questions and deserves large-scale studies. Nevertheless, it appears that the treatment of opioid toxicity (i.e. confusion, myoclonus, sedation) will benefit from the switch of one opioid to another. The underlying theory is based on the non-cross-tolerance between opioids and their intrinsic activity on sub-classes of opioid receptors [19]. Side-effects such as nausea or constipation, although usually moderate, have to be prevented because of their incidence and their implication in treatment failure. The risk of sedation or respiratory depression has to be considered in relation to the clinical situation. Pain is certainly the best antidote to those complications that rarely occur with correct drug management [1]. If such a complication is present, investigations should be performed to exclude other aetiologies before stopping opioid administration or administering naloxone (an opioid antagonist) [20].

The fear of addiction or toxicomany is often associated with morphine and is deeply prevalent among patients. Our role is to inform the patient, family and relatives that morphine may be the drug of choice to control pain and to provide a better quality of life [6]. Guidelines for the use of opioids are proposed in Table 34.6.

Co-analgesics

Co-analgesics may be used in specific circumstances, such as neuropathic pain. The use of antidepressants, e.g. amitriptyline, imipramine or sertraline, and anticonvulsants, e.g. valproate or carbamazepine, has been

Table 34.5.   Recommended opioids for cancer pain

Drug	Route	Equianalgesic dose (mg)*	Starting dose (mg)	Duration of effect (h)	Agonist/ Antagonist	Comments
Codeine	p.o., i.m.	100	60 (p.o.)	4	Agonist	Not superior to NSAIDs/constipation
Tramadol	p.o. (+s.r.) i.m., i.v., rectal	100	50 (p.o.)	4–6	Agonist	Amine reuptake inhibition/equivalent to codeine but with fewer side-effects
Morphine	p.o. (+s.r.) i.m., i.v., s.c., rectal	30–60	10 (p.o.)	4–6	Agonist	First choice for moderate to severe cancer pain
Methadone	p.o., i.v., i.m.	10 (?)	1–5	8–10	Agonist	Not a first choice/useful in opioid rotation programme/risk of drug accumulation/10 times more potent than morphine (?)
Fentanyl	t.d., (i.v., i.m.)	0.1 (?)	25 µg	48–72 (t.d.)	Agonist	Potent opioid/transdermal system/ same side-effects as morphine/useful in opioid rotation programme
Hydro-morphone	p.o. (s.r.), i.v., i.m.	5–7.5	2	3–4	Agonist	High solubility/useful in opioid rotation programme

Adapted from Lossignol [24]. *, Potency relative to 10 mg parenteral morphine; i.v., intravenous; i.m., intramuscular; s.r., sustained release; t.d., transdermal; p.o., per os (taken orally); s.c., subcutaneous.

Table 34.6.   Guidelines for the use of opioids

Start with a short-acting molecule to titrate the pain	Morphine 5 mg (s.c.) or 10 mg (p.o.) every 6 hours ("around the clock")
Evaluate side-effects	Prevention of nausea (metoclo-pramide or haloperidol) Prevention of constipation (laxative regimen)
Favour oral medications	For long-term treatment, move to sustained-release preparations
Prescribe rescue dose	One "rescue dose" is about 10% of the total daily dose
Use a diary to collect information on pain control/pain relief	Use VAS, NS, etc.
Educate the patient and family members	Prevent withdrawal, explain that toxicomany or respiratory depression is uncommon
Change from one opioid to another when side-effects are too severe	Opioid rotation programme

Table 34.7.   Co-analgesics

Amitriptyline	25–75 mg once a day
Carbamazepine	200–600 mg once a day
Clonazepam	0.5 mg once a day
Gabapentine	300 mg × 3
Biphosphonates	Various dosages
Methylprednisolone	Various dosages

Table 34.8.   Pharmacological treatment of bone pain

Paracetamol or NSAID (COX-2?)	500 mg 4–6 b.i.d.
Oral or s.c. morphine	10 mg 4–6 b.i.d. 5 mg 4–6 b.i.d.
Co-analgesic medications according to pain characteristics	
Consider radiation therapy, surgery or biphosphonates	
Consider analgesia before any diagnostic procedures: CT, MRI	Oral or s.c. morphine
Consider sustained-release medications for long-term treatment	

supported by results from controlled trials in painful conditions such as plexopathy, neuropathy and phantom limb syndrome and may be used in association with other analgesics.

Recently, gabapentine, an adjunctive agent for the treatment of epilepsy, has been introduced for the treatment of neuropathic pain [21]. In cancer patients,

gabapentine is associated with a reduction in the need of opioids and could therefore be proposed as the first choice for the management of neuropathic cancer pain [22].

Corticosteroids, e.g. dexamethasone, prednisone, provide pain relief in specific situations, such as soft tissue infiltration or nerve compression or in the case of hepatic metastases. They should not be considered to be the first choice for pain management.

As co-analgesics, biphosphonates and isotopes (e.g. strontium) are described in another chapter (see Table 34.7 for doses).

For all of these drugs, the physician has to be aware of their pharmacological properties and effectiveness to avoid undesirable side-effects or iatrogenic complications. Furthermore, close follow-up with repeated pain evaluation and quantification of side-effects is essential. We estimate that optimal pain relief is obtained if the VAS remains below 3/10, with a pain relief of more than 50% in 24 h. Other interventions may be considered in each case but always in association with pharmacological procedure. The first steps for bone pain treatment are proposed in Table 34.8.

CONCLUSIONS

Adequate pain management requires knowledge in different fields: oncology, neurology, pharmacology and psychology. Pain must be completely evaluated before any diagnostic and therapeutic procedures are undertaken. Complete information should be given to the patient regarding the cause of pain and the nature of treatment. Close and prolonged follow-up of pain and prevention of the potential side-effects related to treatment will provide compliance and trust between the patient and the physician.

REFERENCES

1. Foley KM. The treatment of cancer pain. N Engl J Med 1985; 313: 84–95.
2. Levin DN, Cleland DS, Dar R. Public attitude toward cancer pain. Cancer 1985; 56: 2337–9.
3. Bonica JJ, Ventafridda V, Twycross RG. Cancer Pain. In Bonica J (ed.), Management of Pain. Lea Springer: Philadelphia, 1990; 400–60.
4. Grossman SA. Undertreatment of cancer pain: barriers and remedies. Support Care Cancer 1993; 1: 74–8.
5. Ad Hoc Committee on Cancer Pain of the American Society of Clinical Oncology. Cancer pain assessment and treatment curriculum guidelines. J Clin Oncol 1992; 10: 1976–82.
6. Zens M. Morphine myths: sedation, tolerance, addiction. Postgrad Med J 1991; 67(2). 100–2.
7. Levin AM. Bone metastasis. In Moosa AR, Schimpff SC, Robson MC (eds), Comprehensive Textbook of Oncology, 2nd edn. Williams & Wilkins: Baltimore, MD, 1991: 1638–52.
8. Grossman SA, Lossignol DA. Diagnosis and treatment of epidural metastases. Oncology 1990; 4: 47–54.
9. Mercadante S. Malignant bone pain: pathophysiology and treatment. Pain 1997; 69: 1–18.
10. Bruera E, MacMillan D, Hanson J, MacDonald RN. The Edmonton Staging system for cancer pain: preliminary report. Pain 1989; 37: 203–10.
11. Body JJ. Overview of Osteoclast Inhibitors: In Jasmin (ed.), Textbook of Bone Metastases. John Wiley: Chichester, 2005; 291–300.
12. World Health Organization. Cancer Pain Relief. World Health Organization: Geneva, 1986.
13. Ventafridda V, Fochi C, De Conno D et al. Use of nonsteroidal anti-inflammatory drugs in the treatment of pain in cancer. Br J Clin Pharm 1980; 10(suppl): 343–6S.
14. Brooks PM, Day RO. Nonsteroidal antiinflammatory drugs—differences and similarities. N Engl J Med 1991; 24: 1716–25.
15. Eisenberg E, Berkey CS, Carr DB et al. Efficacy and safety of non-steroidal antiinflammatory drugs for cancer patients. J Clin Oncol 1994; 12: 2756–65.
16. Emery P, Zeidler H, Kvien TK et al. Celecoxib vs. diclofenac in long-term management of rheumatoid arthritis: randomized double-blind comparison. Lancet 1999; 354: 2106–11.
17. Langman DJ, Jensen DM, Watson DJ et al. Adverse upper gastrointestinal effects of rofecoxib compared with NSAIDs. J Am Med Assoc 1999; 282: 1929–33.
18. Wilder-Smith CH, Schimke J, Osterwalder B, Senn HJ. Oral tramadol, a non-opioid agonist and monoamine reuptake blocker and morphine for strong cancer-related pain. Ann Oncol 1994; 5: 141–6.
19. Mancini I, Lossignol DA, Body JJ. Opioid switch to oral methadone in cancer pain. Curr Opin Oncol 2000; 12: 308–13.
20. Lossignol DA. Pitfalls in the use of opiates in the treatment of cancer pain. Support Care Cancer 1993; 1: 256–8.
21. Backonja M, Beydoun A, Edwards KR et al. Gabapentine for the symptomatic treatment of painful neuropathy in patients with diabetes mellitus. J Am Med Assoc 1998; 280: 1837–42.
22. Lossignol DA, Mancini I, Plehiers B et al. Successful treatment of neuropathic cancer pain with gabapentine. Support Care Cancer 2000; 8(abstr): 245.
23. Houston SJ, Rubens RD. Metastatic bone pain. Pain Rev 1994; 1: 138–52.
24. Lossignol DA, Razavi D, Delvaux N. Douleur et analgésie. In Razavi D (ed.), Psycho-Oncologie. Masson: Paris, 1998; 193–218.
25. Koshy RC, Grossman SA. Treatment of bone pain. In Body JJ (ed.), Tumor Bone Diseases and Osteoporosis in Cancer Patients. Marcel Dekker: New York 2000; 245–61.

35

Specific Approaches to Cancer in the Elderly

Lodovico Balducci

H. Lee Moffitt Cancer Center and Research Institute, Tampa, FL, USA

INTRODUCTION

Cancer in the older person has become an increasingly common problem [1,2]. Currently in the USA, 60% of all neoplasms occur in persons aged 65 and older. This proportion is expected to increase if the current demographic trend continues. Presently, persons aged 65 and older represent 12% of the US population; by the year 2020 they are expected to represent 20% of the total population, due to simultaneous prolongation of life expectancy and decline of natality [1,2].

The management of cancer in the older-aged person involves specific questions [3], such as:

- Is the patient going to die of cancer or with cancer?
- Will the cancer affect the patient's function and quality of life during his/her lifetime?
- Is the patient able to tolerate antineoplastic treatment?

These questions stem from two considerations:

1. Ageing is associated with a progressive decline in the functional reserve of multiple organ systems, increased prevalence of co-morbid conditions and of socioeconomic, emotional and cognitive limitations that altogether lead to decreased life expectancy and enhanced vulnerability to stress [4].
2. The process of ageing is highly individualised and poorly reflected in chronological age [3].

Thus, the management of cancer is directed by a form of clinical assessment capable of predicting life expectancy and tolerance of stress. In this chapter the evaluation of the older-aged person with cancer is outlined after summarising the physiological changes of ageing.

PHYSIOLOGICAL AGEING

Ageing is associated with a progressive decline in the functional reserve of many organ systems. As one can see in Figure 35.1, the rate of this decline varies within different systems. For example, there is no appreciable difference in the control of fasting blood sugar between ages 30 and 80, but the maximal respiratory capacity drops more than 40% during the same time span [5]. Of special interest to the management of cancer with cytotoxic chemotherapy are changes in body composition, decline in glomerular filtration rate (GFR) and decline in hepatic phase I reactions. Due to a progressive loss of water and proteins and increment in adipose tissue, the volume of distribution of water-soluble drugs declines and that of fat-soluble drugs expands [6]. Reduced excretion of drugs and of their active metabolites ensues decline in GFR [7], while decline in hepatic phase I reactions may alter the activation and deactivation of drugs and make the patient more susceptible to drug interactions [8].

Haematopoiesis is of special concern because the haematopoietic system is an almost universal target of cytotoxic agents. Haematopoiesis involves the commitment of a pluripotent haematopoietic stem cell (PHSC) into haematopoietic progenitors and the differentiation

Textbook of Bone Metastases. Edited by C. Jasmin, R. E. Coleman, L. R. Coia, R. Capanna and G. Saillant

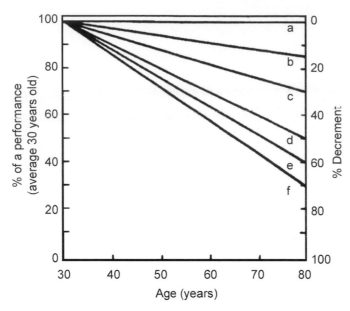

Figure 35.1. Age decrements in physiological performance

of these progenitors into the haematopoietic precursors of the bone marrow, from which the circulating blood elements are derived [9]. The stem cell has low proliferation rate, high self-replicating potential and ability to commit itself into different haematopoietic lines. The committed progenitors have higher proliferation rate than the PHSC but more limited self-replicating potential, and are able to differentiate only into one haematopoietic line. These processes of self-replication, commitment, differentiation and maturation are modulated by a number of cytokines, and require an intact haematopoietic microenvironment. Cytokines may include substances that stimulate haematopoiesis, such as granulocyte-macrophage colony stimulating factor (GM-CSF); granulocyte-colony stimulating factor (G-CSF) and erythropoietin, and substances that may inhibit haematopoiesis, such as interleukin 6 (IL-6) and tumour necrosis factor (TNF). The function of the microenvironment includes homing of PHSC and committed progenitors that is mediated by specific receptors for these elements and production of haematopoietic cytokines. Each haematopoietic area, including reserve of PHSC, balance between stimulatory and inhibitory cytokines, and haematopoietic microenvironment, may become altered with ageing. A number of observations suggests that haematopoiesis becomes restricted with age:

- Progressive loss of active haematopoietic tissue [10].

- Shortened telomeres in haematopoietic stem cells from ageing mammals [11], suggesting that the self-replicating potential of these elements is limited and that ageing may be associated with PHSC depletion.
- Impaired response to haematopoietic stress in both ageing mammals and humans [12].
- Increased incidence of anaemia with age [13].

The gastrointestinal mucosae are also a common target of cytotoxic chemotherapy. The proliferative rate of the cryptal cell increases, while the concentration of mucosal stem cells may decrease with age. This combination of factors may lead to enhanced risk and severity of mucositis [14].

Ageing is also associated with systemic changes that include decline in the production of sexual hormones [15], decreased rate of protein synthesis [16], increased production of inflammatory cytokines [17] and immune-senescence [18]. The increased production of cytotoxic cytokines, combined with lower secretion rate of growth hormone, leads to a prevalently catabolic status known as somatopause [19], which may become a clinical landmark of ageing, beyond which ability to repair injuries is progressively and irreversibly impaired.

The clinical translation of somatopause is still elusive. For clinical purposes, it is necessary to establish the nature of the consistent changes of somatopause and the systemic consequences of these changes, in the same way as menopause is caused by declining ovarian secretions and portends reproductive, cardiovascular and osseous effects.

CLINICAL ASSESSMENT OF AGEING

Ageing is highly individualised [3]. The clinical assessment of the older person must account for this diversity, to predict individual life expectancy and treatment tolerance. Table 35.1 lists current methods of assessing ageing. None of the current laboratory tests can precede clinical findings and provide accurate measurements of each person's functional reserve and life expectancy. The serum concentration of IL-6 is increased in the final stages of ageing, which are also called "frailty" and "near-death" (see below) [20], conditions that are easily recognised by clinical observation. The ratio between circulating cysteine and thiolic groups (s:d), reflects a person's lean body weight and the degree of oxidative damage, and increases progressively with ageing [21]. Cancer and malnutrition may also increase the s:d ratio. Serial determination of s:d may reveal the ageing rate of different individuals, but cross-sectional studies of s:d cannot reveal the different physiological ages of different persons. This test may prove useful in pharmacokinetic studies to estimate the volume of distribution of water-soluble drugs. The circulating levels of D-dimer may also increase with age, but are affected by any form of intravascular coagulation [22]. The laboratory determination of somatopause with circulating levels of growth hormone is undergoing clinical evaluation.

Assessment of neuromuscular function, including strength of upper and lower extremities and time necessary to perform simple tasks (such as getting up from a chair and walking a short distance) are useful to predict specific disabilities but have not proved able to distinguish the physiological age of different persons [23].

Table 35.1. Clinical assessment of ageing

Laboratory assessment	
Serum creatinine	Non-specific
Serum osmolality	Non-specific
Circulating levels of cytokines (IL-6, TNF)	Non-sensitive to early stages of ageing
Cysteine:circulating thiolic groups ratio (s:d)	Non-specific; may be altered by cancer and malnutrition
D-Dimer levels	Non-specific
Serum growth hormone/insulin-like growth factor 1 levels	Experimental
Physical assessment	
Stature	Non-specific; may be influenced by nutrition and osteoporosis
Hand-grasp	In individual situation may predict development of functional disability
Lower extremities strength	Experimental
Rising from a chair	Useful to establish certain movement difficulty; no relationship to functional dependence or life expectancy
Comprehensive Geriatric Assessment (CGA)	
Functional status	
Activities of daily living (ADL) and instrumental activities of daily living (IADL)	Relation to life expectancy, tolerance of chemotherapy, dependence
Co-morbidity	
Number of co-morbid conditions and co-morbidity indices	Relation to life expectancy and tolerance of treatment
Mental status	
Folstein Mini-Mental Status	Relation to life expectancy and dependence
Emotional conditions	
Geriatric Depression Scale (GDS)	Relation to survival; may indicate motivation to receive treatment
Nutritional status	
Mini-Nutritional Assessment (MNA)	Reversible condition; possible relationship to survival
Polypharmacy	Risk of drug interactions
Geriatric syndromes	Relationship to survival
Delirium, dementia, depression, falls, incontinence, spontaneous bone fractures, neglect and abuse, failure to thrive	Functional dependence

A comprehensive geriatric assessment (CGA) is currently the most accurate determination of the age of a person in terms of life expectancy and tolerance of stress [24]. Other advantages of the CGA include detection of conditions that may be reversible and may interfere with cancer treatment, such as co-morbidity, mild dementia, subclinical depression, malnutrition, functional dependence, social isolation and inadequate access to care. Activities of daily life (ADLs) are those activities necessary to maintain one's viability; instrumental ADLs (IADLs) are those needed to maintain one's independence. ADLs include transferring, bathing, dressing, feeding, toileting and grooming; and IADLs include use of transportation, shopping, banking, use of telephone, use of medications, ability to provide one's own meals, laundering and housekeeping. Dependence in one or more ADLs establishes the diagnosis of frailty, a condition in which a person's functional reserve is nearly exhausted, and is associated with a three-fold increase in the short-term (2–3 years) mortality [25]. Dependence in IADLs is associated with a two-fold short-term mortality increase [25] and with increased risk of dementia [26] and of chemotherapy-related complications [27].

The number and seriousness of co-morbid conditions is also associated with increased short-term mortality [28,29]. Piccirillo and Feinstein demonstrated that co-morbidity is an independent risk factor for mortality for patients with head and neck cancer, and proposed that co-morbidity be included in the current disease staging systems [29]. The assessment of co-morbidity is evolving. Initial studies used a number of selected co-morbid conditions as a measurement of co-morbidity. A more precise estimate of the impact of co-morbidity on cancer treatment may be obtained with a score derived from grading the seriousness of each condition. Both the Charlson and the CIRS-G (Concomitant Illness Related Symptoms— Geriatrics) scales have been validated to predict mortality [30]. The Charlson scale is user-friendly but overlooks a number of important conditions; the CIRS-G is more time-consuming, but more comprehensive and more sensitive to variations in symptom severity. Ongoing studies compare the value of these scales in the practice of oncology.

A clear relation exists between survival and mental status, depression, even subclinical depression, and other geriatric syndromes, including falls, delirium, failure to thrive, neglect and abuse, spontaneous fractures and complete incontinence [31–38]. The presence of one or more geriatric syndrome indicates that the patient is frail and cannot live alone, and suggests need of special support for prevention of

chemotherapy-related complications and for treatment compliance. The current definition of geriatric syndromes requires qualifications. For example, delirium should be considered a geriatric syndrome when it complicates mild infections or treatment with non-psychotropic drugs; falls must be spontaneous and occur three times or more in a month. Failure to thrive is absence of weight gain and functional recovery in spite of adequate nutritional support. Although experienced geriatricians may recognise failure to thrive and neglect and abuse, the clinical definition of these conditions is elusive.

The main goal of social assessment is to establish whether a caregiver is needed, is available and is adequate [39]. The functions of the caregiver include:

- Prompt availability for timely management of home emergencies and for providing around-the-clock access to care.
- Emotional support of the patient.
- Acting as a spokesperson for the family, able to provide bridging communication between the family and the provider. In this capacity, the caregiver may spare the practitioner from discordant communication with different family members and at the same time may avoid the stress of conflicting treatment decisions within the family.
- Management of family conflicts, likely to arise during the serious disease of an older parent.

The choice of the caregiver requires tact and expertise. The majority of older people, especially older men, are cared for by an older spouse who may have health problems and functional dependence of her/his own, but who may be unaware of her/his own inadequacy. Generally, if the spouse is not available, caregiving is bestowed on an adult child who may have preexisting family and professional commitments. The management of the caregiver is one of the distinctive aspects of geriatric medicine and includes training and emotional support.

Older patients are at increased risk of malnutrition, especially during stress, due to a reduced rate of protein synthesis. The main role of nutritional assessment is to recognise those patients for whom preventive nutritional interventions may be useful. The Mini-Nutritional Assessment (MNA) is a self-administered and sensitive screening tool [40]. Polypharmacy implies the assumption of more than three daily drugs [41]. The risk of polypharmacy increases with age. Although polypharmacy may be appropriate in face of multiple co-morbid conditions, it still represents a risk factor for overdosing, prescription duplication and drug interactions. Periodic review of medications of older individuals is advisable, especially those who are cared for by different practitioners.

The National Cancer Center Network (NCCN) in the USA has recently convened a panel for guidelines for the management of older individuals. This panel has recognised the following benefits of medicine:

- Gross estimate of life-expectancy.
- Gross estimate of functional reserve and tolerance of chemotherapy.
- Recognition of reversible co-morbid conditions that may interfere with cancer treatment.
- Recognition of special social, economic and nutritional needs that may interfere with cancer treatment.
- Adoption of a common language in the management of older cancer patients. This common language is essential both for retrospective evaluation of quality of care and for prospective assessment of outcome in clinical trials.

After emphasising the diversity of the geriatric population and the need for a comprehensive assessment of the aged, it is important to recognise at least two chronological landmarks: age 70 and age 85. As the prevalence of age-related changes increases steeply between age 70 and 75, it is reasonable to institute some form of comprehensive geriatric assessment (CGA) for persons aged 70 and older. Age 85 may be considered a warning sign of frailty, because by this age more than 50% of the population present some form of geriatric syndrome [42], and are functionally dependent due to poor eyesight or hearing [43].

STAGES OF AGEING

Based on the CGA, some investigators have tried to identify stages of ageing, i.e. groups of persons with different life expectancy and functional reserve. Rockwood et al. showed that faecal incontinence or severe co-morbidity set apart a group of persons with average life expectancy of less than 2 years [44]. Hamermann has proposed four stages of ageing [45]. These stages are defined by the opportunity for preventive interventions and include:

- Opportunities for primary prevention, regarding persons who are fully independent and for whom the main goal is maintenance of this independence.
- Opportunities for secondary prevention regarding persons in need of some rehabilitation.

- Need for tertiary prevention. In this status, which the author calls "frailty", the main goal of prevention is delay of further functional deterioration, while rehabilitation is close to impossible.
- Near death, a condition of progressive deterioration unlikely to benefit from prevention or rehabilitation.

For the oncological patient, it is reasonable to collapse the last two stages of the Hamermann classification into frailty, which implies critical reduction of functional reserve; for practical purposes, the frail person is unable to stand minimal stress and is not a candidate for aggressive cytotoxic chemotherapy [46]. A reasonable clinical definition of frailty includes at least one of the following:

- Dependence in one or more ADL.
- Presence of one or more geriatric syndrome.
- Presence of three or more moderately severe co-morbid conditions or of a serious, life-threatening co-morbid condition.

In Figure 35.2 a decisional model is proposed for the oncological older patient in need of cancer chemotherapy. This model recognises three stages of ageing: full independence and absence of severe co-morbidity, for whom full doses of treatment may be safely used; frail, for whom the main goal of treatment is palliation; and a condition in between. For patients in the latter condition, special provisions may be necessary, such as initial reduction of doses of chemotherapy, assurance of social support and of availability of a caregiver. Of course, newly recognised medical, emotional and social conditions should also be aggressively treated and reversed when that is feasible.

The decisional model represents an attempt to apply the principles of geriatric medicine to the practice of oncology. This model, that has been adopted for more than 6 years at the H. Lee Moffitt Cancer Center and Research Institute, may be fine-tuned with a deeper understanding of ageing and with the development of new clinical and laboratory tests.

CONTROVERSIES RELATED TO THE GERIATRIC ASSESSMENT

The CGA involves a substantial investment of time and resources. It is legitimate, therefore, to study ways to minimise the cost and improve the efficiency of this process. Prior to addressing individual controversies, however, it is important to underline that the CGA is

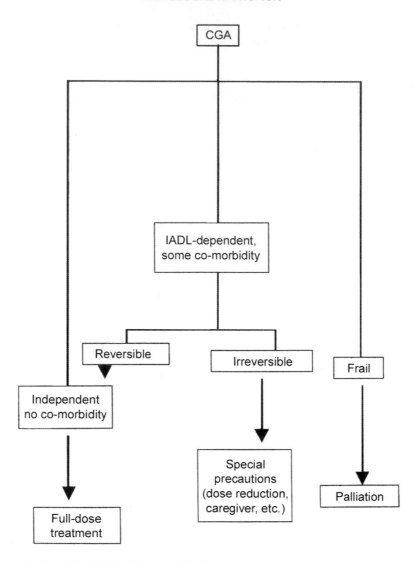

Figure 35.2. Proposed decisional model for older oncological patients in need of cancer chemotherapy

one of the most cost-effective interventions in geriatric assessment. The benefits of a CGA have been clearly demonstrated in several areas of geriatrics and include: prolongation of life and prevention of hospitalisation or of admission to adult living facilities; prevention of falls and in-hospital delirium; and detection of unsuspected conditions that may influence cancer treatment in more than 50% of cancer patients aged 70 and older [47]. The cost of the geriatric assessment per year of life saved is lower than the cost of accepted interventions, such as screening mammography for women aged 50–70.

The controversies related to the CGA include:

- Need of a full assessment for all patients aged 70 and older.
- The person who should perform the assessment.
- The cost of the assessment.

Two approaches have been used to reduce the time burden of the CGA. One approach is to use short screening instruments and to perform a full assessment only for the persons who screen positive [48,49]. Although a number of screening instruments have been validated, the risk still exists that important information may be missed. The second approach is to try to limit the assessment of some parameters, such as functional status and co-morbidity. This approach is not warranted by facts. Extermann et al. have studied the correlation between functional status, measured as performance status and ability to perform ADL and IADL, co-morbidity assessed according to the Charlson and the CIRS-G scales, and mental status of cancer patients aged 70 and older, and found an inadequate correlation among these parameters [47].

Ideally, older individuals should have a primary care provider who performs a geriatric assessment on a regular basis and who communicates the results to other specialists as part of the coordination of the patient's care. The assessment and its periodic updates should become part of the permanent patient record and be available to all practitioners involved in the care of the patient. In the absence of a primary care provider, however, the oncologist should be able to obtain the essential information.

In relation to cost, it is logical to assume that the management of the older person is more costly than the management of the younger person, given the higher prevalence of co-morbidity and functional dependence. Thus, the cost of the geriatric assessment should be examined in the light of two questions: does the geriatric assessment improve the safety of cancer treatment in older persons? Does the geriatric assessment reduce the cost of managing older cancer patients by avoiding costly complications?

CONCLUSIONS

Based on this review, one may draw the following conclusions:

- The geriatric population is highly diverse in terms of life expectancy, tolerance of stress and personal needs. This diversity is poorly reflected in chronological age.
- A CGA is currently the most reliable guide to the management of the older cancer patient. In addition to predicting life expectancy and tolerance of stress, the CGA may also reveal conditions that may compromise cancer treatment, such as unsuspected co-morbidity, cognitive, emotional and social dysfunctions, risk of malnutrition and polypharmacy.
- Some form of geriatric assessment is indicated for persons aged 70 and older. When a full assessment cannot be performed at least some form of screening appears desirable. Although the assessment is best performed by the primary care provider, the oncologist must be able to perform and interpret this assessment when necessary.
- The CGA is evolving with our understanding of age.

REFERENCES

1. Yancik R, Ries LAG. Aging and cancer in America: demographic and epidemiologic perspectives. Hematol/Oncol Clin N Am 2000; 14: 17–24.
2. Yancik RM, Ries L. Cancer and age: magnitude of the problem. In Balducci L, Lyman GH, Ershler WB (eds), Comprehensive Geriatric Oncology. Harwood Academic: London, 1998.
3. Balducci L, Extermann M. Cancer and aging: an evolving panorama. Hematol Oncol Clin N Am 2000; 14: 1–12.
4. Balducci L. The value of the comprehensive geriatric assessment in the management of the older cancer patient. Eur J Gerontol 2000 (in press).
5. Duthie E. Physiology of aging: relevance to symptom perceptions and treatment tolerance. In Balducci L, Lyman GH, Ershler WB (eds), Comprehensive Geriatric Oncology. Harwood Academic: London, 1998: 247–62.
6. Melton LJ, Khosla S, Crowson CS et al. Epidemiology of sarcopenia. J Am Geriat Soc 2000; 48: 625–30.
7. Levey AS, Bosch JP, Lewis JB et al. A more accurate method to estimate glomerular filtration rate from serum creatinine: a new prediction equation. Ann Intern Med 1999; 130: 461–70.
8. Schmucker DL. Aging and the liver: an update. J Gerontol Biol Sci 1998; 53A: B315–20.
9. Balducci L, Hardy CL, Lyman GH. Hemopoietic reserve in older cancer patients: clinical and economical considerations. Cancer Control, JHLMCC, 2000.
10. Moscinsky LC. Hemopoiesis and aging. In Balducci L, Lyman GH, Ershler WB (eds), Comprehensive Geriatric Oncology. Harwood Academic: London, 1998: 399–412.
11. Van Zant G. Stem cells and genetics in the study of development, aging and longevity. Results and Problems in Cell Differentiation, vol 29. Springer-Verlag: Berlin, 2000: 203–35.
12. Chatta GS, Price TH, Allen RC et al. Effects of in vivo recombinant methionyl human granulocyte colony-stimulating factor on the neutrophil response and peripheral blood colony-forming cells in healthy young and elderly adult volunteers. Blood 1994; 84: 2923–9.
13. Ania BJ, Suman VJ, Fairbanks VF et al. Incidence of anemia in older people: an epidemiologic study of a well-defined population. J Am Ger Soc 1997; 45: 823–31.
14. Atillasoy E, Holt PR. Gastrointestinal proliferation and aging. J Gerontol 1993; 48: B43–9.
15. Morley JE, Kaiser FE. Sexual function with advancing age. Med Clin N Am 1989; 73: 1483–95.
16. Short KR, Nair KS. The effect of age on protein metabolism. Curr Opin Clin Nutr Metab Care 2000; 3: 39–44.
17. Hamermann D, Berman JW, Albers GW et al. Emerging evidence for inflammation in conditions frequently affecting older adults: report of a symposium. J Am Ger Soc 1999; 47: 995–9.
18. Burns EA, Goodwin JS. Immunological changes of aging. In Balducci L, Lyman GH, Ershler WB (eds),

Comprehensive Geriatric Oncology. Harwood Academic: Amsterdam, 1998; 213–22.

19. Rosen CJ. Growth hormone and aging. Endocrine 2000; 12: 197–201.

20. Rink L, Cakman I, Kirchner H. Altered cytokine production in the elderly. Mech Ageing Dev 1998; 102: 199–209.

21. Hack V, Breitkreutz R, Kinscherf R et al. The redox status as a correlate of senescence and wasting and as a target for therapeutic intervention. Blood 1998; 54: 59–67.

22. Hager K, Platt D. Fibrin degeneration product concentration (D-dimer) is the source of aging. Gerontology 1995; 41: 159–65.

23 Guralnick JM, Ferrucci L, Pieper CF et al. Lower extremity function and subsequent disability: consistency across studies, predictive models, and value of gait speed alone compared with the short physical performance battery. J Gerontol Med Sci 2000; 55A: M221–31.

24. Alessi CA, Stuck AE, Aronow HU et al. The process of care in preventive "in-home" comprehensive geriatric assessment. J Am Geriat Soc 1997; 45: 1044–50.

25. Reuben DB, Rubenstein LV, Hirsch SH et al. Value of functional status as predictor of mortality. Am J Med 1992; 93: 663–9.

26. Barbeger-Gateau P, Fabrigoule C, Helmer C et al. Functional impairment in instrumental activities of daily living: an early clinical sign of dementia? J Am Geriat Soc 1999; 47: 456–62.

27. Monfardini S, Ferrucci L, Fratino L et al. Validation of a multidimensional evaluation scale for use in elderly cancer patients. Cancer 1996; 77: 395–401.

28. Satariano WA, Ragland DR. The effect of co-morbidity on 3-year survival of women with primary breast cancer. Ann Intern Med 1994; 120: 104–10.

29. Piccirillo JF, Feinstein AR. Clinical symptoms and comorbidity: significance for the prognostic classification of cancer. Cancer 1996; 77: 834–42.

30. Extermann M. Measurement of comorbidity. CRC Hematol Oncol 2000.

31. Manton K. A longitudinal study of functional change and mortality in the United States. J Gerontol 1988; 43: S153–61.

32. Eagles JM, Beattie JAG, Restall DB et al. Relationship between cognitive impairment and early death in the elderly. Br Med J 1990; 300: 239–40.

33. Bruce ML, Hoff RA, Jacobs SC et al. The effect of cognitive impairment on 9-year mortality in a community sample. J Gerontol 1995; 50B: P289–96.

34. Folstein ME, Folstein SE, McHugh PR. Mini Mental State: a practical method for grading the cognitive status of patients for the clinician. J Psychiatr Res 1975; 12: 189–98.

35. Covinsky KE, Kahana E, Chin MH et al. Depressive symptoms and 3 year mortality in older hospitalized medical patients. Ann Int Med 1999; 130: 563–9.

36. Bruce ML, Leaf PJ, Rozal GP et al. Psychiatric status and 9 year mortality data in the New Haven Epidemiologic Catchment Area Study. Am J Psychiat 1994; 151: 716–21.

37. Lyness JM, Ling DA, Cox C et al. The importance of subsyndromal depression in older primary care patients. Prevalence and associated functional disability. J Am Geriat Soc 1999; 47: 647–52.

38 Lyness JM, Noel TK, Cox C et al. Screening for depression in elderly primary care patients: a comparison of the Center for Epidemiologic Studies Depression Scale and the Geriatric Depression Scale. Arch Intern Med 1997; 157: 449–54.

39. Weitzner MA, Haley WE, Chen H. The family caregiver of the older cancer patient. Hematol Oncol Clin 2000; 14: 269–82.

40. Guigoz Y, Vellas B, Garry PJ. Mininutritional assessment: a practical assessment tool for grading the nutritional state of elderly patients. In Facts, Research, Interventions in Geriatrics. Serdi: New York, 1997: 15–60.

41. Corcoran MB. Polypharmacy in the older patient. In Balducci L, Lyman GH, Ershler WB (eds), Comprehensive Geriatric Oncology. Harwood Academic: London, 1998: 525–32.

42. Cassel CK. Money, Medicine and Methusalah. Mt Sinai J Med 1998; 65: 237–45.

43. Hogan DB, Ebly EM, Fung TS. Disease, disability, and age in cognitively intact seniors: results from the Canadian Study of Health and Aging. J Gerontol 1999; 54A: M77–82.

44. Rockwood K, Stadnyk K, Macknigt C et al. A brief instrument to classify frailty in elderly people. Lancet 1999; 353: 205–6.

45. Hamermann D. Toward an understanding of frailty. Ann Intern Med 1999; 130: 945–50.

46. Balducci L, Extermann M. Cancer in the older person: a practical approach. Curr Opin Oncol 2001 (in press).

47. Extermann M, Overcash J, Lyman GH et al. Comorbidity and functional status are independent in older cancer patients. J Clin Oncol 1998; 16: 1582–7.

48. Lachs MA, Williams CS, O'Brien S et al. Mortality of elder mistreatment. J Am Med Assoc 1998; 280: 428–32.

49. Balducci L, Yates G. Guidelines for the management of the older person with cancer. Oncology (2000).

36

Psychological and Social Aspects

Ora Gilbar

University of Haifa, Haifa, Israel

INTRODUCTION

Cancer in general, and cancer with bone metastases specifically, are causes of stress for the patient and the family. Bone metastases, as discussed elsewhere in this volume, is often one of the first signs of disseminated disease in cancer patients and tends to occur in patients with breast, prostate and lung cancer and melanoma [1]. Although the prognosis for these patients is generally poor and treatment is primarily palliative, few studies focus on the psychological responses or coping strategies of patients with bone metastases. Moreover, the extant research bunches patients with bone metastases with patients with metastases in other sites (e.g. lung, brain and liver) and cancer patients with recurrence, despite the fact that patients with bone metastases differ somewhat in terms of prognosis (survival rates are higher compared to patients with metastases in other sites) and psychological and psychosocial state (fewer symptoms of hopelessness and depression; more symptoms of helplessness).

This chapter will discuss the distinctive psychological distress of cancer patients with bone metastases, based on the coping with stress model, relevant studies on advanced cancer patients' clinical experience and qualitative research, which includes interviews of cancer patients with bone metastases carried out for this chapter [2].

STRESS AND COPING MODEL

This is one of the cognitive models developed by Lazarus and Folkman [3], which has become the core model of stress and coping in the area of personal encounters with stress and includes four classes of variables that affect a person who is in a stressful transaction with the environment: appraisals, coping modes, environmental variables and personal variables. These key components, in combination, are assumed to affect adaptation outcomes that include short-term distress, mood and emotion, as well as long-term consequences such as physical health, well-being and social functioning.

Primary appraisal is the assessment of the meaning of the person–environment encounter for the well-being of the individual. Once an event is judged to be stressful, it will be evaluated in terms of conveying harm/loss, threat or challenge. Secondary appraisal is the evaluation of one's coping capability, with the assessment of personal resources being the main determinant of one's ability to overcome the threat the event entails or to adapt to the harm/loss already done [4]. In addition, a reappraisal process is also assumed, by which the meaning of the threat or loss is changed depending on the two types of appraisals and the coping strategies used.

The coping process represents behavioural and cognitive efforts to deal with stressful encounters. Such coping strategies were classified by Lazarus and Folkman [3] and Lazarus [4] as either problem-focused or emotion-focused, thereby delineating the two main functions of coping as dealing with the problem, or with its emotional and physiological outcomes, respectively. In addition, two main groups of antecedents of appraisal were described: environmental variables and personal variables. The main environmental variables include the demands of the situation, constraints on

Textbook of Bone Metastases. Edited by C. Jasmin, R. E. Coleman, L. R. Coia, R. Capanna and G. Saillant
© 2005 John Wiley & Sons Ltd: ISBN 0 471 87742 5

coping and external resources, such as social support. Furthermore, formal aspects of the situation, such as its novelty, ambiguity and controllability, may affect both appraisal and coping efforts. The personal variables include such factors as personal goals, values and beliefs, as well as personal resources that affect the stress and coping process.

Appraisal and coping during acute stressful encounters have been extensively studied, but relatively little research has been devoted to chronic stress and how people cope with it [5]. Lazarus [4] makes a distinction between chronic and acute stress: acute stress is characterised by harmful or threatening time-limited events. In contrast, "chronic stress arises from harmful or threatening, but stable, conditions of life, and from the stressful roles people continually fulfil at work and in the family".

In the context of chronic or terminal illness, patients have the opportunity to develop a more complete understanding of the efficacy of various kinds of appraisals and to acquire a meaningful structure for these appraisals by placing them in a framework of coping goals. Ideally, the coping goals patients set for themselves are reflected in their evaluations of their progress in coping with the illness and in their appraisals of effective ways of coping. However, a key aspect of chronic illness is that it is generally impossible to bring about an improvement in the patient's condition. In addition, many types of disease have ambiguous aspects of duration and symptoms that are difficult to deal with. In many cases, therefore, coping with the disease situation is more a question of tolerating and managing it than eliminating or mastering it [4,6]. For this reason, the types of coping with chronic illness, such as those described by Gignac and Gottlieb [7], are mostly emotion-focused (e.g. acceptance, positive framing, avoidance), with only a few problem-focused coping strategies, such as help-seeking, cited.

Chronically ill patients and their families use a variety of resources to aid them in the coping and adjustment process. Lazarus and Folkman [3] and Moos and Schaefer [8] cite external resources, such as finances and social support, and internal resources, such as education, energy, intelligence and personality disposition. These external and internal resources are vital in the coping and adjustment process in the case of chronic illness such as cancer [9].

CANCER AS A CAUSE OF STRESS

In light of the widespread perception of the illness as a death sentence [10], cancer is generally defined as a stressful situation for both the patient and the family, relying on the stress model by Lazarus and Folkman [3] and Lazarus [4]. This perception affects the quality of life of the cancer patient *a priori*: often, the illness has a less severe effect than anticipated, yet the patient still describes his/her quality of life as poor [11].

Recent research on differences between acute and chronic stress has raised the question of which type of stress is engendered by cancer. One way to distinguish between stress type is by the frequency or duration of stressful events, circumstances or conditions. However, according to Baum et al. [12], this distinction is problematical, as individuals may habituate or adapt to a persistent stressor with repeated exposure; an acute stressor can lead to long-lasting appraisals of stress even after the event itself has ended; and a distinction based on the duration of acute and chronic stress is often arbitrary. Compas et al. [13] posit two processes, one exogenous and the other endogenous, by which acute events can lead to chronic stress. "Exogenous" processes refer to ongoing demands and threats emanating from the environment, e.g. the diagnosis of cancer itself represents an acute traumatic event for patients and their families that is associated with significant short-term psychological distress, as reflected in disruptions in the daily routines and family roles, and threats to the goals and values of the patients and their families. "Endogenous" processes refer to the persistent cognitive and affective re-experiencing of the stressor by patients and family members. Intrusive and uncontrollable thoughts and concerns about the disease, and reminders of it, perpetuate the sense of threat and a state of emotional arousal. Involuntary negative thoughts are part of the response system that unwittingly prolongs stress.

Clearly, cancer engenders both acute and chronic stress. The acute stress is caused by an exogenous process involving a series of time-limited major or minor events related to the specific phases of the illness, which are harmful or threatening for a relatively brief period, e.g. diagnosis, surgery and adjuvant treatment [4]. An individual who is aware of suspect symptoms is in a stressful situation caused by a threat to his/her life. Upon diagnosis, this threat becomes integral in his/her life, although it may decrease or increase in severity with each phase of the illness [14]. Chronic stress, conversely, is caused by an endogenous process stemming from a threat to life from the moment of diagnosis and a threat to the individual's role in the workplace and in the family. Each phase, however, also instigates another type of threat [15]. During the diagnosis process, for example, the patient's stressful feelings stem from uncertainty—is it cancer or is it not? If the diagnosis is cancer, the uncertainty becomes—am I going to die or not? [16].

The surgical intervention phase, which is a central part of cancer treatment, brings with it a threat to the sense of personal invulnerability; concern that one's life is being entrusted largely to strangers; separation from the familiar environment of home and family; fears of loss of control or death while under anaesthesia; and fears of damage to body parts, such as in a mastectomy, colostomy or amputation. Although these pre-operative reactions occur in all surgical patients to some degree, significantly greater stress is involved when cancer is the suspected or the *a priori* diagnosis [17,18].

Similarly, menacing threats are implicit in the medical treatment phases, which consist of radiotherapy, chemotherapy, hormonal therapy or immunotherapy. These threats are present before, during and at the termination of treatment. Before treatment, patients continue to deal with their emotional responses to the diagnosis while being further challenged by the need to choose, or assent to, a systematic, often painful and sometimes dangerous therapy, all within a relatively short period of time [19]. This period is characterised by anxiety related to the uncertainty and unpredictability endemic in the disease and its treatment; the scheduling of treatments; complicated decision-making regarding the most beneficial therapy; and often inadequate information. Even the issue of active participation in the decision-making process is uncertain: some research shows greater emotional distress for active participants in the process than for more passive patients [20–22]. During the medical treatments, patients are threatened by both the outcome and the side-effects [19,23]. Treatment may result in subjective symptom distress, or it may produce toxicity that interferes with the patient's functional abilities and level of independence. Procedures such as intravenous access or dependency on the health care provider for scheduling of treatments are also a source of threat to patients.

The most common distressing physical symptoms of treatment procedures are fatigue, nausea, vomiting, weight change and hair loss, while anxiety is the most prevalent non-physical symptom. Several studies suggest that the severity of the symptoms may depend on the amount of information the patient gets about the potential side-effects, i.e. adequate information may reduce the severity of side-effects [19,24,25]. Often, the side-effects of chemotherapy continue even 6 months after the cessation of treatment [26], impacting on daily functioning, body image, family relationships and sexual relationships. Several drugs have a neurotoxic side-effect as well.

Radiotherapy presents a threat to body image in terms of burns, fear that the release of the radiation will not be accurate, or fear that the toxicity of radiation will be too great. Many patients are concerned about disrobing, type of machine and being alone in the room. Others worry about the duration of exposure and the danger of coughing, breathing or moving during an exposure. These threats have an obvious impact on the psychological well-being of the patient [27].

Although upon completing medical treatment patients feel less threatened, they also have a sense of loss of regular medical surveillance, loss of the security of being under treatment, and loss of support related to ongoing communication with, and availability of, health care providers. Moving into the follow-up phase, cancer patients are in a stressful situation arising from the fear of the spread or recurrence of the illness. The first year is the most stressful. Every symptom is interpreted as a sign that the illness is progressing, and every laboratory test evokes the fear of positive results (i.e. a high score in the marker test, which is evidence of active illness). Often, patients have less family and social support as coping resources in this phase than previously. Family and friends are often criticised by patients for expecting the patient to resume acting "normally" once the treatment stage is over, while the patients continue to struggle with the reality of the risk of recurrence and possible mortality. Information about other patients they know who have had recurrences and have died exacerbates their emotional distress [19].

Patients with recurrence or metastases, a particularly vulnerable group, face new stressors [28]. They are threatened by the evidence that the cancer is not curable, that the length of their survival time is limited, and that death is near and real. At the same time they are threatened by the outcomes of ongoing aggressive medical treatment and, in most cases, pain, which causes a decrease in daily functioning and increased dependency. The most common psychological responses are anxiety and depression. Patients with severe symptoms of anxiety may display tension, restlessness, shortness of breath, numbness and worry. Patients with severe symptoms of depression feel hopelessness and even a suicidal tendency, sleep a lot, cry easily and perceive everything as meaningless.

In the terminal phase, when all medical treatment for halting the progress of the illness has failed, patients suffer from severe physical symptoms, such as pain, anorexia, weakness and specific symptoms related to each type of cancer, e.g. uncontrolled coughing from lung cancer, head pain from brain and neck cancer, etc. They may have difficulty in eating, controlling elimination, focusing attention and escaping pain or discomfort. They are threatened by the loss of valued activities and friendships and begin to anticipate the loss of further activities and relationships. Patients must also deal with their deteriorating appearance, which affects self-image. According to Kübler-Ross [29], patients in this phase are terrified of near-death. They may ask family members not to leave them alone, and are afraid to sleep.

One of the main issues for families of patients with recurrence or metastases, or in the terminal phase, is communication. As long as the patient's outlook is favourable, communication is usually open. However, as the prognosis worsens and the therapy becomes more drastic, communication may start to break down. Medical staff may become evasive when questioned about the patient's status. Family members may be cheerfully optimistic with the patient, but confused and frightened when they try to elicit information from medical staff. The potential for a break in communications as illness advances can be traced to several factors. First, death itself is still very much a taboo topic in our society. The issue is generally avoided in polite conversation, little research is conducted on death and, when death occurs, the survivors often try to bear their grief alone. The proper thing to do, many people feel, is not to bring up the subject.

A second reason that communication breaks down with advancing illness relates to assumptions—possibly faulty—about what others want to hear. Each of the parties—medical staff, patient and family—believes that the others do not want to talk about death. Patients fear upsetting their families or the medical staff by asking questions about death. Family members may not bring up the issue because they fear that the patient's prognosis is poor, and that any discussion of death will be stressful to the patient, exacerbating the medical condition. Physicians and other medical staff do not bring up the issue of death for fear of stressing both the patient and the family.

Patient Coping with the Threat of the Illness

The chronic stressful situation caused by the threat to life, and the acute stress in each phase of the illness, engender a coping process that is unstable. The primary and secondary appraisal by the patient of his/her situation begins again with each phase or,

according to some stress theories, the process is one of reappraisal [4].

A primary threat is posed by having to make decisions about how to treat the disease, especially in the event of conflicting opinions by physicians over what course of action to take. The patient in this situation assesses coping options, focusing on both problem-solving strategies, such as active coping planning, suppression or instrumental support, and emotion-focused strategies such as ventilation, denial or behavioural disengagement [30]. In most cases the patient uses both types, although in differing proportions in each reappraisal. For example, seeking a second medical opinion may be viewed as an active coping strategy, yet may partially involve denial of the diagnosis. Denial is common in the early stages of the disease. The patient seeks another opinion because he/she hopes the physician has erred in the diagnosis, and at the same time believes that this step is necessary in making the best decision for a cure. Following successful surgery, patients may adopt avoidance of the fact that the surgery was an outcome of a cancer diagnosis. Some patients deny that the diagnosis is life-threatening. Denial may also mean denial of an emotional reaction to the threat, e.g. avoiding thinking about the situation, or active efforts at self-distraction from feelings of distress. However, when the illness progresses, the patient's ability to use denial or avoidance as a strategy is more limited. Instead, he/she uses more problem-focused strategies, such as emotional and instrumental support, or emotion-focused strategies such as ventilation, religion and restraint, which are helpful in coping with threat in this phase of the illness.

Extant research assesses the association between appraisal, coping process and psychological distress on the part of the cancer patient. Stanton and Snider's [31] study of 117 women before a breast biopsy, after diagnosis, and, for those who had cancer, after surgery, focuses on personality, cognitive appraisal, coping and mood variables. The findings indicate that, consistent with Lazarus and Folkman's stress theory [3], personal attributes, cognitive appraisals and coping processes are all associated with pre-biopsy mind-set. Subjects who were younger, less optimistic, felt more threatened and used more cognitive avoidance to cope were in greater distress before diagnosis. In the same vein, Epping et al. [32], examining the psychological adjustment of 80 breast cancer patients upon diagnosis and at 3 and 6 month follow-ups, found that symptoms of depression at diagnosis were predicted by low dispositional optimism. Their depression was partially mediated by the use of emotion-focused disengagement coping. At 3 months, changes in anxiety–depression symptoms were predicted by intrusive thought only. At 6 months, low dispositional optimism re-emerged as a significant predictor of change in anxiety/depression and was again partially mediated by the use of emotion-focused disengagement coping. Similar findings are reported by Osowiecki and Compas [33,34]: problem-focused engagement coping was related to fewer anxiety/depression symptoms at diagnosis and emotion-focused disengagement coping was related to more anxiety/depression symptoms at 6 months. Two studies by Nezu et al. [35] on the association between problem solving as a coping mechanism and psychological distress revealed similar findings: recently diagnosed cancer patients who were less effective problem solvers reported a high level of anxiety and depression as well as more cancer-related problems, and a weaker problem-solving ability on the part of breast cancer patients was a significant predictor of psychological distress. This was borne out in research by Maguire [36], showing that patients with a greater number of severe concerns who felt unable to resolve them were most likely to develop depression and symptoms of anxiety. Additionally, the onset of depression was linked to the perception by patients that the information they had been given about their disease was inadequate for their needs, whether in terms of too little or too much information.

Cancer Patients with Bone Metastases: Do They Differ from Patients with Metastases in Other Sites?

The answer to this question is problematic. Most of the extant research analyses mixed cancer patient samples which combine all types of metastases. Moreover, most of these studies focus on the psychological aspect of quality of life stemming from the site of the cancer, i.e. impotence, incontinence (prostate cancer) or breathlessness (lung cancer) [38] as predictors of psychological distress [37–40]. The lack of research on bone metastasis is surprising in light of the frequency of this development in cancer patients, i.e. in more than half of all cancer patients [41].

Based on clinicians' impressions and on preliminary research carried out for this chapter, the tentative conclusion is that the psychological distress of patients with bone metastases is mainly similar to that of patients with other types of cancer. The psychological distress of cancer patients with bone metastases, therefore, will be discussed as part of the broader

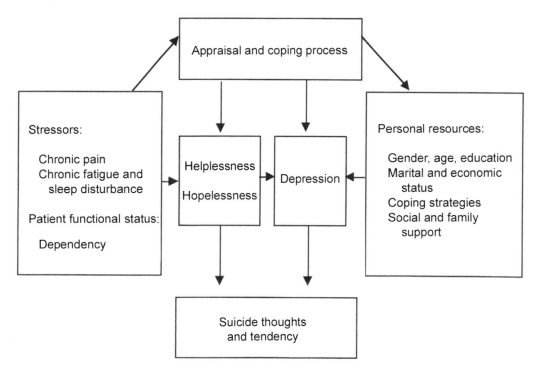

Figure 36.1. Bone metastases coping model

population of cancer patients in the advanced phase who receive palliative care, with differences discussed accordingly.

CANCER PATIENTS WITH METASTASES COPING MODEL

Based on the coping process, cancer patients who have suspected physical symptoms that may be diagnosed as metastases, feel threatened by the possibility of recurrence. Patients who use emotional coping strategies, such as avoidance or denial, in reappraising the new situation may interpret the symptom as related to other health problems: long periods of coughing may be explained as a 'flu symptom, stomach pain related to a virus, back bone pain the result of prolonged work at the computer or unusual physical effort. These patients delay seeking medical advice. In contrast, patients who use active coping or suppression strategies will more readily interpret the symptoms as a sign of metastases and will seek medical advice immediately. When the symptoms are diagnosed as metastases, however, they realise that their survival time is limited and feel hopelessness, helplessness, depression and even suicidal tendencies [42].

Figure 36.1 presents the variables that predict depression in cancer patients with bone metastases. The extent of depression that such patients feel depends on the threat of pathological fracture, reduction in physical ability, chronic fatigue and bone pain, all of which affect hopelessness, helplessness and suicide tendencies. Additionally, the amount of personal and social support has an important effect on the severity of depression. The only difference between these patients and patients with cancer in other sites is the threat of pathological fracture and bone pain.

EVALUATION OF CLINICAL DEPRESSION

The response to the spread of the disease (metastases) is depressive symptoms, ranging from sadness to adjustment disorder with a depressed mood, interfering with daily activity, major depression, loss of interest, weight loss, insomnia, hypersomnia, decreased concentration, etc. [36]. The clinical evaluation, however, requires careful assessment, as some somatic symptoms of depression, such as chronic fatigue, anorexia and weight loss, or decreased interest in sex, may be caused by the medical treatment being administered to the patient (chemotherapy, radio-therapy and hormone therapy) or by pain-control medication. The latter may include glucocortico-steroids, prednisone or dexamethasone, which are widely used in cancer pain management as well as to reduce oedema from brain and spinal cord tumours, or steroids, which may cause an organic–affective syndrome that mimics psychotic depression. In sum, depression in cancer patients generally, and in patients with metastases specifically, is best evaluated, whether clinically or in research, by the degree of the findings of hopelessness, helplessness and suicidal tendency rather than by physical symptoms [43,45].

Considerable research has been done on the role of hope/hopelessness in the individual's well-being generally and in coping with adverse life events in particular (e.g. [46,47]). Hopelessness is believed to contribute negatively to mental health and to predict depression and suicide [48]. It is also believed to have a negative impact on physical health [49]. Conversely, hopefulness is viewed as an element of spiritual and existential well-being [50] and psychosocial well-being [51]. Persons with little hope for the future have been found to be significantly less interested in activity of any sort and, eventually, to have more psychiatric symptoms, including alcoholism and depression [49]. Not surprisingly, cancer patients have been found to be more hopeless about the future and, as a result, more depressed, or to perceive themselves and the world more negatively [52,53].

Both depression and hopelessness are risk factors for suicidal thoughts or tendencies. Beck and Steer [54] have shown that a significant variable in the cognitive process affecting the inclination toward suicide is depression; viz. inactivity, withdrawal and avoidance, along with self-criticism, non-adaptability and painful emotions, all of which overwhelm the individual and erode his/her ability to cope. Suicidal thinking, however, and the tendency to suicide also result from negative inclinations and irrational thought processes, most conspicuously hopelessness regarding the future and helplessness [18,54].

CANCER PATIENTS WITH BONE METASTASES: WHICH PATIENTS DO BEST?

Research on cancer patient distress, and cancer patients with metastases in particular, emphasise that the amount of stressors, as well as the amount of personal and social support, impact on the extent of the patient's psychological distress.

Stressors

Illness variables, such as chronic pain, pathological fracture and fatigue, as well as functional status have an effect on cancer patients' distress.

Chronic Pain

Despite increased pain-control medication upon the onset of metastases, chronic pain and symptoms of depression are found to occur in tandem in cancer patients diagnosed with metastases. A review of the available findings suggests that of patients with metastases of all types of cancer, 70% have significant pain at some time during the course of the illness [55]. Such pain is enervating and demoralising for the patient. It is also profoundly affective, evoking behavioural changes that heighten the suffering of both the patient and his/her family. Cancer patients who are in pain show a greater degree of psychological disturbance, the main responses being depression symptoms that affect daily activity. Psychological distress becomes greater in the case of chronic pain from tumour progression, i.e. metastases, rather than from surgery. Pain plays an important role in vulnerability to suicide. It is associated with psychological distress and mood disturbance as essential cofactors in heightening the risk of suicide in cancer patients [55,56].

Classifying such pain may be carried out by examining the physical, mental, social and spiritual responses of the patient. Overwhelming physical pain evokes mental consequences, such as the inability to concentrate (such a patient has no wish to read or even watch TV); social consequences, such as the absence of any desire to talk (the patient may just turn away); and spiritual consequences, especially a sense of despair [57]. Not only do these patients endure pain, they also deal constantly with the significance of the pain, i.e. the progression of the illness, the time limit for their survival, disability and dependence, all of which engender feelings of helplessness, hopelessness, depression and, in extreme cases, suicidal thoughts.

Patients' assessments of amount of pain are dissimilar, as shown by a study [58] of 125 patients diagnosed with primary lung cancer or bone metastasis. Only 14% of the patients reported that present pain intensity was distressing, horrible or excruciating, while 83% reported that their worst pain reached such levels. The patients reported that they had experienced significantly more intense pain with their worst toothache than either present pain intensity or their worst cancer pain; significantly more intense pain with their worst headache than their present pain intensity; and significantly more intense pain with their worst stomach ache than their present pain. However, they reported that their worst cancer pain was significantly more intense than their worst headache or stomach ache.

By contrast, all the patients in the author's preliminary study reported a high severity of pain, as described by Avi, aged 65, a prostate cancer patient with bone metastases:

> At the beginning of the treatment I had intense pain, primarily in my legs, pain like, how should I describe it, like a blow from a hammer or like bumping into something hard and hurting your bone. But it was even stronger, the sort of pain that isn't concentrated in a specific place. It would start at a specific point but it would pass on to somewhere else, sometimes here, sometimes here, sometimes here, all over. It was very nerve-wracking, it's primarily nerve-wracking; sometimes it wasn't as painful as it was nerve-wracking, because you can't do anything about it. You take a pill, it's supposed to kill the pain, you wait for the pain to subside . . . . Later, as the treatment progressed, the pain gradually lessened, but the burning began . . . as if from salicyclic acid, burning, burning, or the leg was numb altogether, totally numb. If I moved, it [the burning] would start again . . . .

or:

> When I had haemorrhoid pain, for example, I had a solution—using ice. It would soothe [the pain]. I wouldn't walk around, I would sit, or lie, but it wouldn't hurt, until the next time, and the next. Here you have pains that you don't know what to do for them, you take a pill, you take another pill, and it still hurts. You can't put ice on it or whatever, say, exercising. Once I had backaches, so I went to the doctor and he told me: Listen, you have to do physiotherapy, stretching, things like that, so I went and did it and everything was okay. They told me I had a slipped disc or things like that, it hurts, you get old, what can you do? . . . .

As illustrated by the respondents, freedom from pain, or pain control in cancer patients with bone metastases is particularly difficult to achieve. This is so because bone pain responds poorly to opioids [59].

Research on the association between pain and psychological symptoms such as mood disturbance, depression or anxiety has produced varied findings. A study of 70 patients with advanced cancer [60] found that depression does not correlate with severity of pain. A study of three groups of patients [61], 137 with metastastic cancer, 47 with local or regional cancer and 105 with chronic non-cancerous pain of at least 6 months' duration, showed minimal differences in psychological adaptation to pain between the three groups. However, cancer patients with metastases, interpreting the pain as the progression of the illness, reported significantly higher levels of disability and inactivity due to pain than patients whose pain was of a non-malignant origin. In contrast, a study of 40 patients with metastatic cancer in which 47% of the patients had bone metastases reported remarkably low levels of mood disturbance [62]. The means of all negative mood scales were under 2.0, which is categorised as "moderate" (Profile of Mood Scales [POMS], 0–4). Moreover, only a minority of the patients ranked the pain associated with the disease or the treatment as their primary concern. Most ranked pain as their second or third concern behind the disruption caused by the disease in daily life and uncertainty about the future.

Fatigue

Fatigue has been found to be one of the most frequent and significant problems associated with cancer, cancer treatment and chronic distress from the illness [63]. Major depression disorder is the main cause of fatigue in cancer patients. With this, loss of energy is a criterion for depression. Clinical depression and fatigue, in short, are closely associated. Fatigue, moreover, has also been found to be a risk factor for suicide [64].

Cancer patients may experience fatigue from a variety of causes, including preexisting conditions, the direct effects of the disease, symptoms related to the cancer and/or the effects of the cancer treatment. A variety of mechanisms have been suggested to explain cancer-related fatigue, including sleep disturbance, biochemical changes secondary to medical treatment, death thoughts, changes in activity and loss of appetite. Advanced cancer patients who are in chronic stress, undergoing aggressive medical treatment and suffering from pain may experience greater fatigue. Stone et al. [63] found that a combination of dyspnoea

(laboured breathing), psychological distress, pain and overall disease burden accounted for 56% of the variance in fatigue scores. Fatigue was also found to be significantly associated with severity of psychological symptoms, viz. anxiety and depression. Findings by Miaskoski and Lee [65] indicate that approximately three-quarters of a group of 24 cancer patients with bone metastases undergoing radiotherapy reported moderate amounts of fatigue and pain and a significant amount of sleep disturbance and depressive symptoms. A study by Calais da Silva [66] found that fatigue and reduced social and sexual life played important roles in the overall psychological well-being of 76 prostate carcinoma patients with metastases.

Bone metastasis patients in the research sample interviewed for the chapter reported on the major effect of fatigue on their daily life and their feelings. Malka, aged 60, explained:

> Naturally, we don't go out, we don't go over to the children, I'm at home all the time. He [Malka's husband] goes out to do the chores, I don't. I'm here. Lots of things have changed completely. It affects the whole family. The children say to me: there's a child's birthday, or whatever, a grandchild, come. But I'm not up to it. My daughter lives with me for the time being. She says come, let's take a walk. My feet don't function, they don't walk. I get halfway down the street and I say to her, come, I have no strength.
>
> I lie down, and when I think, I feel weak, a weakness that settles in my shoulders, in my back. I told my oncology doctor about it and she said it's emotional and things like that, I don't know, depression from the illness. I don't want to think, heaven forbid. It's depressing. So I do everything, [but] like it or not, the illness is there...

Patient's Functional Status

Functional status has an impact not only on the patient's quality of life but on body image and self-esteem and is, therefore, one of the risk factors for sense of helplessness and depression. In extreme cases, it is a risk factor for suicide. Patients with metastases in the bone in particular are often disfigured because of medical treatments, pathological fracture or paraplegia [67]. Such disability heightens the sense of loss of control and helplessness that most cancer patients feel in all phases of the illness. Rebecca, aged 60, describes her feelings thus:

> I used to be very active.... I worked in child care, everyone loved me.... Everything has died in me, to my regret. The house was lively, I liked working, I liked earning money, helping my children, my grandchildren, I liked to grow those little flowers, to see them grow; all that is finished for me.... Today, I don't have the strength that I had before the illness, it's finished. I do something, I get tired and I lie down. I lie down and then get up. I still have the energy in my heart to help myself, but my body.... And thoughts in my head all the time about what will be, what will be, what will be....

Avi says:

> I have no patience for a lot of things, things I like to do. I don't talk, I don't discuss the fact that there are physical things I can't do. What you can't do you can't do, but even smaller things that I like to do, often I have no patience for. It's a kind of process....

> You fall down, you get up. For example, sometimes we go out to dance Friday night.... Sometimes we would go out to dance and I would feel that my feet wouldn't move, what's there to do, they don't move....

A study by Fulton [68] of 80 breast cancer patients with metastases, 40% of whom, found strong and significant correlations between physical rehabilitation status and mood. Similar findings by Breitbart [42] showed that incidence of depression increased with level of disability, advanced illness and pain. Additionally, reduced social life as the illness progresses plays an important role in overall psychological well-being, as reported by Calais da Silva [66]. In contrast, Sze et al. [60] found no differences in level of disability between 70 depressed and non-depressed cancer patients with advanced impairment. The activity of daily living in these patients was not related to depression, although they suffered from pain.

10–30% of patients with bone metastases develop fractures of the long bones and a loss of the ability to walk in the case of bone involvement of the lower extremities. The resultant dependency involved causes stress to the patients and to the family, may evoke feelings of helplessness, and exacerbates depression symptoms that the patient already has in reaction to the progression of the disease [59].

Personal Resources

Gender, Age, Education, Marital and Economic Status

Based on the coping with stress model generally and its application to cancer patients in an advanced phase specifically [4], such personal resources as age, gender, education, marital status and economic status play an important role in psychological adjustment and quality of life [38]. Little research, however, has been devoted to this area, and findings are divergent. Most extant studies do not confirm the importance of the role of personal resources [4]. Sze et al. [60] reported no difference in age, gender or educational level between depressed and non-depressed patients with advanced cancer. Similar findings were indicated by Brady and Helgesson [69] in a study of 30 breast cancer patients in recurrence. No association was found between age, education and income in an initial interview and 6 months later, although women with a higher family income had a less positive outlook than women with lower family incomes. Kugaya et al. [70] found that advanced stage of cancer, unmarried status and feelings of helplessness/hopelessness were significantly associated with depression. Similar findings by Alisson et al. [71] pointed to unemployment, older age, female gender and more advanced disease stage as predicting a worse quality of life.

The author's study of cancer patients with bone metastases indicated differences associated with gender and unmarried status only. Female patients described more feelings of guilt and concern regarding their reduced ability to manage the household and carry out their role as a housewife. The focus for male patients was impotence arising from the medical treatments for prostate cancer. For some male patients, their divorced status engendered greater feelings of loneliness and anger. Eli, age 50, a divorced patient, reported:

> I left the hospital on Friday after the examination. I was told to return on Sunday for the surgery. I came home to an empty house. When the house is empty and I'm in good health, it's a pleasure, but when there's a [health] problem, this kind of silence is pressurising and frightening.... So I came in, closed myself up in the house, was tense, and waited....

I have a large family, but no one came to visit me, so I'm angry at them, I'm filled with anger....Of course, no one owes me anything, but when I was in good health, I called, I went over, I visited. I too had problems, but with this, I took an interest [in them]. That's it. Lots of water has flowed under the bridge, as they say, and I'm paying for it now.

Coping Strategy

While coping strategy is an important aspect affecting adjustment to illness, only a single extant study deals with the association between coping strategy and psychological state of patients with advanced cancer. Research by Classen et al. [72] on 101 women diagnosed with metastatic or recurrent cancer, 40% of whom had bone metastases, indicates that a fighting spirit and emotional expressiveness were found to be associated with better emotional state. The choice of coping strategy, however, was evaluated as relating to pain outcomes by Lin [73], studying 88 patients with chronic cancer pain and 85 patients who had chronic lower back pain, respectively. They found that the strategies used most frequently by patients with chronic cancer pain were prayer/hope and pain medication.

Social Support

Social support has been found to reduce or buffer negative psychological responses to a variety of stressful life events, including life-threatening illness. Social support is most commonly defined as functions performed for an individual under stress by family members, significant others, friends or professionals. These functions are generally classified as: (a) instrumental aid (e.g. goods and services); (b) expressive aid (e.g. caring, listening); or (c) informational aid (e.g. education or advice) [9]. Following the coping with stress model [4], social support may be viewed as a form of coping assistance or as active participation by significant others in an individual's stress-management efforts.

Support needs may change over the course of the illness. For example, in the early stage, support may involve the provision of information to help a patient decide upon treatment after diagnosis (informational aid). Patients hospitalised for long periods or in an advanced phase may require assistance with household tasks to meet their family responsibilities (instrumental aid). At various points, the patient's fears may increase the need for reassurance that others will continue to demonstrate love and emotional support/emotional aid (expressive aid) [74].

Little research has been carried out on the impact of social support on the adjustment to advanced cancer (metastases and recurrence). An early study by Bloom and Spiegel [75] of 86 advanced metastatic breast cancer patients found that emotional support was related to the patient's outlook; greater social activity had a positive effect on the patient's adjustment and social functioning. A more recent cross-sectional study of 81 women who rated their social support and adjustment across a variety of domains [76] indicated that emotional support from various sources was associated with less emotional distress but was not associated with adjustment. Research by Brady and Helgesson [69] on 30 patients with a recurrence of breast cancer showed that emotional support from a partner and informational support from an oncologist related to decreased physical problems over time, but this was not related to psychological distress over time.

Family support greatly affected coping with the illness in the author's study of cancer patients with bone metastases [2], although the subjects reported having a high level of guilt toward their relatives. Annie, a 60-year-old breast cancer patient with bone metastases, describes these feelings thus:

> It's true that I didn't want this [to happen], it's true that I'm not to blame for it, but the fact is that I feel guilty [that it happened]. My daughter sits in the house and doesn't live her life because of me, and I'm the cause because I became ill, you understand.

Avi says:

> I don't really want to bother, or burden my family. I must say that this is a big dilemma. I have always said one for all and all for one, no matter what the circumstances. I must say that up to now it has worked. What will happen next, I don't know, but I know that it works.

Rebecca says:

> I have a wonderful family, I have exceptional grandchildren, and it's so painful to me that I have burdened them, as if I betrayed them, the whole future I had with them. It does something

to my heart.... I simply have no solution.... It grabs the whole family...

Women with breast cancer also have greater feelings of guilt involving the passing on of a high risk for breast cancer to their daughters, as described by Annie:

Not only have I done this to them [to the family] at this time, but I also know that cancer is hereditary. Perhaps I have passed it on to my daughter? That's a very difficult thought. To endow such a terrible thing to the person I love most and who is closest to me.

CONCLUSION

Little research has been devoted to the coping with illness of cancer patients with bone metastases. The studies that have been carried out on cancer patients with metastases in various sites indicate that feelings of helplessness and hopelessness contribute to depression caused by the threat to life and medical outcomes. In the case of cancer patients with bone metastases, however, extant research focuses on the coping with symptoms of depression that appear to stem mainly from reduced physical ability, chronic pain, fatigue and pathological fracture. Surprising findings in the author's study [2] revealed that the patients did not have suicidal tendencies, although such thoughts did appear. Conceivably, cancer patients with bone metastases feel less hopeless than other patients with metastases because they still believe that the medical treatment will help stop the progression of the disease. The study also confirms family support as an important element in coping during the advanced stage of the illness. With this, patients often feel guilt caused by their reduced functioning and their distress at burdening spouses, daughters, sisters, etc. The most common feeling described by the patients, however, related to their uncertainty about the process of their imminent death, which caused tremendous stress to them and their families.

In addition to the need for more prospective research to assess the psychosocial distress of cancer patients with bone metastases, there is a need for special caring programmes that coordinate specialists in onco-orthopaedics and pain control with the oncology nurse and psycho-oncologist. This will lead to reduced depressive symptoms and an improved quality of life.

REFERENCES

1. Nielsen OS. Palliative treatment of bone metastases. Acta Oncol 1996; 35(suppl 5): 58–60.
2. Winstok Z, Gilbar O. Cancer patients with bone metastases: coping with illness (unpublished qualitative study, 2000).
3. Lazarus RS, Folkman S. Stress Appraisal and Coping. Springer: New York, 1984.
4. Lazarus RS. Stress and Emotion: A New Synthesis. Free Association Books: London, 1999.
5. Gignac MAM, Gottlieb BH. Caregivers' appraisals of efficacy in coping with dementia. Psychol Aging 1996; 11(2): 214–25.
6. Folkman S. Psychosocial effects of HIV infection. In Goldberger L, Breznitz S (eds), Handbook of Stress: Theoretical and Clinical Aspects. Free Press: New York, 1993: 658–81.
7. Gignac MAM, Gottlieb BH. Changes in coping with chronic illness: the role of caregivers' appraisals of coping efficacy. In Gottlieb BH (ed.), Coping with Chronic Illness. Plenum: New York, 1997: 245–67.
8. Moos RH, Schaefer JA. Coping resources and process: current concepts and measures. In Goldberger L, Berznitz S (eds), Handbook of Stress: Theoretical and Clinical Aspects, 2nd edn. Free Press: New York, 1993: 234–57.
9. Spencer SM, Carver CS, Price AA. Psychological and social factors in adaptation. In Holland J (ed.), Psycho-oncology. Oxford University Press: New York, 1998: 211–22.
10. Garcia HB, Lee PCY. Knowledge about cancer and use of health care services among Hispanic and Asian-American older adults. J Psychosoc Oncol 1989; 6: 157–77.
11. Wagner MK, Armstrong D, Laughlin JE. Cognitive determinants of quality of life after onset of cancer. Psychol Rep 1995; 77: 147–54.
12. Baum C, Cohen L, Hall M. Control and intrusive memories as possible determinants of chronic stress. Psychosom Med 1993; 55: 274–86.
13. Compas BC, Connor J, Osowiecki D, Welch A. Effortful and involuntary responses to stress. In Gottlieb BH (ed.), Coping with Chronic Stress. Plenum: New York, 1997: 105–30.
14. Watson M. Psychological care for cancer patients and their families. J Ment Health 1994; 3: 456–65.
15. Taylor SE. Health Psychology. McGraw-Hill: New York, 1991.
16. David HP. Coping with cancer. A personal odyssey. Patient Educ Couns 1999; 37: 293–7.
17. Gottesman D, Lewis MS. Differences in crisis reactions among cancer and surgery patients. J Consult Clin Psychol 1982; 50: 381–8.
18. Jacobsen PB, Roth AJ, Hollau J. Surgery. In Holland JC (ed.), Psycho-oncology. Oxford University Press: New York, 1998: 257–68.
19. Knobf MT, Pasacreta JV, Valentine A, McCorkle R. Chemotherapy, hormonal therapy, and immunotherapy. In Holland JC (ed.), Psycho-oncology. Oxford University Press: New York, 1998: 277–88.
20. Fallowfield L, Ford S, Lewis S. No news is not good news: information preferences of patients with cancer. Psycho-oncology 1995; 4: 197–202.

21. McHugh P, Lewis S, Ford S et al. The efficacy of audiotapes in promoting psychological well-being in cancer patients: a randomized, controlled track. Br J Cancer 1995; 71: 388–92.

23. Greenberg DB. Radiotherapy. In Holland JC (ed.), Psycho-oncology. Oxford University Press: New York, 1998: 269–76.

24. Tierney AJ, Taylor J, Closs SJ. Knowledge, expectations and experiences of patients receiving chemotherapy for breast cancer. Cancer Scand J Ca Sci 1992; 6(2): 75–80.

25. Campora E, Naso C, Vitullo MT et al. The impact of chemotherapy on the quality of life of breast cancer patients. J Chemo 1992; 4(1): 59–63.

26. Beisecker AE, Cook MK, Ashworth J et al. Side effects of adjuvant chemotherapy: perceptions of node negative breast cancer patients. Psycho-Oncol 1997; 6(2): 85–93.

27. Chandra PS, Chaturvedi SK, Channabasavanna SM et al. Psychological well-being among cancer patients receiving radiotherapy: a prospective study. Qual Life Res 1998; 7(6): 495–500.

28. Breitbart W, Jaramillo JR, Chochinov HM. Palliative and terminal care. In Holland JC (ed.), Psycho-oncology. Oxford University Press: New York, 1998: 437–49.

29. Kübler-Ross E. On Death and Dying. Macmillan: New York, 1969.

30. Carver CS, Scheier MF, Weintraub JK. Assessing coping strategies: a theoretically-based approach. J Pers Soc Psychol 1989; 56: 267–88.

31. Stanton AL, Snider PR. Coping with breast cancer diagnosis: a prospective study. Health Psychol 1993; 1 16–23.

32. Epping J, JoAnne E, Compas BE et al. Psychological adjustment in breast cancer: process of emotional distress. Health Psychol 1999; 18(4): 325–6.

33. Osowiecki DM, Compas BE. Psychological adjustment to cancer: control beliefs and coping in adult cancer patients. Cog Ther Res 1998; 22(5): 483–99.

34. Osowiecki DM, Compas BE. A prospective study of coping, perceived control, and psychological adaptation to breast cancer. Cog Ther Res 1999; 23(2): 169–80.

35. Nezu CM, Nezu AM, Friedman SH et al. Cancer and psychological distress: two investigations regarding the role of social problem-solving. J Psychosoc Oncol 1999; 16(3–4): 127–40.

36. Maguire P. Depression and cancer. In Robertson MM, Katona CLE (eds), Depression and Physical Illness. Wiley: Chichester, 1997: 429–41.

37. Esper P, Redman BG. Supportive care, pain management, and quality of life in advanced prostate cancer. Urol Clin N Am 1999; 26(2): 375–89.

38. Montazeri A, Cillis CR, McEwen J. Quality of life in patients with lung cancer: a review of literature from 1970–1995. Chest 1998; 113(2): 467–81.

39. DeAntoni EP, Crawford D. Pretreatment of metastatic disease. Cancer 1994; 74(7, suppl): 2182–7.

40. Clark JA, Wray N, Brody B et al. Dimensions of quality of life expressed by men treated for metastatic prostate. Soc Sci Med 1997; 45(8): 1299–309.

41. Body JJ, Cossignol D, Ronson A. The concept of rehabilitation of cancer patients. Curr Opin Oncol 1997; 9(4): 332–40.

42. Breitbart W. Psycho-oncology: depression, anxiety, delirium. Semin Oncol 1994; 21: 754–69.

43. Spiegel D, Giese-Davis J. Biol Psychiatry 2003; 54(3): 269–82.

44. Billings JA, Block S. Depression. J Palliat Care 1995; 11(1): 48–54.

45. Lynch ME. The assessment and prevalence of affective disorders in advanced cancer. J Palliat Care 1995; 11(1): 10–18.

46. Farran CJ, Herth KK, Popovich JM (eds). Hope and Hopelessness. Sage: Thousand Oaks, California, 1995

47. Scheier MF, Carver CS. Dispositional optimism and physical well-being. The influence of generalized outcome expectation on health. J Personality 1987; 55: 169–210.

48. Beck AT, Steer RA, Newman CF. Hopelessness, depression, suicidal ideation and clinical diagnosis of depression. Suicide Life-Threat Behav 1993; 28: 139–45.

49. Everson SA, Goldberg DE, Kaplan GS et al. Hopelessness and risk of mortality and incidence of myocardial infarction and cancer. Psychosom Med 1996; 58: 113–21.

50. Mickley JR, Soeken K, Belcher A. Spiritual well-being, religiousness and hope among women with breast cancer. IMAGE: J Nurs Scholar 1992; 24(4) 267–72.

51. Miller JF. Hope-inspiring strategies of the critically ill. Appl Nurs Res 1989; 2(1): 23–9.

52. DeVellis BN, Blalock SJ. Illness attributions and hopelessness depression: the role of hopelessness expectancy. J Abnorm Psychol 1992; 101(2) 257–64.

53. Klauer T, Filipp SH. Life-change perceptions in cognitive adaptation to life-threatening illness. Eur Rev Appl Psychol 1997; 47(3) 181–8.

54. Beck AT, Steer RA. Beck Depression Inventory Manual. The Psychological Corporation. Harcourt Brace, Jovanovich: Philadelphia, PA, 1987.

55. Breitbart W, Payne DK. Pain. In Holland J (ed.), Psycho-oncology. Oxford University Press: New York, 1998: 450–67.

56. Massie M, Gagnon P, Holland J. Depression and suicide in patients with cancer. J Pain Sympt Manag 1994; 9: 325–31.

57. Hanrathy JF. Palliative Care of the Terminally Ill. Radcliffe Medical Press: Oxford, 1989.

58. Berry DL, Wilkie DJ, Hung H-Y, Blumenstein BA. Cancer pain and common pain: a comparison of patient-reported intensities. Oncol Nurs Forum 1999; 26(4): 721–6.

59. Mercadante S. Malignant bone pain pathophysiology and treatment. Pain 1997; 69: 1–18.

60. Sze FK, Wong E, Lo R, Woo J. Do pain and disability differ in depressed cancer patients? Palliat Med 2000; 11(1): 11–17.

61. Turk DC, Sist TC, Okifugi A et al. Adaptation to metastatic cancer pain, regional/local cancer pain and non-cancer pain: role of psychological and behavioral factors. Pain 1998; 74: 247–56.

62. Dar R, Beach CM, Borden PL, Cleeland S. Cancer pain in the marital system: a study of patients and their spouses. J Pain Sympt Manag 1992; 7(2): 87–93.

63. Stone P, Richards MA, Hern R, Hardy J. A study to investigate the prevalence, severity and correlates of fatigue among patients with cancer in comparison with a control group of volunteers without cancer. Ann Oncol 2000; 11(5): 561–7.

64. Hopwood P, Howell A, Maguire P. Psychiatric morbidity in patients with advanced cancer of the breast: prevalence

measured by two self-rating questionnaires. Br J Cancer 1991; 64: 349–52.

65. Miaskowski C, Lee KA. Pain, fatigue, and sleep disturbances in oncology outpatients receiving radiation therapy for bone metastasis: a pilot study. J Pain Symptom Manag 1999; 17(5) 320–32.

66. Calais da Silva F. Quality of life in prostatic carcinoma. Eur Urol 1993; 24(suppl 2): 113–17.

67. Kornblith AB. Psychosocial adaptation of cancer survivors. In Holland JC (ed.), Psycho-oncology. Oxford University Press: New York, 1998.

68. Fulton C. Patients with metastatic breast cancer: their physical and psychological rehabilitation needs. Intern J Rehab Res 1999; 22: 291–301.

69. Brady SS, Helgesson VS. Social support and adjustment to recurrence of breast cancer. J Psychosoc Oncol 1999; 17(2): 31–5.

70. Kugaya A, Tatsuo A, Hitoshi O et al. Correlates of depressed mood in ambulatory head and neck cancer patients. Psycho-oncology 1999; 8(6): 494–9.

71. Alisson PJ, Locker D, Dauphinee S et al. Correlates of health-related quality of life in upper aerodigestive tract cancer patients. Qual Life Res 1998; 7(8): 713–22.

72. Classen C, Koopman C, Angell K, Spiegel D. Coping style associated with psychological adjustment to advanced breast cancer. Health Psychol 1996; 15(6): 434–7.

73. Lin EC. Comparison of the effects of perceived self-efficacy on coping with chronic cancer pain and coping with chronic low back pain. Clin J Pain 1998; 14: 4.

74. Nelles WB, McCaffrey RJ, Blanchard CG, Ruckdeschel JC. Social support and breast cancer: a review. J Psycho Oncol 1991; 9(2): 21–34.

75. Bloom JR, Spiegel D. The relationship of two dimensions of social support to the psychological well-being and social functioning of women with advanced breast cancer. Soc Sci Med 1984; 19: 831–7.

76. Northouse LL, Darris G, Charrou-Moore C. Factors affecting couples' adjustment to recurrent breast cancer. Soc Sci Med 1995; 41: 69–76.

37

Metabolic Bone Diseases in Childhood Cancer

Vallo Tillman, Helena Davies and Nick Bishop

The Sheffield Children's Hospital, Sheffield, UK

INTRODUCTION

By the age of 15, about 1/650 children in the UK will have developed childhood cancer [1]. Of these, about two-thirds can now expect to be cured [2–4]. This means that currently about 1/900 young adults in the UK is a survivor of childhood cancer. Brain tumours and leukaemia are the commonest of the childhood cancers, representing about 24% and 33%, respectively (Figure 37.1).

Acute lymphoblastic leukaemia (ALL) is the commonest childhood leukaemia representing about 25% of all childhood cancers. There is a peak age of incidence between 3 and 6 years of age and it is slightly more common in boys than girls, with boys comprising about 55–60% of cases [5]. Bone pain is a common presenting symptom in children with leukaemia [6] and a significant proportion will have fractures and/or evidence of osteoporosis at diagnosis [7,8].

Possible aetiological factors for osteoporosis include the leukaemia *per se*, chemotherapy, particularly steroids and methotrexate, and radiotherapy, directly or through growth hormone (GH) deficiency. Studies to date have failed to reach a consensus on key factors in aetiology. In particular, the importance of chemotherapy remains controversial.

Bone density in childhood is most often assessed using dual-energy X-ray absorptiometry (DXA). Lumbar spine bone density and total body bone density are most commonly measured. The bone mineral content is divided by area to give "areal bone density" (aBMD). The results from DXA are influenced by bone size. The growth of a child can increase the areal BMD, although there would be no actual increase in the true volumetric BMD. A child with larger bones will have a higher areal BMD than a child of the same age with smaller bones. Adjustment for bone size is thus particularly important in longitudinal studies in children, where growth variation can affect the result.

Different methods have been developed to adjust BMD for body size [9–11] or calculate "apparent volumetric" BMD [12–14]. It remains unclear whether adjusting areal BMD for body size using the relationship derived from measurements in healthy children improves prediction of fracture risk in childhood cancer survivors. However, it does provide a further method of comparison with the healthy population.

BONE ABNORMALITIES AT THE DIAGNOSIS OF ALL

Fever and bone pain are classical presenting symptoms in the child with ALL. Radiological changes in bones, such as metaphyseal lines, lysis, periostal reaction, osteoporosis and pathological fracture, are found at the time of diagnosis [15,16]. Of children with ALL, 14/40 (36%) had musculoskeletal pain at the time of diagnosis, whereas 12% and 10% had radiographic evidence of osteopenia and fractures [17]. In a separate study, up to 58% of children with ALL had some type of radiological lesion in bone at the time of diagnosis [16].

Textbook of Bone Metastases. Edited by C. Jasmin, R. E. Coleman, L. R. Coia, R. Capanna and G. Saillant
© 2005 John Wiley & Sons Ltd: ISBN 0 471 87742 5

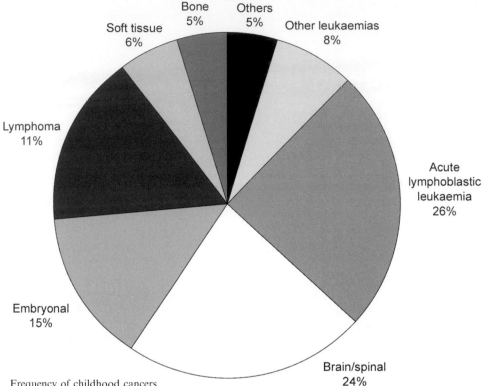

Figure 37.1. Frequency of childhood cancers

The mechanism of these lesions is not well established, but they may result from leukaemic infiltration of the bone marrow or from secretion of PTH-related peptides (PTHrP) and tumour-related cytokines [18,19]. There are many cytokines produced by lymphocytes and monocytes that induce osteoclast formation and thus facilitate bone resorption: these include interleukin-1 (IL-1) and IL-6, colony-stimulating factors, tumour necrosis factor-α (TNFα) and lymphotoxin. Increased serum PTHrP levels have been found in adult T cell leukaemia/lymphoma [20]. However, the role of these cytokines in the pathogenesis of bone lesions in childhood leukaemia is much less certain. However, the majority of clinical data suggest that resorption is not increased at the time of diagnosis in ALL [16,17,21,22]. In addition, studies of leukaemic cells themselves have failed to show increased cytokine mRNA for IL-6 or TNFα, two specific candidates for activating bone resorption in pathological states.

Disturbances in vitamin D metabolism that may impair bone metabolism have been seen at an early stage of the disease. Low 1,25-(OH)$_2$D levels were seen at the diagnosis of ALL and remained low through the treatment period, while 25-(OH)$_2$D levels were normal, indicating that this was not due to primary vitamin D deficiency [17]. Authors suggested that low 1,25-(OH)$_2$D serum levels might be due to receptor-mediated binding of 1,25-(OH)$_2$D to leukaemic lymphoblasts and to the requirement for 1,25-(OH)$_2$D in the differentiation of cells in myeloid cell lineage. Binding of 1,25-(OH)$_2$D to receptors on immature lymphoid leukaemic cells is significantly higher than that of normal mature lymphocytes [23]. Abnormally low circulating 1,25-(OH)$_2$D levels associated with hypercalciuria may result in calcium and phosphate depletion, thus limiting bone mineralisation. However, in some children primary vitamin D deficiency as evidenced by low serum levels of 25-(OH)$_2$D [24] should be considered as a possible cause of reduced bone mineralisation.

There have been many studies of bone turnover using markers of bone formation and bone resorption. Various studies report a reduction in markers of bone formation, such as alkaline phosphate (ALP), osteocalcin (OC), and type I collagen amino-terminal (PINP) and carboxy-terminal (PICP) propeptides in children with ALL at the time of diagnosis

[16,17,21,22,25]. Four of the above studies also found reduced bone resorption, indicating that children with ALL are in a low bone turnover state caused by the disease itself. Only Arikoski et al. [25] reported slightly increased bone resorption at diagnosis; they measured type I collagen carboxy-terminal telopeptide (ICTP), but in their cohort there were only 11/46 patients with ALL. As ICTP is not a specific marker of type I collagen resorption, the significance of this observation is unclear.

RADIOTHERAPY

Cranial Irradiation and GH Deficiency

Cranial irradiation as prophylaxis against central nervous system (CNS) relapse was used in standard treatment protocols until the late 1980s. Most reported studies examining bone density have thus consisted mainly of children who have received cranial irradiation as their CNS-directed therapy [8,17,26–31]. Because of concerns about long-term effects, cranial irradiation was removed from the standard UK ALL treatment protocol in 1990 (UKALL XI). Cranial irradiation is currently used in the UK only in children with proven CNS disease; standard-risk children receive intrathecal methotrexate alone. Internationally, cranial irradiation is no longer used as prophylaxis for standard-risk ALL but details of CNS-directed therapy vary from country to country.

Gilsanz et al. [32] studied 42 survivors of ALL (29 had cranial irradiation) who had the trabecular bone density of the spine evaluated by quantitative computed tomography (QCT) at an average of 3.5 years after completion of chemotherapy. The ALL survivors had significantly lower bone density than age-, gender- and race-matched non-leukaemic control subjects and this decrease was accounted for solely by the subset of patients who had received cranial irradiation. The irradiated patients had significantly lower volumetric BMD than the non-irradiated group (-0.93 vs. $+0.21$ SDS). The effects on bone density of 18 Gy and of 22.5–25.2 Gy were indistinguishable. The authors postulated that cranial radiation may cause growth hormone (GH) deficiency, resulting in growth retardation and reduced BMD. Male gender [26] and older age at time of investigations (>19 years old) [33] have been found to be related to reduced areal BMD also.

GH plays an important role in bone growth, skeletal maturation and development of bone mass [34]. Children with GH deficiency have reduced BMD [35,36] even after adjusting for bone size. In adults with childhood-onset GH deficiency, osteopenia is more severe than adult-onset GH deficiency [37]. This is likely to be due to failure to achieve a normal peak bone mass, rather than accelerated bone loss [35]. Survivors of ALL who were GH-deficient and not treated with GH had significantly reduced areal BMD at femoral neck, lumbar spine and Ward's triangle than those survivors with normal GH status or those treated with GH [30]. Patients treated with GH or those without GH deficiency had areal BMD similar to the controls. The authors concluded that GH deficiency during childhood leads to reduced accumulation of peak bone mass and predisposes these patients to increased risk of osteoporosis later in adulthood. However, Brennen et al. [28] did not find that current GH status had influenced BMD in survivors of childhood ALL, all treated with cranial radiation. Vertebral (T12–L3) BMD measured by QCT in patients with severe GH deficiency did not differ from those with normal GH status [28]. The discrepancy between these two studies might be because in the former study [30] BMD was not corrected for body size (mean height SDS in the non-treated GH deficiency group was -2.2), whereas in the latter BMD was measured by QCT, which gives volumetric BMD (g/cm^3).

Total Body Irradiation (TBI)

Total body irradiation is used as conditioning treatment prior to bone marrow transplantation. Irradiation may cause direct bone loss at the site of the irradiation, particularly at trabecular bone sites. In addition, TBI may directly damage gonadal function, affecting the production of sex hormones, which may lead to impaired BMD. Other mechanisms involve the effects on the hypothalamic–pituitary axis, leading to GH deficiency, which is a known risk factor for osteoporosis.

Nysom et al. [38] measured bone mass in 25 survivors of childhood leukaemia or lymphoma (21 with ALL) who had received TBI and allogeneic bone marrow transplant (BMT) a median of 8 years prior to study. Whole-body bone mineral content (BMC) and areal BMD were reduced (-0.8 and -0.5 SDS, respectively). However, the low BMC was influenced by a reduced height for age, and therefore the size-adjusted bone mass (BMC for bone area) was normal.

Patients who had childhood acute myeloid leukaemia (AML) have been reported to have low areal BMD SDS [39]. However, the areal BMD values were not adjusted for height or bone area and therefore could be affected by bone size.

CHEMOTHERAPY

The majority of bone mass studies in childhood cancer patients have been cross-sectional and included children who have received cranial irradiation (CI) (reviewed in Table 37.1). It has therefore been difficult

to clarify the impact of chemotherapy alone on bone metabolism and BMD.

There have been three prospective studies of longitudinal changes in BMD in newly diagnosed children with cancer (reviewed in Table 37.2). In the first study [40], 40 children with newly diagnosed ALL were monitored at 6 monthly intervals throughout 24 months of chemotherapy, of whom 29 completed the study. Radiographic evidence of osteopenia was observed in 10%, 64%, and 76% at diagnosis, 12 and 24 months, respectively. Fractures occurred in

Table 37.1. Cross-sectional studies on bone health in survivors of childhood cancer

Reference	No. of cancer subjects	Methods	Key results
Arikoski et al. [26]	29 ALL, 2–20 years after chemotherapy	DXA, lumbar, femoral BMD	Lumbar, femoral BMDs reduced. Male gender and cranial irradition associated with low BMD
Arikoski et al. [59,60]	48 (22 ALL) at completion of chemotherapy	DXA, lumbar, femoral volumetric BMD, serum ICTP, OC, PICP, vit D metabolites	ALL: lumbar (−0.8 SDS), femoral (−1.0 SDS) BMDs ↓. Other tumours: femoral BMD ↓ (−0.8 SDS). Whole group: ICTP ↑; 25(OH)D, 1,25(OH)D and Ca all ↓; PICP and OC not changed
Aisenberg et al. [42]	40 (10 ALL) ~13 years (mean) after chemo- and radio- therapy	DXA, lumbar, femoral, total body BMD	Femoral (−0.7 SDS), total body (−0.3 SDS) BMDs ↓, but not lumbar BMD. Gonadal dysfunction correlated to reduced BMD
Brennan et al. [28]	31 ALL, 18 years after DXT	Vertebral (T12–L3) BMD by QCT, lumbar and femoral BMD by DXA	Vertebral (−1.3 SDS), lumbar (−0.7 SDS), femoral (−0.4 SDS) BMDs ↓. BMD was not correlated to GH status
Gilsanz et al. [32]	42 ALL, mean 3.5 years off chemotherapy; 29/42 had CI	QCT, lumbar spine BMD	Lumbar spine BMD SDS was ↓ in those with CI (−0.93 vs. +0.21 SDS in non-CI)
Henderson et al. [61]	60 (30 ALL), mean 4 years off chemotherapy	DXA, lumbar spine BMD	Mean BMD was normal (−0.28 SDS). Weight SDS was the major determinant of BMD SDS
Hesseling et al. [62]	97 (22 ALL), 5–23 years after diagnosis	DXA, lumbar BMD	45% had low BMD (< −1.0 SDS). Increased radiation dose was correlated with lower BMD (also true for ALL)
Nussey et al. [30]	64 (43 ALL), 40/44 had DXT	DXA, lumbar, femoral BMD	Only patients with ALL and GH deficiency not treated with GH (n=14) had low BMDs
Nysom et al. [63]	185 (130 ALL), 67 had CI and 25 had TBI, median 11 years from diagnosis	DXA, lumbar, whole-body BMC and BMC for bone area	Whole body BMC (−0.65), BMC for bone area (−0.53) SDS ↓, lumbar BMC (−0.5), BMC for bone area (−0.55) SDS ↓. CI and older age at follow-up were risk factors for reduced BMC
Nysom et al. [38]	25 ALL with BMT, 4–13 years previously	DXA, whole-body BMC, BMC for bone area	BMC was 0.8 SDS less than predicted, while BMC for bone area was normal. Low BMC was related to additional cranial DXT and age >20 years at follow-up
Vassilopoulou-Sellin et al. [64]	26, median 18 years after diagnosis	DXA, lumbar, hip BMD	Lumbar (−1.4), femoral neck (−1.1), total hip (−1.1) BMD SDS. Low BMD was related to cranial DXT
Warner et al. [31]	66 (35 ALL)	DXA, whole-body, lumbar spine, hip BMC % from predicted	In ALL, lumbar spine and hip BMC (%) ↓. Exercise capacity and levels of physical activity were correlated to BMC (%) at hip

For abbreviations, see text.

39% of children during treatment (expected fracture incidence over 2 years would be 7%). Lumbar spine BMC was measured by dual-photon absorptiometry. Reduction in BMC occurred in 64% of patients and was most severe in those greater than 11 years of age at diagnosis. By 6 months of therapy, 84% children were hypomagnesaemic, of whom 52% were hypermagnesuric. Plasma osteocalcin, which was subnormal at diagnosis, increased to normal by 6 months of treatment. Urinary cross-link N-telopeptide became elevated in 58% of children by the end of therapy. The authors concluded that skeletal morbidity and a reduction in bone mineral mass become more prevalent during treatment, with increased bone resorption, which was probably due to corticosteroid administration. However, the BMD was not corrected for body size, which is particularly important in longitudinal studies and in children with short stature [11]. Apparent volumetric BMD of lumbar spine and femoral neck was longitudinally measured by DXA in 18 children with solid tumours and in 10 children with ALL [24,25]. Femoral apparent volumetric BMD fell by -11.3% during the first year of treatment, whereas age- and sex-matched controls showed annual increments of $+0.7\%$. The markers of bone formation (PICP and OC), which were decreased at diagnosis, returned to normal by the end of the follow-up, whereas the marker of bone resorption (ICTP) increased above normal. Reduced levels of 25-hydroxyvitamin D, 1,25-dihydroxyvitamin D and IGF-binding protein-3 were observed during the study. The authors concluded that:

. . . increased bone resorption and impaired development of femoral bone density were observed in children with cancer during chemotherapy. Deficient accumulation of bone mass may lead to impaired development of peak bone mass and predispose children with cancer to increased risk of osteoporosis and diminished skeletal resistance to fractures later in life.

Longitudinal changes in whole-body BMD in ALL have been studied by Boot et al. [21], who found normal total body BMD at diagnosis that decreased significantly during the first year of treatment, whereas lumbar spine BMD SDS did not change significantly. Parameters of bone turnover increased to normal during the treatment period. The authors concluded that total-body BMD decreased significantly during treatment and remained low in 4/9 patients 1 year after completion of the treatment. The key results of prospective studies are summarised in Table 37.2. The changes in BMD and bone turnover have been largely attributed to steroid treatment.

Glucocorticoid-induced Osteoporosis

Glucocorticoids (GC) are universally used in the treatment regimens for leukaemia. Osteoporosis is a well-recognised complication of long-term use of GC. Children are particularly at risk for steroid-induced osteoporosis because of their more rapid bone turnover [41].

The mechanisms of steroid-induced osteoporosis are multiple. The classical view of the effect of GCs has been that they induce renal calcium efflux and inhibit calcium uptake from the intestine, leading to a fall in serum calcium and secondary hyperparathyroidism. Hyperparathyroidism has been observed in patients with ALL during remission induction (mostly

Table 37.2. Prospective/longitudinal studies on bone health in children with ALL

Reference	No. of cancer subjects	Methods	Key results
Arikoski et al. [24]	28 (10 ALL)	1 year, DXA, lumbar, femoral volumetric BMD	During first year of therapy: femoral (-11%) vol BMD ↓. PICP and OC ↓ at diagnosis, but normalised during the study. During study, ICTP ↑; 25(OH)D, 1,25(OH)D and Ca all ↓
Atkinson et al. [7]	16 ALL	2.5 years, single-photon absorptiometry, radius BMC	During therapy: Ca ↓, Mg ↓, 1,25(OH)D ↓, hypercalciuria, hypomagnesiuria. BMC ↓ $(-2.3\,\text{SDS})$; 6 months after therapy: all above normalised except 1,25 (OH)D and BMC $(-2.4\,\text{SDS})$
Boot et al. [21]	14 ALL	3 years, DXA, lumbar, total body BMD	Total body BMD ↓ during study. 4/9 had low total body BMD at 3 years
Halton et al. [8]	40 ALL	2 years, X-ray, dual-photon absorptiometry, lumbar BMC	At 24 months: 76% had osteopenia (by X-ray), BMC ↓ in 64% and urinary N-telopeptide ↑ during study

prednisolone or dexamethazone) [7,24,25,27]. The consequences of continuously elevated PTH levels will be to increase bone resorption and reduce bone formation. This pattern of effects has been widely reported immediately after initiating GC therapy, but the increase in bone resorption does not usually continue. Sorva et al. [16] evaluated bone formation and degradation rates at diagnosis, during induction and during consolidation treatment in 35 children with ALL, using two serum markers of bone collagen formation (PINP and PICP) and a marker of degradation (ICTP). Type I collagen turnover (i.e. both synthesis and degradation) was remarkably low at diagnosis. The PICP and PINP levels declined further during the first week of therapy, whereas the ICTP levels had risen by the end of the induction phase. By the end of the 12 week interval, the concentrations of the formation and degradation markers had returned to normal.

There are additional effects of GCs on systems that modulate bone remodelling:

- *Pituitary*—inhibition of secretion of GH; although serum GH and IGF1 levels are normal, IGF1 bioreactivity is reduced, possibly due to increased IGFBP-1. Also, inhibition of LH/FSH and ACTH secretion.
- *Gonadal function*—inhibition of synthesis of oestrogen by the ovary and testosterone by the testes; note that the adverse effects of GCs are seen in both eugonadal and hypogonadal individuals, and that the largest reported changes in bone mass are seen in older children whose gonadal function might be expected to contribute to bone mass accretion [33,42].
- *Adrenal*—decrease in secretion (due to suppression of ACTH) of DHEA and androstenedione.
- *Cellular transport*—decrease in transport of calcium and phosphate.

GC Direct Effects on Bone Cells

It is important to distinguish between the developmental and regulatory effects of GCs on bone formation—GCs may enhance differentiation of osteoblastic cells thus providing more cells to contribute to new bone formation (but also see below) but in the complete organ will also inhibit the functions of the differentiated cells and may also provoke apoptosis.

In the normal bone remodelling cycle, bone resorption (which lasts about 2 weeks in any individual site) is followed by bone formation (which lasts about 2.5 months). In children the amount of bone replaced in each "packet" is 3% more than that removed, thus maintaining an increase in bone mass as part of linear skeletal growth [43].

In GC-induced bone disease in animals and humans, bone resorption is initially increased for about a week after starting therapy, but then continues at the normal rate. However, the amount of new bone formed to "fill in" the defects created by resorption is reduced, reflecting both an apparent reduction in osteoblastogenesis and increased apoptosis of osteoblasts.

Increased osteoblast and osteocyte apoptosis have been widely reported in sections of bone from GC-treated humans and animals. Recent data concerning the speed of onset/offset of fracture risk associated with steroid therapy [44] has suggested that preservation of the integrity of the osteocyte network is a critical factor in preventing fractures in GC-treated patients.

Previous studies have failed to show a clear benefit of the use of calcium and vitamin D in the prevention of fractures in GC-treated adult patients. There is some evidence for beneficial effects with calcitriol and calcium in combination and for drugs of the bisphosphonate family. There are no data available for children that indicate either the preferred mode of treatment of established osteoporosis caused by GCs, or prophylaxis in this vulnerable group.

Methotrexate Osteopathy

Methotrexate is a common antineoplastic drug used in the treatment of childhood malignancies. It is the backbone of antimetabolite therapy during post-remission (maintenance) therapy for ALL. Methotrexate osteopathy has been found during maintenance therapy in children with ALL and in infants with intracranial tumours treated with high doses of methotrexate [45–47]. Methotrexate osteopathy is characterised by severe lower extremity pain and by osteoporosis particularly involving the lower extremities. In addition, thick dense provisional zones of calcification and growth arrest lines resembling scurvy have been also described [46]. Fractures may occur. The appearance must be distinguished from recurrent or metastatic disease. The mechanism by which methotrexate affects bone is not clear, but it has been suggested that it may be related to methotrexate's antifolic acid effects [46] and to inhibition of osteoblast proliferation seen in cultured human osteoblasts [48]. The inhibitory effect of methotrexate on bone proliferation may be further potentiated by low 1,25

(OH)-D levels [46]. Histomorphometric studies in rats showed that short-term administration of methotrexate decreased trabecular bone volume by almost a quarter and bone formation rate diminished by more than half [49].

OTHER MALIGNANCIES

Osteosarcoma

Osteosarcoma is the commonest malignant bone tumour of childhood. About 4–5% of all childhood cancers are osteosarcomas, with the long bones of the lower limbs being the commonest primary site [50,51]. It is also the commonest secondary tumour to occur as a consequence of treatment for a solid tumour during childhood, usually within the region of previous radiation therapy [52]. In addition, there is a significantly increased risk of osteosarcoma in patients with hereditary retinoblastoma and Li–Fraumeni syndrome [53,54]. About 20–25% of children with osteosarcoma will have metastatic disease at presentation, with approximately 10% of these children having bony metastases [52].

Ewing's Sarcoma

Ewing's sarcoma is the second most common cancer of bone in childhood [55]. It belongs to the heterogeneous group of small-round-cell tumours that also includes neuroblastoma and primitive neuroectodermal tumours [56]. The commonest primary sites are the pelvis and upper femur [50,51]. The overall incidence of metastases at presentation is similar to osteosarcoma, with about 20–25% of patients having metastatic disease at presentation. However, bony metastases are more common, with about 25% of these children having bony metastases [55]. Both osteosarcoma and Ewing's sarcoma have a peak incidence in the second decade of life [51].

Rhabdomyosarcomas and Neuroblastoma

Rhabdomyosarcomas constitute over half of all soft-tissue sarcomas in children and about 4% of all childhood cancers. As in Ewing's tumours, skeletal metastases are common and occur in about 25% of all patients with rhabdomyosarcomas [57].

Neuroblastoma is the commonest solid tumour of childhood, representing about 6% of all childhood

cancers. Like Ewing's tumour, it is a small-round-cell tumour but has a peak incidence in the first decade of life, with most cases occurring in the first 5 years. In a series of 648 patients with Stage IV and Stage IVS disease, bony metastases were present in 55% at diagnosis [58].

SUMMARY

The principal cancerous disease affecting bone in children is acute lymphoblastic leukaemia. The available evidence indicates that there is low bone mass at diagnosis, with low bone turnover, and that survivors have reduced bone mass for size at final height. Insufficient numbers of survivors are available in other groups to comment on the long-term skeletal outcome for less common tumours. Studies are needed to assess the role of specific interventions in preserving bone mass following treatment for cancer in children, who may face life-long skeletal complications.

REFERENCES

1. Davies HA. Late problems faced by childhood cancer survivors. Br J Hosp Med 1993; 50: 137–40.
2. Stiller CA, Chessells JM, Fitchett M. Neurofibromatosis and childhood leukaemia/lymphoma: a population-based UKCCSG study [see comments]. Br J Cancer 1994; 70: 969–72.
3. Stiller CA, Eatock EM. Patterns of care and survival for children with acute lymphoblastic leukaemia diagnosed between 1980 and 1994. Arch Dis Child 1999; 81: 202–8.
4. Stiller CA, Benjamin S, Cartwright RA et al. Patterns of care and survival for adolescents and young adults with acute leukaemia—a population-based study. Br J Cancer 1999; 79: 658–65.
5. Lilleyman JS. Childhood Leukaemia: the Facts. Oxford University Press: Oxford, 1994.
6. Jonsson OG, Sartain P, Ducore JM, Buchanan GR. Bone pain as an initial symptom of childhood acute lymphoblastic leukemia: association with nearly normal hematologic indexes. J Pediatr 1990; 117: 233–7.
7. Atkinson SA, Fraher L, Gundberg CM et al. Mineral homeostasis and bone mass in children treated for acute lymphoblastic leukemia. J Pediatr 1989; 114: 793–800.
8. Halton JM, Atkinson SA, Fraher L et al. Altered mineral metabolism and bone mass in children during treatment for acute lymphoblastic leukemia. J Bone Min Res 1996; 11: 1774–83.
9. Warner JT, Cowan FJ, Dunstan FD et al. Measured and predicted bone mineral content in healthy boys and girls aged 6–18 years: adjustment for body size and puberty. Acta Paediatr 1998; 87: 244–9.
10. Molgaard C, Thomsen BL, Prentice A et al. Whole body bone mineral content in healthy children and adolescents [see comments]. Arch Dis Child 1997; 76: 9–15.

11. Prentice A, Parsons TJ, Cole TJ. Uncritical use of bone mineral density in absorptiometry may lead to size-related artifacts in the identification of bone mineral determinants. Am J Clin Nutr 1994; 60: 837–42.

12. Kroger H, Vainio P, Nieminen J, Kotaniemi A. Comparison of different models for interpreting bone mineral density measurements using DXA and MRI technology. Bone 1995; 17: 157–9.

13. Katzman DK, Bachrach LK, Carter DR, Marcus R. Clinical and anthropometric correlates of bone mineral acquisition in healthy adolescent girls. J Clin Endocrinol Metab 1991; 73: 1332–9.

14. Sievanen H, Kannus P, Nieminen V et al. Estimation of various mechanical characteristics of human bones using dual energy X-ray absorptiometry: methodology and precision. Bone 1996; 18: 17S.

15. Rogalsky RJ, Black GB, Reed MH. Orthopaedic manifestations of leukemia in children. J Bone Joint Surg Am 1986; 68: 494–501.

16. Sorva R, Kivivuori SM, Turpeinen M et al. Very low rate of type I collagen synthesis and degradation in newly diagnosed children with acute lymphoblastic leukemia. Bone 1997; 20: 139–43.

17. Halton JM, Atkinson SA, Fraher L et al. Mineral homeostasis and bone mass at diagnosis in children with acute lymphoblastic leukemia. J Pediatr 1995; 126: 557–64.

18. Bertolini DR, Nedwin GE, Bringman TS et al. Stimulation of bone resorption and inhibition of bone formation in vitro by human tumour necrosis factors. Nature 1986; 319: 516–18.

19. Manolagas SC, Jilka RL. Bone marrow, cytokines, and bone remodeling. Emerging insights into the pathophysiology of osteoporosis. N Engl J Med 1995; 332: 305–11.

20. Roodman GD. Mechanisms of bone lesions in multiple myeloma and lymphoma. Cancer 1997; 80: 1557–63.

21. Boot AM, van den Heuvel-Eibrink MM, Hahlen K et al. Bone mineral density in children with acute lymphoblastic leukaemia. Eur J Cancer 1999; 35: 1693–7.

22. Crofton PM, Ahmed SF, Wade JC et al. Effects of intensive chemotherapy on bone and collagen turnover and the growth hormone axis in children with acute lymphoblastic leukemia. J Clin Endocrinol Metab 1998; 83: 3121–9.

23. Feldman J, Federico MH, Sonohara S et al. Vitamin D3 binding activity during leukemic cell differentiation. Leuk Res 1993; 17: 97–101.

24. Arikoski P, Komulainen J, Riikonen P et al. Alterations in bone turnover and impaired development of bone mineral density in newly diagnosed children with cancer: a 1-year prospective study. J Clin Endocrinol Metab 1999; 84: 3174–81.

25. Arikoski P, Komulainen J, Riikonen P et al. Impaired development of bone mineral density during chemotherapy: a prospective analysis of 46 children newly diagnosed with cancer [see comments]. J Bone Min Res 1999; 14: 2002–9.

26. Arikoski P, Komulainen J, Voutilainen R et al. Reduced bone mineral density in long-term survivors of childhood acute lymphoblastic leukemia. J Pediatr Hematol Oncol 1998; 20: 234–40.

27. Atkinson SA, Halton JM, Bradley C et al. Bone and mineral abnormalities in childhood acute lymphoblastic leukemia: influence of disease, drugs and nutrition. Int J Cancer 1998; 11(suppl): 35–9.

28. Brennan BM, Rahim A, Adams JA et al. Reduced bone mineral density in young adults following cure of acute lymphoblastic leukaemia in childhood. Br J Cancer 1999; 79: 1859–63.

29. Hoorweg-Nijman JJ, Kardos G, Roos JC et al. Bone mineral density and markers of bone turnover in young adult survivors of childhood lymphoblastic leukaemia. Clin Endocrinol (Oxf) 1999; 50: 237–44.

30. Nussey SS, Hyer SL, Brada M et al. Bone mineralization after treatment of growth hormone deficiency in survivors of childhood malignancy [published erratum appears in Acta Paediatr Suppl 1995 Jun; 84(6): 620]. Acta Paediatr Suppl 1994; 399: 9–15.

31. Warner JT, Evans WD, Webb DK et al. Relative osteopenia after treatment for acute lymphoblastic leukemia. Pediatr Res 1999; 45: 544–51.

32. Gilsanz V, Carlson ME, Roe TF, Ortega JA. Osteoporosis after cranial irradiation for acute lymphoblastic leukemia. J Pediatr 1990; 117: 238–44.

33. Nysom K, Holm K, Michaelsen KF et al. Bone mass after treatment for acute lymphoblastic leukemia in childhood. J Clin Oncol 1998; 16: 3752–60.

34. Arikoski P, Komulainen J, Riikonen P, Kroger H. Skeletal problems in children with malignancies. In Schönau E, Matkovic V (eds), Paediatric Osteology. Prevention of Osteoporosis—a Paediatric Task? Elsevier Science: Singapore, 1998: 137–41.

35. Kaufman JM, Taelman P, Vermeulen A, Vandeweghe M. Bone mineral status in growth hormone-deficient males with isolated and multiple pituitary deficiencies of childhood onset. J Clin Endocrinol Metab 1992; 74: 118–23.

36. Shore RM, Chesney RW, Mazess RB et al. Bone mineral status in growth hormone deficiency. J Pediatr 1980; 96: 393–6.

37. Holmes SJ, Economou G, Whitehouse RW et al. Reduced bone mineral density in patients with adult onset growth hormone deficiency. J Clin Endocrinol Metab 1994; 78: 669–74.

38. Nysom K, Holm K, Michaelsen KF et al. Bone mass after allogeneic BMT for childhood leukaemia or lymphoma. Bone Marrow Transpl 2000; 25: 191–6.

39. Bhatia S, Ramsay NK, Weisdorf D et al. Bone mineral density in patients undergoing bone marrow transplantation for myeloid malignances. Bone Marrow Transpl 1998; 22: 87–90.

40. Halton JM, Atkinson SA, Fraher L et al. Altered mineral metabolism and bone mass in children during treatment for acute lymphoblastic leukemia. J Bone Min Res 1996; 11: 1774–83.

41. Joseph JC. Corticosteroid-induced osteoporosis. Am J Hosp Pharm 1994; 51: 188–30.

42. Aisenberg J, Hsieh K, Kalaitzoglou G et al. Bone mineral density in young adult survivors of childhood cancer. J Pediatr Hematol Oncol 1998; 20: 241–5.

43. Parfitt AM, Travers R, Rauch F, Glorieux FH. Structural and cellular changes during bone growth in healthy children. Bone 2000; 27(4): 487–94.

44. Van Staa TP, Leufkens HG, Abenhaim L et al. Use of oral corticosteroids and risk of fractures. J Bone Min Res 2000; 15(6): 993–1000.

45. O'Regan S, Melhorn DK, Newman AJ. Methotrexate-induced bone pain in childhood leukemia. Am J Dis Child 1973; 126: 489–90.

46. Schwartz AM, Leonidas JC. Methotrexate osteopathy. Skel Radiol 1984; 11: 13–16.

47. Meister B, Gassner I, Streif W et al. Methotrexate osteopathy in infants with tumors of the central nervous system. Med Pediatr Oncol 1994; 23: 493–6.

48. Scheven BA, van der Veen MJ, Damen CA et al. Effects of methotrexate on human osteoblasts in vitro: modulation by 1,25-dihydroxyvitamin D3. J Bone Min Res 1995; 10: 874–80.

49. Friedlaender GE, Tross RB, Doganis AC et al. Effects of chemotherapeutic agents on bone. I. Short-term methotrexate and doxorubicin (adriamycin) treatment in a rat model. J Bone Joint Surg Am 1984; 66: 602–7.

50. Arndt CA, Crist WM. Common musculoskeletal tumors of childhood and adolescence. N Engl J Med 1999; 341: 342–52.

51. Widhe B, Widhe T. Initial symptoms and clinical features in osteosarcoma and Ewing sarcoma. J Bone Joint Surg Am 2000; 82: 667–74.

52. Le Vu B, de Vathaire F, Shamsaldin A et al. Radiation dose, chemotherapy and risk of osteosarcoma after solid tumours during childhood. Int J Cancer 1998; 77: 370–7.

53. Birch JM. Genes and cancer. Arch Dis Child 1999; 80: 1–3.

54. Link MP, Eilber F. Osteosarcoma. In Pizzo PA, Poplack DG (eds), Principles and Practice of Pediatric Oncology, vol 3. Lippincott-Raven: Philadelphia, PA, 1993: 889–920.

55. Grier HE. The Ewing family of tumors. Ewing's sarcoma and primitive neuroectodermal tumors. Pediatr Clin N Am 1997; 44: 991–1004.

56. Triche TJ. Pathology of pediatric malignancies. In Pizzo PA, Poplack DG (eds), Principles and Practice of Pediatric Oncology, vol 2. Lippincott-Raven: Philadelphia, PA, 1993: 115–52.

57. Yoshikawa H, Ueda T, Mori S et al. Skeletal metastases from soft-tissue sarcomas. Incidence, patterns, and radiological features. J Bone Joint Surg Br 1997; 79: 548–52.

58. DuBois SG, Kalika Y, Lukens JN et al. Metastatic sites in stage IV and IVS neuroblastoma correlate with age, tumor biology, and survival [see comments]. J Pediatr Hematol Oncol 1999; 21: 181–9.

59. Arikoski P, Komulainen J, Riikonen P et al. Reduced bone density at completion of chemotherapy for a malignancy. Arch Dis Child 1999; 80: 143–8.

60. Arikoski P, Kroger H, Riikonen P et al. Disturbance in bone turnover in children with a malignancy at completion of chemotherapy. Med Pediatr Oncol 1999; 33: 455–61.

61. Henderson RC, Madsen CD, Davis C, Gold SH. Bone density in survivors of childhood malignancies. J Pediatr Hematol Oncol 1996; 18: 367–71.

62. Hesseling PB, Hough SF, Nel ED et al. Bone mineral density in long-term survivors of childhood cancer. Int J Cancer 1998; 11(suppl): 44–7.

63. Nysom K, Molgaard C, Holm K et al. Bone mass and body composition after cessation of therapy for childhood cancer. Int J Cancer 1998; 11(suppl): 40–3.

64. Vassilopoulou-Sellin R, Brosnan P, Delpassand A et al. Osteopenia in young adult survivors of childhood cancer. Med Pediatr Oncol 1999; 32: 272–8.

8

Bone Metastases in Specific Tumours

Section Editor: Lawrence R. Coia

38

Breast Cancer

William F. Hartsell

Advocate Good Samaritan Cancer Center, Downers Grove, IL, USA

INTRODUCTION

Bone metastases may occur from many types of cancer, but the overall impact of metastatic disease to bones is probably greatest in women with breast cancer, which is the most common malignancy of women in many areas of the world, including Europe and North America. Bones are a common site of metastases, and may be the only site of metastatic disease in a substantial number of women. These patients may have a relatively long duration of survival. Because of the prevalence of breast cancer, the frequency with which it metastasises to bone and the length of time that patients may live with bone metastases, this group of patients comprises the largest cohort of patients with bone metastases. In retrospective evaluations of patients with bone metastases, breast cancer patients usually comprise the largest proportion of patients studied. In addition, there are more prospective studies evaluating patients with bone metastases from breast cancer than from any other primary site.

In autopsy series, as many as 85% of women have evidence of bone metastases [1]. As would be expected, the risk of osseous metastases is somewhat lower in clinical series. Bones are one of the most common sites of metastases, second only to local/regional recurrence. Approximately 30% of all women diagnosed with invasive breast cancer will eventually develop bone metastases. The majority of women with metastatic breast cancer have involvement of the bones as well: 70% of women with metastatic breast cancer develop bone metastases [2]. There may be a long interval between initial diagnosis and the appearance of bone metastases. Patients entered on International Breast Cancer Study Group trials had an 8.2% risk of bone metastases at 2 years and a 27.3% risk at 10 years. Although the rate was somewhat higher in the first 2 years after diagnosis, there was still a substantial risk of developing clinically overt bone metastases at 8–10 years after diagnosis [3].

The clinical course of women with bone metastases as the first site of breast cancer relapse is significantly different from that of women with visceral metastases. The median survival for women after discovery of bone metastases is 24 months, compared to only 12 months for those with visceral metastases [2]. Patients with bone metastases have more stable, indolent disease. There is a subgroup of patients with metastatic disease that remains confined to the bones (with no visceral metastases). The clinical course in this group of patients is even more indolent and protracted, with median survival times of 4 years [4].

The primary tumour characteristics associated with bone metastases include oestrogen and progesterone receptor positivity, low tumour grade and low proliferative indices (S-phase fraction $< 5\%$) [2]. These are indicators of more indolent disease in general. In contrast, patients with negative receptors and higher proliferative indices tend to develop visceral metastases. Nodal status is also an important predictor of risk for the development of bone metastases. The risks of bone metastases in patients with $\geqslant 4$ positive axillary nodes are $> 40\%$ at 10 years. Patients with local or regional recurrence also have a relatively high risk of bone metastases, with more than 35% developing clinical evidence of bone disease by 10 years.

Textbook of Bone Metastases. Edited by C. Jasmin, R. E. Coleman, L. R. Coia, R. Capanna and G. Saillant
© 2005 John Wiley & Sons Ltd: ISBN 0 471 87742 5

The more indolent course and longer survival times have a strong impact on the choice of therapy in these patients. Surgical fixation of weakened bones, control of disease (in addition to pain control) and prevention of further osseous metastases are thus more important for patients with breast cancer than most other primary sites. Prevention of complications from bone metastases, such as hypercalcaemia or spinal cord compression, are more important because of the long window of opportunity for these complications to occur. There is a wide selection of effective therapies in breast cancer, including multiple hormonal therapies, multiple chemotherapeutic drugs and drug combinations, bisphosphonates, external beam radiation therapy, radionuclides and monoclonal antibodies. This wide range of therapeutic options makes the selection of the most appropriate therapy more complicated. To ensure that the most appropriate treatments are offered, a multimodality approach to these patients is essential.

EVALUATION AND IMAGING

Any bone may be involved, but the axial skeleton is the most commonly detected site of disease. Thoracic vertebral bodies, lumbar spine, pelvis and ribs are the predominant sites of disease [5,6]. The bones of the skull are more commonly involved by metastatic breast cancer than by malignancies from other primary sites.

Plain radiographs of bone metastases from breast cancer most commonly show osteolytic disease, but osteoblastic processes or combinations of both appearances may be detected as well [5]. The appropriate use of imaging studies depends upon the clinical situation. In general, imaging for bone metastases should be done only in symptomatic or high-risk patients. Bone scintigraphy is neither cost-effective nor clinically useful in asymptomatic patients at the time of diagnosis, and is typically not useful as a routine follow-up study [7,8]. For symptomatic patients, bone scintigraphy is useful as the initial screening tool for bone metastases. Bone scans are typically sensitive but not specific markers of osseous metastases. If there are multiple lesions, there is a high likelihood that these actually represent metastatic disease [9]. However, with only a single abnormal hot spot on bone scintigraphy, there is a significantly higher likelihood that this is a false positive, and additional studies to confirm the presence of metastases may be required. Magnetic resonance imaging (MRI) is especially useful in the vertebral column [10]. Positron emission tomography (PET) is useful for lesions with high metabolic activity but is less accurate in osteoblastic lesions [11]. The accuracy of PET is less in bone than in other organs, with a higher rate of false negative results in bone than in visceral organs. This may be due to the lower metabolic activity of the tumours that metastasise to bone, compared to the more metabolically active and aggressive tumours that are more likely to involve liver, lungs and other viscera.

Because of the potential for lengthy survival in patients with bone metastases from breast cancer, it is important to evaluate weight-bearing bones to ensure that the risk of pathological fracture is low. Plain radiographs of weight-bearing bones (especially femurs) are essential, both in patients with symptoms of hip pain and in asymptomatic patients with bone scans that show increased uptake in the hips.

Two other complications of bone metastases merit special consideration during the initial evaluation of subsequent clinical course of patients with metastatic breast cancer. Hypercalcaemia occurs in approximately 10–15% of women with bone metastases from breast cancer, but is extremely rare in women without evidence of bone metastases [12,13]. Hypercalcaemia may occur in as many as 30% of women with both liver and bone metastases, and is usually seen in patients with extensive metastatic disease [13]. Treatment of hypercalcaemia is discussed in detail in Chapter 27. Because of the long potential clinical course in patients with bone metastases, and because of the frequent involvement of the thoracic and lumbar spine, spinal cord compression may occur in 10% of patients with bone metastases from breast cancer. The index of suspicion should be high in patients with back pain, with a low threshold for imaging of potential areas of cord compression.

SURGERY

Surgical management of bone metastases is covered in more detail elsewhere. Surgical intervention is more important in metastatic breast cancer than most other malignancies for several reasons. The potentially lengthy duration of survival allows metastatic foci greater time to cause problematic cortical destruction. Any complication that does occur may negatively impact quality of life for a longer period of time than would be the case with other malignancies.

Complications of metastatic breast cancer that may require surgical management include pathological fractures, cortical bone destruction with impending pathological fracture, and spinal cord compression. Pathological fractures are found more commonly in patients with breast cancer than in all other malignancies combined [14,15]. Most of these occur with osteolytic disease, although osteoblastic lesions can also cause pathological fractures [15]. All patients with metastatic disease to the hips and other weight-bearing bones should be evaluated with appropriate imaging. Patients with evidence of cortical destruction require evaluation by an orthopaedic surgeon to allow timely surgical intervention in patients with a significant risk of fracture. This multidisciplinary approach will decrease the likelihood of significant skeletal complications and thus allow for better quality of life. Patients with cortical destruction that is not deemed sufficient to warrant prophylactic fixation may need routine orthopaedic follow-up.

For patients found to have a pathological fracture, factors that influence the decision of whether or not to use surgical intervention include life expectancy and general physical condition [14,15]. With more indolent course of disease, younger age of patients and lower risk of co-morbid conditions compared to other malignancies, patients with breast cancer are more likely to tolerate and benefit from surgical intervention. Depending on the type of operative procedure, radiation therapy may be required post-operatively to prevent further skeletal complications from progressive disease.

MEDICAL THERAPY

The primary goal of treatment with chemotherapy or hormones is to palliate symptoms and improve quality of life. In most studies of chemotherapy for metastatic breast cancer, the measures of outcome have been response rather than quality of life indices. Response is used as a proxy for palliation, but this may not be appropriate. The International Union Against Cancer (UICC) response criteria require objective measures of response to therapy [16]. For bone lesions, this requires resolution of bone abnormalities. For lytic lesions, this means evidence of healing with recalcification of the lytic lesions, which may take 6 months. With bone scintigraphy, there can be a "flare" with increase in intensity of abnormalities, and these changes may last for 3–6 months following chemotherapy [17,18]. Thus, a lesion may look worse on bone scan but actually be responding. More appropriate measures of response include pain relief, amount of narcotic pain medication required and general quality of life assessments. The difficulty of assessing response for palliative therapy is highlighted by a study from Hainsworth. Four patients with painful bone metastases received chemotherapy. None of these patients had a response by radiographic

criteria, but two had pain relief for 6 and 8 months (thus accomplishing the goals of treatment) [19].

The response rates of metastatic breast cancer depend on site of disease. Osseous metastases show much lower response rates than soft tissue disease, and often have lower response rates than visceral disease [17,18,20]. This probably reflects the insensitivity of current imaging methods to detect tumour response in bone, but other factors may be responsible as well.

Hormonal Therapy

Approximately one-third of unselected patients with metastatic breast cancer will respond to endocrine therapy [21]. The response rate is much higher in patients with oestrogen receptor-positive disease (50–60%) and highest in patients with both oestrogen and progesterone receptor-positive disease (65–75%). Patients with oestrogen and progesterone receptors that are negative have only a 5–10% response rate to hormonal therapy. The receptor levels in metastatic lesions tend to reflect the status of the primary lesion, with similar receptor levels in both the primary and metastatic sites [21]. As discussed previously, bone metastases occur more frequently in patients with receptor-positive disease. Thus, hormonal therapy is the mainstay of systemic therapy for bone metastases.

Surgical endocrine manipulation has been used for many years, but has for the most part been supplanted by medical therapy. Oophorectomy gives immediate effects, with a complete response rate of 20–30% in patients with metastatic breast cancer. Radiation therapy has also been used to effectively eliminate ovarian hormonal function. Doses of 20 Gy given in 1 week will cause hormonal levels to diminish, although it may require 2–10 weeks to reach minimal levels. Surgical adrenalectomy and surgical or radiotherapeutic hypophysectomy were used in the past, but are now obsolete because the same effect can be obtained with medications.

The most commonly used hormonal treatment for metastatic breast cancer is tamoxifen. This is a non-steroidal anti-oestrogen that inhibits the effects of oestrogen by competing for binding sites [22]. It may also augment tumour inhibition. Although tamoxifen has long been presumed to be cytostatic only, there is some evidence that it may also exert cytotoxic effects. The standard dose used is 20 mg/day. There is no evidence that higher doses are more effective. With this dose, side-effects are minimal and typically transient. Hot flashes occur in 10% of patients. In patients with significant bone disease, a flare reaction may occur in approximately 5%. Nausea, vomiting, significant weight gain and mood disturbances occur in < 5% of patients. There may be transient eye abnormalities in less than 1% of patients. Other anti-oestrogens have been compared to tamoxifen for treatment of metastatic disease, and thus far there is no clear evidence that any of these agents are more effective (or less toxic) than tamoxifen.

Progestins are also used for treatment of metastatic breast cancer. Two agents have been used extensively: medroxyprogesterone acetate (MPA) and megestrol acetate (MA). A randomised comparison of these two agents was reported by Willemse et al. [23]. The dose of MPA was 1000 mg/day, and MA was 160 mg/day. The study group included post-menopausal patients with advanced breast cancer, with 44 patients receiving MPA and 48 patients receiving MA. The response in bone was significantly better in the MPA group (45% vs. 12%), but there were significantly more side-effects with MPA (increases in body weight, systolic blood pressure, serum creatinine, hot flashes, sweating and tremors). Muss et al. compared tamoxifen and high-dose MPA as the initial hormonal therapy for patients with metastatic breast cancer [24]. The response rate in bone was higher with the MPA (33% vs. 13%), although survival and time to treatment failure were not significantly different. At the time of disease progression, patients were switched to the other regimen. There was only a 12–14% response to the second therapy, not significantly different between the two regimens. Toxicity was minimal for both arms, although weight gains of more than 20 pounds were common on the MPA arm (35% of patients vs. 2% with tamoxifen).

Aminoglutethimide suppresses adrenal function, acting as a medical adrenalectomy. It is an effective treatment of metastatic breast cancer, including bone metastases. Response rates of 25% may be seen in patients who have failed first-line hormonal therapy [25]. Typically, a glucocorticoid is given concomitantly with the aminoglutethimide to prevent Addisonian symptoms [25].

The new aromatase inhibitors appear to be effective in treatment of metastatic breast cancer, including metastatic disease to the bones. Anastrazole is a non-steroidal aromatase inhibitor that produces significant oestrogen suppression. Two large multicentre international trials have shown anastrazole to be at least equivalent to tamoxifen as first-line therapy for women with metastatic breast cancers in terms of overall response rates, time to progression and survival [26,27]. In both of these trials, substantial numbers of patients (45–65%) had metastatic disease to bone,

including 15–25% with bone as the only site of metastatic disease. Site-specific responses from these studies have not yet been reported, but anastrazole is likely to be used with increasing frequency as initial therapy for patients with metastatic breast cancer. A combined analysis of two randomised trials showed anastrozole to be superior to megestrol acetate for women with metastatic breast cancer who had failed prior tamoxifen therapy [28]. This analysis showed not only a better response rate, but also an overall survival advantage for the women receiving anastrozole.

Chemotherapy

Chemotherapy is effective in the treatment of metastatic breast cancer, but the appropriate use of chemotherapy depends on many factors. In general, patients with rapidly growing disease, disease-free interval of less than 2 years, poor response (or progression) with hormone therapy, and/or negative oestrogen and progesterone receptors are appropriate candidates for chemotherapy [25]. Age is not a strict selection criterion, although younger patients are more likely to be given chemotherapy. Younger patients are more likely to have the risk factors listed above, and older patients are more likely to have co-morbid conditions, limiting their ability to receive chemotherapy. Treatment is more effective when the principles of dose intensity are followed, and thus adequate renal, hepatic, cardiac and bone marrow function is required. The function of these organs should be adequately evaluated prior to beginning chemotherapy.

The response rates seen with single-agent chemotherapy for bone metastases are usually quite low. Degardin and colleagues found a 16% overall response rate in patients treated with vinorelbine for metastatic breast cancer, but no response in bone [29]. Karapetis et al. evaluated continuous-infusion 5-fluorouracil for treatment of patients with metastatic breast cancer [30]. Some responses were seen in patients with visceral or soft tissue disease, but there were no responses in bone lesions. Doxorubicin as a single agent has a higher response than other single agents for metastatic breast cancer, including in bone [31]. Liposomal doxorubicin may accumulate preferentially in bone lesions as well. Two patients who were treated with liposomal doxorubicin developed pathological fractures in the femur. At the time of surgical repair of the fracture, biopsies were taken not only from the bone but also from adjacent skeletal muscle. The concentrations of doxorubicin in the nuclei of breast cancer cells in the bone were approximately 10 times greater than the concentration in muscle cells [32]. The taxanes may also be useful in systemic treatment of bone metastases. Schneider et al. found radiographic responses in 33% (7/21) of patients receiving paclitaxel for bone metastases from breast cancer [33]. Of interest is the fact that three of those seven patients had "flare" reactions seen on bone scintigraphy 3 months after the start of the taxane treatment; these areas showed decreased signal intensity on subsequent scans.

Multiple drug combinations are associated with much higher response rates than single agents in the treatment of bone metastases. Objective responses are seen in 20–60% of lytic bone lesions using standard regimens of cyclophosphamide, methotrexate, and 5-fluorouracil (5-FU) (CMF) or cyclophosphamide, doxorubicin and 5-FU (CAF) [17]. Various combinations have been used, but the most effective seem to be based on an anthracycline antibiotic or a taxane. A review by Kamby confirms the higher response rates in soft tissue disease (55–60%) compared to bone (31–44%) [20]. The combination of vincristine, doxorubicin and prednisolone was one of the most active regimens in soft tissue and visceral disease, with 64–78% response rates, but achieved only a response rate of 26% for bone metastases. Ardavanis et al. obtained a 50% partial response rate in bone using vinorelbine, cyclophosphamide and 5-FU [34]. Although with smaller numbers, Iino et al. obtained responses in 67% (8/12) patients with bone metastases using mitoxantrone, doxifluridine and medroxyprogesterone [35].

The optimal duration of therapy is unclear. Radiographic response in the bone may take 6 months, to allow recalcification of osteolytic lesions. This makes it difficult to make decisions about duration of treatment early in the course of therapy. For patients who appear to have stable or responding disease, should the chemotherapy be prolonged until disease progression? Continuous chemotherapy results in prolongation of the median time to progression but does not appear to impact overall survival time.

The use of high-dose chemotherapy with autologous peripheral stem cell rescue for metastatic breast cancer remains controversial [36]. Recent evidence from randomised trials suggests that high-dose therapy is not likely to provide significant improvements in survival for patients with metastatic disease. The patterns of failure following high-dose therapy show recurrent disease in areas of known bulky disease prior to the high-dose chemotherapy. The addition of local therapy to the high-dose chemotherapy appears to increase the long-term control in those areas [37].

Most of the cytotoxic therapy used for treatment of breast cancer is non-specific, directed simply at rapidly dividing cells. New agents are being developed that are targeted specifically to tumour cells or the tumour microenvironment. This exciting concept offers the possibility of effective treatment with significantly fewer side-effects than non-targeted approaches. The first of these agents in clinical use is a monoclonal antibody directed at the Her-2/neu growth factor receptor. Trastuzumab (Herceptin) has been used in patients with metastatic breast cancer as a single agent, with responses of 15–20% [38]. The response rates are higher when given in combination with chemotherapeutic agents [39–41]. It is not yet clear whether these agents will be effective in treatment of bone metastases. Other new agents are being developed that inhibit angiogenesis or induce apoptosis.

BISPHOSPHONATES

The exact mechanism by which bisphosphonates influence bone and bone metastases is not certain; it is likely that there are multiple actions on different cells that inhibit tumour progression in bone and allow healing. Bisphosphonates inhibit osteoclast-mediated bone resorption, and may exert effects on osteoblasts as well [42]. There are also effects on macrophages, inducing apoptotic cell death [43]. There is recent information suggesting that the bisphosphonates may induce apoptotic cell death in certain tumour types, including breast carcinoma cells [44]. These compounds also influence cytokine production: clodronate inhibits IL-1β, IL-6 and TNFα, while pamidronate stimulates cytokine production [45]. Finally, these compounds inhibit adhesion of tumour cells to the bone matrix [46].

The compounds that have been studied most extensively in clinical trials are clodronate pamidronate, and zoledronic acid. The dose of clodronate used in many of these studies is 1600 mg/day, given orally. The duration of treatment has been 2–3 years. Pamidronate has been given both orally and by intravenous administration. The intravenous route is more commonly used, with doses of 90 mg given over 2 h, once per month. Zoledronic acid is given as a dose of 4 mg intravenously over 15–30 minutes.

Bisphosphonates were first used clinically for the treatment of known osteolytic bone metastases. Multiple Phase II reports of bisphosphonates as the sole treatment for osteolytic metastases showed positive effects, with relief of pain in 50% of patients and radiographic evidence of bone healing in 25% [47,48].

Paterson et al. reported a trial of clodronate for patients with metastatic breast cancer [49]. This was a

Table 38.1.   Randomised trials of bisphosphonates for treatment of osseous metastases from breast cancer

Reference	Treatment	Patients (*n*)	Time to skeletal complications	Bone complications	Response rate
[52]	Pamidronate 90 mg i.v.	382	13.1 Months	43%	
	Placebo		7 Months	56%	
[53]	Pamidronate 90 mg i.v.	374	10.4 Months	56%	
	Placebo		6.9 Months	67%	
[54]	Chemotherapy	152	168 Days	46 Events	28%
	Chemotherapy + pamidronate 45 mg i.v. q 3 weeks	143	249 Days	53 Events	33%

randomised, double-blind, placebo-controlled trial of clodronate 1600 mg/day orally given for 2 years. There was a significant reduction in the frequency of hypercalcaemic episodes and in the incidence of vertebral fractures.

Van Holten-Verzantvoort reported a similar trial using pamidronate [50]. Patients with breast cancer with bone metastases were randomised to oral pamidronate 300 mg/day for 2 years vs. placebo. A significant reduction in skeletal problems was noted with the pamidronate: fewer episodes of hypercalcaemia (65% decrease), less bone pain (30%), fewer cases of symptomatic impending fracture (50%) and decreased need for palliative radiotherapy (35%). However, there was considerable gastrointestinal toxicity, and 23% of patients on the pamidronate arm stopped treatment because of toxicity. Although the pamidronate was effective, it appears that intravenous infusion is superior because of the problems with gastrointestinal toxicity using oral pamidronate.

At least three randomised trials using intravenous pamidronate have been completed which evaluated patients with bone metastases from breast cancer. Two consecutive trials from the same group compared intravenous pamidronate to placebo in 750 patients with metastatic breast cancer. Patients given pamidronate 90 mg i.v. every month for 12 months had significantly fewer skeletal complications, less bone pain and better performance status than patients who received placebo. The time to the first skeletal complication was significantly longer as well [51,52]. In contrast, the study reported by Conte et al. did not show these same benefits to pamidronate [53]. The patients on this study all received chemotherapy and were randomised to receive concomitant pamidronate 45 mg i.v. every 3 weeks vs. no additional therapy. There was no reduction in the number of new bone metastases, and responses in bone were the same between the two groups. The duration of response was longer in the pamidronate group, with time to bone

progression of 249 days compared to 168 days in the group that received chemotherapy alone (Table 38.1). Zoledronic acid may be more effective than the other bisphosphonates in treatment of bone metastases. Rosen et al. performed a randomized comparison of zoledronic acid to pamidronate in 1130 patients with bone metastases from breast cancer [54]. The time to first skeletal-related event was significantly prolonged with zoledronic acid (301 vs. 174 days) and overall there were fewer skeletal-related events in the zoledronic acid group, especially in the subset of patients with osteolytic disease.

An exciting avenue of current research is in the use of bisphosphonates as adjuvant therapy for high-risk patients with no evidence of bone metastases. The mechanisms of action of the bisphosphonates suggest that these compounds may be useful in preventing the development of bone metastases. Multiple trials evaluating this hypothesis have been recently completed. There have been somewhat conflicting results from these studies. The group from Helsinki randomly assigned patients with lymph node-positive breast cancer to receive placebo or clodronate 1600 mg orally each day for 3 years [55]. Thus far, no benefit has been seen, with similar numbers of patients developing bone metastases in the two groups. A collaborative group from Canada, UK and Scandinavia evaluated oral clodronate 1600 mg vs. placebo for 2 years, and found a decreased incidence of bone metastases in the patients receiving the clodronate [56]. There was no difference in survival or on other metastatic sites between the two groups. Diel et al. reported the results of a study from Heidelberg [57]. Patients with metastatic breast cancer cells detected in the bone marrow by immunohistochemical studies (but with no evidence of metastases on radiographic studies) were randomised to receive clodronate 1600 mg orally for 2 years vs. placebo. A total of 302 patients were randomised on the study. In the clodronate group, the incidence of osseous metastases was significantly decreased. In addition, metastases to non-osseous sites were also decreased. Because of this, there was improvement in disease-free survival and in overall survival for the clodronate group.

The role for bisphosphonates is evolving, and information from ongoing trials will help delineate the appropriate role for this therapy. The National Surgical Adjuvant Breast Project has initiated an adjuvant trial of clodronate in high-risk patients with no evidence of bone metastases. The planned accrual for this study is more than 2000 women, so it should be large enough to determine whether bisphosphonates can prevent the development of bone metastases.

Radiation Therapy

External Beam Irradiation

External beam radiation therapy is an effective and commonly used treatment for palliation of bone metastases. The primary goals of local field radiation are pain relief, improvement of quality of life, maintenance of function (and improvement of mobility) and prevention of skeletal complications such as pathological fracture. Since breast cancer is the primary site responsible for the highest incidence of painful osseous metastases, there is a broad experience with palliative radiation therapy. Indeed, in randomised trials of radiotherapy for bone metastases, breast cancer patients comprise the majority of patients enrolled.

The first (and largest) of these trials was performed by the Radiation Therapy Oncology Group (RTOG) in the 1970s [58]. In this study, patients with painful bone metastases from any solid tumour primary site were randomised based upon the number of metastatic sites; 39% of the patients on this study had breast primaries. Patients with a single painful metastatic osseous site were randomised to receive 40.5 Gy in 15 fractions or 20 Gy in five fractions. Those with multiple painful sites were randomised to 15 Gy in five fractions, 20 Gy in five fractions, 25 Gy in five fractions or 30 Gy in 10 fractions. Measures of pain relief were relatively crude, with the treating physician rating the patient's pain as mild, moderate or severe. There was no significant difference in pain relief in any of the groups. For the patients with solitary metastases, 57% of patients experienced complete pain relief and an additional 26% had partial pain relief. For those with multiple metastatic sites, completed pain relief was achieved in 53% and another 30% had partial pain relief. These results indicated that the shorter-course schedules were as effective in achieving pain relief as the longer-course, higher-dose schedules. The magnitude and duration of response were higher in breast and prostate cancers than in other primaries.

Blitzer, using the combined endpoints of complete pain and narcotic relief and absence of retreatment, reanalysed the data from RTOG 74-02 [59]. This analysis showed that the longer, more protracted courses of treatment were more effective at producing this combined pain/narcotic/retreatment endpoint. In this analysis, patients with solitary metastatic sites had complete combined pain relief in 55% with the longer-course treatment (40.5 Gy in 3 weeks) compared to 37% for the shorter treatment (20 Gy in 1 week). In a similar fashion, the patients with multiple metastases had 46% complete relief with 30 Gy in 2 weeks compared to 28% in patients receiving 25 Gy in 1 week.

Both the original study and the reanalysis are flawed. The criteria for multiple vs. solitary lesions were not well defined; thus, most of the patients with "solitary" metastases actually had a solitary painful site but multiple metastases. The measures of outcome were crude assessments of pain as determined by the treating physician, rather than the patient. In the reanalysis, randomised strata were regrouped by number of treatments in a fashion that was not consistent with the original study design, nor was it consistent with radiobiological principles: in terms of effective radiobiological dose to tumour, 25 Gy given in five fractions is equivalent to 30 Gy in 10 fractions.

There have been multiple other prospective randomised trials evaluating the efficacy of different dose/fractionation regimens of local field radiation therapy for bone metastases. The specific treatment parameters have varied from study to study, and the pain assessment instruments have differed as well. However, the common theme among these studies is that there is no significant difference in pain control whether a short-course, low-dose scheme or higher-dose, protracted schedule is utilised. There does appear to be a threshold dose below which the treatment is less effective. Hoskin et al. performed a prospective randomised trial of single treatments of 8 Gy vs. 4 Gy [60]. The response rate (complete plus partial relief) was significantly higher for the 8 Gy arm (69%) compared to the 4 Gy treatment (44%), and retreatment was required more often in the 4 Gy group. The complete response rate and duration of response were not significantly different between the two groups. In this study, there was no difference in magnitude or duration of response for breast cancers compared to other tumours.

Most patients have minimal pain relief within 2 weeks, but best pain relief is not achieved until 4 weeks or more after treatment. Price et al. found that 32% of patients with breast primaries had pain relief 8 days after treatment, but 82% had pain relief at 4 weeks and 88% had pain relief by 8 weeks [61].

The optimal dose and fractionation schedule for palliation of bone metastases remains controversial. Powers and Ratanatharathorn argue that there is enough evidence in the literature to support a dose–response relationship, with higher doses providing better pain relief and longer duration of palliation [62]. Retreatment is more frequently required after shorter-course, lower-dose radiotherapy schedules (Table 38.2). Using the data from the RTOG study, Porter et al. calculated the effective doses using the linear quadratic method (biologically effective dose, or BED) [63]. Using pain response and freedom from retreatment as endpoints, the treatment schedules using higher BED were associated with better pain relief and decreased need for retreatment.

It is apparent that there is no consensus on the optimal dose and fractionation scheme for palliative radiation therapy. Because of the multiple variables to be considered, including location and extent of the bone metastases, age and performance status of the patient, extent of other disease and co-morbid factors, it is probably appropriate to avoid a single dogmatic, constricted regimen for these patients. A clinical decision based on the overall condition of the patient will yield several scenarios. For patients with poor performance status and multiple co-morbid conditions, 8 Gy in a single fraction or 15 Gy in five treatments is appropriate. For patients with a solitary metastatic site, excellent performance status, and no other co-morbid conditions, consideration may be given to a protracted course of therapy using low doses per treatment to a relatively high total dose. The majority of patients will likely fall into an intermediate

category. For these patients, 30 Gy in 10 fractions or 35 Gy in 14 fractions may be appropriate.

While the primary goal of radiation therapy for bone metastases is to provide palliation of pain, there are additional endpoints that are important. RTOG 9714 was a randomised, prospective trial of patients with breast or prostate primaries, and one to three painful osseous metastases [64]. The patients were randomised to 8 Gy in a single fraction vs. 30 Gy in 10 fractions. There was no difference between the two dose fractionation schemes in terms of pain relief, the primary endpoint of the study. Multiple other outcome indices are being evaluated, including narcotic usage, quality of life (Functional Assessment of Cancer Therapy), and the Health Utilities Index. An important part of this study is a comparison of the economic impacts of each of the treatment schedules. These additional studies may help to determine the most appropriate dose schedule.

For patients with some cortical destruction of bone, radiation therapy is effective at preventing pathological fracture. Some component of reossification and healing is seen in 65–85% of lytic lesions following external beam irradiation [65,66].

Hemi-body Irradiation and Systemic Radionuclides

Radiotherapy may also be used as a "systemic" therapy. These methods are most useful in patients with diffuse bone metastases. Patients with one or two painful metastatic sites are more appropriately treated with local field external beam irradiation. Indications for the use of systemic or wide-field radiation include the presence of multiple painful bone metastases, the

Table 38.2. Retreatment of bone metastases with local field radiation therapy

Reference	Dose/fractions	Retreatment (%)	Comments
[69]	8 Gy/1	25	39% With breast primaries
	24 Gy/6	7	
[61]	8 Gy/1	11	37% With breast primaries
	30 Gy/10	3	
[60]	4 Gy/1	20	
	8 Gy/1	9	
[58]	15 Gy/5	23	39% With breast primaries
	20 Gy/5	15	
	25 Gy/5	16	
	30 Gy/10	12	
	20 Gy/5	24	
	40.5 Gy/15	11	

development of new painful sites shortly after local field treatment of other sites, diffuse skeletal involvement, and disease that is insensitive to hormone therapy or chemotherapy [67]. There are two methods of treating large areas of the body, and both are targeted primarily at bone metastases: wide-field external beam radiation therapy (hemi-body irradiation) and systemic radionuclide therapy.

Hemi-body irradiation (HBI) involves the use of external beam radiation therapy designed to cover a large area of the skeleton; the actual fields cover approximately one-half to one-third of the skeleton. It is targeted to the axial and proximal appendicular skeleton.

HBI is effective in providing pain relief for patients with metastatic breast cancer, and is used for patients with disease in multiple sites. In the RTOG 78-10 study, nearly 90% of patients experienced pain relief, with approximately 30% achieving complete pain relief [68].

One of the disadvantages of HBI is that it covers all of the bones (not just those with metastatic disease) plus the surrounding normal tissues and organs within a large field of the body, and is not targeted to specific areas of disease involvement. Systemic radionuclides have the advantage of more selective targeting of disease [67]. The compounds currently used are calcium analogues, and typically are concentrated in areas of most significant bone activity. Phosphorus-32 (^{32}P) was initially used to treat bone pain nearly 50 years ago. However, it causes myelosuppression, and also is taken up in significant quantities by the liver and other normal tissues outside of the bone. Strontium-89 (^{89}Sr) selectively accumulates in the bone (especially in osteoblastic lesions), and emits low-energy β particles (electrons). This gives high doses of treatment to the bone with relative sparing of the bone marrow. Responses in patients with metastatic breast cancer are seen in 80–90% of patients, with 10–20% achieving complete pain relief and 50% experiencing a partial response. Samarium-153 (^{153}Sm) has a shorter half-life than ^{89}Sr and is rapidly cleared from the body. An additional advantage is that it has a small γ component and thus γ-ray images (similar to ^{99m}Tc bone scans) can be obtained to evaluate the localisation of the isotope. Other isotopes, such as rhenium-186 (^{186}Re), are currently being evaluated for treatment of bone metastases.

Ongoing studies are evaluating the potential for prophylactic usage of systemic radionuclides in patients with asymptomatic or minimally symptomatic bone metastases—to decrease the risk of progression of osseous metastases.

SUMMARY

Breast cancer is common, and bone is one of the most common sites of metastatic deposits. The clinical course is slower and more indolent than for most other primary sites, and the duration of survival for patients with metastatic breast cancer may be relatively long. For these reasons, aggressive treatment of bone metastases is more important in breast cancer than in other malignancies.

A thorough evaluation of the extent of disease in patients found to have bone metastases is important. Patients with bone disease in the weight-bearing bones should have radiographic evaluation of bone scan abnormalities, and orthopaedic consultation if there is evidence of cortical destruction. Orthopaedic stabilisation of the weight-bearing bones should be aggressively pursued in many of these patients to prevent pathological fractures.

Patients with receptor-positive primary tumours typically should receive hormonal or endocrine manipulation as the initial systemic treatment. Tamoxifen is the most frequently used hormonal treatment, but medroxyprogesterone acetate and the new aromatase inhibitors appear to be as effective as tamoxifen for osseous metastases. Patients with receptor-negative tumours and those with progression of bone disease on hormonal therapy should be considered for chemotherapy. Multiple drug combinations that are either anthracycline- or taxane-based are most likely to be effective. If only a single chemotherapeutic agent is used, an anthracycline such as doxorubicin or a taxane such as paclitaxel appear to be the best choices. The UICC criteria for assessment of response is not a sufficiently sensitive measure of clinical improvement in patients with bone metastases, and alternative assessments (such as quality of life and pain indices) may be better indicators of the efficacy of systemic treatment.

The role of bisphosphonates as an adjuvant for prevention of bone metastases is not yet clearly defined. In patients with overt bone metastases, the bisphosphonates clearly reduce the incidence and severity of skeletal complications and should be used routinely.

Radiation therapy is effective in palliating painful osseous metastases. Patients with one or two painful sites should be treated with external beam radiotherapy. The most appropriate treatment schedule remains controversial, but a rational guideline is to use short treatment courses (one or a few treatments) for patients with poor performance status, and more extended courses (10–15 treatments) for patients with better performance status. Radiation therapy is more effective at providing complete and durable pain relief when the pain is less than severe; thus, radiotherapy should be considered early in the clinical course rather than as a final effort at palliation of pain. Patients with breast cancer frequently have multiple bone metastases. For these patients, treatment with systemic radionuclides (^{89}Sr, ^{153}Sm, ^{186}Re) is effective in both palliating pain and preventing the development of new painful sites.

In summary, patients with breast cancer metastatic to bone may have a long duration of survival, and there are many effective treatments to improve quality of life in these patients. The best approach to these patients is with a multidisciplinary approach.

REFERENCES

1. Nielsen OS, Munro AJ, Tannock IF. Bone metastases: pathophysiology and management policy. J Clin Oncol 1991; 9: 509–24.
2. Solomayer EF, Diel IJ, Meyberg GC et al. Metastatic breast cancer: clinical course, prognosis and therapy related to the first site of metastasis. Breast Cancer Res Treat 2000; 59: 271–8.
3. Colleoni M, O'Neill A, Goldhirsch A et al. Identifying breast cancer patients at high risk for bone metastases. J Clin Oncol 2000; 18: 3925–35.
4. Sherry MM, Greco FA, Johnson DH, Hainsworth JD. Metastatic breast cancer confined to the skeletal system. An indolent disease. Am J Med 1986; 81: 381–6.
5. Scheid V, Buzdar AU, Smith TL et al. Clinical course of breast cancer patients with osseous metastasis treated with combination chemotherapy. Cancer 1986; 58: 2589–93.
6. Tubiana-Hulin M. Incidence, prevalence and distribution of bone metastases. Bone 1991; 12(suppl 1): S9–10.
7. Wikenheiser KA, Silberstein EB. Bone scintigraphy screening in stage I–II breast cancer: is it cost-effective? Cleve Clin J Med 1996; 63: 43–7.
8. Yeh KA, Fortunato L, Ridge JA et al. Routine bone scanning in patients with T1 and T2 breast cancer: a waste of money. Ann Surg Oncol 1995; 2: 319–24.
9. Jacobson AF, Stomper PC, Jochelson M et al. Association between number of sites of new bone scan abnormalities and presence of skeletal metastases. J Nucl Med 1990; 31: 387–92.
10. Traill ZC, Talbot D, Golding S et al. Magnetic resonance imaging vs. radionuclide scintigraphy in screening for bone metastases. Clin Radiol 1999; 54: 448–51.
11. Cook GJ, Houston S, Rubens R et al. Detection of bone metastases in breast cancer by 18FDG PET: differing metabolic activity in osteoblastic and osteolytic lesions. J Clin Oncol 1998; 16: 3375–9.
12. Brada M, Rowley M, Grant DJ et al. Hypercalcemia in patients with breast cancer. Acta Oncol 1990; 29: 577–80.
13. Coleman RE, Rubens RD. The clinical course of bone metastasis from breast cancer. Br J Cancer 1987; 55: 61–6.
14. Higinbotham NL, Marcove RC. The management of pathologic fractures. J Trauma 1965; 5: 792–8.

15. Healey JH, Brown HK. Complications of bone metastases: surgical management. Cancer 2000; 88(12, suppl): 2940–51.
16. Ayward JL, Carbone PP, Heuson JC. Assessment of response to therapy in advanced breast cancer. A project of the Programme on Clinical Oncology of the International Union Against Cancer Eur J Cancer 1977; 13: 89–94.
17. Harvey HA. Issues concerning the role of chemotherapy and hormonal therapy of bone metastases from breast carcinoma. Cancer 1997; 80: 1646–51.
18. Schneider JA, Divgi CR, Scott AM. Flare on bone scintigraphy following Taxol chemotherapy for metastatic breast cancer. J Nucl Med 1994; 35: 1748–52.
19. Hainsworth JD, Andrews MB, Johnson DH, Greco FA. Mitoxantrone, fluorouracil, and high-dose leucovorin: an effective, well-tolerated regimen for metastatic breast cancer. J Clin Oncol 1991; 9: 1731–5.
20. Kamby C, Vestlev PM, Mouridsen HT. Site-specific effect of chemotherapy in patients with breast cancer. Acta Oncol 1992; 31: 225–9.
21. Osborne CK, Yochnowitz MG, Knight WA. The value of estrogen and progesterone receptors in the treatment of breast cancer. Cancer 1980; 46: 2884–8.
22. Henderson IC. Endocrine therapy of metastatic breast cancer. In Breast Diseases, 2nd edn. Lippincott: Philadelphia, PA, 1991: 564–73.
23. Willemse PH, van der Ploeg E, Sleijfer DT et al. A randomized comparison of megestrol acetate (MA) and medroxyprogesterone acetate (MPA) in patients with advanced breast cancer. Eur J Cancer 1990; 26: 337–43.
24. Muss HB, Case LD, Atkins JN. Tamoxifen vs. high-dose oral medroxyprogesterone acetate as initial endocrine therapy for patients with metastatic breast cancer: a Piedmont Oncology Association study. J Clin Oncol 1994; 12: 1630–8.
25. Harris JR, Morrow M, Bonadonna G. Cancer of the breast. In Cancer: Principles and Practice of Oncology, 4th edn. Lippincott: Philadelphia, PA, 1993: 1264–332.
26. Bonneterre J, Thurlmann B, Robertson JFR et al. Anastrazole vs. tamoxifen as first-line therapy for advanced breast cancer in 668 postmenopausal women: results of the tamoxifen or arimidex randomized group efficacy and tolerability study. J Clin Oncol 2000; 18: 3748–57.
27. Nabholtz JM, Buzdar A, Pollak M et al. Anastrazole is superior to tamoxifen as first-line therapy of advanced breast cancer in postmenopausal women: results of a North American multicenter randomized trial. J Clin Oncol 2000; 18: 3758–67.
28. Buzdar AU, Jonat W, Howell A et al. Anastrazole vs. megestrol acetate in the treatment of postmenopausal women with advanced breast carcinoma: results of survival update based on a combined analysis of data from two mature phase III trials. Cancer 1998; 83: 1142–52.
29. Degardin M, Bonneterre J, Hecquet B et al. Vinorelbine (navelbine) as a salvage treatment for advanced breast cancer. Ann Oncol 1994; 5: 423–6.
30. Karapetis CS, Patterson WK, Pittman KB et al. Treatment of metastatic breast cancer with continuous infusional 5 fluorouracil. Aust NZ J Med 1999; 29: 517–22.

31. Jones RB, Holland RF, Bhardway S. A phase I–II study of dose-intensive Adriamycin for advanced breast cancer. J Clin Oncol 1987; 5: 172–7.

32. Symon Z, Peyser A, Tzemach D et al. Selective delivery of doxorubicin to patients with breast carcinoma metastases by stealth liposomes. Cancer 1999; 86: 72–8.

33. Schneider JA, Divgi CR, Scott AM et al. Flare on bone scintigraphy following Taxol chemotherapy for metastatic breast cancer. J Nucl Med 1994; 35: 1748–52.

34. Ardavanis A, Extra JM, Espie M et al. Phase II trial of a combination of vinorelbine, cyclophosphamide and 5-fluorouracil in the treatment of advanced breast cancer. In Vivo 1998; 12: 559–62.

35. Iino Y, Yokoe T, Sugamata N et al. A combination chemoendocrine therapy of mitoxantrone, doxifluridine, and medroxyprogesterone acetate for anthracycline-resistant advanced breast cancer. Cancer Chemother Pharmacol 1998; 41: 243–7.

36. Gale RP, Park RE, Dubois R et al. Delphi-panel analysis of appropriateness of high-dose chemotherapy and blood cell or bone marrow autotransplants in women with breast cancer. Clin Transpl 2000; 14: 32–41.

37. Shah AB, Hartsell WF, Ghalie R, Kaizer H. Patterns of failure following bone marrow transplantation for metastatic breast cancer: the role of consolidative local therapy. Int J Radiat Oncol Biol Phys 1995; 32: 1433–8.

38. Cobleigh MA, Vogel CL, Tripathy D et al. Efficacy and safety of herceptin (humanized anti-HER2 antibody) as a single agent in 222 women with HER2 overexpression who relapsed following chemotherapy for metastatic breast cancer. Proc Am Soc Clin Oncol 1998; 17: 97a.

39. Norton L, Slamon D, Leyland-Jones B et al. Overall survival (OS) advantage to simultaneous chemotherapy (CRx) plus the humanized anti-HER2-overexpressing (HER2+) metastatic breast cancer (MBC). Proc Am Soc Clin Oncol 1999; 18: 127a.

40. Slamon D, Leyland-Jones B, Shak S et al. Addition of herceptin (humanized anti-HER2 antibody) to first line chemotherapy for HER2 overexpressing metastatic breast cancer (HER2+/MBC) markedly increases anticancer activity: a randomized, multinational controlled Phase III trial. Proc Am Soc Clin Oncol 1998; 17: 98a.

41. Pegram MD, Lipton A, Hayes DF et al. Phase II study of receptor-enhanced chemosensitivity using recombinant humanized anti-p185[HER2/new] monoclonal antibody plus cisplatin in patients with HER2/new-overexpressing metastatic breast cancer refractory to chemotherapy treatment. J Clin Oncol 1998; 16: 2659–71.

42. Fleisch H. Bisphosphonates: mechanisms of action. Endocr Rev 1998; 19: 80–100.

43. Reitsma PH, Teitelbaum SL, Bijvoet OLM et al. Difference action of the biophosphates (3-amino-1-hydroxypropylidene)-1-1biphosphonate (APD) and disodium dichloromethylidene Bisphophate (Cl$_2$MDP) on rat macrophage-mediated bone resorption in vitro. J Clin Invest 1982; 70: 927–33.

44. Busch M, Rave-Frank M, Hille A, Duhmke E. Influence of clodronate on breast cancer cells in vitro. Eur J Med Res 1998; 3: 427–31.

45. Sauty A, Pecherstorfer M, Zimmer-Roth I et al. Interleukin-6 and tumour necrosis factor α levels after bisphosphonates treatment in vitro and in patients with malignancy. Bone 1996; 18: 133–9.

46. Van der Pluijm G, Vloedgraven H, van Beek E et al. Biophosphates inhibit the adhesion of breast cancer cells to bone matrices in vitro. J Clin Invest 1996; 98: 698–705.

47. Coleman RE, Whitaker KD, Moss DW et al. 3-Amino-1,1 hydroxypropylidene bisphosphonate (APD) for the treatment of bone metastases from breast cancer. Br J Cancer 1988; 58: 621–5.

48. Morton AR, Cantrill JA, Pillai GV et al. Sclerosis of lytic bone metastases after disodium aminohydroxypropylidene bisphosphonate (APD) in patients with breast cancer. Br Med J 1988; 297: 772–3.

49. Paterson AHG, Powles TJ, Kanis JA et al. Double-blind controlled trial of oral clodronate in patients with bone metastases from breast cancer. J Clin Oncol 1993; 11: 59–65.

50. Van Holten-Verzantvoort ATM, Kroon HM, Bijvoet OLM et al. Palliative pamidronate treatment in patients with bone metastases from breast cancer. J Clin Oncol 1993; 11: 491–8.

51. Hortobagyi GN, Theriault RL, Lipton A et al. Long-term prevention of skeletal complications of metastatic breast cancer with pamidronate. J Clin Oncol 1998; 16: 2038.

52. Theriault RL, Lipton A, Hortobagyi GN et al. Pamidronate reduces skeletal morbidity in women with advanced breast cancer and lytic bone lesions: a randomized, placebo-controlled trial. J Clin Oncol 1999; 17: 846–54.

53. Conte PF, Latreille J, Mauriac L et al. Delay in progression of bone metastases in breast cancer patients treated with intravenous pamidronate: results from a multinational randomized controlled trial. J Clin Oncol 1996; 14: 2552–9.

54. Rosen LS, Gordon DH, Dugan W Jr et al. Zoledronic acid is superior to pamidronate for the treatment of bone metastases in breast carcinoma patients with at least one osteolytic lesion. Cancer 2004; 100: 36–43.

55. Saarto T, Blomqvist C, Virkkunen P et al. No reduction of bone metastases with adjuvant clodronate treatment in node-positive breast cancer patients. Proc Am Soc Clin Oncol 1999; 18: 128a.

56. Powles TJ, Paterson A, Nevantaus S et al. Adjuvant clodronate reduces the incidence of bone metastases in patients with primary operable breast cancer. Proc Am Soc Clin Oncol 1998; 17: 123a.

57. Diel IJ, Solomayer EF, Costa SD et al. Reduction in new metastases in breast cancer with adjuvant clodronate treatment. N Engl J Med 1998; 339: 357–63.

58. Tong D, Gillick L, Hendrickson FR. The palliation of symptomatic osseous metastases. Final results of the Radiation Therapy Oncology Group. Cancer 1982; 50: 893–9.

59. Blitzer PH. Reanalysis of the RTOG study of the palliation of symptomatic osseous metastasis. Cancer 1985; 55: 1468–72.

60. Hoskin PJ, Price P, Easton D et al. A prospective randomized trial of 4 Gy or 8 Gy single doses in the treatment of metastatic bone pain. Radiother Oncol 1992; 3: 74–8.

61. Price P, Hoskin PJ, Easton D et al. Prospective randomized trial of single and multifraction radiotherapy

schedules in the treatment of painful bony metastases. Radiother Oncol 1986; 6: 247–55.

62. Powers WE, Ratanatharathorn V. Palliation of bone metastases. In Principles and Practice of Radiation Oncology, 3rd edn. Lippincott-Raven: Philadelphia, PA, 1997.

63. Porter AT, Benda R, Ben-Josef E. Palliation of metastases: bone and spinal cord. In Clinical Radiation Oncology. Churchill Livingstone: Philadelphia, PA, 2000.

64. Hartsell WF, Scott C, Bruner DW et al. Phase III randomized trial of 8 Gy in 1 fraction vs. 30 Gy in 10 fractions for palliation of painful bone metastases: preliminary results of RTOG 97-14. Int J Radiat Oncol Biol Phys 57 (2 Suppl): S124, 2003.

65. Body JJ. Metastatic bone disease: clinical and therapeutic aspects. Bone 1992; 13(suppl 1): S57–62.

66. Garmaitis CJ, Chu FCH. The effectiveness of radiation therapy in the treatment of bone metastases from breast cancer. Radiology 1978; 126: 235–7.

67. Perez CA, Sartor O, Janjan N, Ratanatharathorn V. Management of painful bone metastases with emphasis on the use of radiopharmaceuticals. Princip Pract Radiat Oncol 2000; 1: 2–22.

68. Salazar OM, Rubin P, Hendrickson FR et al. Single dose half-body irradiation for palliation of multiple bone metastases from solid tumors. Cancer 1986; 58: 29–36.

69. Steenland E, Leer JW, van Houwelingen H et al. The effect of a single fraction compared to multiple fractions on painful bone metastases: a global analysis of the Dutch Bone Metastasis Study. Radiother Oncol 1999; 52: 101–9

39

Prostate Cancer

Edward Chow,[1] Malcolm J. Moore,[2] Jackson Wu,[3] Padraig Warde[2] and Carlos A. Perez[4]

[1]*Toronto Sunnybrook Regional Cancer Centre, Toronto, ON, Canada*
[2]*Princess Margaret Hospital, Toronto, ON, Canada*
[3]*Tom Baker Cancer Centre, Calgary, AB, Canada*
[4]*Radiation Oncology Center, Saint Louis, MO, USA*

INTRODUCTION

Prostate cancer is the most prevalent cancer in North American men and ranks the second most common among European males [1,2]. In 2002, 189 000 new cases of prostate cancer were expected, accounting for 30% of new cancer diagnoses in the USA. Prostate cancer is the second most common cause of cancer-related deaths, with estimated deaths of 30 200 (10% of all estimated cancer deaths in the USA) in 2002 [1]. Even though the sensitive serum marker prostatic specific antigen (PSA) has improved detection of subclinical disease and helps to properly select patients for more aggressive treatments, both the detection of curable disease and the overall cure rates remain at about 70%. It becomes obvious that only half (70% × 70%) of men diagnosed with prostate cancer can be cured, leaving a large number who may eventually require palliative treatment [3]. Bone metastasis is the most frequent cause of morbidity in men with advanced prostate cancer.

Eight percent of White American males and 14% of African–American males have bone metastases at presentation [4]. Patients who progress following initial curative treatments often develop bone metastases and 85–100% of patients who die of prostate cancer have bone metastases [5].

DEVELOPMENT OF BONE METASTASES AFTER INITIAL THERAPY

Most of the observational studies on patients managed by a "watchful waiting" approach are retrospective but support the correlation of initial PSA, clinical stage and Gleason score at diagnosis with the long-term incidence of bone metastases. Patients with T1/T2 or T3/T4 disease develop metastases at 10 years in 3–41% and 12–55% of cases, respectively. Patients with well, moderately or poorly differentiated tumours develop metastases at 10 years in 3–10%, 13–57% and 42–80% of cases, respectively [6–10].

The development of metastatic disease among patients with early stages of cancer treated by radical prostatectomy (RP) or radical radiation therapy is relatively infrequent, especially if radical treatment is followed by adjuvant systemic therapy [11]. Pound and associates reported 15% biochemical recurrence rate (rising PSA) and 5% bone metastases rate among 1997 clinical stage T1–2 patients treated by RP, after a median follow-up of 5 years. The median time from time of PSA failure to metastases was 8 years. Risk factors for progression to bone metastases after RP included Gleason score $\geq$ 7, presence of seminal vesicle invasion or lymph node involvement, or biochemical failure within 2 years of prostatectomy [11].

Textbook of Bone Metastases. Edited by C. Jasmin, R. E. Coleman, L. R. Coia, R. Capanna and G. Saillant
© 2005 John Wiley & Sons Ltd: ISBN 0 471 87742 5

Zagars et al. reported that, in 938 clinical stage T1–3 men treated with radiation therapy with a mean follow-up of 45 months, 29% of patients developed biochemical failure and 20% of these patients (6% of the total) developed bone metastases [12]. The risk factors for developing bone metastases after radiation therapy include Gleason score $\geq$ 8, pretreatment PSA > 20 ng/dl, clinical T3 or T4 disease, clinically positive lymph nodes, or failure to achieve PSA nadir below 4.0 ng/dl after radiation therapy [13,14]. The likelihood of developing bone metastases is much greater if biochemical failure occurs during hormonal therapy, especially when the hormones are used for salvage. In this situation, bone metastases are usually detectable within 1.5–3 years. Furthermore, when established metastatic disease becomes unresponsive to hormonal treatment, new bone lesions often appear within 11–52 weeks [15].

DISTRIBUTION OF BONE METASTASES

The most common site of distant bone metastases in prostate cancer patients is the axial skeleton. Significant controversy exists over the exact aetiology of this preferential spread. Batson proposed the generally accepted theory that prostate cancer metastasises to the spine and pelvis through the Batson's plexus, an extra-peritoneal system of valveless veins in the posterior torso, preferentially draining to the bones of the pelvis and the spine through the vertebral veins, followed later by involvement of the long bones and skull [16]. Dodds and associates offered their counter-argument, since the distribution of skeletal metastases from prostate cancer is comparable with that of other primary tumours [17]. The preponderance of metastases to the axial skeleton and proximate long bones may be a function of regional arterial blood flow and not of any specific venous drainage [18].

On a microscopic level, metastatic bone generally contains areas of both bone destruction (osteoclastic process) and bone formation (osteoblastic process). In prostate cancer, the osteoblastic process predominates and gives rise to the typical radiographic appearance often referred to as blastic or sclerotic lesions. Despite an increase in bone density, the new bone formation triggered by prostate cancer often lacks the strength of normal bone, resulting in increased risk of pathological fractures, albeit to a lesser extent than bone metastases that are predominantly lytic. This osteoblastic reactivity to the presence of prostate cancer can facilitate radiographic detection by bone-seeking radioisotope tracers, which preferentially bind to areas of new bone

formation. Hence the bone scan has a much greater sensitivity to detect asymptomatic bone metastases than plain radiographs. This preferential uptake of tracers is also exploited for treatment with systemic radioisotopes, using calcium analogues such as strontium-89 (^{89}Sr) to deliver therapeutic doses of radiation to these areas of tumours that trigger new bone deposition.

EVALUATION OF PATIENTS WITH BONE METASTASES

Bone metastases are frequently symptomatic, significantly affecting the quality of life in patients with advanced disease. Symptoms include intermittent or constant bone pain, bone marrow suppression, hypercalcaemia, pathological fractures and spinal cord/nerve roots compression. Clinical evaluation typically includes a thorough history, physical examination, bone scan, plain radiographs and serum alkaline phosphatase. However, benign processes such as healing fractures, arthritis, Paget's disease, other bony infectious diseases and inflammatory diseases may lead to false positives on a bone scan [19]. For this reason, suspicious areas on bone scan should be confirmed by plain radiographs and a biopsy if necessary.

In very advanced cases, the entire skeleton may appear abnormal. Although this is sometimes confused with a normal scan, patients with a superscan do not demonstrate renal excretion of the radionuclide because of extensive uptake in bone. If spinal cord compression is suspected clinically, a CT scanning myelogram or MRI imaging is of urgent importance. In a study by Bayley et al., prostate cancer patients with bone metastases without neurological signs were screened for occult spinal cord compression using MRI. The extent of disease on bone scan and the duration of continuous hormonal therapy were found to predict the presence of occult spinal cord compression [20].

RADIATION THERAPY IN ADVANCED PROSTATE CANCER

Localised External Beam Radiation Therapy

External beam radiation therapy remains one of the most effective and cost-efficient methods of relieving pain of bone metastases. Despite numerous trials, there is still no uniform consensus on the optimal dose fractionation scheme.

Retrospective series have documented prompt improvement in pain in 80–90% of cases [21–29] with various dose fractionations without inducing serious haematological or gastrointestinal toxicity [30–33]. Prostate cancer patients contributed a significant proportion in those trials. The Radiation Therapy Oncology Group (RTOG) conducted a prospective randomised trial (RTOG 74-02) on patients with bone metastases. They concluded that the low-dose short-course schedules were as effective as the more aggressive high-dose protracted regimens in pain relief. The only notable difference by treatment group was in the solitary metastases group, with an 18% rate of fracture in those patients receiving 4050 cGy/15 fractions compared with 4% in the group receiving 2000 cGy/5 fractions [34]. However, fracture risk was not assessed pre-irradiation. This study was also criticised because it dealt only with the physicians' evaluations of treatment efficacy.

What further complicates this trial is that a re-analysis of the data, grouping solitary and multiple bony metastases, using the endpoint of pain relief, taking into account narcotic score and retreatment, concluded, contrary to the initial report, that the number of radiotherapy fractions was significantly associated with complete pain relief [35]. This clearly demonstrates the importance of endpoint definition in such studies.

Subsequent to the RTOG trial, there have been several prospective randomised trials evaluating different dose-fractionation schemes. Price et al. reported results on 288 patients randomised to either 8 Gy given in a single fraction or 30 Gy given in 10 daily fractions. Pain was monitored using a self-assessed diary, along with a record of analgesic intakes. The median survival for all patients was 5 months and there was no difference between 8 Gy and 30 Gy in overall or duration of response at 1 year. However, a large proportion of patients was lost to follow-up evaluation in their study [36]. The same group later conducted another study on 270 patients randomising to either a single 4 Gy or a single 8 Gy treatment. The median survival for all patients was 8 months, but treatment with a single 4 Gy produced a lower overall response rate (53%) than the 8 Gy (76%) [37].

Two other large-scale multi-centre trials also compared the efficacy of 8 Gy single treatment against multiple treatments. The Bone Pain Working Party in the UK studied 765 patients and found no difference in the degree and duration of pain relief between single treatment and five fractionated treatments [38]. The Dutch Bone Metastases study included 1171 patients and found no difference in pain relief as well as quality of life following 8 Gy or 24 Gy treatments [39] (Table 39.1) [34,36–43].

However, in the Bone Pain Trial Working Party trial [38], retreatment was more frequent in the single-dose group (76/329, 29.1%) than in the multifraction group (32/327, 9.8%) (Figure 39.1) and in the study by Steenland et al. [39] the number of patients requiring retreatment was 147 (25%) in the 8 Gy group and 41 (7%) in the 24 Gy treatment group.

One critical review on the subject of dose-fractionation concluded that protracted fractionated radiotherapy, given over 2–4 weeks, results in more complete and durable pain relief [44]. Recent surveys in North America suggest that radiation oncologists prefer a protracted treatment scheme, despite evidence showing similar effectiveness between a single treatment of 8 Gy and multiple fractionations [45–48]. On the other hand, European oncologists have now adopted single treatment of 8 Gy as standard practice for patients with uncomplicated metastatic bone pain [49]. Debate continues over what may be best treatment for subgroups of patients with favourable characteristics and prolonged survival [49–52]. These patients typically present with solitary or limited number of bone metastases after a long disease-free interval following initial radical treatment for breast or prostate cancer. In this group of patients, higher doses of radiation fractionated over 2–4 weeks may provide more durable pain relief [52]. The current RTOG 97-14 bone metastases trial will specifically address this question. Some studies have suggested that prostate cancer patients responded better compared to patients with other primaries [34,36–38,53] but this observation has yet to be confirmed by on-going studies.

Wide-field/Half-body External Beam Radiation (HBI)

HBI is useful for patients with multiple painful bone metastases. Single-fraction HBI has been shown in retrospective and prospective Phase I and II studies to provide pain relief in 70–80% of patients [54–57]. Pain relief is apparent within 24–48 h [57,58]. Toxicities include minor bone marrow suppression and gastro-intestinal side-effects such as nausea and vomiting following upper abdominal radiation, and may be controlled with ondansetron or dexamethasone [33,58,59]. Pulmonary toxicity is minimal, provided that the lung dose is limited to 6 Gy (corrected dose) [60]. Fractionated HBI was investigated in a Phase II study that compared a single fraction (n=14) with fractionated HBI (25–30 Gy in nine or ten fractions)

Table 39.1. Selected fractionation trials of treatment of painful bone metastases

Author/institution (treatment arms)	Total no. of patients	Proportion with prostate cancer (%)	CR or PR (%)		Frequency of re-irradiation (%)	
			Low dose	High dose	Low dose	High dose
Bone Pain Working Party (UK) [38] (8 Gy vs. 20 Gy/5#)	765	34	57 CR 78 PR	58 CR 78 PR	23	10
Dutch Bone Metastasis Study [39] (8 Gy vs. 24 Gy/6#)	1171	23	37 CR 72 PR	33 CR 69 PR	25	7
Nielson et al. [40] (8 Gy vs. 20 Gy/5#)	241	33	12 CCR* 15 CR 62 PR	12 CCR* 17 CR 74 PR	20	12
Jeremic et al. [41] (4 Gy (vs. 6 Gy) vs. 8 Gy)	327	16	21 CR 59 Min	32 CR 78 Min	42	38
Gaze et al. [42] (10 Gy vs. 22.5 Gy/5#)	280	20	15 CCR 39 CR 84 Min	14 CCR 42 CR 89 Min	N/A	N/A
Niewald et al. [43] (20 Gy/5# vs. 30 Gy/15#)	100	10	33 CR 77 Min	31 CR 86 Min	N/A	N/A
Hoskin et al. [37] (4 Gy vs. 8 Gy)	270	13	36 CR 44 PR	39 CR 69 PR	20	9
Price et al. [36] (8 Gy vs. 30 Gy/10#)	288	8	35 CR 84 Min	27 CR 84 Min	$n=15$	$n=4$
Radiation Therapy Oncology Group 74-02 [34] (20 Gy/5# vs. 30 Gy/10#) (vs. others)**	($n=186$ vs. $n=202$)	15	37 CCR 56 CR 89 Min	46–55 CCR 57 CR 87 Min	Overall 16	

* CCR, complete combined relief, 0 pain score, 0 narcotic score.
** Two of four arms from multiple metastases group selected for purpose of illustration only.
CR, complete response; PR, partial response; Min, minimal response; N/A, not available.

($n=15$). Pain relief was achieved in over 94% of patients. At 1 year, 70% in the fractionated and 15% in the single fraction group had pain control, and retreatment was required in 71% and 13% for the single and fractionated group respectively [61]. Poulter and colleagues reported results of a randomised trial of 499 patients comparing local radiation alone vs. local radiation plus a single fraction of HBI. The study documented a lower incidence of new bone metastases (50% vs. 68%) and fewer patients requiring further local radiotherapy at 1 year after HBI (60% vs. 76%) [32]. The choice of dose-fractionation schedule for HBI was explored by Salazar et al. [62]. Fifty of the 156 randomised patients from six countries had prostate cancer. Among the three trial arms, of 15 Gy in five fractions over 5 days, 8 Gy in two fractions over 1 day, and 12 Gy in four fractions over 2 days, the 15 Gy/five fractions/5 days regimen provided not only pain relief as much as the other regimens, but also a longer survival duration compared with the other regimens. More prostate cancer patients are planned to be entered into the study to confirm this unexpected finding.

Radionuclides

Patients with metastatic prostate cancer often present with multiple bone metastases requiring external beam radiation to several parts of the skeleton, some of which require more than one course of palliative radiotherapy. Systemic radiotherapy using radionuclides has been increasingly recognised as an important contributor to improvements in quality of life for this group of patients. ^{89}Sr (Metastron) or ^{153}Sm-EDTMP (Quadramet) have an affinity for bone and concentrate in areas of bone turnover in association with hydroxyapatite. They accumulate in osteoblastic lesions at a greater rate than in normal bone with a lesion:normal bone ratio of approximately 5 [63]. The mechanism of action of radiopharmaceuticals in relieving pain of bone metastases is not known, but is assumed to be the result of destruction of carcinogenic tumour cells in the bone. Table 39.2 summarises the physical characteristics of various radiopharmaceuticals available.

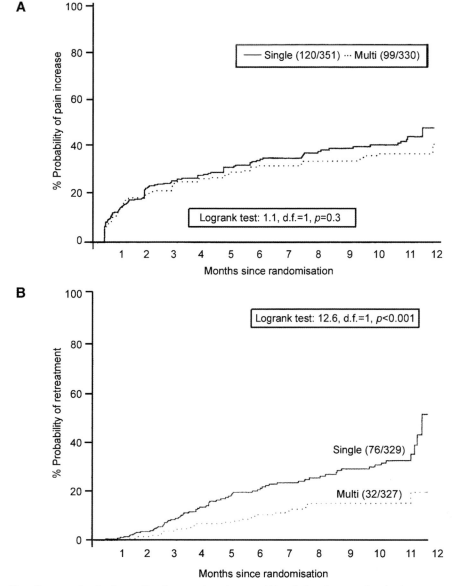

Figure 39.1. Time from randomisation to first increase in pain score (A) and time from randomisation to retreatment of painful site by radiation therapy (B) in 761 patients randomised to single- or multiple-fraction radiation therapy

Contraindications to bone-seeking radiopharmaceuticals [64] include:

1. Karnofsky performance $\leqslant 50$.
2. Extensive soft tissue metastases.
3. Platelet count $< 60\,000 \times 10^6$.
4. Recent rapid fall in platelet count, even if $> 60\,000 \times 10^6$.
5. White count $< 2.5 \times 10^6$.
6. Disseminated intravascular coagulation.

7. Myelosuppressive chemotherapy within previous month.
8. Projected survival of less than 2 months.
9. Half-body irradiation (HBI) within previous 2 months.
10. Impending or established pathological fractures and cord compressions.

Impending or established pathological fractures and cord compressions are to be managed by surgical or

Table 39.2. Radionuclides for treatment of painful bone metastases

	^{153}Sm	^{89}Sr	^{32}P
Particles	β/γ	β	β
Energy (maximum/average) (MeV)	0.81/0.29	1.46/0.58	1.7/0.69
Physical half-life (days)	1.9	50.6	14.3
Dose	1 mCi/kg	4 mCi	5 mCi
Chemical background	Diphosphonate	Ca analogue	DNA
Penetration in tissue (mm)	2–3	4–6	4–8

radiation oncology team as acute emergencies. Once the fracture or compression is stabilised, radionuclides may be appropriate therapy for on-going palliation of pain [64].

^{89}Sr has been evaluated in Phase III studies involving patients with hormone-refractory disease [30,31]. It is an injectable, non-sealed radionuclide with a physical half-life of 50.5 days. It decays with the emission of β-particles (free electrons with maximum energy of 1.5 MeV) which have a range of 0.8 cm in tissue. ^{89}Sr is preferentially taken up and retained by sites of osteoblastic metastases, but is washed out of normal healthy bone with a biological half-life of 14 days. The differential distribution and retention of the nuclide result is a therapeutic advantage through targeted delivery of radiation to metastatic bony sites [65–67]. This selective distribution also limits haematological adverse effects, and the dose-limiting factors seen with other agents, such as phosphorus-32 (^{32}P).

Several studies have been conducted using ^{89}Sr in the treatment of bone metastasis. Pain relief occurs in 50–70% of patients within 3 months following treatment [30,59,68]. Porter et al. [30] reported on a multi-centre study in which 126 patients with painful metastasis from carcinoma of the prostate were refractory to hormonal therapy. Patients were treated with local field radiation therapy and either 10.8 mCi ^{89}Sr or a placebo. In the ^{89}Sr-treated group, 17% of the patients stopped taking analgesics as compared to 2% in the placebo group. At 3 months after randomisation, 59% of the ^{89}Sr group were free of new painful metastasis in comparison to 34% in the placebo group. The median time to further radiotherapy was 35 weeks in the treated group compared to 20 weeks in the placebo group. Quality of life, pain relief and improvement in physical activity were statistically significantly superior in the patients treated with ^{89}Sr.

Quilty and colleagues [59] described the results in 284 patients with metastatic prostate cancer and painful bone metastasis who were randomised to receive either external beam local or HB radiation

therapy or ^{89}Sr (200 MBq). HBI resulted in pain relief in 64%, compared to 66% in the ^{89}Sr group. Local irradiation provided pain relief in 61% compared to 66% in the comparable ^{89}Sr group. However, fewer patients reported new painful metastatic sites after ^{89}Sr treatment than after HBI or local field irradiation.

Randomised controlled trials of ^{89}Sr in the palliation of patients with metastatic prostate cancer are listed in Table 39.3 [30,59,68,69]. ^{89}Sr is recommended for use in patients with hormone-refractory prostate cancer who have multiple uncontrolled painful sites of bone metastases, on both sides of the diaphragm, not adequately controlled with conventional analgesic therapy, and in whom the multiple fields of external beam radiation may cause unacceptable toxicity. However, it has not been shown to lengthen the average duration of patient survival. Two articles have shown the cost-effectiveness of ^{89}Sr in lifetime management costs when compared with standard patterns of care in patients with advanced progressive disease [70,71].

An unexpected finding in the study reported by Porter et al. was a significant fall in PSA values in the group treated with ^{89}Sr. This finding raises the speculation that treatment with bone-seeking radio-pharmaceuticals may exert a significant tumoricidal effect above that of mere pain relief [30]. This observation should be treated with caution, however, since data were not consistently collected for all patients as a secondary treatment endpoint [64].

^{89}Sr can cause reversible bone marrow suppression, particularly thrombocytopenia, but clinically significant sequelae are uncommon. Platelet and leukocyte counts may drop by 30–40% [30,59,69]. The nadir is seen 4–6 weeks after injection, and recovery is usually complete by 6–10 weeks. The severity of the myelosuppression is related to metastatic burden and may also be dependent on the physical/biological half-life and the energies of emitted β particles. Occasionally, patients experience a transient increase in bone pain. This "pain flare" seems to occur a few days after ^{89}Sr administration. According to some

Table 39.3. Randomised controlled trials of strontium-89 in prostate cancer patients with bone metastases

Trials	Treatment arms	Palliative outcome	Comment
Quilty et al. [59] (n=148)	Local XRT vs. 200 MBq	Pain relief 8–12 weeks after treatment	No significant difference in pain relief at index sites; significantly more patients free of new painful sites and fewer patients required further XRT in ^{89}Sr group
Quilty et al. [59] (n=157)	Hemi-body XRT vs. 200 MBq	As above	No significant difference in pain relief at index sites; significantly more patients free of new painful sites in ^{89}Sr group
Lewington et al. [68] (n=32)	Placebo vs. 150 MBq at week 1 or week 6 if needed	Pain relief at week 5	Significantly more patients in ^{89}Sr group showed improvement in score
Buchali et al. [69] (n=49)	Placebo vs. 75 MBq monthly for 3 months	Pain relief 1–3 years after treatment	No significant difference in pain relief
Porter et al. [30] (n=126)	Local XRT and placebo vs. local XRT and 400 MBq	Pain relief 12 weeks after treatment	No significant difference in pain relief. Significantly fewer new painful sites and significant difference favouring ^{89}Sr in terms of need for analgesics, time to further XRT and quality of life

XRT, radiotherapy.

investigators, pain flare may be associated with subsequent pain relief. A flushing sensation, particularly facial, after injection of ^{89}Sr has been noted in some patients but is self-limited.

Samarium-153 ([153]Sm)-EDTMP is an alternative agent licensed for routine use in the USA. It is a therapeutic agent consisting of radioactive [153]Sm and a tetraphosphonate chelator, EDTMP, formulated as a sterile, non-pyrogenic, clear, colourless to light amber isotonic solution for intravenous administration.

The β particle of [153]Sm-EDTMP penetrates an average of 3.1 mm in soft tissue and 1.7 mm in bone. Physical half-life is 46.3 h (1.93 days). The physical characteristics of [153]Sm may offer less bone marrow morbidity and allow for prompt recovery of blood counts.

In patients with metastatic bone lesions, the presence or absence of [153]Sm-EDTMP uptake is similar to that of ^{99m}Tc diphosphonate uptake in bone scan examination. The recommended dose of Quadramet is 1.0 mCi/kg (37 MBq/kg) administered intravenously over a period of 1 min through a secure indwelling catheter and followed with a saline flush. The dose to be administered should be measured by a suitable radioactivity calibration system, such as a radionuclide dose calibrator, immediately before administration. The dose of radioactivity to be administered and the identity of the patient should be verified before administering Quadramet, as required by the Nuclear Regulatory Commission. Patients should not be released until their radioactivity levels and exposure rates comply with federal and local regulations. This procedure can be performed as an outpatient.

Overdosage with Quadramet has not been reported, and an antidote for Quadramet overdosage is not known. However, supportive care for bone marrow suppression or hypocalcaemia and cardiac arrhythmias secondary to the EDTMP should be instituted symptomatically. Quadramet is contraindicated in patients with known hypersensitivity to EDTMP or similar phosphonate compounds.

Finkelstein and Veldkamp evaluated the effect of external beam irradiation on the pharmacokinetics of [153]Sm-EDTMP (Quadramet) uptake and distribution [72]. In theory, external beam irradiation may inhibit the uptake of [153]Sm and decrease its usefulness. Ten patients with histologically proven breast or prostate cancer and painful bone metastasis were enrolled in a trial in which a split-dose technique was used, with external radiation sandwiched between two half-doses of [153]Sm (0.5 mCi/kg, external beam, and a second dose of [153]Sm at 0.5 mCi/kg). The patients were scanned with a GE Starcam 2000 system at 3 and 24 h after each dose. The external beam consisted of 3000–4000 cGy over 2–4 weeks. Each patient served as his/her own control. Average whole body uptake was within 2% between the first and second dose of [153]Sm. The average interval between the first and second dose of [153]Sm was 28 days. Involved bones had two to 20 times the uptake of uninvolved bones. Involved irradiated bones took up 96% of the Quadramet on the second dose compared to their first dose. Involved unirradiated bones took up 94% of the Quadramet on the second dose compared to their first dose uptake. There was no significant difference between these two uptakes ($p=0.92$). Thus, external beam irradiation had no significant effect on the uptake of ^{153}Sm-EDTMP during the 28 day average time course studied. Thus, either external beam or Quadramet may be given first, depending on the clinical situation.

Collins et al. reported on a Phase I/II trial in which 52 prostate cancer patients were given ^{153}Sm-EDTMP, increasing the doses in 0.5 mCi/kg increments from 1 to 3 mCi/kg. Pain response was 76%; there was a significant difference favouring the 2.5 mCi/kg dose level from baseline in pain relief as well as decreased opioid use ($p=0.024$ and 0.015, respectively) compared with the 1 mCi/kg group. Increasing haematologic toxicity was observed with higher doses of the radio-pharmaceutical [73].

Tian et al. reported on a study in which 105 patients with painful bone metastases were treated with either 37 MBq/kg or 18.5 MBq/kg ^{153}Sm-EDTMP; 58/70 (83%) patients in Group I and 30/35 (86%) patients in Group II had a positive pain relief response. Pain relief was approximately equivalent in both dose groups. No serious side-effects were noted [74]. There is good evidence of a therapeutic benefit that is comparable to ^{89}Sr in patients with osteoblastic bone metastases.

Dickie and Macfarlane [75] reported a non-randomised comparison in 57 patients who received ^{89}Sr (38 patients) or ^{153}Sm-EDTMP (19 patients) for prostate cancer metastatic to bone. Forty patients had radionuclide therapy alone, and 28/40 (or 70%) responded in terms experiencing a beneficial effect on pain. In the other 17 patients, the effect of the radionuclide on pain could not be assessed because they received external beam radiotherapy concomitant with a therapeutic radionuclide. There were no different response rates between the ^{153}Sm and ^{89}Sr groups as measured by them on pain or in the time to progression. The median time to progression for all patients was 2–3 months. Decreased platelet counts were slightly higher in the ^{89}Sr group. Results of this study are summarised in Table 39.4. No clinically significant toxicity, including myelosuppression, has been observed.

Sartor et al. [76] evaluated repeat administration of ^{153}Sm in the treatment of painful bone metastases. Multiple 1.0 mCi/kg doses of ^{153}Sm-lexidronam were administered to patients, based on recurrence of painful symptoms. Fifty-four administrations were given to 18 prostate or breast cancer patients (15 males, three females). All patients received at least two doses and four received three or more doses (range, 2–11 doses/patient). The mean administered

Table 39.4. Strontium and samarium for bone metastases from prostate carcinoma

	^{89}Sr	^{153}Sm
Total patients	38	19
Evaluable for pain relief	25	15
Analgesic effect	15 (60%)	13 (86%)
Flare	5 (13%)	6 (31%)
Platelet nadir ($\times 1000$)	24	61
Grade 3 (25–50)	3	0
Grade 4 (< 25)	1	0
Time to progression (median months)	2	3

^{89}Sr vs. ^{153}Sm; $p=$n.s. From Dickie and Macfarlane [75].

dose was 81 ± 17 mCi (range, 52–113 mCi), and the median interval between doses was 133 days. A transient decrease in white blood cells (WBCs) and platelets (PLTs) to approximately 50% of baseline levels was the only toxicity observed (Table 39.5). Median time to nadir for both WBCs and PLTs was 4–5 weeks, regardless of the number of administrations, with recovery generally by week 8. There was no trend toward increasing marrow toxicity with increasing numbers of administrations. Grade 4 toxicities of WBCs or PLTs occurred in only one patient (after three doses). These data demonstrate that multiple 1.0 mCi/kg doses of ^{153}Sm-lexidronam can be safely administered with haematologic toxicity similar to that observed following a single dose.

Three prospective randomised placebo-controlled Phase III trials have been performed with ^{153}Sm-EDTMP in palliation of pain for patients with bone metastases. Two studies have been published in the peer-reviewed literature [77,78]; the other has been published only in abstract form [79].

A randomised double-blind placebo-controlled trial using ^{153}Sm-EDTMP was reported by Serafini et al. [78]; patients with painful bone metastases (prostate, breast, lung, and others) were randomised, 36 patients

Table 39.5. White blood cell and platelet levels

	Dose 1 ($n=18$)	Dose 2 ($n=18$)	Dose $\geqslant 3$ ($n=18$)
WBC Nadir $\pm$ SD	3.7 ± 1.0	3.5 ± 1.0	3.6 ± 1.0
($\times 1000/\mu$l) (% of baseline)	(54%)	(54%)	(56%)
PLT Nadir $\pm$ SD ($\times 1000/\mu$l)	114 ± 36	105 ± 46	97 ± 30
(% of baseline)	(47%)	(47%)	(53%)

From Sartor et al. [76].

to be treated with a placebo, 36 with 0.5 mCi/kg ^{153}Sm, and 35 with 1.0 mCi/kg ^{153}Sm. Four weeks after initial injection, patients with no improvement in pain scores were unblinded; patients receiving placebo were eligible for active treatment with 1 mCi/kg. Data were available for statistical analysis only for the first 4 weeks of the study. All patients had bone pain and a bone scan positive for metastases. A majority of patients had a diagnosis of prostate cancer (68%) and had failed hormone therapy; the second most common diagnosis was breast cancer (18%) and had failed chemotherapy. The majority of patients (74%) were taking narcotics for pain control. Most patients had previously received external beam irradiation.

When both patient- and physician-derived data were analysed, the 1.0 mCi/kg dose of ^{153}Sm-EDTMP was associated with a statistically significant reduction in pain, beginning 1 week after injection (Figure 39.2). Pain relief continued to be statistically significantly improved over the 4 week period of the blinded study; these findings were consistent for patients with prostate cancer, breast cancer or miscellaneous cancers. For patients achieving pain relief in the 1.0 mCi/kg arm of the study, approximately half continued to experience relief 16 weeks later. Of patients treated with the 1.0 mCi/kg dose, 72% experienced some pain relief compared with 43% in the placebo group (Figure 39.3). Patients in the placebo group had increasing analgesic consumption; patients in the active-treatment group had a relative decline in analgesic consumption.

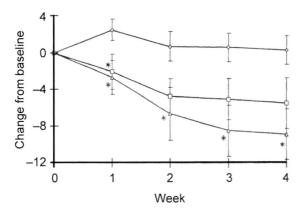

Figure 39.2. Change from baseline in area under the pain curve–visual analogue scale during the first 4 weeks for patients who received placebo, 0.5 mCi/kg of ^{153}Sm-EDTMP, or 1.0 mCi/kg of ^{153}Sm-EDTMP. ($\diamond$), placebo; ($\square$), 0.5 mCi/kg; ($\triangle$), 1.0 mCi/kg. *Designates a statistically significant difference from placebo. From Buchali et al. [69]

No grade IV decreases in either white counts or platelets were observed. The average platelet and white count nadirs were 118 000/µl and 3100/µl in the 1.0 mCi/kg group. Platelet and white counts recovered approximately 8 weeks after injection. Pain flare was noted in about 7.5% in the active-treatment groups in contrast to about 5% in the placebo group.

In the second placebo-controlled trial evaluating ^{153}Sm-EDTMP in bone pain palliation, 150 patients with hormone-refractory prostate cancer were enrolled [79] using a 2:1 randomisation scheme (the majority of patients were treated with the putatively active agent). Less than 10% of these patients had a soft tissue metastasis; 80% were taking narcotic analgesics at the time of study entry. As in the previous study, patients could be unblinded if there was no pain improvement 4 weeks after the initial injection; thus statistically valid comparison could be obtained only during the first 4 weeks of the study. The majority of patients (approximately 60%) had previously received external beam irradiation.

As with the other placebo-controlled studies using ^{153}Sm-EDTMP, participants in the placebo group had a relatively increased analgesic consumption as compared with participants receiving the active therapy; this reached statistical significance at 3 and 4 weeks after injection. Pain was statistically significantly reduced at 1–2 weeks after injection (depending on the pain scale used) and remained lower than with placebo during 4 weeks of the statistically valid follow-up period. Adverse events were similar between the two treatment groups, except for mild decreases in platelet and white blood cell counts. The average platelet nadir was 127 000/µl; the average nadir for white cells was 3.8/µl.

Resche et al. [77] reported on 114 patients with painful bone metastases (the majority from prostate or breast cancer), 55 of whom were randomised to receive 0.5 mCi/kg and 59 to receive 1.0 mCi/kg in a single dose. Imaging studies performed 24–72 h after administration of the ^{153}Sm-EDTMP showed excellent visualisation of bone metastases, which had been demonstrated on pre-treatment ^{99m}Tc scans. At baseline only 33% of patients in each dose group were able to sleep through the night. The frequency increased to 45% and 59% for the 0.5 and 1.0 mCi/kg groups, respectively; the change was statistically significant for the 1.0 mCi/kg patients ($p=0.026$). Pain relief as judged by the physicians at week 4 after treatment was 55% in the patients receiving 0.5 mCi/kg and 70% in the patients treated with 1.0 mCi/kg. At week 4, 22% and 33% of patients, respectively, were either much better or completely improved. In the 0.5 mCi/kg group, 6/15

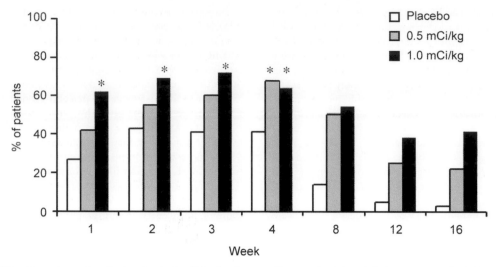

Figure 39.3. Percentage of patients who had relief of pain according to physician global assessment. Includes categories of "slight", "moderate", "marked" and "complete" pain relief. Percentages based on the number of patients at baseline. *Designates a statistically significant difference from placebo during the first 4 weeks. From Buchali et al. [69]

patients (40%) with breast cancer were responders compared with 16/20 (80%) in the 1.0 mCi/kg group.

The mean decreased platelet count from baseline was 56% with 0.5 mCi/kg and 43% with 1.0 mCi/kg ^{153}Sm administration. The corresponding values for white blood counts were 60% and 49%, respectively.

Rhenium-186-HEDP (^{186}Re) has been evaluated for the treatment of painful osseous metastasis. In an early report by Maxon and colleagues [80], 20 patients received 33 mCi ^{186}Re intravenously for skeletal metastasis from hormone-resistant prostate cancer. Thirteen patients were evaluable. Six received ^{186}Re(Sn) followed by a placebo, and seven were treated initially by placebo followed by the rhenium injection. The group initially treated with ^{186}Re experienced a 22% decrease in pain compared with 39% increase in pain in the control group treated initially by placebo ($p < 0.05$). In a follow-up study performed by Maxon and associates [81], they reported the results of a double-blind cross-over comparison with placebo in the treatment of painful osseous metastasis with 30–35 mCi ^{186}Re. About 80% of patients experienced pain relief. Treatment with ^{186}Re resulted in more significant pain relief when compared to placebo.

de Klerk and colleagues [82] performed a dose escalation study of ^{186}Re(Sn)-HEDP in 24 patients with metastatic hormone-resistant prostate cancer. Patients were treated with administered activity starting at 3.5 mCi, escalated at 1.5 mCi increments to a maximum activity of 9.5 mCi. Thrombocytopenia was

the dose-limiting toxicity and the authors concluded that 8.0 mCi was the maximally tolerated dose.

Whether ^{89}Sr or ^{153}Sm-EDTMP or HBI provide similar degree of palliation on painful bone metastases remains undetermined. HBI affects both osseous and extra-osseous tumours, whereas ^{89}Sr and ^{153}Sm-EDTMP affect only osseous tumours with adequate radioisotope uptake. Local field RT combined with adjuvant HBI or ^{89}Sr appears to be superior to local field therapy alone for patients with multiple bone metastases [83].

HORMONAL THERAPY OF PROSTATE CANCER

Patients who are symptomatic from bone metastases should be first treated with hormonal therapy if the tumour is not hormone-refractory and there is no radiographic evidence of an impending fracture or spinal cord compression. About 80% of men will respond initially to androgen ablation. The appropriate initial management is either medical or surgical castration. The former can be achieved by LHRH agonists, such as buserelin or goserelin and leuprolide, which are now available in depot injectable forms with duration of action lasting up to 4 months per injection. After an initial surge of testosterone due to the agonistic effect, downregulation of LH receptors in the pituitary gland diminishes the stimulation of testosterone production in the testis, resulting in castrate levels of testosterone. To prevent the "flare" of the disease from initial stimulatory action of LHRH agonist, it is advisable to start patients with a 7–10 day course of a non-steroidal peripheral androgen-receptor antagonist, such as flutamide or bicalutamide. These treatments will lead to rapid relief of symptoms in the majority of patients, although appropriate analgesia should be given during the time that the patient first presents with bone pain [84].

The concept of total androgen blockade (TAB) was first introduced in the early 1980s as a novel therapy for the treatment of metastatic prostatic cancer. The adrenal glands contribute 15–20% of the total circulating serum testosterone, and therefore the concept of TAB theoretically is superior to testicular hormonal ablation. This has spawned multiple randomised clinical trials in which monotherapy was compared with TAB. Although some individual trials demonstrate a positive result with improved survival, a published meta-analysis by the Prostate Cancer Trialists' Collaborative Group has shown, at most, very small effects in favour of TAB [85]. Moreover, the largest North American trial that compared orchidectomy plus flutamide vs. orchidectomy alone found no improvement in survival and poorer quality of life of patients in the TAB arm [86,87]. The combined treatment is also more costly. Thus, the cost-effectiveness of TAB does not justify its routine use as initial treatment for men with metastatic prostate cancer [84].

Steroidal antiandrogens such as oestrogen and megoestrol have fallen out of favour as hormonal therapy, as they carry cardiovascular side-effects and are associated with sometimes debilitating lethargy, fatigue and weight gain. Non-steroidal antiandrogens, such as flutamide and bicalutamide, do not have steroid side-effects, although flutamide in particular may cause gastrointestinal side-effects. The only advantage of these agents is that they may allow preservation of potency in some men who are potent prior to therapy, although a recent study has suggested that there is slow loss of potency in patients who are treated with these agents [88]. Evidence from randomised trials suggest that there is a small deficit in both the probability of relief of symptoms and in survival from the use of monotherapy with a peripheral antiandrogen, as compared to that with orchidectomy or an LHRH agonist [89] and this cannot, therefore, be regarded as standard therapy. The strategy of using a peripheral antiandrogen alone should be discussed with men who regard preservation of potency as important for their quality of life [84].

Disease progression during hormonal monotherapy with orchidectomy or LHRH analogue may yet respond to additional peripheral antiandrogen such as flutamide or bicalutamide (Casodex). About one-third of the patients will respond to this additional treatment but responses, unfortunately, are rather short—they are typically in the order of 3 months, as compared to an initial response to hormonal therapy of about 1 year or greater.

Casodex is a steroid antiandrogen that binds to cytosol androgen receptors, producing decreased testosterone levels and elevation of gonadotropins by inhibiting the binding of testicular and adrenal androgens to the androgen receptor in the prostate [90,91]. Because of the higher binding affinity and longer half-life (7–10 days), it has improved oral potency in comparison with flutamide [90,92–94]. The Casodex dose of 50 mg daily was found to be equivalent to 750 mg daily of flutamide [95]. As monotherapy, the daily dose is 150 mg [96]. This formulation in 2002 was under review by the FDA in the USA.

Iversen et al. reported on two randomised multi-institutional trials, in which the efficacy and toxicity of a 150 mg daily dose of Casodex monotherapy was compared to castration or 3.6 mg goserelin acetate (Zoladex) every 28 days for treatment of patients with non-metastatic advanced prostate cancer. With median follow-up of 202 and 205 weeks in both studies, the data were merged; survival with 150 mg Casodex monotherapy was equivalent to surgical or medical castration. In one study, median time to tumour progression was 1368 days in the bicalutamide and 836 days in the castration group; however, in the other study, median progression times were 918 and 1054 days, respectively. This discrepancy may be related to the tumour characteristics in the treatment groups or variations in disease assessment. Breast pain/tenderness and gynaecomastia were more frequent in the patients treated with bicalutamide (47% vs. 3.8%); hot flashes were more common with castration (50% vs. 13.4% with Casodex). In quality of life assessment, patients treated with bicalutamide had a significant benefit in sexual interest and better physical capacity [96].

Finasteride is a steroid analogue that specifically blocks prostatic 5α-reductase activity in androgen-sensitive tissue [97]. The usual dose is 10 mg daily. Patients treated with finasteride showed a delayed increase in prostate-specific antigen (PSA) of approximately 9 months in the first year and 14 months in the second year, compared with a placebo group. Fewer recurrences occurred in the finasteride group, but the differences were not statistically significant [98].

If there is a further relapse after response to the added antiandrogen therapy, the antiandrogen should be withdrawn. Such "withdrawal" responses have been documented in about 20% of prior responders [99].

It is unclear whether a LHRH agonist should be continued in a patient who appears to be resistant to hormonal therapy. In most areas of cancer treatment, an ineffective agent is stopped when failure is evident. That is the policy in the UK, for example. In North America, there is the impression that some patients may have a flare in their disease when LHRH agonist is stopped, but such impressions can be misleading, since many patients are experiencing a general progression of their disease at this time. The standard treatment in North America is to continue the agent, although it is reasonable to discuss the possibility of withdrawal with patients. There is little data to indicate whether recovery of testosterone levels and sexual function is likely to occur following cessation of antiandrogen treatment [84].

Whether patients with asymptomatic metastatic disease should receive hormonal therapy remains unclear. Crawford et al. have documented an increased survival advantage for medically or surgically castrated patients with minimal metastatic disease compared to those with more extensive bone metastases [100]. A large trial conducted by the British Medical Research Council showed a small improvement in survival and fewer cancer-related complications in men whose hormonal therapies were initiated at the time of diagnosis rather than the time of disease progression. The survival gain, however, was mainly seen for those with locally advanced disease without clinical metastases [101]. The gains of hormonal therapy are counterbalanced by the side-effects of androgen ablation, which usually includes impotence, hot flashes and loss of bone density. It is important to discuss this trade-off with patients, since some patients may prefer to defer such treatment.

An alternative to continuous hormonal therapy still under investigation is the use of intermittent androgen suppression. Intermittent hormonal therapy was first introduced in 1986 by Klotz et al., who demonstrated the potential use of this approach in 19 patients treated with diethylstilboestrol and one patient with flutamide [102]. Crook et al. later reported the feasibility of this approach and its impact on the quality of life in prostate cancer patients [103]. Experiments with animal models have shown that this approach delays the time at which animals will become resistant to further hormonal therapy [104]. Intermittent androgen suppression is increasingly used in urological practice; it aims to maintain androgen responsiveness of tumour cells by regular cycles of treatment cessations and tumour regrowth to specific PSA limits. Intermittent androgen suppression improves the quality of life in patients with primarily hormone-dependent tumours without adverse effects and seems to be most effective in patients with prostate cancer with asymptomatic biochemical progression and low tumour burden. Patients should be treated to maintain castrate testosterone levels within the framework of randomised trials and characterised for survival and prognostic factors associated with response to intermittent androgen suppression treatment.

Goldenberg et al., in 47 patients with locally advanced prostate cancer, initiated combined androgen blockade and continued for at least 6 months until PSA nadir level was observed. Medication was withheld until PSA increased from 10 to 20 ng/ml. Combined androgen blockade was repeated until PSA regulation became androgen-independent. Mean time to tumour progression was 128 weeks, and mean survival was 210 weeks [105].

While the approach may seem attractive from the point of view of cost savings and minimising side-effects, some have warned about potential selection of androgen-independent tumour clonogens, which may have a potentiating effect on otherwise quiescent disease. Longer follow-up of patients treated with this approach is necessary, while ongoing randomised clinical trials comparing intermittent with continuous therapy in the setting of both early and metastatic disease will hopefully prove a definitive role of intermittent androgen suppression [84].

Unfortunately, almost all patients will eventually become hormone-resistant unless they succumb to other illnesses. About 20% of patients are hormone-resistant de novo and in others, the median time to development of hormone resistance is 1–2 years, although there is wide variability and some patients may respond to hormonal treatment for many years. In general, patients who have high-grade disease tend to develop hormone-resistant disease more quickly. Once the disease achieves the state of hormone resistance, the range of expected survival times is short, with a mean survival time of about 1 year [84].

CHEMOTHERAPY IN ADVANCED PROSTATE CANCER

While hormonal therapy is often effective in controlling advanced disease, all patients will eventually become hormone-resistant. Hormone-refractory prostate cancer (HRPC) is a more difficult problem, with no clear consensus about the optimal management strategy. Older studies of systemic chemotherapy were largely disappointing, leading many reviewers to conclude that it had little role in the standard management of these patients [106]. HRPC is characterised by a median survival of approximately 1 year and a system complex of pain from bony metastases, a decreasing functional status, fatigue and eventually bone marrow failure. Once symptoms develop, their disease significantly disables most patients. These patients are intolerant of aggressive cytotoxic therapies because of their age, poor performance status and limited marrow reserve. Intensive investigational therapies, studied in selected patients at a tertiary care centre, are often not suitable for the majority of those with HRPC seen in routine practice.

A stringent description of HRPC would require disease progression in the presence of optimal hormonal management with castrate levels of testosterone, along with the lack of response to antiandrogen withdrawal or any other hormonal therapies. Disease progression may be demonstrated by a sequential elevation in PSA levels, new or worsening metastatic lesions, or increasing symptoms related to tumour growth. In the past, most patients would be identified on the basis of symptomatic progression. Recently, more asymptomatic patients are being identified on the basis of a rising PSA. The criteria to define HRPC and the proportion of patients who are symptomatic will influence outcome in clinical studies. An apparent increase in median survival from approximately 9–12 months in older studies of chemotherapy, to 15–18 months in more recent ones may be more a reflection of differences in the population treated than any improvements in therapy. There are a number of useful non-cytotoxic approaches for the treatment of bone pain in patients to HRPC that have been reviewed earlier in the chapter. However, there is now convincing evidence that the use of chemotherapy can also be very useful in the palliative management of bone pain in patients with HRPC [107].

Older trials in HRPC examined overall survival as a study endpoint, but few in the past have included quality of life assessments in their analyses. However, when treating a non-curable illness like HRPC with potentially toxic therapy a balance must be sought between the amelioration of disease-related symptoms if a treatment is successful, and the side-effects created by the treatment. It is only recently that palliative endpoints such as quality of life analyses, pain indices and analgesic scores have been formally evaluated in clinical trials in HRPC. As most patients with prostate cancer have non-measurable disease, changes in serum PSA have been proposed as a surrogate measure of activity of treatment. Reductions in PSA may represent evidence of antitumour activity of the treatment, although PSA may only be produced by a small component of the tumour and there have been reports of patients with falling PSA values in the setting of disease progression. The Prostate-Specific Antigen Working Group has defined a PSA response as a decline from pre-treatment baseline of at least 50%, confirmed at least 4 weeks later without clinical or radiographic evidence of progression [108]. PSA changes do not meet the criteria for surrogacy, in that they cannot substitute for a true endpoint of clinical benefit. However, standardisation of the PSA response is necessary to help decide what agents should be investigated further in Phase III trials.

Mitoxantrone Plus Prednisone in HRPC

Mitoxantrone is a semi-synthetic anthracenedione with some structural similarities to doxorubicin (Figure 39.4). Early studies with mitoxantrone in HRPC showed that it had modest activity using conventional response criteria but was well tolerated, with improvements in disease-related symptoms, particularly bone pain. A multi-centre Phase II study of mitoxantrone plus prednisone found that 9/25 (36%) achieved a significant improvement in pain that was associated with other improvements in quality of life [109]. This led to a larger study by Tannock et al. randomising patients between mitoxantrone plus prednisone and prednisone alone using palliative endpoints and quality of life analyses. This study showed superior palliation from mitoxantrone plus prednisone, with an overall palliative pain response rate of 38%, as defined by a stringent reduction in pain without an increase in analgesic medication, or by a $\geqslant 50\%$ reduction in analgesia without increase in pain. This is compared to a palliative pain response rate of 21% in patients receiving prednisone alone ($p < 0.025$). In addition, the duration of palliation and the time to symptomatic progression in all patients was substantially and

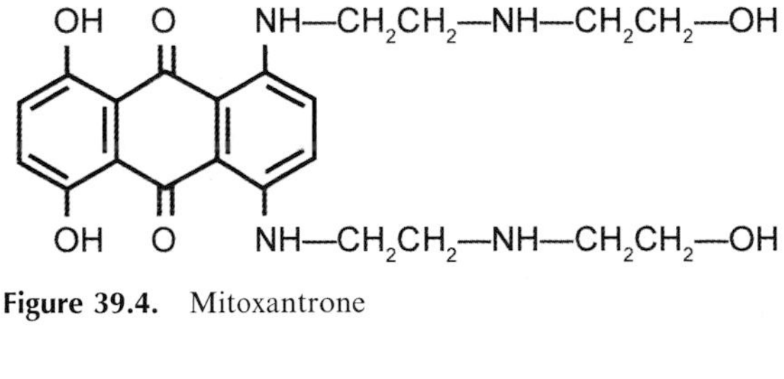

Figure 39.4. Mitoxantrone

significantly longer in the patients receiving the chemotherapy (medians of 43 weeks vs. 18 weeks, $p < 0.0001$). The patients who met the criterion for palliative response also had improvements in most domains of quality of life, including highly significant improvements in overall well-being. Unfortunately, there was no significant difference in overall survival. The trial also showed a PSA response rate of 44% on mitoxantrone as compared to 23% on prednisone alone. Time to progression was also delayed in patients receiving chemotherapy [105]. Two additional Phase III trials of mitoxantrone with steroids in patients with HRPC have been conducted. The Cancer and Leukaemia Group B (CALGB) study randomised 242 patients (both symptomatic and asymptomatic) to either mitoxantrone plus hydrocortisone or to hydrocortisone alone. Similar to the Canadian study, this trial showed improved pain, PSA response and time to progression with chemotherapy but no impact upon overall survival [110]. The US Oncology Group conducted a similar trial in 124 asymptomatic patients and demonstrated improvements in PSA response (48% vs. 24%) time to progression (10.5 vs. 3.8 months) without any impact on overall survival [111] (Table 39.6).

The Phase III trials of mitoxantrone are the first definitive evidence of the palliative benefits of chemotherapy in HRPC. There are a number of other drugs being evaluated in Phase II trials. Many involve the combination of estramustine, which is an oestrogen linked to an alkylating agent, with another cytotoxic agent. Estramustine has been extensively tested in HRPC patients, and as a single agent its benefits are minimal. The more recent trials of estramustine use in HRPC involve its combination with other chemotherapeutic agents, especially those that provide synergistic cytotoxicity *in vitro*. The current emphasis is to determine which combinations and what schedules

are worthy of evaluation in Phase III trials. Combinations of estramustine with vinca alkaloids and taxanes have reported PSA responses in the range of 40–60% in Phase II trials. There is the potential for gastrointestinal and haematological toxicity with these combinations and the overall impact upon disease-related symptoms, as well as quality of life, have yet to be assessed. The contribution of estramustine to the efficacy of some of these combinations has also been questioned. Studies of docetaxel (taxotere) have consistently shown PSA responses in the range of 60% both with and without estramustine. Several Phase III studies comparing docetaxel-based treatments to mitoxantrone plus prednisone have recently been completed. These trials will include quality of life measures as well as the power to detect potentially modest but important improvements in survival. The Southwest Oncology Group (SWOG 9916) is comparing estramustine + docetaxel + dexamethasone to mitoxantrone + prednisone as first- or second-line therapy for HRPC. Each arm will accrue about 300 patients with a power to detect a 33% increase in median survival. Other endpoints include time to progression, PSA response, toxicity and quality of life. Docetaxel plus prednisone in two dosing schedules is being compared to mitoxantrone plus prednisone in a large international study which completed accrual in 2002 and will be reported in 2003. Endpoints will be survival (powered to detect a 33% improvement), palliation and quality of life.

In recent years there has been a tremendous surge in the development of biological targets for cancer therapy. Given the relative insensitivity of prostate cancer to cytotoxic agents, this area holds much promise. Various types of gene therapy and immune therapy based on antigen-presenting cells are under evaluation in laboratory models and early phase trials.

Table 39.6. Phase III trials of mitoxantrone + steroids in hormone-refractory prostate cancer

Reference	Therapy	No. of patients	PSA response* (%)	Pain improved (%)	TTP (months)	OS (months)
Tannock et al. [107]	Mitoxantrone + prednisone	80	44	38	5.5	12.1
	Prednisone alone	81	23	21	2.3	11.8
Kantoff et al. [110]	Mitoxantrone + hydrocortisone	119	38	Not reported	3.7	12.3
	Hydrocortisone alone	123	22	Not reported	2.2	12.6
Gregurich [111]	Mitoxantrone + prednisone	56	48	N/A**	10.5	No difference
	Prednisone alone	63	24	N/A**	3.8	No difference

* Denotes > 50% decline from baseline.
**All patients in this study were free of pain at baseline.
TTP, time to progression; OS, overall survival.

Similarly, antiangiogenesis therapies, differentiation therapies, pro-apoptotic therapies and matrix metalloproteinase inhibitors are under early investigation in a number of tumour sites, including HRPC. While impact of all these agents have been minimal to date, the appropriate clinical settings and combinations in which to use these agents remains an area of active research.

CHEMOTHERAPY IN EARLIER STAGE PROSTATE CANCER

The clinical use of chemotherapy in prostate cancer is currently restricted to patients with hormone-refractory disease. However there is an increased interest in studying the benefits of chemotherapy earlier in the course of the illness. This has been stimulated by results in other tumours, such as breast and colorectal cancer, where the benefits of chemotherapy have been greatest when used in the setting of clinically localised disease (i.e. adjuvant therapy). To date the only data available are from older studies where the chemotherapy used may not have been optimal and in addition the sample size did not provide sufficient power to detect modest differences in outcome. Recently two very large Phase III studies examining the role of chemotherapy in earlier stage disease have been opened. The Southwest Oncology Group will randomise 1360 patients with defined high-risk characteristics following radical prostatectomy to either androgen therapy for 2 years or to androgen therapy plus six cycles of mitoxantrone plus prednisone. The RTOG will randomise 1440 patients to receive either radiotherapy plus hormones or to the same regimen plus four cycles of estramustine, paclitaxel and oral etoposide. Both studies have sufficient power to detect a 15–20% improvement in median or 5 year survival, although it will be at least 10 years until results are sufficiently mature to answer this question.

In summary, chemotherapy has value in the palliative management of hormone-refractory prostate cancer. Mitoxantrone plus prednisone provides improvements in pain and quality of life for approximately 40% of those treated. Other promising regimens, such as the estramustine combinations or docetaxel, are currently undergoing further testing in randomised trials. There is a general increase in investigation into understanding the mechanisms of hormonal resistance and in developing more novel strategies to prevent or treat this problem. These

should eventually translate into better systemic therapies for the treatment of this difficult problem.

BISPHOSPHONATES IN PROSTATE CANCER

Bisphosphonates are the treatment of choice for malignant hypercalcaemia and bone metastases in multiple myeloma and breast cancer. The predominant osteoblastic metastases in prostate cancer question the use of bisphosphonates, which have been shown to be most effective in osteolytic bone metastases. The objective endpoints used in clinical trials are hypercalcaemia and pathological fractures usually associated with osteolytic bone metastases, which are relatively uncommon in prostate cancer [112].

There is nonetheless some data to suggest benefits of bisphosphonates in prostate cancer. In prostate cancer with bone metastases, the immediate biochemical changes following bisphosphonate treatment are very similar to those observed in patients with predominately lytic bone disease. Potent bisphosphonates can cause progressive decreases in urinary calcium and hydroxyproline excretion as well as serum calcium concentration in prostate cancer [113]. Suppression of bone resorption is associated with significant decrease in bone pain and analgesic consumption.

Adami et al. reported sustained relief of pain in prostate cancer patients treated with clodronate, with improved mobilisation of otherwise bedridden patients [114]. Percival et al. also reported a case of reversal of paraplegia in a patient treated with clodronate and mithramycin [115].

Adami and associates further reported on another study of 56 patients allocated randomly to four single-blind dose-finding controlled studies employing a visual analogue scale and the assessment of analgesic consumption. The initial comparison of intravenous clodronate ($n=7$) with placebo ($n=6$) showed a striking difference in response, favouring clodronate, resulting in placebo being discontinued for ethical reasons [116]. Vorruether et al. reported significant reduction in pain after clodronate in 64/85 patients (75%) with bone metastases secondary to prostate cancer. Nineteen patients became completely pain-free [117]. Experience with intravenous pamidronate and alendronate has been similar in limited studies [101,118–121]. In contrast, results of studies with less potent bisphosphonates, such as etidronate, or with oral clodronate, are rather disappointing [122,123].

Factors that can affect the response of bisphosphonates include potency of the agent, mode of administration, dose and duration of treatment. To achieve successful responses, initial high doses of potent bisphophonates are followed by maintenance treatment at doses sufficient to suppress bone resorption effectively without affecting the mineralisation of newly formed bone. The latter can be achieved by either repeated infusions or continuous oral administration [112,124].

There is some evidence that bisphosphonates may prevent the development of bone metastases from prostate cancer. Boissier et al. demonstrated that bisphosphonates *in vitro* can inhibit the adhesion of prostate cancer cells to unmineralised as well as mineralised bone extracellular matrices [125]. A histomorphometric study of iliac crest bone biopsies in 18 patients with metastatic prostate cancer on clodronate compared with 12 control patients confirmed its antiresorptive properties, with decreased ratios of eroded surface to bone surface as well as decreased ratios of osteoclast number to bone surface [126].

There have been four randomised, double-blind placebo-controlled clinical trials of the use of bisphosphonates in patients with metastatic prostate cancer. Smith randomly assigned 57 patients with hormone-refractory prostate cancer and symptomatic bone metastases to receive intravenous and/or oral sodium etidronate or placebo. He found no difference in the symptomatic response rate or analgesic requirement [127]. A British trial led by the MRC Clinical Trials Unit randomly assigned 311 patients with hormone-sensitive prostate cancer to oral sodium clodronate or placebo [128]. They reported in an abstract a delay in the time to symptomatic bone progression with the use of clodronate.

A Canadian study coordinated by NCIC Clinical Trials Group randomly assigned 208 patients with hormone-resistant prostate cancer to receive intravenous clodronate or placebo in addition to palliative chemotherapy with mitoxantrone and prednisone [129]. They reported no differences in the primary endpoint of palliative response, defined by improvement in pain and/or decrease in analgesic intake. A secondary analysis did suggest that in a small subset of patients who received clodronate, there was improvement in moderate or severe pain.

Saad et al. attempted to explore the role of the potent bisphosphonate zoledronic acid in patients with hormone-refractory prostate cancer and symptomatic bone metastases [130]. The authors conclude that zoledronic acid reduced skeletal-related events in prostate cancer patients with bone metastases. However, there were no differences in disease progression, performance status or quality of life scores among the treatment arms. This study adds to the evidence that bisphophonates have some activity in reducing the incidence of skeletal-related events but also with some added toxicity (renal dysfunction). Zoledronic acid is a reasonable choice to offer to patients who fail standard therapies and who are at high risk for bone fractures or spinal cord compression, but currently bisphosphonates, including zoledronic acid, cannot be recommended as a standard therapy for men with prostate cancer and metastases to bone [131].

Better understanding of the cellular and molecular mechanisms underlying bone metastases in prostate cancer will aid the design of treatment protocols, and perhaps support the notion of "adjuvant" therapy with bisphosphonates—administering bisphosphonates before the development of metastatic disease. A number of trials are currently under way.

PROGNOSTIC FACTORS IN METASTATIC PROSTATE CANCER

While more research is needed for effective systemic therapies, recognition of factors that correlate survival is important for the palliative management. Emrich and colleagues, in analysis of 1940 patients with untreated and hormone-refractory cancers found that anorexia, elevated acid and alkaline phosphatase, pain, obstructive symptoms and poor performance status were the most important factors associated with poorer survival [132].

The extent and distribution of bone metastases influence prognosis too. The worst prognosis is seen in men with axial plus appendicular metastases, as compared with axial only; prognosis worsens for men with 0 vs. 6+ to < 20 vs. > 20 sites of skeletal involvement [133]. Men with low pre-treatment testosterone have a shortened survival compared with normal or high testosterone. Bone pain, poor performance status and increased alkaline phosphatase indicate poor prognosis in patients with bone metastases. The median survival is 16–24 months from ablative therapy for this group of patients [134]. Clinical management and future clinical trials should consider these prognostic variables.

FUTURE DIRECTIONS

Insights into the mechanism underlying the initiation and progression of prostate cancer could provide new ways to develop therapeutic interventions, including design of agents that may block signal transduction pathways or cytokine interactions that lead to disease progression. There has been progress in active specific immunotherapeutic approaches in the treatment of metastatic prostate cancer [135–141]. Future studies including novel prostate cancer-specific antigen discovery, optimisation of vaccine delivery and combination therapies between conventional and immunotherapy, may bring new strategies to existing treatment modalities [142]. The efficacy or combination of radionuclides and bisphosphonates needs to be compared. Enhancements of radiation response that may be obtained by the use of cisplatin as a radiosensitiser will need to be evaluated. Whether the use of radiopharmaceuticals in early metastatic disease with the commencement of hormonal therapy will result in more therapeutic benefit remains to be investigated. More efforts are required to test the efficacy of bisphosphonates in the treatment and prevention of progression of metastatic disease.

The advent of intermittent hormonal therapy may reduce the toxicity on prolonged continuous use. The real challenge is to develop better means to avert hormone-refractory prostate cancer and better treatments for patients with hormone-refractory disease when it occurs. Chemotherapy, which has been previously considered ineffective in advanced prostate cancer, is now demonstrating new promise, as randomised trials have defined clear improvements in palliative endpoints. Although survival benefit has not yet been shown in a randomised trial, the increasing rates of response to combination therapy seen in multiple Phase II studies gives the hope that one day chemotherapy may impact on survival [143]. Combinations of chemotherapy with newer biological treatments may represent an opportunity to improve outcomes with non-cross-reactive toxicity, although this area of study has been minimally explored to date.

REFERENCES

1. CA. A cancer journal for clinicians. Cancer J Clin 2002: 52(1).
2. Office of Population Consensus and Survey. Cancer Statistics. England and Wales. HMSO: Series MB1:96/1, 1996.
3. Farkas A, Schneider D, Perrotti M et al. National trends in the epidemiology of prostate cancer, 1973–1994: evidence for the effectiveness of prostate specific antigen screening. Urology 1998; 52: 444–8.
4. Landis S, Murray T, Bolden S et al. Cancer statistics. CA Cancer J Clin 1999; 49: 8–29.
5. Whitmore WJ Jr. Natural history and staging of prostate cancer. Urol Clin N Am 1984; 11: 209–20.

6. Chodak G, Thisted R, Gerber G et al. Results of conservative management of clinically localized prostate cancer. N Engl J Med 1994; 330: 242–8.
7. Adolfsson J, Steineck G, Hedlund P. Deferred treatment of locally advanced nonmetastatic prostate cancer: a long-term follow-up. J Urol 1999; 161: 505–8.
8. Lerner S, Seale-Hawkins C, Carlton C et al. The risk of dying of prostate cancer in patients with clinically localized disease. J Urol 1991; 146: 1040–5.
9. Johansson J, Holmberg L, Johansson S et al. Fifteen-year survival in prostate cancer: a prospective, population-based study in Sweden. J Am Med Assoc 1997; 277: 467–71.
10. Albertsen P, Hanley J, Gleason D et al. Competing risk analysis of men aged 55–74 years at diagnosis managed conservatively for clinically localized prostate cancer. J Am Med Assoc 1998; 280: 975–80.
11. Carlin B, Andriole G. The natural history, skeletal complications, and management of bone metastases in patients with prostate carcinoma. Cancer 2000; 88: 2989–94.
12. Pound C, Partin A, Eisenberger M et al. Natural history of progression after PSA elevation following radical prostatectomy. J Am Med Assoc 1999; 281: 1591–7.
13. Zagars G, Pollack A, von Eschenbach A. Serum testosterone: a significant determinant of metastatic relapse for irradiated localized prostate cancer. Urology 1997; 49: 327–34.
14. Schellhammer P, El-Mahidi A, Kuban D et al. Prostate specific antigen after radiation therapy. Urol Clin N Am 1997; 24: 407–14.
15. Newling D, Denis L, Vermeylen K. Orchidectomy vs. goserelin and flutamide in the treatment of newly diagnosed metastatic prostate cancer. Analysis of the criteria of evaluation used in the European Organization for Research and Treatment of Cancer Genitourinary Group Study 30853. Cancer 1993; 72: 3793–8.
16. Batson O. The function of the vertebral veins and their role in the spread of metastases. Ann Surg 1940; 112: 138–49.
17. Dodds P, Caride V, Lytton B. The role of vertebral veins in the dissemination of prostatic carcinoma. J Urol 1981; 126: 753–5.
18. Perez C. Prostate. In Perez C, Brady L (eds), Principles and Practice of Radiation Oncology. Lippincott-Raven: Philadelphia, PA, 1997: 1583–694.
19. McCarthy P, Pollack H. Imaging of patients with stage D prostatic carcinoma. Urol Clin N Am 1991; 18(1): 35–53.
20. Bayley A, Milosevic M, Bland R et al. A prospective study of factors predicting clinically occult spinal cord compression in patients with metastatic prostate carcinoma. Cancer 2001; 92(2): 303–10.
21. Allen K, Johnson T, Hibbs G. Single-dose irradiation of bone metastases. Acta Radiol Ther Phys Biol 1976; 15: 337–9.
22. Arcangeli G, Micheli A, Arcangeli G et al. The responsiveness of bone metastasis to radiotherapy: the effect of site, histology and radiation dose on pain relief. Radiother Oncol 1989; 14: 95–101.
23. Garmatis C, Chu F. The effectiveness of radiation therapy in the treatment of bone metastases from breast cancer. Radiology 1978; 16: 235–7.

24. Gilbert R, Kim J, Posner J. Epidural spinal cord compression from metastatic tumor: diagnosis and treatment. Ann Neurol 1978; 3: 40–51.

25. Jensen N, Roesdahl K. Single-dose irradiation of bone metastases. Acta Radiol Ther Phys Biol 1976; 15: 337–9.

26. Kumar P, Bahrassa F, Espinoza M. The role of radiotherapy in management of metastatic bone disease. J Natl Med Assoc 1978; 70: 909–11.

27. Schocker J, Brady L. Radiation therapy for bone metastases. Clin Orthop 1982; 169: 38–43.

28. Vargha Z, Glicksman A, Beland J. Single-dose radiation therapy in the palliation of metastatic disease. Radiology 1969; 93: 1181–4.

29. Qasim M. Single-dose palliative irradiation for bony metastases. Strahlentherapie 1977; 153: 531–2.

30. Porter A, McEwan A, Powe J. Results of a randomized Phase III trial to evaluate the efficacy of strontium-89 adjuvant to local field external beam irradiation in the management of endocrine resistant metastatic prostate cancer. Int J Radiat Oncol Biol Phys 1993; 25: 805–13.

31. Porter A, McEwan A. Strontium-89 as an adjuvant to external beam radiation improves pain relief and delays disease progression in advanced prostate cancer: results of a randomized controlled trial. Semin Oncol 1993; 20: 38–43.

32. Poulter C, Cosmatos D, Rubin P et al. A report of RTOG 8206: A phase III study of whether the addition of single-dose hemibody irradiation to standard fractionated local field irradiation is more effective than local field irradiation alone in the treatment of symptomatic osseous metastases. Int J Radiat Oncol Biol Phys 1992; 23: 207–14.

33. Priestman T, Roberts J, Lucraft H et al. Results of a randomized, double-blind comparative study of ondansetron and metoclopramide in the prevention of nausea and vomiting following high-dose upper abdominal irradiation. Clin Oncol 1990; 2: 71–5.

34. Tong D, Gillick L, Hendrickson F. The palliation of symptomatic osseous metastases: final results of the study by the Radiation Therapy Oncology Group. Cancer 1982; 50: 893–9.

35. Blitzer P. Reanalysis of the RTOG study of the palliation of symptomatic osseous metastases. Cancer 1985; 55: 1468–72.

36. Price P, Hoskin P, Easton D et al. Prospective randomized trial of single and multi-fraction radiotherapy schedules in the treatment of painful bony metastases. Radiother Oncol 1986; 6: 247–55.

37. Hoskin PJ, Price P, Easton D et al. A prospective randomized trial of 4 Gy or 8 Gy single doses in the treatment of metastatic bone pain. Radiother Oncol 1992; 23: 74–8.

38. Bone Pain Trial Working Party. 8 Gy single fraction radiotherapy for the treatment of metastatic skeletal pain: randomized comparison with multi-fraction schedule over 12 months of patient follow-up. Radiother Oncol 1999; 52: 111–21.

39. Steenland E, Leer J, van Houwelingen H et al. The effect of a single fraction compared to multiple fractions on painful bone metastases: a global analysis of the Dutch Bone Metastasis Study. Radiother Oncol 1999; 52: 101–9.

40. Nielsen O, Bentzen S, Sandberg E et al. Randomized trial of single dose versus fractionated palliative radiotherapy of bone metastases. Radiother Oncol 1998; 47: 233–40.

41. Jeremic B, Shibamoto Y, Acimovic L et al. A randomized trial of three single-dose radiation therapy regimens in the treatment of metastatic bone pain. Int J Radiat Oncol Biol Phys 1998; 42: 161–7.

42. Gaze M, Kelly C, Kerr G et al. Pain relief and quality of life following radiotherapy for bone metastases: a randomized trial of two fractionation schedules. Radiother Oncol 1997; 45: 109–16.

43. Niewald M, Tkocz H, Abel U et al. Rapid course radiation therapy vs. more standard treatment: a randomized trial for bone metastases. Int J Radiat Oncol Biol Phys 1996; 36: 1085–9.

44. Ratanatharathorn V, Powers W, Moss W et al. Bone metastasis: review and critical analysis of random allocation trials of local field treatment. Int J Radiat Oncol Biol Phys 1999; 44: 1–18.

45. Chow E, Danjoux C, Wong R et al. Palliation of bone metastases: a survey of patterns of practice among Canadian radiation oncologists. Radiother Oncol 2000; 56: 305–14.

46. Duncan G, Duncan W, Maher EJ. Patterns of palliative radiotherapy in Canada. Clin Oncol 1993; 5: 92–7.

47. Ben-Josef E, Shamsa F, Williams A et al. Radiotherapeutic management of osseous metastases: a survey of current patterns of care. Int J Radiat Oncol Phys 1998; 40: 915–21.

48. Hartsell W, Shah A, Graney M et al. Palliation of bone metastases in the USA: a survey of patterns of practice. Support Care Cancer 1998; 6: 175(abstr 45).

49. Bentzen S, Hoskin P, Roos D et al. Fractionated radiotherapy for metastatic bone pain: evidence-based medicine or . . .? Int J Radiat Oncol Biol Phys 2000; 46: 681–2.

50. Chow E, Danjoux C, Connolly R et al. Bone metastasis: review and critical analysis of random allocation trial of local field treatment: regarding Ratanatharathorn et al. Int J Radiat Oncol Biol Phys 2000; 46: 517–18.

51. Ratanatharathorn V, Powers W, Moss W et al. Response to the letter from Dr Edward Chow and associates to the editor. Int J Rad Oncol Biol Phys 2000; 46: 518.

52. Ratanatharathorn V, Powers W, Moss W et al. In response to Dr. Bentzen et al. Int J Rad Oncol Biol Phys 2000; 46: 682–3.

53. Needham P, Mithal N, Hoskin P. Radiotherapy for bone pain. J R Soc Med 1994; 87: 503–5.

54. Fitzpatrick P, Rider W. Half body irradiation. Int J Radiat Oncol Biol Phys 1976; 1: 197–207.

55. Hoskin P, Ford H, Harmer C. Hemibody irradiation (HBI) for metastatic bone pain in two histologically distinct groups of patients. Clin Oncol 1989; 1: 67–9.

56. Kuban D, Delbridge T, El-Mahdi A et al. Half-body irradiation for treatment of widely metastatic adenocarcinoma of the prostate. J Urol 1989; 141: 572–4.

57. Salazar O, Rubin P, Hendrickson F et al. Single-dose half-body irradiation for palliation of multiple bone metastases from solid tumors. Final radiation therapy oncology group report. Cancer 1986; 58: 29–36.

58. Dearnaley D, Bayly R, A'Hern R et al. Palliation of bone metastases in prostate cancer. Hemibody irradiation or strontium-89? Clin Oncol 1992; 4: 101–7.

59. Quilty P, Kirk D, Bolger J et al. A comparison of the palliative effects of strontium-89 and external beam radiotherapy in metastatic prostate cancer. Radiother Oncol 1994; 31: 33–40.

60. Van Dyk J, Keane T, Kan S et al. Radiation pneumonitis following large single dose irradiation: a re-evaluation based on absolute dose to lung. Int J Radiat Oncol Biol Phys 1981; 7: 461–7.

61. Zelefsky M, Scher H, Forman J et al. Palliative hemiskeletal irradiation for widespread metastatic prostate cancer: a comparison of single dose and fractionated regimens. Int J Radiat Oncol Biol Phys 1989; 17: 1281–5.

62. Salazar O, Sandhu T, Da Motta N et al. Fractionated half-body irradiation (HBI) for the rapid palliation of widespread, symptomatic, metastatic bone disease: a randomized phase III trial of the international atomic energy agency (IAEA). Int J Radiat Oncol Biol Phys 2001; 50(3): 765–75.

63. Eary J, Collins C, Stabin M et al. Samarium-153–EDTMP biodistribution and dosimetry estimation. J Nucl Med 1993; 34: 1031–6.

64. McEwan A. Use of radionuclides for the palliation of bone metastases. Semin Radiat Oncol 2000; 10: 103–14.

65. Blake G, Zivanovic M, Blaquiere R et al. Strontium-89 therapy: measurement of absorbed dose to skeletal metastases. J Nucl Med 1988; 29: 549–57.

66. Breen S, Powe J, Porter A. Dose estimation of strontium-89 radiotherapy of metastatic prostatic carcinoma. J Nucl Med 1992; 33: 1316–23.

67. Blake G, Wood J, Wood P et al. Sr therapy: strontium plasma clearance in disseminated prostatic carcinoma. Eur J Nucl Med 1989; 15: 49–54.

68. Lewington V, McEwan A, Ackery D et al. A prospective randomized double-blind crossover study to examine the efficacy of strontium-89 pain palliation in patients with advanced prostate cancer metastatic to bone. Eur J Cancer 1991; 27: 954–8.

69. Buchali K, Correns H, Schuerer M et al. Results of a double-blind study of 89-strontium therapy of skeletal metastases of prostatic carcinoma. Eur J Nucl Med 1988; 14: 349–51.

70. McEwan A, Amyotte G, McGowan D et al. A retrospective analysis of the cost effectiveness of treatment with Melastron (^{89}Sr-chloride) in patients with prostate cancer metastatic to bone. Nucl Med Commun 1994; 15: 499–504.

71. Malmberg I, Persson U, Ask A et al. Painful bone metastases in hormone-refractory prostate cancer: Economic costs of strontium-89 and/or external radiotherapy. Urology 1997; 50: 747–53.

72. Finkelstein E, Veldkamp L. Effect of external beam irradiation on the uptake and distribution of samarium-153 EDTMP. Int J Radiat Oncol Biol Phys 2001; 51(suppl 1): 237–8.

73. Collins C, Eary J, Donaldson G et al. Samarium-153–EDTMP in bone metastases of hormone-refractory prostate carcinoma: a phase I/II trial. J Nucl Med 1993; 34: 1839–44.

74. Tian J, Zhang J, Hou Q et al. Multi-centre trial on the efficacy and toxicity of single-dose samarium-153–ethylene diamine tetramethylene phosphonate as a palliative treatment for painful skeletal metastases in China. Eur J Nucl Med 1999; 26: 2–7.

75. Dickie GJ, Macfarlane D. Strontium and samarium therapy for bone metastases from prostate carcinoma. Australas Radiol 1999; 43(4): 476–9.

76. Sartor O, Bushnell D, Reid R, Quick D. Repeated administration of ^{153}Sm-lexidronam in the treatment of

77. Resche I, Chatal J-F, Pecking A et al. A dose-controlled study of 153 SM-ethylene diamine tetramethylene phosphonate (EDTMP) in the treatment of patients with painful bone metastases. Eur J Cancer 1997; 33: 1583–91.

78. Serafini AN, Houston SJ, Resche I et al. Palliation of pain associated with metastatic bone cancer using samarium-153 lexidronam: a double-blind placebo-controlled clinical trial. J Clin Oncol 1998; 16: 1574–81.

79. Sartor O, Quick D, Reid R et al. A double blind placebo-controlled study of 153-samarium–EDTMP for palliation of bone pain in patients with hormone-refractory prostate cancer. 92nd Annual Meeting of the American Urological Association, 1997: abstr 1252.

80. Maxon HR, Schroder LE, Thomas SR et al. Re-186 (Sn) HEDP for treatment of painful osseous metastasis: initial clinical experience in 20 patients with hormone-resistant prostate cancer. Radiology 1990; 176: 155–9.

81. Maxon HR, Schroder LE, Hertzberg VS et al. Rhenium-186 (Sn) HEDP for treatment of painful osseous metastases: results of a double-blind crossover comparison with placebo. J Nucl Med 1991; 32: 1877–81.

82. deKlerk JM, Zonnenberg BA, van-get Schip AD et al. Dose escalation study of rhenium-186 hydroxyethylidene diphosphonate in patients with metastatic prostate cancer. Eur J Nucl Med 1994; 21: 1114–20.

83. Powers W, Ratanatharathorn V. Palliation of bone metastases. In Perez C, Brady L (eds), Principles and Practice of Radiation Oncology. Lippincott-Raven: Philadelphia, PA 1997: 2199–217.

84. Tannock I. Management of metastatic prostate cancer. Oncol Rounds 2000; 2(3).

85. Prostate Cancer Trialists' Collaborative Group. Maximum androgen blockade in advanced prostate cancer: an overview of 22 randomized trials with 3283 deaths in 5710 patients. Lancet 1995; 346: 265–9.

86. Eisenberger M, Blumenstein B, Crawford E et al. Bilateral orchidectomy with or without flutamide for metastatic prostate cancer. N Engl J Med 1998; 339: 1036–42.

87. Moinpour C, Savage M, Troxel A et al. Quality of life in advanced prostate cancer: results of a randomized therapeutic trial. J Natl Cancer Inst 1998; 90: 1537–44.

88. Schroder F, Collette L, De Reijke T et al. Prostate cancer treated by anti-androgens: Is sexual function preserved? Br J Cancer 2000; 82: 283–90.

89. Bales G, Chodak G. A controlled trial of bicalutamide vs. castration in patients with advanced prostate cancer. Urology 1996; 47: 38–43.

90. Kolvenbag G, Nash A. Bicalutamide dosages used in the treatment of prostate cancer. Prostate 1999; 39: 47–53.

91. Neri R. Antiandrogens: preclinical and clinical studies. Urology 1994; 44: 53–60.

92. Furr B. Relative potencies of flutamide and Casodex. Endocr Rel Cancer 1997; 4: 197–202.

93. Sarosdy M. Which is the optimal antiandrogen for use in combined androgen blockade of advanced prostate cancer? The transition from a first- to second-generation antiandrogen. Anti-Cancer Drugs 1999; 10: 791–5.

94. Teutsch G, Goubet F, Battmann T et al. Non-steroidal antiandrogens: synthesis and biological profile of high-

affinity ligands for the androgen receptor. J Steroid Biochem 1994; 48: 111–19.

95. Schellhammer PF, Sharifi R, Block NL. Clinical benefits of bicalutamide compared with flutamide in combined androgen blockade for patients with advanced prostatic carcinoma: final report of a double-blind, randomized, multicenter trial. Urology 1997; 50: 330–6.

96. Iversen P, Tyrrell C, Kaisary A et al. Casodex (bicalutamide) 150 mg monotherapy compared with castration in patients with previously untreated non-metastatic prostate cancer: results from two multi-center randomized trials at a median follow-up of 4 years. Urology 1998; 51: 389–96.

97. Stoner E. The clinical development of a 5-α reductase inhibitor, finasteride. J Steroid Biochem Mol Biol 1990; 37: 375–8.

98. Andriole G, Lieber M, Smith J et al. Treatment with finasteride following radical prostatectomy for prostate cancer. Urology 1995; 45: 491–7.

99. Scher H, Zhang Z, Nanus D et al. Hormone and anti-hormone withdrawal: implications for the management of androgen-independent prostate cancer. Urology 1996; 47: 61–9.

100. Crawford E, Smith J, Soloway M et al. A randomized controlled clinical trial of leuprolide and Anandron vs. leuprolide and placebo for advanced prostate cancer. J Urol 1990; 143: 221A.

101. The Medical Research Council Prostate Cancer Working Party Investigators Group. Immediate vs. deferred treatment for advanced prostatic cancer: initial results of the Medical Research Council trial. Br J Urol 1997; 79: 235–46.

102. Klotz L, Herr H, Whitmore W. Intermittent DES therapy for symptomatic, metastatic prostate cancer. Cancer 1986; 58: 2456–60.

103. Crook J, Szumaker E, Malone S et al. Intermittent androgen suppression in the management of prostate cancer. Urology 1999; 53: 530–4.

104. Sato N, Gleave M, Bruchovsky N et al. Intermittent androgen suppression delays progression to androgen-independent regulation of prostate-specific antigen gene in the LNCaP prostate tumour model. J Steroid Biochem Mol Biol 1996; 58: 139–46.

105. Goldenberg S, Bruchovsky N, Gleave M et al. Intermittent androgen suppression in the treatment of prostate cancer: a preliminary report. Urology 1995; 45: 839–44.

106. Tannock IF. Is there evidence that chemotherapy is of benefit to patients with carcinoma of the prostate? J Clin Oncol 1985; 3: 1013–21.

107. Tannock I, Osoba D, Stockler M et al. Chemotherapy with mitoxantrone plus prednisone or prednisone alone of symptomatic hormone-resistant prostate cancer. A Canadian randomized trial with palliative endpoints. J Clin Oncol 1996; 14: 1756–64.

108. Bubley G, Carducci M, Dahut W et al. Eligibility and response guidelines for phase II clinical trials in androgen-independent prostate cancer: recommendations from the Prostate-Specific Antigen Working Group. J Clin Oncol 1999; 17: 3461–7.

109. Moore M, Osoba D, Murphy K et al. Use of palliative endpoints to evaluate the effects of mitoxantrone and low-dose prednisone in patients with hormonally resistant prostate cancer. J Clin Oncol 1994; 12: 689–94.

110. Kantoff P, Halabi S, Conaway M et al. Hydrocortisone with or without mitoxantrone in hormone-refractory prostate cancer: results of the cancer and leukemia group B 9182 study. J Clin Oncol 1999; 17: 2506–13.

111. Gregurich M. Phase III study of mitoxantrone/low-dose prednisone vs. low-dose prednisone alone in patients with asymptomatic hormone-refractory carcinoma of the prostate. Proc Am Soc Clin Oncol 2000; 19: 336(abstr 1321).

112. Papapoulos S, Hamdy N, van der Pluijm G. Bisphosphonates in the management of prostate carcinoma metastatic to the skeleton. Cancer 2000; 88: 3047–53.

113. Pelger R, Lycklama A, Nijeholt A et al. Short-term metabolic effects of pamidronate in patients with prostatic carcinoma and bone metastases. Lancet 1989; ii: 865.

114. Adami S, Salvagno G, Guarrera G et al. Dichloro-methylene-diphosphonate in patients with prostate carcinoma metastatic to the skeleton. J Urol 1985; 134: 1152–4.

115. Percival R, Watson M, Williams J et al. Carcinoma of the prostate: remission of paraparesis with inhibitors of bone resorption. Postgrad Med J 1985; 61: 551–3.

116. Adami S, Mian M. Clodronate therapy of metastatic bone disease in patients with prostatic carcinoma. Recent Results Cancer Res 1989; 116: 67–72.

117. Vorreuther R. Bisphosphonates as an adjunct to palliative therapy of bone metastases from prostate cancer. Br J Urol 1993; 72: 792–5.

118. Adami S. Bisphosphonates in prostate carcinoma. Cancer 1997; 80: 1674–9.

119. Clarke N, Holbrook I, McClure J et al. Osteoclast inhibition by pamidronate in metastatic cancer: a preliminary study. Br J Cancer 1991; 63: 420–3.

120. Clarke N, McClure J, George N. Disodium pamidronate identifies differential osteoclastic bone resorption in metastatic prostate cancer. Br J Urol 1992; 69: 64–70.

121. Lipton A, Glover D, Harvey H et al. Pamidronate in the treatment of bone metastases: results of two dose-ranging trials in patients with breast or prostate cancer. Ann Oncol 1994; 5(suppl 7): S31–5.

122. Carey P, Lippert M. The treatment of painful prostatic bone metastases with oral etidronate sodium. Urology 1988; 32: 403–7.

123. Elomaa I, Kylmala T, Tammela T et al. Effect of clodronate on bone pain. A controlled study in patients with metastatic prostate cancer. Int Urol Nephrol 1992; 24: 159–61.

124. Coleman R, Purohit O, Black C et al. Double-blind, randomised, placebo-controlled, dose-finding study of oral ibandronate in patients with metastatic bone disease. Ann Oncol 1999; 10: 311–16.

125. Boissier S, Magnetto S, Frappart L et al. Bisphosphonates inhibit prostate and breast carcinoma cell adhesion to unmineralized and mineralized bone extracellular matrices. Cancer Res 1997; 57: 3890–4.

126. Fernandex-Conde M. Skeletal response to clodronate in prostate cancer with bone metastases. Am J Clin Oncol 1997; 20: 471–6.

127. Smith JA Jr. Palliation of painful bone metastases from prostate cancer using sodium etidronate: results

of a randomized, prospective, double-blind, placebo-controlled study. J Urol 1989; 141: 85–7.

128. Dearnaley DP, Sydes MR, on behalf of the MRC PR5 Collaborators. Preliminary evidence that oral clodronate delays symptomatic progression of bone metastases from prostate cancer: first results of the MRC PR5 Trial. Proc Am Soc Clin Oncol 2001; 20: 174a.

129. Ernst DS, Tannock IF, Venner PM et al. Randomized placebo controlled trial of mitoxantrone/prednisone and clodronate mitoxantrone/prednisone alone in patients with hormone refractory prostate cancer (HRPC) and pain: National Cancer Institute of Canada Clinical Trials Group Study. Proc Am Soc Clin Oncol 2002; 21: 177a.

130. Saad F, Gleason D, Murray R et al. A randomized, placebo-controlled trial of zoledronic acid in patients with hormone-refractory metastatic prostate carcinoma. J Natl Cancer Inst 2002; 94(19): 1458–68.

131. Canil C, Tannock I. Should bisphosphonates be used routinely in patients with prostate cancer metastatic to bone? J Natl Inst 2002; 94(19): 1422–3.

132. Emrich L, Priore R, Murphy G et al. The investigators of the National Prostatic Cancer Project: prognostic factors in patients with advanced stage prostate cancer. Cancer Res 1985; 45: 5173–9.

133. Soloway M, Hardeman S, Hickey D et al. Stratification of patients with metastatic prostate cancer based on extent of disease on initial bone scan. Cancer 1987; 61: 195–202.

134. Chodak G, Vogelzang N, Caplan R et al. Independent prognostic factors in patients with metastatic (stage D2) prostate cancer. Zoladex Study Group. J Am Med Assoc 1991; 265: 618–21.

135. Murphy G, Tjoa B, Ragde H et al. Phase I clinical trial: T-cell therapy for prostate cancer using autologous dendritic cells pulsed with HLA-A0201-specific peptides from prostate-specific membrane antigen. Prostate 1996; 29: 371 80.

136. Tjoa B, Simmons S, Bowes V et al. Evaluation of phase I/II clinical trials in prostate cancer with dendritic cells and PSMA peptides. Prostate 1998; 36: 39–44.

137. Murphy G, Tjoa B, Simmons S et al. Infusion of dendritic cells pulsed with HLA-A2-specific prostate-specific membrane antigen peptides: a phase II prostate cancer vaccine trial involving patients with hormone-refractory metastatic disease. Prostate 1999; 38: 73–8.

138. Murphy G, Tjoa B, Simmons S et al. Phase II prostate cancer vaccine trial: report of a study involving 37 patients with disease recurrence following primary treatment. Prostate 1999; 39: 54–9.

139. Tjoa B, Erickson S, Bowes V et al. Follow-up evaluation of prostate cancer patients with autologous dendritic cells pulsed with PSMA peptides. Prostate 1997; 32: 272–8.

140. Simmons S, Tjoa B, Rogers M et al. GM-CSF as systemic adjuvant in a phase II prostate cancer vaccine trial. Prostate 1999; 39: 291–7.

141. Tjoa B, Simmons S, Elgamal A et al. Follow-up evaluation of a phase II prostate cancer vaccine trial. Prostate 1999; 40: 125–9.

142. Tjoa B, Murphy G. Progress in active specific immunotherapy of prostate cancer. Semin Surg Oncol 2000; 18: 80–7.

143. Oh WK. Chemotherapy for patients with advanced prostate carcinoma. A new option for therapy. Cancer 2000; 88: 3015–21.

40

Multiple Myeloma

Robert A. Kyle

Mayo Clinic, Rochester, MN, USA

INTRODUCTION

Multiple myeloma (MM) most likely has been present for centuries, but the first well-documented case was reported by Samuel Solly in 1844. Six years later, Thomas MacIntyre described the illness of Thomas Alexander McBean, who had severe bone pain and at autopsy was found to have cells in the bone marrow consistent with those of MM. MacIntyre noted that when heated, the urine was found to "abound in animal matter" but it "underwent complete solution" when boiled and reappeared on cooling. He sent a sample of the urine to Henry Bence Jones, a 31-year-old physician at St. George's Hospital who had already established a reputation as a chemical pathologist. Jones confirmed the findings of MacIntyre and concluded that the protein represented a deutoxide of albumen; however, Jones recognised the significance of the protein when he advised "seeking for this oxide of albumen in other cases of mollities osium" [1].

The term "multiple myeloma" was introduced by J. von Rustizky in 1873, and 16 years later Otto Kahler described a case involving a 46 year-old physician named Dr. Loos. He had an 8 year course of progressive pain, recurrent fractures, loss of height and severe kyphosis. His urine contained the typical protein as described by Jones, and his bone marrow contained large cells consistent with myeloma. J. H. Wright, who described the peripheral blood stain of the same name, reported a patient with MM in 1898. Radiographs showed changes in multiple ribs (Roentgen rays had been discovered only 3 years before). Wright emphasised the presence of numerous thin-walled blood vessels (increased angiogenesis) in the tumours and concluded that the cells represented plasma cells or their immediate descendants. The diagnosis of MM was facilitated by the use of bone marrow aspiration in 1927 and 12 years later by electrophoresis, which demonstrated the tall, narrow-based "church spire" peak.

Immunoelectrophoresis was introduced in 1953, and immunofixation was first described 11 years later. Urethane was introduced as specific therapy for MM in 1947 but was subsequently shown to be ineffective. Sarcolysin (L-phenylalanine mustard, melphalan) was introduced in 1958 and continues to be a useful agent for treatment of this disease [1]. Currently, large doses of melphalan are used as the preparative regimen for autologous or allogeneic transplantation.

DEFINITION AND EPIDEMIOLOGY

MM is characterised by the neoplastic proliferation of a single clone of plasma cells producing a monoclonal (M-) protein. The proliferation of this clone of plasma cells often results in skeletal destruction, with punched-out lytic lesions or pathological fractures producing pain or hypercalcaemia. The annual incidence of MM is 4/100 000 [2]. The reported increased incidence during the past few decades is probably related more to the increased availability of medical facilities for the elderly and to improved diagnostic techniques rather than to an actual increased incidence. MM accounts for more than 10% of haematological malignancies but only 1% of all malignant diseases. It occurs in all races, but rates are lower in Asian populations and higher in African–Americans. The median age of patients is 65 years, and only 2% are younger than

Textbook of Bone Metastases. Edited by C. Jasmin, R. E. Coleman, L. R. Coia, R. Capanna and G. Saillant
© 2005 John Wiley & Sons Ltd: ISBN 0 471 87742 5

40 years. The cause of MM is unknown, but exposure to radiation, herbicides or insecticides, and *Human herpesvirus-8* may play a role in some cases.

CLINICAL MANIFESTATIONS

Bone pain is frequent and is usually the major concern of the patient. It is present at the time of diagnosis in two-thirds of patients and most often involves the back or chest. It is aggravated by movement, and the patient is frequently pain-free if movement is avoided. Nocturnal pain is usually not a feature unless the patient changes position. Spasms of back pain are often induced by movement. Sudden, severe back pain from a compression fracture may occur after a fall or lifting an object, even when trauma is minimal. The patient's height may decrease 4–6 inches during the course of the disease because of vertebral compression. Sudden pains in the ribs followed by localised tenderness indicate a rib fracture, even though the radiograph may be negative. Involvement of the mandible is not infrequent, and a pathological fracture can occur while eating. Weakness and fatigue are common, but fever does not occur unless the patient has an infection. The liver is palpable in about one-sixth of patients, but splenomegaly is rare. Extra-medullary plasmacytomas may occur during the course of the disease.

Skeletal involvement is common; three-quarters of patients have lytic lesions, osteoporosis or fractures on conventional radiographs at diagnosis. The vertebrae, skull, ribs and thoracic cage, pelvis and proximal humeri and femora, which are the sites of the red marrow, are the bones most frequently involved. Osteosclerotic lesions are rare [3]. Technetium-99m (^{99m}Tc) bone scanning is inferior to conventional radiography and is not advised. Large lytic lesions may be overlooked because bone formation does not occur. Computed tomography (CT) is helpful in patients who have bone pain but no abnormalities on radiography. Magnetic resonance imaging (MRI) is useful for diagnosis. In one series, the thoracolumbar MRI was normal in patients with monoclonal gammo-pathy of undetermined significance (MGUS) and abnormal in more than 80% of patients with overt MM [4]. In another report, the MRI pattern was abnormal in 82% of 61 patients with MM [5]. The role of MRI in evaluation of spinal cord compression has been the subject of an extensive review [6].

Radiculopathy and compression of the nerve root by an extramedullary plasmacytoma may produce severe radicular pain. Compression of the spinal cord from an extramedullary plasmacytoma occurs in 5% of patients.

Renal insufficiency (serum creatinine $\geqslant 2$ mg/dl) occurs in 20% of patients at diagnosis. Acute renal failure can be the presenting finding in some patients. The two major causes of renal failure are "myeloma kidney", in which large casts in the distal and collecting tubules occur, and hypercalcaemia, which is present in 15% of patients at diagnosis.

LABORATORY FINDINGS

Anaemia is present in approximately 70% of patients at diagnosis and occurs in most during the course of the disease [7]. It is normocytic and normochromic and results from marrow replacement by plasma cells, chronic renal insufficiency, and myelosuppression from chemotherapy. Hypercalcaemia occurs in 15% of patients, and serum creatinine levels are 2 mg/dl or more in 20%. Electrophoresis of the serum shows a spike or a localised band in 80% of patients at diagnosis. Approximately 10% have hypogammaglob-ulinaemia. An M-protein is found in the serum with immunofixation in nearly 90% of patients. IgG occurs in about 50%, IgA is present in 20%, and nearly one-fifth of patients have only a free monoclonal light chain (Bence Jones proteinemia). Immunofixation of the urine reveals an M-protein (κ or λ) in 75% of patients. The κ:λ ratio is 2:1. An M-protein is found in the serum or urine at the time of diagnosis in 97% of patients with MM. Plasma cells generally account for more than 10% of all nucleated bone marrow cells. Immunoperoxidase staining of the cytoplasm is helpful for differentiating a monoclonal plasma cell prolifera-tion from a polyclonal plasmacytosis caused by a metastatic carcinoma, chronic infections, liver disease or autoimmune diseases.

DIAGNOSIS AND DIFFERENTIAL DIAGNOSIS

The diagnosis of MM often is not difficult because most patients present with typical symptoms or laboratory abnormalities. Minimal criteria for the diagnosis include a bone marrow with more than 10% plasma cells or a tissue biopsy specimen demonstrating monoclonal plasmacytosis plus one of the following: M-protein in serum (usually > 3 g/dl), M-protein in urine, or lytic lesions. The usual clinical features of MM must be present. Metastatic carci-noma, connective tissue disorders or lymphoma must be considered in the differential diagnosis. Monoclonal gammopathy of undetermined significance (MGUS), smouldering multiple myeloma (SMM) and primary amyloidosis (AL) must be differentiated from MM. Patients with MGUS have an M-protein value $<3\,g/dl$, bone marrow with $<10\%$ plasma cells, and no anaemia, lytic lesions, hypercalcaemia, renal insufficiency or Bence Jones proteinuria. Patients with SMM have a serum M-protein value $>3\,g/dl$ and $>10\%$ plasma cells in the bone marrow but no other features of MM. Patients with MGUS or SMM should not be treated until symptoms of MM develop or laboratory abnormalities progress, because these patients may remain stable for many years. The size of the serum M-protein and the urine M-protein and the number of bone marrow plasma cells are helpful in the differential diagnosis. The level of uninvolved serum immunoglobulins is not reliable, because almost 40% of patients with MGUS have a reduction of one or more uninvolved immunoglobulins.

Measurement of the synthesis of DNA by the plasma cell labelling index is useful for differentiating MGUS or SMM from MM [8]. An increased labelling index indicates active myeloma. Monoclonal plasma cells with the same isotype can be detected in the peripheral blood of 80% of patients with active MM, whereas patients with MGUS or SMM have few or no circulating plasma cells. The β_2-microglobulin level is of no help for differentiating benign from malignant plasma cell proliferative disorders. Differentiation of AL from MM is arbitrary, because both diseases are plasma cell proliferative disorders with different manifestations. In AL there are no lytic lesions, bone marrow plasma cells are usually $<20\%$, and the amount of monoclonal light chain in the urine is modest. AL will develop during the course of MM in approximately 10% of patients, but MM develops rarely in patients who present with AL.

No single test reliably differentiates a patient with MGUS from one in whom MM or other malignant disease will subsequently develop. One must follow the patient who has MGUS or SMM with measurements of the M-protein value in the serum and urine and periodic evaluation of the pertinent clinical and laboratory parameters.

TREATMENT

Although most patients with MM have symptomatic disease at diagnosis and require therapy, some are asymptomatic and should not be treated. Patients with SMM or MGUS should be observed until progression occurs. All symptoms, physical findings and laboratory data must be considered in the decision to treat. If there is doubt about beginning therapy, it is best to re-evaluate the patient in 2–3 months and delay therapy until progressive disease is evident. There is no evidence that early treatment of MM is advantageous.

Radiotherapy

Palliative radiation in a dose of 20–30 Gy should be limited to patients with disabling pain who have a well-defined focal process that has not responded to chemotherapy or analgesics. Analgesics in combination with chemotherapy usually can control the pain. This approach is preferred to focal radiation, because pain frequently occurs in another site. Radiation therapy may be repeated, but it is ultimately limited by the development of neutropenia or thrombocytopenia, which in turn may restrict the use of chemotherapy. Radiation therapy in MM is limited and should be used only for discrete lesions, because it does not benefit the patient with systemic disease.

Autologous Stem Cell Transplantation

If the patient is aged <70 years, the physician should discuss the possibility of autologous peripheral blood stem cell transplantation with the patient. The haematopoietic stem cells should be collected before the patient is exposed to alkylating agents. Chemotherapy, consisting of melphalan and prednisone or a combination of chemotherapeutic agents, is generally advisable for patients aged >70 years or in younger patients in whom transplantation is not feasible.

Autologous peripheral blood stem cell transplantation has virtually replaced autologous bone marrow transplantation because engraftment is more rapid and there is less contamination with tumour cells. Autologous peripheral stem cell transplantation is applicable for more than half of patients with MM. The absolute number of $CD34^+$ cells per kilogram is the most reliable and practical method for determining the adequacy of a stem cell collection. The two major shortcomings are that: (a) myeloma is not eradicated even with large doses of chemotherapy or total body radiation; and (b) autologous peripheral stem cells are contaminated by myeloma cells or their precursors.

The mortality rate with autologous transplantation is currently 1–2%.

Most physicians initially treat the patient with vincristine and doxorubicin (Adriamycin) intravenously for 96 h and dexamethasone orally (VAD) for 3–4 months to reduce the number of tumour cells in the bone marrow and peripheral blood. Dexamethasone, with or without thalidomide, is being evaluated for initial therapy [9,10]. Peripheral blood stem cells are collected after administration of granulocyte colony-stimulating factor (G-CSF), with or without high-dose cyclophosphamide. One can proceed with the transplantation after high-dose chemotherapy or total body radiation, followed by infusion of the peripheral blood stem cells. The other choice is to treat the patient with alkylating agents after stem cell collection until a plateau is reached, and then give the patient α_2-interferon or no therapy until early relapse. At that time, the patient is given high-dose melphalan and the previously collected peripheral blood stem cells are infused. Both early and late transplantation are reasonable options. In one study, 185 patients were treated with three or four courses of VAD and then randomised to high-dose chemotherapy and autologous stem cell transplantation or to conventional chemotherapy and then autologous transplantation when their disease progressed. There was no difference in the median survival of the two groups (65 vs. 64 months). The main advantage of early transplantation was a shorter period of chemotherapy [11].

A randomised trial by the French Myeloma Group compared high-dose chemotherapy followed by autologous bone marrow transplantation with conventional chemotherapy in 200 previously untreated patients with myeloma who were <65 years [12]. Data were analysed on an intention-to-treat basis; 25% of the patients randomised to transplantation did not receive a transplant. The response rate (81% vs. 57%) and complete response rate (22% vs. 5%) were superior in the transplant group. The 5 year event-free survival (28% vs. 10%) and overall survival rates (52% vs. 12%) were higher in the transplant group. It must be kept in mind that patient selection plays an important role in response and survival. In this regard, a group of 77 patients with MM who fulfilled the criteria for transplantation (age <65 years, stage II or III, good performance status, and disease responsive to initial chemotherapy) but who were treated with conventional chemotherapy had a survival of 5 years, which is similar to that with autologous stem cell transplantation [13]. Patients refractory to VAD have the same overall survival as those who respond to

VAD [14]. In an effort to prolong survival, highly purified $CD34^+$ cells did not influence the achievement of clinical or molecular complete remission, remission duration, or overall survival [15]. Thus, tumour cell purging does not appear to be beneficial.

The role of total body irradiation (TBI) in the preparative regimen is controversial. When melphalan ($140 \, mg/m^2$) plus TBI was compared with melphalan ($200 \, mg/m^2$), there was no difference in response rate, event-free survival or overall survival. Toxicity with melphalan ($200 \, mg/m^2$) was significantly less than that with melphalan plus TBI [16]. Consequently, most investigators have discontinued the use of TBI and give only melphalan ($200 \, mg/m^2$) as the preparative regimen. In an effort to improve the preparative regimen, studies are being done of holmium-166 (^{166}Ho)-DOTMP or samarium-153 (^{153}Sm)-EDTMP in conjunction with melphalan.

The role of double or tandem autologous stem cell transplants is controversial. In an uncontrolled series of 231 patients with newly diagnosed MM who received a second transplant, 51% achieved a complete response and 95% had a complete or partial response. The authors believed that the double transplant extended both event-free and overall survival, even in patients with unfavourable cytogenetics and increased β_2-microglobulin values [17]. In a randomised trial of 400 patients from France, there was no difference in event-free or overall survival between the single and double autologous stem cell transplant groups when evaluated at 2 years. The two groups were similar from the standpoint of age, sex, stage, Ig isotype, β_2-microglobulin value, C-reactive protein level, and bone marrow plasmacytosis. The complete response rate was 32% with a single transplant and 33% with a double transplant. At 2 years, the event-free survival rates were 54% and 57%, respectively, whereas the overall survival rates were 71% and 67% [18]. In a subsequent evaluation, patients with a double transplant had a greater 7 year survival (42% vs. 21%) [19].

Almost all patients will have relapse after an autologous stem cell transplantation. In a preliminary analysis of a randomised trial of 85 patients with MM, treatment with high-dose melphalan and autologous bone marrow transplantation followed by α_2-interferon maintenance therapy suggested both a prolongation of relapse-free survival and an overall survival benefit. However, the final analysis of this trial demonstrated no significant difference in relapse-free or overall survival among patients randomised to maintenance therapy with α_2-interferon [20]. Idiotype-treated autologous dendritic cells are being used to prolong response duration [21].

Allogeneic Bone Marrow Transplantation

The major advantage of allogeneic transplantation is that the graft contains no tumour cells that lead to a relapse. Unfortunately, more than 90% of patients with MM are ineligible because of their age, lack of an HLA-matched sibling donor, or inadequate renal, pulmonary or cardiac function. Furthermore, there is a mortality rate of approximately 25%. In a report of 266 patients from the European Blood and Bone Marrow Transplantation Registry, 51% obtained a complete response. The overall treatment-related mortality rate was approximately 40%. The actuarial survival was 30% at 4 years and 20% at 10 years [22]. In a comparison of the Registry data for transplantations performed in 1983–1993 with those performed in 1994–1998, median overall survival was 10 months and 50 months, respectively, and transplant-related mortality at 6 months was 38% and 21%, respectively [23].

It is obvious that the mortality rate for allogeneic transplantation must be reduced before it can assume a major role in the treatment of MM. Promising approaches are a "mini-allogeneic" transplant [24] or depletion of T cells in an effort to reduce transplant-related mortality. Graft-vs.-myeloma effect has been noted after donor peripheral blood mononuclear cells were given for relapse following allogeneic transplantation. Eight of 13 patients with relapsed myeloma following an allogeneic bone marrow transplantation responded to donor lymphocyte infusions [25]. Conventional allogeneic transplantation currently cannot be recommended because of the excessive mortality.

Chemotherapy

Chemotherapy is the preferred initial treatment for overt, symptomatic MM in patients aged > 70 years or in younger patients in whom transplantation is not feasible. Melphalan and prednisone, given orally, produce an objective response in only 50–60% of patients. Melphalan must be given when the patient is fasting, because food interferes with absorption. Leukocyte and platelet counts should be determined at 3 week intervals after beginning therapy, because the melphalan dosage must be altered until mid-cycle neutropenia or thrombocytopenia occurs. The melphalan and prednisone regimen should be repeated at 6 week intervals. The usual course of MM is one of progression, and if the patient's pain is alleviated and there is no evidence of progressive disease, the therapy may be beneficial despite the failure to reach an objective response.

Because of the obvious shortcomings of melphalan and prednisone, various combinations of therapeutic agents have been used. In an overview of individual data for 4930 persons from 20 randomised trials comparing melphalan and prednisone with various combinations of therapeutic agents, response rates were significantly higher with combination chemotherapy (60%) than with melphalan and prednisone alone (53%) ($p < 0.00001$). However, there was no significant difference in duration of response or overall survival. In addition, there was no evidence that any group of patients benefited from receiving combination chemotherapy [26].

Chemotherapy should be continued for at least 1 year or until the patient is in a plateau state, which is defined as stable serum and urine M-protein levels and no evidence of progression of disease. Continued alkylating agent chemotherapy may lead to the development of a myelodysplastic syndrome or acute leukaemia [27]. Patients should be followed closely during the plateau state, and the same chemotherapy should be reinstituted if relapse occurs after 6 months.

REFRACTORY MULTIPLE MYELOMA

Cure rarely occurs; therefore, almost all patients who respond to chemotherapy will eventually relapse if they do not die of another disease. In addition, at least one-third of patients treated initially with vincristine–Adriamycin–dexamethasone (VAD) do not obtain an objective response. The highest response rates reported for patients with MM resistant to alkylating agents have been with VAD. Approximately 80% of the activity of VAD is from dexamethasone, and it has therefore been used as a single agent.

Thalidomide, in an initial dosage of 200 mg daily with a gradual increase to 800 mg daily if needed, produces a response in about one-third of patients refractory to therapy [28,29]. A combination of thalidomide and dexamethasone has shown promise. Constipation, weakness or fatigue, sleepiness, rash and peripheral neuropathy are undesirable side-effects. In most patients, response occurs within 6 weeks and with only 400 mg thalidomide daily. Promising approaches for the treatment of patients with refractory myeloma include the use of immunomodulatory agents, such as CC5013 (Revlimid) [30] and the proteasome inhibitor bortezomib (PS-341; Velcade) [31].

Treatment of Skeletal Complications

Skeletal involvement often leads to pain, pathological fractures or hypercalcaemia [32]. These complications result from increased osteoclastic bone resorption. The increase in osteoclastic activity in MM is mediated by the release of osteoclastic-stimulating factors, including interleukin-1 (IL-1), interleukin-6 (IL-6) and tumour necrosis factor (TNF).

Bisphosphonates are specific inhibitors of osteoclastic activity and have been evaluated as conjunctive therapy to chemotherapy for MM. In a prospective study, 377 patients with stage III MM with at least one lytic lesion were randomised to receive pamidronate (90 mg intravenously every 4 weeks) or placebo [33]. The patients were stratified at entry into those receiving first-line chemotherapy (stratum 1) and those who failed first-line chemotherapy and were receiving subsequent therapy regimens (stratum 2). Skeletal events were defined as pathological fractures, need for operation to treat or prevent pathological fractures, need for radiation to bone, or spinal cord compression. Patients receiving pamidronate had a significant reduction in both the proportion experiencing skeletal events and the number of skeletal lesions per year. The pamidronate group also had a reduction in the number of patients with development of new pathological fractures and requiring radiation therapy, a significant decrease in bone pain, a decreased requirement for analgesic drugs, and improved quality of life. Bisphosphonates may induce apoptosis in human myeloma cell cultures and thus exert a direct effect on MM [34]. Therefore, patients with MM who have lytic lesions or osteopenia should receive pamidronate (90 mg intravenously over 2 h every 4 weeks). Pamidronate is well tolerated, but cost is a factor [35]. The American Society of Clinical Oncology clinical practice guidelines for the use of bisphosphonates recommend either pamidronate or zoledronic acid, 4 mg intravenously over 15 min every 3–4 weeks, in patients who have lytic lesions on skeletal radiographs [36]. Creatinine levels must be determined and evaluation done for proteinuria periodically during bisphosphonate therapy.

Patients should be encouraged to be as active as possible, but they must avoid undue trauma. Fixation of fractures or pending fractures with an intramedullary rod and methylmethacrylate has produced good results. Bone pain should be treated with analgesics or narcotics as necessary.

Hypercalcaemia occurs in 15% of patients with MM. It should be suspected in the presence of unexplained anorexia, nausea, vomiting, polyuria, polydypsia, constipation, confusion or stupor. Hydration and prednisone (25 mg four times a day) are effective in most cases. If not, a bisphosphonate such as pamidronate or zoledronic acid should be given.

SOLITARY PLASMACYTOMA

The diagnosis is based on histological evidence of a tumour consisting of monoclonal plasma cells identical to those in MM. In addition, complete skeletal radiographs must show no additional lytic lesions, the bone marrow aspirate must contain no evidence of MM, and immunofixation of serum and concentrated urine should show no M-protein. Exceptions to the last-mentioned criterion occur, but therapy for the solitary lesion often results in disappearance of the M-protein. The uninvolved or background immunoglobulins are usually normal. There should be no evidence of anaemia, hypercalcaemia or renal insufficiency.

Solitary plasmacytoma of bone is uncommon and occurs in 3–5% of patients with plasma cell neoplasms. It occurs more commonly in men than women (65% vs. 35%), and the median age is about a decade younger than that of patients with MM (55 vs. 65 years). The most common symptom at presentation is pain at the site of the skeletal lesion. Severe back pain or spinal cord compression may be the presenting feature of solitary plasmacytoma involving the vertebrae. A pathological fracture may be the first clue. Soft tissue extension of a plasmacytoma, as in a rib, may result in a palpable mass. The axial skeleton is more commonly involved than the appendicular skeleton [37]. Thoracic vertebrae are more commonly involved than lumbar or cervical vertebrae. Involvement of the distal axial skeleton below the elbows or knees is extremely rare.

Therapy

Tumoricidal radiotherapy is the treatment of choice for patients with solitary plasmacytoma of bone. The patient should receive a dose of 40–45 Gy over approximately 4 weeks. If the plasmacytoma has been excised for diagnostic purposes, radiotherapy should also be given. On the basis of the available data, Dimopoulos et al. [38] concluded that adjuvant chemotherapy should not be administered to patients with solitary plasmacytoma of bone. The use of alkylating agents prophylactically may lead to existence of the residual plasma cells or to myelo-dysplasia or secondary acute leukaemia.

Natural History

Three patterns of failure may occur: (a) development of MM; (b) local recurrence; and (c) development of new solitary bone lesions in the absence of MM. Overt MM develops in approximately 50% of patients with solitary plasmacytoma of bone. For most patients who have progression, it occurs within 3–4 years. However, progression may occur as many as 15 years later. Local recurrence is rare if the patient has had tumoricidal radiation. Multiple solitary plasmacytomas without evidence of MM occur in up to 5% of patients. If the recurrent lesion appears more than 2 years after recognition of the solitary plasmacytoma, it should be treated with tumoricidal radiation. If repeated solitary lesions occur at shorter intervals, systemic therapy, such as autologous stem cell transplantation, should be given. Some patients may remain stable for long periods despite the persistence of an M-protein after tumoricidal radiation.

Prognostic Factors

The presence of marrow involvement on MRI is associated with a higher rate of relapse. In a group of 23 patients with solitary plasmacytoma of the thoracolumbar spine, MM developed in 7/8 patients with a solitary lesion on plain radiographs alone but in only 1/7 patients who also had negative results on MRI [39]. Ten-year myeloma-free survival was 91% in patients whose M-protein resolved at 1 year after radiation therapy and 29% in those whose M-protein persisted [40]. Patients with high-grade angiogenesis in the plasmacytoma are more likely to have progression to multiple myeloma [41].

CONCLUSION AND FUTURE DIRECTIONS

Patients with SMM should not be treated until there is evidence of progressive disease. If the patient is younger than 70 years, autologous peripheral blood stem cell transplantation should be seriously considered. Unfortunately, the procedure is not curative and most patients have relapse. Allogeneic transplantation is associated with a high mortality rate, and approaches such as mini-allogeneic transplantation or T cell depletion are being addressed. Thalidomide is a promising new agent for the treatment of refractory myeloma.

The preparative regimen for both autologous and allogeneic transplantation must be improved. Currently, residual myeloma in the patient is the major cause of relapse. Efforts must be made to remove the tumour cells or, more importantly, their precursors from the peripheral blood before reinfusion of the haematopoietic stem cells. New agents for therapy include analogues of thalidomide, TNFα inhibitors, and bortezomib (PS-341) (a proteasome inhibitor).

REFERENCES

1. Kyle RA. Multiple myeloma: an odyssey of discovery. Br J Haematol 2000; 111: 1035–44.
2. Kyle RA, Beard CM, O'Fallon WM, Kurland LT. Incidence of multiple myeloma in Olmsted County, Minnesota: 1978 through 1990, with a review of the trend since 1945. J Clin Oncol 1994; 12: 1577–83.
3. Lacy MQ, Gertz MA, Hanson CA, et al. Multiple myeloma associated with diffuse osteosclerotic bone lesions: a clinical entity distinct from osteosclerotic myeloma (POEMS syndrome). Am J Hematol 1997; 56: 288–93.
4. Bellaiche L, Laredo JD, Liote F et al. Magnetic resonance appearance of monoclonal gammopathies of unknown significance and multiple myeloma. The GRI Study Group. Spine 1997; 22: 2551–7.
5. Kusumoto S, Jinnai I, Itoh K et al. Magnetic resonance imaging patterns in patients with multiple myeloma. Br J Haematol 1997; 99: 649–55.
6. Moulopoulos LA, Dimopoulos MA. Magnetic resonance imaging of the bone marrow in hematologic malignancies. Blood 1997; 90: 2127–47.
7. Kyle RA, Gertz MA, Witzig TE et al. Review of 1027 patients with newly diagnosed multiple myeloma. Mayo Clin Proc 2003; 78: 21–33.
8. Greipp PR, Witzig TE, Gonchoroff NJ et al. Immunofluorescence labeling indices in myeloma and related monoclonal gammopathies. Mayo Clin Proc 1987; 62: 969–77.
9. Rajkumar SV, Hayman S, Gertz MA et al. Combination therapy with thalidomide plus dexamethasone for newly diagnosed myeloma. J Clin Oncol 2002; 20: 4319–23.
10. Weber D, Rankin K, Gavino M et al. Thalidomide alone or with dexamethasone for previously untreated multiple myeloma. J Clin Oncol 2003; 21: 16–19.
11. Fermand JP, Ravaud P, Chevret S et al. High-dose therapy and autologous peripheral blood stem cell transplantation in multiple myeloma: up-front or rescue treatment? Results of a multicenter sequential randomized clinical trial. Blood 1998; 92: 3131–6.
12. Attal M, Harousseau JL, Stoppa AM et al. A prospective, randomized trial of autologous bone marrow transplantation and chemotherapy in multiple myeloma. Intergroupe Français du Myélome. N Engl J Med 1996; 335: 91–7.
13. Bladé J, San Miguel JF, Fontanillas M et al. Survival of multiple myeloma patients who are potential candidates

for early high-dose therapy intensification/autotransplantation and who were conventionally treated. J Clin Oncol 1996; 14: 2167–73.

14. Rajkumar SV, Fonseca R, Lacy MQ et al. Autologous stem cell transplantation for relapsed and primary refractory myeloma. Bone Marrow Transpl 1999; 23: 1267–72.

15. Lemoli RM, Martinelli G, Zamagni E et al. Engraftment, clinical, and molecular follow-up of patients with multiple myeloma who were reinfused with highly purified CD34$^+$ cells to support single or tandem high-dose chemotherapy. Blood 2000; 95: 2234–9.

16. Moreau P, Facon T, Attal M et al. for the Intergroupe Francophone du Myélome. Comparison of 200 mg/m^2 melphalan and 8 Gy total body irradiation plus 140 mg/m^2 melphalan as conditioning regimens for peripheral blood stem cell transplantation in patients with newly diagnosed multiple myeloma: final analysis of the Intergroupe Francophone du Myélome 9502 randomized trial. Blood 2002; 99: 731–5.

17. Barlogie B, Jagannath S, Desikan KR et al. Total therapy with tandem transplants for newly diagnosed multiple myeloma. Blood 1999; 93: 55–65.

18. Attal M, Payen C, Facon T et al. Single vs. double transplant in myeloma: a randomized trial of the "Inter Groupe Français du Myélome" (IFM). Blood 1997; 90(suppl 1, abstr): 418a.

19. Attal M, Harousseau J-L, Facon T et al. Double autologous transplantation improves survival of multiple myeloma patients: final analysis of a prospective randomized study of the "Intergroupe Francophone du Myélome" (IFM 94). Blood 2002; 100(abstr): 5a.

20. Cunningham D, Powles R, Malpas J et al. A randomized trial of maintenance interferon following high-dose chemotherapy in multiple myeloma: long-term follow-up results. Br J Haematol 1998; 102: 495–502.

21. Valone FH, Lacy MQ, Mackenzie M et al. Immunotherapy of multiple myeloma using idiotype-loaded dendritic cells (APC8020). Proc Am Soc Clin Oncol 2000; 19(abstr): 453a.

22. Gahrton G, Tura S, Svensson H et al. for the European Group for Blood and Marrow Transplantation (EBMT). Allogeneic bone marrow transplantation in multiple myeloma—an update of the EBMT Registry. In VI International Workshop on Multiple Myeloma: Syllabus, Boston, 14–18 June 1997.

23. Gahrton G, Svensson H, Cavo M et al. Progress in allogenic bone marrow and peripheral blood stem cell transplantation for multiple myeloma: a comparison between transplants performed 1983–93 and 1994–8 at European Group for Blood and Marrow Transplantation centres. Br J Haematol 2001; 113: 209–16.

24. Kroger N, Schwerdtfeger R, Kiehl M et al. Autologous stem cell transplantation followed by a dose-reduced allograft induces high complete remission rate in multiple myeloma. Blood 2002; 100: 755–60.

25. Lokhorst HM, Schattenberg A, Cornelissen JJ et al. Donor leukocyte infusions are effective in relapsed

multiple myeloma after allogeneic bone marrow transplantation. Blood 1997; 90: 4206–11.

26. Myeloma Trialists' Collaborative Group. Combination chemotherapy versus melphalan plus prednisone as treatment for multiple myeloma: an overview of 6633 patients from 27 randomized trials. J Clin Oncol 1998; 16: 3832–42.

27. Kyle RA, Gertz MA. Second malignancies after chemotherapy. In Perry MC (ed.), The Chemotherapy Source Book. Williams & Wilkins: Baltimore, MD, 1992: 689–702.

28. Singhal S, Mehta J, Desikan R et al. Antitumor activity of thalidomide in refractory multiple myeloma. N Engl J Med 1999; 341: 1565–71.

29. Rajkumar SV, Fonseca R, Dispenzieri A et al. Thalidomide in the treatment of relapsed multiple myeloma. Mayo Clin Proc 2000; 75: 897–901.

30. Richardson PG, Schlossman RL, Weller E et al. Immunomodulatory drug CC-5013 overcomes drug resistance and is well tolerated in patients with relapsed multiple myeloma. Blood 2002; 100: 3063–7.

31. Richardson PG, Barlogie B, Berenson J et al. Phase II study of the proteasome inhibitor PS-341 in multiple myeloma (MM) patients (pts) with relapsed/refractory disease (abstract). Proc Am Soc Clin Oncol 2002; 21: 11a.

32. Kyle RA. Multiple myeloma: review of 869 cases. Mayo Clin Proc 1975; 50: 29–40.

33. Berenson JR, Lichtenstein A, Porter L et al. Long-term pamidronate treatment of advanced multiple myeloma patients reduces skeletal events. Myeloma Aredia Study Group. J Clin Oncol 1998; 16: 593–602.

34. Shipman CM, Rogers MJ, Apperley JF et al. Bisphosphonates induce apoptosis in human myeloma cell lines: a novel anti-tumour activity. Br J Haematol 1997; 98: 665–72.

35. Kyle RA. The role of bisphosphonates in multiple myeloma (editorial). Ann Intern Med 2000; 132: 734–6.

36. Berenson JR, Hillner BE, Kyle RA et al. American Society of Clinical Oncology clinical practice guidelines: the role of bisphosphonates in multiple myeloma. J Clin Oncol 2002; 20: 3719–36.

37. Frassica DA, Frassica FJ, Schray MF et al. Solitary plasmacytoma of bone: Mayo Clinic experience. Int J Radiat Oncol Biol Phys 1989; 16: 43–8.

38. Dimopoulos MA, Moulopoulos LA, Maniatis A, Alexanian R. Solitary plasmacytoma of bone and asymptomatic multiple myeloma. Blood 2000; 96: 2037–44.

39. Liebross RH, Ha CS, Cox JD et al. Solitary bone plasmacytoma: outcome and prognostic factors following radiotherapy. Int J Radiat Oncol Biol Phys 1998; 41: 1063–7.

40. Wilder RB, Ha CS, Cox JD et al. Persistence of myeloma protein for more than one year after radiotherapy is an adverse prognostic factor in solitary plasmacytoma of bone. Cancer 2002; 94: 1532–7.

41. Kumar S, Fonseca R, Dispenzieri A et al. Prognostic value of angiogenesis in solitary bone plasmacytoma. Blood 2003; 101: 1715–17.

41

Malignant Non-Hodgkin's Lymphoma

O. Reman

Service d'Hématologie Clinique, CHU de Caen, France

INTRODUCTION

The incidence of non-Hodgkin's lymphoma (NHL) is rising, not only in the USA but also worldwide [1–2]. Several systems have been developed in an attempt to classify the lymphoma. The most recent is the Revised European American Lymphoma (REAL) classification [3]. Three groups of NHL were individualised: low-grade lymphoma (one-third of lymphomas), aggressive lymphoma (approximately 20%) and intermediate lymphoma. A multicentre 1993 study established a five-feature prognostic model including age, stage (Ann Arbor; see Table 41.1), performance status, number of extranodal sites of disease and lactico-dehydrogenase (LDH) level [4]. The primary treatment is chemotherapy, while radiotherapy, interferon or monoclonal antibodies (anti-CD20 alone or with isotopes) may also be used [5–6].

Lymphoma often involves lymph nodes but up to 50% of non-Hodgkin's lymphomas involve non-nodal sites. The most frequent non-nodal sites are liver, lung, bone marrow or the gastrointestinal tract. The prognosis of lymphoma may be worsened with involvement of non-nodal sites such as the bone marrow. The involvement of bone by lymphoma is rare and appears with a frequency of 1–2% among bone malignancies, while 15% of malignant lymphomas secondarily involve bone [7].

PRIMARY MALIGNANT LYMPHOMA OF BONE

Primary lymphoma of bone (PLB) was first described in 1928 by Oberling [8]. In 1939, Frederic Parker and Henry Jackson described a primary bone tumour that they called "sarcomas with reticulinic cells". The treatment they recommended was radiotherapy after resection [9].

Given its rarity, most reports of primary bone lymphoma include only a small number of cases. There are reports of larger series collected over a long period of time, but these are of limited value because of changes in staging and the use of a variety of treatments.

Definition

Primary lymphoma of bone is defined as single or multiple bone site involvement by lymphoma at presentation. Secondary multiple organ involvement may occur.

Frequency

Primary lymphoma of bone represents less than 5% of primary bone tumours. Heyning et al. found 106 cases out of a total of 11 000 cases of bone tumours reported during 1943–1996 [10]. The registry of malignant bone tumours in Leeds, UK, reported 54 cases (2.6%) out of a total of 2075 cases of malignant bone tumours during 1958–1994 [11].

Primary lymphoma of bone represented only 4.7% of 1467 cases of extranodal lymphomas collected by Freeman et al. [7]. A review published in 1996 by Ostrowsky reports less than 1000 cases [12].

Clinical Presentation

The median age at the time of diagnosis is 50 years. Men are affected slightly more often than women. The

Textbook of Bone Metastases. Edited by C. Jasmin, R. E. Coleman, L. R. Coia, R. Capanna and G. Saillant
© 2005 John Wiley & Sons Ltd: ISBN 0 471 87742 5

Table 41.1. Ann Arbor staging classification

Stage	
I	Involvement of a single lymph node region or lymphoid structure
II	Involvement of two or more lymph node regions or lymphoid structures on the same side of the diaphragm
III	Involvement of lymph node regions or lymphoid structures on both sides of the diaphragm
IV	Involvement of extranodal sites
E	Involvement of single extranodal site contiguous to nodal site
A/B	No symptoms/fever, night sweats, weight loss

Data from Carbone et al. [19].

disease can also occur in children. Three consecutive studies during 1983–1997 published by the Pediatric Oncology Group reported 31 cases of primary lymphoma of bone (5.5%) out of 567 cases of paediatric lymphoma [13].

The main presenting symptoms and signs are bone pain and a palpable mass. Systemic signs, such as night sweats, fever and weight loss, are rare. Long bone involvement is seen in 50% of cases, but any other bone site can also be involved (vertebra, pelvis, ribs, scapula, skull, mandible) [14] (see Table 41.2). A spontaneous fracture may appear at the site of bone involvement. Hypercalcaemia at presentation was noted in a case of multifocal intermediate grade B cell primary lymphoma of bone [15].

Prior bone trauma is sometimes reported to have occurred at the tumour site. Three of 14 patients with primary lymphoma of bone had trauma 4–12 years prior to diagnosis [16]. Significant immunosuppression could be a risk factor for developing primary

lymphoma of bone. A 66 year-old patient with a B cell lymphoma was diagnosed as PLB, 11 months after a liver transplant [17]. Piira et al. also reported a case of PLB in a patient with HIV infection [18].

Most of the patients present with localised disease (Ann Arbor stage I or II) at the time of diagnosis [19]. Patients with stage II PLB have multiple bone involvement (multifocal lymphoma) or disseminated disease.

Other Diagnostic Procedures

In addition to a radiograph, useful diagnostic procedures include bone scintigraphy with technetium or gallium, and magnetic resonance imaging (MRI).

A radiograph often shows a non-specific lytic bone lesion, frequently surrounded by a periosteal reaction. The typical long bone lesion is metaphyseal, a cortical rupture, periosteal reaction and infiltration of adjacent soft tissue (Figure 41.1). A "moth-eaten" appearance of the lytic involvement is sometimes seen in pelvic bone with a frequently associated soft tissue mass. Vertebral lesions may be lytic or sclerotic. Complications such as primary fractures are rare and are occasionally seen after radiation therapy [20].

Scintigraphy with technetium-99 (^{99m}Tc) (Figure 41.2) reveals increased uptake in the tumour periphery and soft tissue uptake. In contrast, gallium-67 (^{67}Ga) scintigraphy reveals both increased central and peripheral tumour uptake with decreased soft tissue uptake. A gallium scan is therefore more sensitive [20] if soft tissue is involved.

Positron emission tomography (PET: ^{18}F fluorodeoxyglucose) is a promising diagnosis tool. It could be useful to confirm the localised nature of the tumour

Table 41.2. Distribution of primary lymphoma of bone by site in a compilation of 242 patients*

References	Upper extremities	Lower extremities	Pelvis	Spine, axial skeleton	Skull, facial bone
Bacci et al. [36]	1/26	12/26	4/26	9/26	
Baar et al. [32]	2/17	9/17	2/17	4/17	
Brousse et al. [26]	2/28	7/28	5/28	14/28	5/28
Christie et al. [35]	13/70	16/70	13/70	25/70	11/70
Dubey et al. [31]	4/45	15/45	3/45	12/45	10/45
Leeson et al. [20]	10/22	7/22	2/22	3/22	
Mendenhall et al. [37]	1/20	14/20	2/20	1/20	2/20
Vassalo et al. [16]	4/14	8/14		2/14	
	37/242 (16%)	89/242 (37%)	31/242 (13%)	69/242 (24%)	28/242 (12%)

* Some patients had more than one bone lymphoma site.

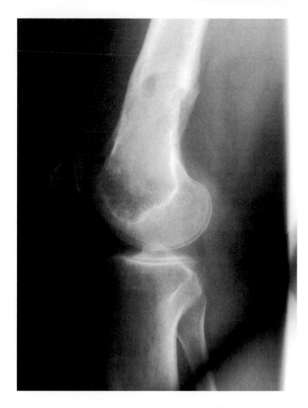

Figure 41.1. Primary bone lymphoma. X-ray image of destructive lesion of the femur with cortical disruption

and also to evaluate the response to treatment. Other prospective complementary studies are suggested to confirm the role of PET in the evaluation of bone tumours [21–22].

MRI is a sensitive method. A Canadian group reported MRI images in 27 patients with primary lymphoma of bone: T1-weighted signals vary in intensity. The T2 signal is mostly heterogeneous (Figures 41.3, 41.4, 41.5). No apparent correlation was found between MRI images and semi-quantitative histopathological features (vascularisation and maturation of tumour fibrosis) [23]. Hermann reported an hypointense signal in T1-weighted and an heterogenous signal in T2-weighted signals. A subcutaneous soft tissue mass is observed in 40% of cases [23–24]. It is important to note that MRI after therapy is not able to distinguish between persistent disease and healing bone.

Pathology

The most common histological type of primary lymphoma of bone is diffuse large cell malignant lymphoma. A few cases of lymphocytic lymphoma have been reported. Immunophenotyping is mostly positive for B cells and the CD20 marker [25]. T cell phenotype is rarely found: only 3/28 cases in a report by Brousse et al. [26], and 3/48 cases in a study reported by Fairbanks et al. [27]. A T cell CD30 large cell phenotype PLB in a 71 year-old male patient was recently described. Fusion transcript NPM/ALK was detected by PCR, and t(2;5)(p23;q35) translocation was detected by the fluorescence *in situ* hybridisation (FISH) technique [28]. Rare T or null cell anaplastic lymphomas have been reported [18,29].

Treatment

The treatment of primary lymphoma of bone had been radiotherapy alone, but today chemotherapy followed by adjuvant radiotherapy is generally considered to be the standard treatment (see Table 41.3).

Dosoretz et al. treated 30 patients by radiotherapy alone and reported a 63% (Table 41.3) overall survival and 53% event-free survival at 5 years. The local 5 year recurrence was 14% if the tumour was treated by less than 50 Gy compared to no recurrence at doses higher than 50 Gy [30].

A retrospective study of 63 patients treated during 1970–1989 with radiotherapy (50 cases), radiation and chemotherapy (10 cases) or chemotherapy alone (two cases) was reported by Fairbanks et al. [27]. Most of the patients (43/63) had a large cell lymphoma. All patients had stage I disease (Ann Arbor classification). The overall 5 year survival was identical but better results were obtained when radiotherapy exceeded 40 Gy. In a univariate analysis, patients treated with chemotherapy and radiation had a longer event-free survival than patients treated with radiotherapy alone.

Dubey et al. reported a series of 45 patients treated in 1970–1992, including 36 patients treated with (CHOP) cyclophosphamide, doxorubicin, vincristine and prednisolone chemotherapy and 40–60 Gy, five patients treated with radiation alone, and four with chemotherapy alone. They did not find any significant difference in the overall survival or event-free survival between patients treated with chemotherapy vs. patients treated with radiotherapy alone or between patients with stage I vs. stage II disease. The overall 5 and 10 year survival rates were 68% and 60%, respectively [31].

Baar et al. reported 17 patients with primary bone lymphoma from 1975 to 1992, including 14 patients with diffuse large cell, two patients with diffuse mixed cell and one case with small non-cleaved cell

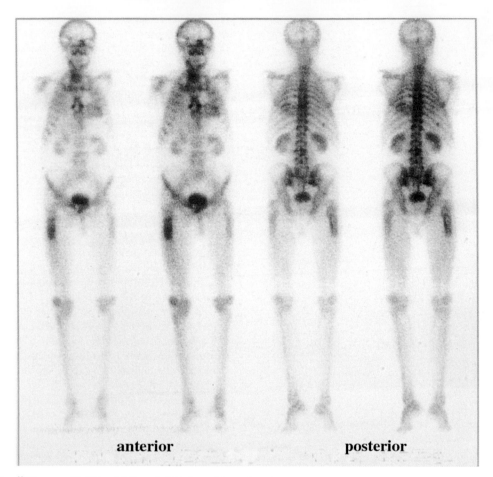

anterior   **posterior**

Figure 41.2. ^{99m}Tc scan. Multifocal (rib and right femur) bone lymphoma

lymphoma. Eleven patients were treated with anthracycline-based multiagent chemotherapy and radiation; five patients were treated with chemotherapy alone and one patient with radiation alone. Thirteen patients had stage I, two patients stage II and the other two patients stage IV disease. An overall response was noted in 94% of patients with 18% having a complete remission, 58% a partial remission and 18% a minor remission. After 29 months of follow-up, 13 patients (76%) continued to be in remission [32].

Heyning et al. reported 60 cases treated with radiotherapy alone (5%); radiotherapy and chemotherapy (40%); radiotherapy, chemotherapy and surgery (18%) and other unspecified associations in 33%. A complete remission was noted in 48% of cases, with an overall 5 year survival of 61% and an event-free 5 year survival rate of 46%. Factors found to be related to worse prognosis were age (overall 5 year survival in patients aged < 60 years was 76% vs. 37% in older patients) and histological type of lymphoma. The overall survival and event-free survival is shorter in patients with immunoblastic lymphoma, representing 16% of patients. In a univariate analysis, LDH level, Ann Arbor stage and tumour size were not demonstrated to be significant prognostic factors. The overall survival was not influenced by type of treatment, but event-free survival was better after CHOP chemotherapy [10].

The Adult Lymphoma Study Group (Groups d'Etude du Lymphome de l'Adulte; GELA) retrospectively analysed 28 cases of primary lymphoma of bone; 86% of the patients were aged < 60 years. Disease confined to bone was noted in 17 cases (61%). Chemotherapy was given in all cases, and was followed by radiotherapy in seven cases. These 28 patients with

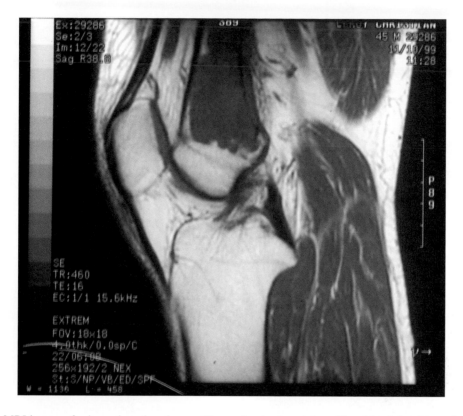

Figure 41.3. MRI images of primary bone lymphoma of femur showing hypointense T1-weighted signal intensity

Table 41.3. Treatment and overall survival of 538 patients with primary bone lymphoma in 15 reports

References	Number of cases	Age average (years)	Treatment	Overall survival
Barr et al. [32]	17	36	RT + CT 11, CT 5, RT 1	82% at 29 months
Bacci et al. [36]	30	NK	RT + CT 26, RT 4	88% at 13 years
Brousse et al. [26]	28	48	CT 21, CT + RT 7	65% at 5 years
Clayton et al. [39]	37	51	CT + RT 18, RT 8, S 8, CT 2	NK
Christie et al. [35]	70	60	RT + CT 39, RT 27	59% at 5 years
Dosoretz et al. [30]	33	58	RT 30	64% at 5 years
Dubey et al. [31]	45	52	CT + RT 36, RT 5, S 4	68% at 5 years
Fairbanks et al. [27]	63	55	RT 50, CT 10, CS 2	57% (RT), 90% (CT + RT) at 5 years
Fidias et al. [42]	37	41	CT + RT 35, CT 2	91% at 5 years, 87% at 10 years
Heyning et al. [10]	60	48	RT 5, CT + RT 35, 20 other associations	46% at 5 years
Lewis et al. [38]	15	42	RT + CT 10, CT 4	NK
Limb et al. [11]	54	35	RT 21, CT + RT 16	46% at 5 years
Mendenhall et al. [37]	21	53	RT 9, CT + RT 11, CT 1	56% at 5 years
Reimer et al. [41]	14	29	RT 1, CT + RT 6, CT 6, S 1	NK
Vassalo et al. [16]	14	39	CT + RT 3, RT 5, CT 1	NK

CT, chemotherapy; RT, radiotherapy; S, surgery alone; NK, not known.

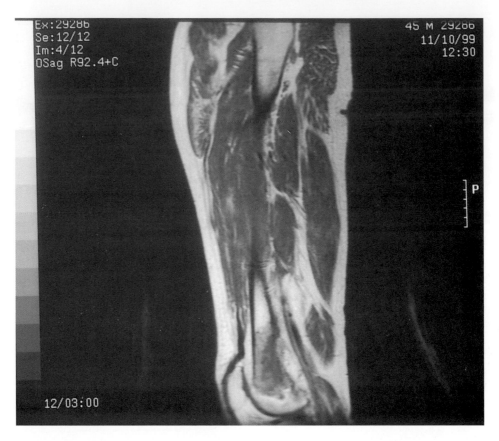

Figure 41.4.   MRI image of primary bone lymphoma of femur showing heterogeneity of T2-weighted signal

primary lymphoma of bone were compared to 2932 patients with non-bone lymphoma treated with the same protocol. Complete response rates were similar in both groups (86% and 84%) but overall survival was better in primary lymphoma of bone (65%) [26].

Relapses can occur at the initial site or in nodal areas [40]. A second complete response is difficult to achieve by chemotherapy. Savage et al. reported the use of rituximab (anti-CD20 monoclonal antibody) in a 58 year-old woman who relapsed after chemo-radiotherapy with a second complete response ongoing at 33 months [33].

Treatment of Paediatric Cases

Among the 31 cases of primary lymphoma of bone published by the Pediatric Oncology Group, 21 were large cell lymphomas, five were lymphoblastic lymphomas, two were small non-cleaved lymphomas

and three were unclassifiable lymphomas. Seven patients were treated by both chemotherapy and radiotherapy and 20 were treated by chemotherapy alone. Overall and event-free survival were estimated to be 100% and 95%, respectively at 5 years. Only one patient relapsed after chemotherapy but a second complete response was achieved in this patient [13].

Prognostic Factors

The Ann Arbor staging classification for lymphoma is a strong prognostic factor for PBL. Involvement of a single bone site is associated with a better prognosis than multifocal PBL or a nodal involvement of PBL [12,26].

Desoretz et al. have analysed the impact of pathology on survival. The probability of survival at 5 years was 64% for PBL with cleaved-cells; 13% for non-cleaved cell lymphomas and 0% for pleomorphic

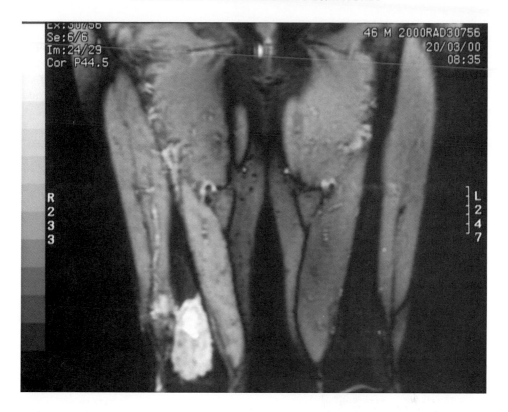

Figure 41.5.   MRI image of primary bone lymphoma of femur showing strong fixation of gadolinium

lymphomas. Recently, anaplastic cell lymphomas were reported to have a more favourable prognosis, but few publications are available [34].

The prognostic value of age is a question of debate: on multivariate analysis of 70 cases of PBL, Christie et al. did not find age to be of prognostic significance [35]. Fidias et al. found that pelvic involvement, a pathological fracture and age are the most important prognostic indicators of overall survival [42]. Indeed, the International Index, based on patient age, LDH level and performance status, is a valid prognostic tool: survival of patients with score 0 was better than survival of those with scores 1 or 2 in a study by Dubey et al., which showed a survival of 85% for score 1 and 43% for score 2 [31].

In conclusion, optimal therapy for PBL is chemotherapy followed by radiotherapy. Chemotherapy alone is active and avoids some of the complications of radiotherapy but it carries a significant risk of local failure. The effectiveness of new drugs such as rituximab with chemotherapy or after relapse needs further investigation.

SECONDARY BONE MALIGNANT LYMPHOMAS

Secondary bone involvement is reported in 15% of malignant lymphomas. Unless clinical symptoms or signs of bone pain or mass are present, the initial staging of lymphoma does not include skeletal X-ray or scintigraphy [42–43].

Contrary to PBL, axial secondary involvement seems to be more frequent than involvement of the extremities. There is no correlation between cortical bone involvement and bone marrow involvement [44].

An interesting report of GELA related a worse prognosis of secondary bone lymphoma among 3179 patients included in an NHL protocol, 219 patients (7%) had bone involvement and the rate of complete response was lower in this group than in patients without bone involvement (respectively, 40% and 50%). The overall 5 year survival rate was also lower (less than 40%), despite treatment with a combination of chemotherapy and radiotherapy [26].

Secondary bone involvement in other types of lymphoma have been reported but they are very rare. African-type Burkitt's lymphoma is typically associated with involvement of the maxilla and is very sensitive to chemotherapy alone [45]. Bone involvement has also been reported in low-grade lymphomas such as lymphocytic lymphoma or lymphoplasmocytic lymphoma [46].

REFERENCES

1. Carli PM, Boutron MC, Maynadie M et al. Increase in the incidence of non-Hodgkin's lymphomas: evidence for a recent sharp increase in France independent of AIDS. Br J Cancer 1994; 70: 713–15.
2. Landis SH, Murray T, Bolden S, Wingo PA. Cancer statistics, 1999. CA Cancer J Clin 1999; 49: 8–31.
3. Harris NL, Jaffe ES, Stein H et al. A revised European–American classification of lymphoid neoplasms: a proposal from the International Lymphoma Study group. Blood 1994; 84: 1361–92.
4. Shipp MA. A predictive model for aggressive non-Hodgkin's lymphoma. N Engl J Med 1993; 329: 987–94.
5. Solal-Celigny P, Lepage E, Brousse N et al. Recombinant interferon-α2b combined with a regimen containing doxorubicin in patients with advanced follicular lymphoma. N Engl J Med 1993; 329: 1608–13.
6. Coiffier B, Haioun C, Ketterer N et al. Rituximab (anti-CD20 monoclonal antibody) for the treatment of patients with relapsing or refractory aggressive lymphoma: a multicenter phase II study. Blood 1998; 92: 1927–32.
7. Freeman C, Berg JW, Cutler SJ. Occurrence and prognosis of extranodal lymphomas. Cancer 1972; 29: 252–60.
8. Oberling C. Les réticulosarcomes et les réticuloendothé-liosarcomes de la moelle osseuse (sarcomes d'Ewing). Bull Assoc Fr Etude Cancer (Paris) 1928; 17: 259–96.
9. Parker F, Jackson H Jr. Primary reticulum cell sarcoma of bone. Surg Gynecol Obstetr 1939; 68: 45–50.
10. Heyning FH, Hogendoorn PC, Kramer MH et al. Primary non-Hodgkin's lymphoma of bone: a clinico-pathological investigation of 60 cases. Leukemia 1999; 13(12): 2094–8.
11. Limb D, Dreghorn C, Murphy JK, Mannion R. Primary lymphoma of bone. Intern Orthop 1994; 18: 180–3.
12. Ostrowski ML, Unni KK, Banks PM et al. Malignant lymphoma of bone. Cancer 1986; 58: 2646–55.
13. Parker BR, Marglin S, Castellino RA. Skeletal manifestations of leukemia, Hodgkin disease, and non-Hodgkin lymphoma. Sem Roentgenol 1980; 4: 302–15.
14. Suryanarayan K, Shuster JJ, Donaldson SS et al. Treatment of localized primary non-Hodgkin's lymphoma of bone in children: a pediatric oncology group study. J Clin Oncol 1999; 17: 456–9.
15. Evron E, Goland S, Klepfish A et al. Primary multifocal lymphoma of bone presenting as hypercalcemic crisis: report of a rare manifestation of extranodal lymphoma. Leuk Lymph 1999; 34: 197–200.
16. Vassalo J, Assuncao M-CGA, Machado JC. Primitive malignant lymphomas of bone. Ann Pathol 1998; 1: 44–8.
17. Hermann G, Abdelwahab IF, Capozzi J et al. Primary non-Hodgkin lymphoma of bone: unusual manifestation of lymphoproliferative disease following liver transplantation. Skel Radiol 1999; 28: 175–7.
18. Piira TA, Ries K, Kjeldsberg CR, Perkins SL. Anaplastic large cell lymphoma presenting primarily in bone in a patient with AIDS. Hematol Pathol 1994; 8: 111–16.
19. Carbone PP, Kaplan HS, Musshoff K et al. Report of the committee on Hodgkin's disease staging classification. Cancer Res 1971; 31: 1860–1.
20. Leeson MC, Makely JT, Carter JR, Krupco T. The use of radioisotope scans in the evaluation of primary lymphoma of bone. Orthop Rev 1989; 18: 410–16.
21. Moog F, Kotzerke J, Reske SN. FDG PET can replace bone scintigraphy in primary staging of malignant lymphoma. J Nucl Med 1999; 40: 1407–13.
22. Carr R, Barrington SF, Madan B et al. Detection of lymphoma in bone marrow by whole-body positron emission tomography. Blood 1998; 91: 3340–6.
23. Salter M, Sollaccio RJ, Bernreuter WK, Weppelmann B. Primary lymphoma of bone: the use of MRI in pretreatment evaluation. Am J Clin Oncol 1989; 12: 101–5.
24. Hermann G, Klein MJ, Abdelwahab IF, Kenan S. MRI appearance of primary non-Hodgkin's lymphoma of bone. Skel Radiol 1997; 26: 629–32.
25. Pettit CK, Zukerberg LR, Gray MH et al. Primary lymphoma of bone. A B cell neoplasm with high frequency of multilobulated cells. Am J Surg Pathol 1990; 14: 329–34.
26. Brousse C, Baumelou E, Morel P. Primary lymphoma of bone; a prospective study of 28 patients. Joint Bone Spine 2000; 67: 446–51.
27. Fairbanks RK, Bonner JA, Inwards CY et al. Treatment of stage IE primary lymphoma of bone. Int J Radiat Oncol Biol Phys 1994; 28: 363–72.
28. Lones MA. Anaplastic large cell lymphoma arising in bone: report of a case of the monomorphic variant with the t(2;5)(p23;q35) translocation. Arch Path Lab Med 2000; 124: 1339–43.
29. Chan JKC, Ng CS, Hui PK et al. Anaplastic large cell Ki-1 lymphoma of the bone. Cancer 1991; 68: 2186–91.
30. Dosoretz DE, Murphy GF, Raymond AK et al. Radiation therapy for primary lymphoma of bone. Cancer 1983; 51: 44–6.
31. Dubey P, Ha CS, Besa PC et al. Localized primary malignant lymphoma of bone. Int J Radiat Oncol Biol Phys 1992; 37: 1087–93.
32. Baar J, Burkes RL, Bell R et al. Primary non-Hodgkin's lymphoma of bone. A clinicopathologic study. Cancer 1994; 73: 1194–9.
33. Savage DG, Staron R. Rituximab for bone lymphoma. Ann Intern Med 2001; 134: 1156–7.
34. Dosoretz DE, Raymond KA, Murphy GF et al. Primary lymphoma of bone. The relationship of morphologic diversity to clinical behavior. Cancer 1982; 50: 1009–14.
35. Christie DR, Barton MB, Bryant G et al. Osteo-lymphoma (primary bone lymphoma): an Australian review of 70 cases. Aust NZ J Med 1999; 29: 214–19.
36. Bacci G, Ferraro A, Casadei et al. Primary lymphoma of bone: long-term results in patients treated with vincristine–adriamycin–cyclophosphamide and local radiation. J Chemother 1991; 3: 189–93.

37. Mendenhall NP, Jones JJ, Kramer BS et al. The management of primary lymphoma of bone. Radiother Oncol 1987; 9: 137–45.

38. Lewis SJ, Bell RS, Fernandes BJ, Burkes RL. Malignant lymphoma of bone. Can J Surg 1994; 37: 43–9.

39. Clayton F, Butler JJ, Ayala AG et al. Non-Hodgkin's lymphoma in bone. Pathologic and radiologic features with clinical correlates. Cancer 1987; 60: 2494–501.

40. Baar J, Burkes RL, Gospodarowicz M. Primary non-Hodgkin's lymphoma of bone. Sem Oncol 1999; 26(3): 270–5.

41. Reimer RR, Chabner BA, Young RC et al. Lymphoma presenting in bone. Results of histopathology, staging and therapy. Ann Intern Med 1977; 87: 50–5.

42. Fidias P, Spiro I, Sobzack ML et al. Long-term results of combined modality therapy in primary bone lymphoma. Int J Radiat Oncol Biol Phys 1999; 45: 1213–18.

43. Rosenberg SA, Diamond HD, Jaslowitz B et al. Lymphosarcoma: a review of 1269 cases. Medicine 1961; 40: 31–84.

44. Braunstein EM, White SJ. Non-Hodgkin lymphoma of bone. Radiology 1980; 135: 59–63.

45. Burkitt D. A sarcoma involving the jaws in African children. Br J Surg 1958; 46: 218–33.

46. Macro M, Bonnefoy C, Loyau G et al. Leucémie lymphoïde chronique avec ostéolyse iliaque. Rev Rheum 1990; 3: 236–7.

42

Lung Cancer

Daniel E. Roos

Royal Adelaide Hospital, Adelaide, South Australia

INTRODUCTION

In the Western world, lung cancer ranks second in cancer incidence behind prostate in men and breast in women, and is the number one cause of cancer death. More than 20% of patients with lung cancer have bone pain at initial presentation [1] and up to 65% will develop bone metastases during the course of their disease [2]. The management of bone metastases from carcinoma of the lung thus constitutes a significant component of oncology practice.

RELATIVE CLINICAL FEATURES OF BONE METASTASES FROM LUNG CANCER

Table 42.1 illustrates that in the context of the common malignancies associated with secondary skeletal involvement, the incidence of bone metastases from lung cancer is intermediate in frequency, but associated (together with melanoma) with the worst prognosis. The median survival with bone metastases from non-small cell lung cancer (NSCLC) is typically 3–6 months [3]. Because of the high incidence and relatively long natural history of breast and prostate cancer, these two malignancies have a much higher prevalence of bone metastases, together accounting for probably 80% of cases [3].

As with most other malignancies, bone metastases from lung cancer most commonly affect the axial skeleton. In a study of 300 patients with newly diagnosed squamous cell carcinoma (SCC) and adenocarcinoma of the lung, 121 with abnormal extra-articular bone uptake on whole body bone scan (WBBS), the commonest site was the spine (53% of patients), followed by rib (45%) and extremity (16%) [1], although the high rate of false positives on WBBS must be borne in mind (see below).

Because of the absence of symptoms early in its course, lung cancer is often disseminated at the time of diagnosis. Indeed, more than 75% of patients are not suitable for surgery because of obvious metastatic disease. Even those who undergo radical resection frequently have undetected metastases, as demonstrated in an autopsy study of 202 patients who died within a month of surgery; 35% of patients had evidence of persistent lung cancer, the pattern varying with histology and 70% of those with small cell lung cancer (SCLC) had dissemination, compared with only 33% for SCC. With the latter cell type, residual local disease was similar in frequency to distant foci, whereas SCLC and adenocarcinoma were much more commonly metastatic, mainly to liver, bone, adrenals and brain [4]. For all histologies combined, bone constitutes the commonest site of involvement at presentation, occurring in approximately 40% of patients with metastases, followed by intrathoracic (contralateral lung, mediastinum and pericardium, 30%), non-regional nodes (20%), liver (15%), brain (15%) and skin (10%) [5]. However, organ involvement varies considerably with histological sub-type. Approximately 70% of patients with disseminated SCLC before treatment have bone metastases, followed by 45% for adenocarcinoma, 25% for large cell undifferentiated carcinoma and 15% for SCC. There is less variation in the rates of bone metastases in lung cancer patients reported at autopsy (25–40%), but again, SCLC and adenocarcinoma have a higher

Textbook of Bone Metastases. Edited by C. Jasmin, R. E. Coleman, L. R. Coia, R. Capanna and G. Saillant
© 2005 John Wiley & Sons Ltd: ISBN 0 471 87742 5

Table 42.1.   Incidence and prognosis of bone metastases

Primary	Incidence in advanced disease (%)	Median survival (months)	5 year survival (%)
Myeloma	95–100	20	10
Breast	65–75	24	20
Prostate	65–75	40	25
Thyroid	60	48	40
Lung	30–40	<6	<5
Kidney	20–25	6	10
Melanoma	15–45	<6	<5

Adapted from Coleman [3].

predilection than large cell undifferentiated carcinoma and SCC [5].

There are clinical differences between involvement of the two components of the skeletal system viz. bone marrow and osseous tissue. The latter causes pain, the former is usually painless but may lead to thrombocytopenia or anaemia. SCLC has the highest propensity for marrow involvement, typically 15–25% at diagnosis, although the rates are about 10% higher if *bilateral* iliac crest aspiration and biopsy are performed [6]. Marrow involvement is approximately half as common for adenocarcinoma and large cell undifferentiated carcinoma, and rare with SCC (3%) [4].

Along with myeloma, breast, melanoma, thyroid, renal and gastrointestinal malignancies, most bone metastastes from lung cancer are lytic (especially SCC), but SCLC is notable for a higher tendency to produce osteoblastic lesions, which also occur with prostate, breast, carcinoid, Hodgkin's/non-Hodgkin's lymphoma and medulloblastoma.

A Japanese study of 112 patients with positive WBBS and cancers of the lung (39 patients), breast (27), stomach (25) and prostate (21) gives some insight into the differing natural histories of these primaries. Prostate and stomach cancers had significantly more bone metastases at the time of detection than lung cancers, but there was no correlation between the survival time and the number of lesions at presentation in the four primary types. Stomach cancer had the highest rate of increase in the number of bone metastases on serial WBBS, but the rate of increase had (negative) prognostic significance only for prostate cancer [7]. On the other hand, Park et al. in the previously mentioned retrospective series of patients with SCC or adenocarcinoma of the lung found a prognostic dichotomy based on WBBS findings. One or two (extra-articular) bone hotspots did not affect overall survival relative to no hotspots (median survival respectively 8.0, 9.5 and 9.1 months), whereas those with three or more bone hotspots had a statistically significant ($p < 0.05$) worse survival (median 3.8 months) (Figure 42.1). Of note, there was no significant difference in survival between (otherwise) stage I–IIIB patients with ⩾ 3 sites of bone uptake and stage IV with other organ metastases, or stage IV with radiologically proven bone metastases at diagnosis. This suggests that patients with ⩾ 3 extra-articular hotspots have a high probability of true bone metastases and should be considered as clinical stage IV, with correspondingly poorer prognosis [1].

DETECTION OF BONE METASTASES FROM LUNG CANCER

Technetium WBBS is well established as superior to screening radiographic bone survey in detecting skeletal metastases in lung cancer, although plain X-rays are useful in symptomatic patients or to further investigate equivocal scintigraphic lesions [4]. Routine staging bone scanning has never been shown to be cost-effective in early stage disease, but is still widely practised because of the potential implications of a positive scan. A joint statement of the American Thoracic Society and the European Respiratory Society on pre-treatment evaluation of NSCLC in 1997 advocates no pre-operative imaging of the skeleton (or brain) in patients with no symptoms or other evidence of distant metastases [8]. This is consistent with the results of a meta-analysis published in 1995, which found median negative predictive values of clinical evaluation relative to bone scan and CT brain in the range 90–95% [9]. However, a case can be made for skeletal imaging if aggressive treatment of a solitary brain metastasis is being considered (along with the lung primary), in view of the association between brain and bone metastases [10].

In SCLC, bone scan and marrow examination are complementary [4]. There is also evidence that MRI scanning further increases the detection rate, as it is

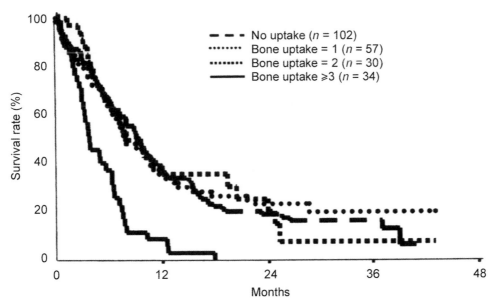

Figure 42.1. Survival curves for 223 lung cancer patients with zero, one, two or more than two extra-articular hotspots on bone scan at presentation. Patients with more than two hotspots vs. other groups ($p < 0.05$). From [1], with permission from Elsevier Science © 2000

more sensitive than WBBS in the spine and pelvis, while WBBS is more sensitive in the skull, ribs and periphery [11]. However, the clinical and cost implications of this finding remain uncertain.

Unfortunately, WBBS is limited by its low specificity, despite high sensitivity. Positron emission tomography (PET) with fluorine-18 (^{18}F) deoxyglucose (FDG-PET) shows great promise in this respect. In one series of 110 consecutive NSCLC patients, 21 with biopsy or radiographically confirmed bone metastases, the false negative rate was identical for WBBS and FDG-PET, but the latter had a far superior false positive rate for an overall accuracy of 96% with FDG-PET and 66% for WBBS (Table 42.2) [12].

This difference can be explained by the increased metabolic activity (glycolysis) of malignant lesions,

which enables them to be distinguished from most normal tissues with FDG-PET, compared with the non-selective uptake of technetium in any area of increased bone turnover (neoplastic, inflammatory, degenerative, etc.) [12]. Although potentially cost-effective in the staging of NSCLC [13], FDG-PET is currently limited by the lack of widespread availability of dedicated PET cameras [14].

EXTERNAL BEAM RADIOTHERAPY FOR BONE METASTASES FROM LUNG CANCER

At the time of writing there have been at least 17 randomised trials (including abstracts) in the English language since 1982, examining the issue of fractionation for metastatic bone pain in well over 5000 patients. Intention-to-treat response rates are approximately 60%, with about half of the responses being complete and half partial. There is little evidence of a dose-response above a single 8 Gy fraction [44]. Lung cancer has been well represented in these trials. Approximately 20% of the randomised patients had lung cancer, with breast (40%) and prostate (20%) as the other two common primaries.

Most trials have found, surprisingly, no statistically significant correlation between response and histology/primary site, although in the Radiation Therapy

Table 42.2. Comparison of technetium bone scan with PET in the detection of bone metastases from a series of 110 consecutive non-small cell lung cancer patients

	Bone scan	FDG-PET
False negative	2/21 (10%)	2/21 (10%)
False positive	35/54 (65%)	2/89 (2%)
Accuracy	73/110 (66%)	106/110 (96%)

FDG-PET, ^{18}F deoxyglucose positron emission tomography. Data from Bury et al. [12].

Oncology Group (RTOG) study, Tong et al. did report more frequent *complete* pain relief and more frequent *minimal* relief for prostate and breast primaries compared with lung or other primaries ($p < 0.001$) [16]. In the three trials from the British group (comprising Yarnold, Hoskin, Price et al.), there was also a suggestion of a lower prospect of pain relief for lung cancer patients (unquantified), regardless of the dose schedule [17].

The issue of fractionation for metastatic bone pain has been the source of considerable debate in the radiation oncology literature [18]. Despite the evidence from the above mentioned randomised trials, surveys of patterns of practice over the past decade have shown continuing reluctance of radiation oncologists (ROs) to use single fractions for metastatic bone pain (summarised in [15]). This is especially the case in the USA, where $< 1\%$ of ROs report using single fractions for bone metastases from breast and prostate cancer [19]. Major factors emerging from the surveys to explain the preference for multiple fractions include training (reflecting the "apprenticeship" nature of the specialty), private practice (reflecting reimbursement issues) and concerns about preventing recurrent pain. Although several trials *have* reported higher retreatment rates after single fractions, this is thought to reflect clinicians' lower threshold to retreat after lower doses [15]. Primary site influences fractionation, at least in Canada and Australia/New Zealand (ANZ), where this variable has been assessed. The percentage of ROs using a single 8 Gy for localised bone pain from breast, lung and prostate primaries was respectively 16%, 16% and 31% ($p = 0.056$) in Canada compared with 15%, 42% and 28% ($p = 0.013$) in ANZ [15]. In the latter survey, the presence of a neuropathic (radicular/dermatomal) component to the bone pain led to decreased use of single fractions (42 vs. 15% for lung primary). A Trans-Tasman Radiation Oncology Group randomised trial (TROG 96.05), which closed in Dec 2002, compared a single 8 Gy with 20 Gy in five fractions for neuropathic pain due to bone metastases. Response rates are of a similar order of magnitude to localised bone pain, with lung cancer accounting for approximately 30% of randomised patients in this trial [20].

WIDE-FIELD RADIOTHERAPY FOR BONE METASTASES FROM LUNG CANCER

Wide-field (so-called "hemi-body") RT can be considered in the setting of multiple/diffuse symptomatic bone metastases. In the numerous studies published over the last two decades on this treatment technique, the majority of primaries were prostate (approximately 50%) and breast (30%), with only about 10% lung cancer (representative sample in [21]). There are relative contraindications which limit its widespread applicability for lung cancer patients, viz. Karnofsky performance status < 70, life expectancy < 6 weeks and previous RT to the lung and mediastinum (for upper hemi-body). The classical doses established by RTOG Study 78-10 [22] are a single 6 Gy (uncorrected lung dose) for upper hemi-body and a single 8 Gy for mid- or lower hemi-body RT, although fractionated treatment has also been investigated (15–30 Gy at 2.5 3 Gy/fraction). Overall response rates for hemi-body RT are typically 70–100%, with pain relief usually more rapid than with focal RT [21]. However, from the limited data on lung cancer, there is some suggestion that bone metastases from this primary may respond less well than prostate and breast cancer, at least with respect to *complete* pain relief [22,23]. This mirrors the experience with localised field RT (see above).

RADIOISOTOPES FOR BONE METASTASES FROM LUNG CANCER

The majority of the literature on the current generation of radiopharmaceuticals for bone metastases, e.g. strontium-89 (^{89}Sr), samarium-153 (^{153}Sm), rhenium-186 (^{186}Re) again relates to the two common primaries with the longest survivals, viz. prostate and breast. Nevertheless, some of the randomised trials have accrued small numbers of patients with other primaries, including lung (e.g. 8/384 = 2% of patients with lung cancer in three trials investigating ^{153}Sm) [24]. There is once again some evidence that the response of lung and other primaries to both ^{89}Sr and ^{153}Sm is not as high as for breast and prostate [25,26]. Robinson reported an approximately 30% response rate to ^{89}Sr for lung cancer compared with 80% for prostate and breast [25]. The relatively limited published experience of these radiopharmaceuticals for bone metastases from lung cancer leaves their role for this indication incompletely defined at the time of writing.

CHEMOTHERAPY FOR BONE METASTASES FROM LUNG CANCER

The effectiveness of cytotoxic chemotherapy in this setting is not well documented. Most studies report overall response rates without specifying response of bone metastases *per se* and in practice, bone pain is often treated with radiotherapy instead of (or as well as) chemotherapy in view of the proven effectiveness of radiation. A survey of North American specialists who treat lung cancer found significant variation in the perceived role of chemotherapy for NSCLC with painful bone metastases—it was controversial in the USA and not recommended in Canada [27]

The focus of chemotherapy trials currently is to combine established agents with novel drugs, such as the taxanes (paclitaxel, docetaxel), camptothecins (irinotecan, topotecan) and newer anti-metabolites (e.g. gemcitabine), in order to develop more active and better-tolerated combinations [28]. However, there appears to be little interest at present in investigating the specific response of skeletal metastases from lung cancer.

There is indirect evidence of activity for chemotherapy in this setting from statistically significant falls in biochemical markers of bone metabolism (serum osteocalcin/alkaline phosphatase, and urine calcium/hydroxypyrole excretion) and decreased WBBS isotope uptake after cisplatin-based chemotherapy for NSCLC [29].

Although best documented for myeloma and breast cancer, there is also some support in randomised trials for the use of bisphosphonates in the pain management of skeletal metastases from other malignancies, including lung cancer. However, once more the number of patients accrued with this primary is relatively limited [2,30], and the benefit for rapidly progressing primaries such as lung may be marginal [31].

HYPERCALCAEMIA AND LUNG CANCER

Estimates of malignancy-associated hypercalcaemia rates vary widely in the literature, depending on the cancer population in question, the definition of hypercalcaemia and whether incidence, prevalence or risk from cancer diagnosis until death is being quoted. The prevalence at presentation to a tertiary centre (approximated by studying newly registered patients who have hypercalcaemia detected within a short period of time after registration) is, in fact, relatively low. For instance, in an MD Anderson Cancer Center study of 7667 patients, the overall rate of moderate to severe hypercalcaemia (total serum calcium ≥ 2.7 mmol/l) was only 1.2%. Lung cancer (all histologies) was the fourth commonest cause (1.9%). Of interest, although NSCLC was the second commonest primary associated with *severe* (calcium > 3.3 mmol/l) hypercalcaemia (7/677 patients), there were no cases of severe hypercalcaemia in SCLC (0/

132). Renal cell carcinoma had the highest rate overall (4.7%), but hypercalcaemia was uncommon at presentation in breast cancer (0.9%) (Table 42.3) [32].

However, a different picture emerges when considering patients with "advanced cancer" who are reported to have rates of hypercalcaemia of 5–10% [3], increasing to 20–40% "at some time during the course of their disease" [32]. Here, lung and breast cancer together may account for nearly half of malignancy-associated hypercalcaemia (Table 42.4) [33]. The reported incidence in lung cancer varies between 12.5% and 35% [34].

There are notable differences in the clinical features of hypercalcaemia as a metabolic complication of lung cancer compared with other malignancies. With lung cancer, the incidence varies with histology (most common with SCC, uncommon with adenocarcinoma, rare with SCLC) and is often unrelated to bone

Table 42.3. Estimated prevalence of moderate/severe hypercalcaemia in 7667 patients newly registered at the MD Anderson Cancer Center

Primary site	Number with hypercalcaemia/ number tested	Prevalence (%)
Urinary tract[1]	17/481	3.5
Myeloma	4/126	3.2
Unknown primary	8/329	2.4
Lung[2]	15/809	1.9
Leukaemia	6/473	1.3
Non-Hodgkin's lymphoma	4/381	1.0
Others	36/5200	0.7
Total	88/7667	1.2

[1]Renal cell carcinoma 10/212=4.7%, others 7/269=2.6%.
[2]Non-small cell carcinoma 13/677=1.9%, small cell carcinoma = 2/132=1.5%.
Data from Vassilopoulou-Sellin et al. [32].

Table 42.4. Relative frequency of malignancy-associated hypercalcaemia in a hospital survey of 219 patients

Primary site	Percentage of cases
Lung	25
Breast	20
Urothelial[1]	10
Head and neck	7
Myeloma	6
Others	32

[1]Kidney 3%, others 7%.
Data from Fisken et al. [33].

metastases, i.e. humeral factors elaborated by the tumour (parathyroid hormone-related protein, PTHrP) play a significant role. Hypercalcaemia may occur at any stage of the disease, but usually not at presentation. On the other hand, hypercalcaemia with breast cancer and myeloma is generally associated with extensive osteolytic bone destruction. In head and neck cancer, it typically occurs in the pre-terminal phase of advanced disease but is seldom related to bone metastases. It is uncommon in lymphoma, with the notable exception of adult T cell and some diffuse large B cell histologies [34].

Initial management for lung cancer-related hypercalcaemia, as for other primaries, is with rehydration and bisphosphonates, which inhibit osteoclast activity and calcium resorption from bone.

PATHOLOGICAL FRACTURE AND LUNG CANCER

Lung cancer ranks behind breast cancer and myeloma in referral rate for management of *extra-spinal* malignant pathological fracture (Table 42.5) [35], although such fractures are rare with SCLC.

However, survival after pathological fracture due to lung cancer is very poor (median 3–4 months) compared with other primaries, e.g. approximately 2 years for prostate and breast cancer, and one year for renal cell carcinoma. Nevertheless, if the patient is expected to survive for at least some weeks, surgical intervention may still be indicated to relieve the debilitating symptoms associated with pathological fracture [35].

Lung cancer also ranks behind breast and prostate cancer with respect to referral for surgical stabilisation of *spinal* fractures (Table 42.6) [36]. The low referral rates for lung cancer are very likely influenced by the

Table 42.5. Relative frequency of various primaries in a series of 239 extra-spinal pathological fractures in 211 patients

Primary site	Percentage of fractures
Breast	49
Myeloma	14
Lung	9
Prostate	9
Kidney	3
Bowel	3
Others	13

Data from Galasko [35].

Table 42.6 Relative frequency of various primaries in a series of 42 patients referred for surgical management of spinal pathological fractures

Primary site	Percentage of fractures
Breast	40
Prostate	14
Lung	7
Kidney	5
Myeloma	5
Others	29

Data from Hatrick et al. [36].

poor performance status and prognosis of these patients.

SPINAL CORD COMPRESSION AND LUNG CANCER

Spinal cord compression occurs in 8–10% of all lung cancer patients [6]. Breast and lung are the commonest causes of malignant spinal cord compression (15–20% of cases each), followed by unknown primary (about 15%) then lymphoma, prostate, sarcoma, myeloma, kidney (5–10% each) [37]. In a series of 131 patients, lung was the commonest cause of cord compression occurring as the first presentation of cancer, comprising about half of such cases. Of interest, there was a higher predilection for upper and mid-thoracic vertebrae than with other tumours. This presumably relates to regional venous drainage patterns, mirroring the increased tendency of pelvic tumours to give rise to cauda equina lesions compared to primaries from other sites [38].

There is no compelling evidence in the literature that the dose of palliative RT should be different from that used for other primaries (usually 30 Gy in 10 fractions or 20 Gy in five fractions), but the effectiveness for lung cancer is poor, typically lasting only 1–3 months [6]. The paucity of randomised data on the relative role of RT and surgical decompression/stabilisation in this setting for all primaries is well recognised. However, in view of the dismal prognosis of metastatic lung cancer, the risks of surgery are less frequently considered justified in these patients.

HYPERTROPHIC OSTEOARTHROPATHY

Approximately 10% of cases of pulmonary malignancy have associated some or all of the features of hypertrophic pulmonary osteoarthropathy (HPOA), a syndrome of digital clubbing and chronic proliferative periostitis with sub-periosteal new bone formation. There may also be arthritis of adjacent joints [39]. As such, it may mimic or occur coincident with bone metastases from lung cancer. However, the symmetrical linear cortical uptake in long bones, and polyarticular uptake in the hands and feet on WBBS, are characteristic (Figure 42.2). The aetiology and pathogenesis are unknown, but presumed to be mediated by neurohumoral factors elaborated by the tumour. HPOA may also occur with chronic pulmonary sepsis and various cardiovascular and gastrointestinal diseases. Some are idiopathic or hereditary. With lung cancer, treatment of the primary can relieve the symptoms of HPOA, but it is unknown whether radiotherapy to the involved bones/joints is effective [39].

FUTURE PROSPECTS

There has been considerable research interest recently in the investigation of biochemical markers of skeletal metastases. Type I collagen constitutes more than 90% of the organic matrix of mineralised bone and serum concentrations of collagen breakdown products (e.g. carboxy-terminal telopeptide of Type I collagen, ICTP) and collagen synthesis by-products (e.g. amino-terminal propeptide of Type I collagen, PINP) may be of value in assessing and managing patients with malignancies that metastasise to bone [40]. For lung cancer in particular, the serum levels of both ICTP and PINP are significantly increased in patients with bone metastases compared to those without distant metastases and with healthy subjects. Furthermore, unlike ICTP, PINP is significantly elevated *only* with bone metastases, not with metastases to other organs. These markers could potentially assist with assessing response to therapy, disease progression and prognosis, and the greater specificity of PINP suggests that it could also be a useful adjunctive tool for the diagnosis of bone metastases in lung cancer [41].

Whilst the clinical role of PET in the evaluation of patients with bone metastases is not yet clearly defined, as mentioned above it also shows great promise. Not only can it detect occult metastases in potentially operable early stage lung cancer, but it may be even more useful in stage III disease under consideration for radical RT or chemo-RT. Here, the pick-up rate might be expected to be higher due to the greater risk of metastases in patients with disease already known to be more advanced. MacManus et al. recently

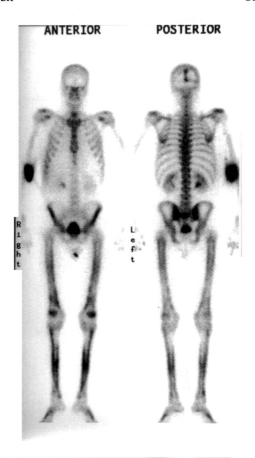

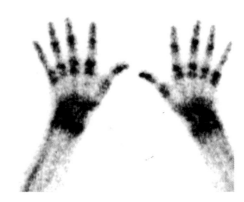

Figure 42.2. Technetium bone scan of a patient with hypertrophic osteoarthropathy due to lung cancer. From [39], with permission

demonstrated this in a series of 167 consecutive lung cancer patients with stages I–III by conventional staging, including CT chest and upper abdomen and WBBS; 32 patients (19%) were found to have distant metastases on PET (including six with bone secondaries), and there was a statistically significant increase in the rate of detection with increasing pre-PET stage ($I = 7.5\%$, $II = 18\%$, $III = 24\%$; $p = 0.016$). The detection rate for bone metastases may have been greater if PET imaging had not been restricted to the thorax and upper abdomen (due to limited availability of PET scanning time) in this study [42]. PET may also have a role in evaluating the response of bone metastases from lung and other cancers to treatment, and it is likely that new tracers, such as labelled amino acids and purine bases, will further broaden its scope in the future [43].

REFERENCES

1. Park JY, Kim KY, Lee J et al. Impact of abnormal uptakes in bone scan on the prognosis of patients with lung cancer. Lung Cancer 2000; 28: 55–62.
2. Bloomfield DJ. Should bisphosphonates be part of the standard therapy of patients with multiple myeloma or bone metastases from other cancers? An evidence-based review. J Clin Oncol 1998; 16: 1218–25.
3. Coleman RE. Skeletal complications of malignancy. Cancer 1997; 80: 1588–94.
4. Hansen HH. Evaluation of skeletal and hepatic metastases in bronchogenic carcinoma. In Muggia F, Rozencweig (eds), Lung Cancer: Prognosis in Therapeutic Research. Raven: New York, 1979: 537–42.
5. Hansen HH. Diagnosis in metastatic sites. In Straus MJ (ed), Lung Cancer: Clinical Diagnosis and Treatment, 2nd edn. Grune and Stratton: New York, 1982: 185–200.
6. Hansen HH, Goldstraw P, Gregor A et al. Tumours of the trachea and lung. In Peckham M, Pinedo H, Veronesi U (eds), Oxford Textbook of Oncology. Oxford University Press: New York, 1995: 1533–57.
7. Ohmori K, Matsui H, Yasuda T et al. Evaluation of the prognosis of cancer patients with metastatic bone tumours based on serial bone scintigrams. Jap J Clin Oncol 1997; 27: 263–7.
8. American Thoracic Society and European Respiratory Society Consensus Report. Pretreatment evaluation of non-small cell lung cancer. Am J Resp Crit Care Med 1997; 156: 320–32.
9. Silvestri GA, Littenberg B, Colice GL. The clinical evaluation for detecting metastatic lung cancer. Am J Resp Crit Care Med 1995; 152: 225–30.
10. Earnest F, Ryu JH, Miller GM et al. Suspected non-small cell lung cancer: incidence of occult brain and skeletal metastases and effectiveness of imaging for detection—pilot study. Radiology 1999; 211: 137–45.
11. Perrin-Resche I, Bizais Y, Buhe T et al. How does iliac crest bone marrow biopsy compare with imaging in the detection of bone metastases in small cell lung cancer? Eur J Nucl Med 1993; 20: 420–5.
12. Bury T, Barreto A, Daenen F et al. Fluorine-18 deoxyglucose positron emission tomography for the detection of bone metastases in patients with non-small cell lung cancer. Eur J Nucl Med 1998; 25: 1244–7.

13. Berlangieri SU, Scott AM. Metabolic staging of lung cancer. Editorial. N Engl J Med 2000; 343: 290–1.
14. Pieterman RM, van Putten JWG, Menzelaar JJ et al. Preoperative staging of non-small cell lung cancer with positron-emission tomography. N Engl J Med 2000; 343: 254–61.
15. Roos DE. Continuing reluctance to use single fractions of radiotherapy for metastatic bone pain: an Australian and New Zealand practice survey and literature review. Radiother Oncol 2000; 56: 315–22.
16. Tong D, Gillick L, Hendrickson FR. The palliation of symptomatic osseous metastases: final results of the study by the Radiation Therapy Oncology Group. Cancer 1982; 50: 893–9.
17. Bone Pain Trial Working Party (UK). 8 Gy single fraction radiotherapy for the treatment of metastatic skeletal pain: randomised comparison with a multi-fraction schedule over 12 months of patient follow-up. Radiother Oncol 1999; 52: 111–21.
18. Bentzen SM, Hoskin PJ, Roos DE et al. Fractionated radiotherapy for metastatic bone pain: evidence-based medicine or...? Letter to the Editor. Int J Radiat Oncol Biol Phys 2000; 46: 681–5.
19. Ben-Josef E, Shamsa F, Williams AO et al. Radiotherapeutic management of osseous metastases: a survey of current patterns of care. Int J Radiat Oncol Biol Phys 1998; 40: 915–21.
20. Roos DE, Turner SL, O'Brien PC et al. Randomised trial of 8 Gy in 1 versus 20 Gy in 5 fractions of radiotherapy for neuropathic pain due to bone metastases (Trans-Tasman Radiation Oncology Group, TROG 96.05). Radiother Oncol (in press).
21. Powers WE, Ratanatharathorn V. Palliation of bone metastases. In Perez CA, Brady LW (eds), Principles and Practice of Radiation Oncology. Lippincott-Raven: Philadelphia, PA, 1998; 2199–217.
22. Salazar OM, Rubin P, Hendrickson FR et al. Single-dose half-body irradiation for the palliation of multiple bone metastases from solid tumours: Final Radiation Therapy Oncology Group report. Cancer 1986; 58: 29–36.
23. Salazar OM, de Motta NW, Bridgman SM et al. Fractionated half-body irradiation (HBI) for pain palliation in widely metastatic cancer: comparison with single dose. Int J Radiat Oncol Biol Phys 1996; 36: 49–60.
24. Serafini AN. Samarium Sm-153 lexidronam for the palliation of bone pain associated with metastases. Cancer 2000; 88: 2934–9.
25. Robinson RG. Strontium-89 for bone pain due to blastic metastatic disease. Appl Radiol Aug 1993: 44–7.
26. Serafini AN, Houston SJ, Resche I et al. Palliation of pain associated with metastatic bone cancer using samarium-153 lexidronam: a double-blind placebo-controlled clinical trial. J Clin Oncol 1998; 16: 1574–81.
27. Palmer MJ, O'Sullivan B, Steele R et al. Controversies in the management of non-small cell lung cancer: the results of an expert surrogate study. Radiother Oncol 1990; 19: 17–28.
28. Anonymous. Importance of established drugs in the new millennium. Editorial. Oncol Commun 2000; 4: 1.
29. Kolaczkowska M, Junik R, Rzymkowska M et al. The effect of chemotherapy on bone metabolism in patients with non-small cell lung cancer [Polish]. Pneumonolgia i Alergolgia Polska 1998; 66: 283–9.

30. Piga A, Bracci R, Ferretti B et al. A double blind randomized study of oral clodronate in the treatment of bone metastases from tumours poorly responsive to chemotherapy. J Exp Clin Cancer Res 1998; 17: 213–7.

31. Elomaa I. Use of bisphosphonates in skeletal metastases. Acta Oncol 2000; 39: 445–54.

32. Vassilopoulou-Sellin R, Newman BM, Taylor SH et al. Incidence of hypercalcaemia in patients with malignancy referred to a comprehensive cancer center. Cancer 1993; 71: 1309–12.

33. Fisken RA, Heath DA, Bold AM. Hypercalcaemia—a hospital survey. Qu J Med 1980; 196: 405–18.

34. Muggia FM. Overview of cancer-related hypercalcaemia: epidemiology and etiology. Semin Oncol 1990; 17(suppl 5): 3–9.

35. Galasko CSB. Pathological fracture. In Peckham M, Pinedo H, Veronesi U (eds), Oxford Textbook of Oncology. Oxford University Press: New York, 1995: 2286–95.

36. Hatrick NC, Lucas JD, Timothy AR et al. The surgical treatment of metastatic disease of the spine. Radiother Oncol 2000; 56: 335–9.

37. Fuller BG, Heiss J, Oldfield EH. Spinal cord compression. In De Vita VT, Hellman S, Rosenberg SA (eds), Cancer: Principles and Practice of Oncology. Lippincott-Raven: Philadelphia, PA, 1997: 2476–86.

38. Stark RJ, Henson RA, Evans SJ. Spinal metastases: a retrospective survey from a general hospital. Brain 1982; 105: 189–213.

39. Roos DE. Hypertrophic pulmonary osteoarthropathy: is there a role for radiotherapy to symptomatic sites? Case report and literature review. Acta Oncol 1996; 35: 101–5.

40. Demers LM, Costa L, Lipton A. Biochemical markers and skeletal metastases. Cancer 2000; 88: 2919–26.

41. Kobayashi T, Gabazza EC, Taguchi O et al. Collagen metabolites as tumour markers in patients with lung carcinoma. Cancer 1999; 85: 1951–7.

42. MacManus MP, Hicks R, Matthews JP et al. High rate of detection of unsuspected distant metastases by PET in apparent stage III non-small cell lung cancer: implications for radical radiation therapy. Int J Radiat Oncol Biol Phys 2001; 50: 287–93.

43. Cook GJ, Fogelman I. The role of positron emission tomography in the management of bone metastases. Cancer 2000; 88: 2917–33.

44. Roos DE, Fischer RJ. Radiotherapy for painful bone metastases: an overview of the overviews. Clin Oncol 2003; 15: 342–4. Erratum 2003; 15: 509.

43

Kidney Cancer

Uzma Malik and Mohammed Mohiuddin

A. B. Chandler Medical Center, Lexington, KY, USA

INTRODUCTION

Renal cell carcinoma is an unusual tumour, both in its biological behaviour and its response to treatment [1]. Approximately 30% of patients present with distant metastases at the time of diagnosis [2,3]. The sites of distribution include lung, soft tissue, bone, liver, skin and central nervous system [4]. The percentage of patients who develop metastases during the course of the disease has been shown to be as high as 90% [5]. Of this group, 25–50% will have osseous metastases [5,6]. Satisfactory palliation of metastatic bone disease is important, not only for pain control and comfort measures, but also to prevent complications which can, potentially, result in high morbidity. Satisfactory palliation is also important because patients with predominantly bone metastases have longer survival than patients with predominantly visceral metastases. The median survival for patients with bone metastases associated with renal cell carcinoma is approximately 12 months [7].

DISTRIBUTION OF BONE METASTASES FROM KIDNEY CANCER

The site of osseous metastasis is most likely to be in the axial skeleton. Common sites of involvement include vertebrae, ribs, humerus, femur, skull and pelvis. By virtue of their number, ribs are often involved and this may be as high as 35–40% of metastatic bone lesions [8]. Thoracic spine and lumbar spine lesions account for approximately 30% each of all metastatic bone disease secondary to kidney cancer [8]. A pelvic metastasis (sacrum, ilium, ischium or pubis) is present in about 40% of all patients. When the long bones are involved, the proximal portion is far more likely to have a lesion than the distal area and the lower arm and lower leg are only involved in < 5% of all patients [8]. The proximal portion of the humerus and femur is involved in 20% and 27% of patients, respectively (Table 43.1).

One of the most notable features of this tumour is the unusual and bizarre pattern of metastatic spread, including such sites as the iris, nose, epididymis, gall bladder, urinary bladder and corpus cavernosum [9]. In terms of bony metastases, another unusual facet of the metastatic pattern of this tumour is its propensity to metastasise to the scapula [10]. Scapular metastasis may be the presenting symptom, is frequently large and, generally, not part of a picture of disseminated disease [10]. The cause of this predilection is not clearly known but is likely related to vascular features. The renal veins have tributaries from the back and abdominal walls and the scapula itself has an extensive anastomosis of veins on its costal and dorsal surfaces, which may connect with the vessels draining the kidney [11,12]. In a review by Gurney and colleagues, 36.6% of patients with metastatic bone disease secondary to kidney cancer had disease in the scapula. These were mostly solitary or associated with a small number of asymptomatic metastases in other bones (Table 43.2). In two patients, the diagnosis of the primary tumour was suspected by the presentation of a patient with a large scapular tumour [10].

The presence of metastatic lesions in hands and feet has also been reported, although infrequently, and has usually been associated with diffuse tumour spread and

Textbook of Bone Metastases. Edited by C. Jasmin, R. E. Coleman, L. R. Coia, R. Capanna and G. Saillant
© 2005 John Wiley & Sons Ltd: ISBN 0 471 87742 5

Table 43.1.   Sites of osseous metastases

Site	Number of patients	Percentage of patients
Skull	41	16.3
Maxilla	2	0.8
Mandible	3	1.2
Spine		
Cervical	22	8.7
Thoracic	84	33.3
Lumbar	80	31.7
Sacrum	23	9.1
Ribs	98	38.9
Clavicle	15	6.0
Scapula	39	15.5
Humerus	52	20.6
Radius	7	2.8
Ulna	2	0.8
Ilium	76	30.2
Ischium	25	9.9
Pubis	9	3.6
Femur	68	27.0
Lower leg	3	1.2

From Swanson et al. [8] Osseous metastases secondary to renal cell carcinoma. Urology 1981; 18: 556–61

Table 43.2.   Scapular metastases in patients with hypernephroma

Metastatic pattern	Number of patients	Patients requiring palliative radiotherapy
Scapula only	6	5
Scapula and two other sites	7	6
Scapula and three other sites	2	0
Total	15	11

From Gurney et al. [10] Bone metastases in hypernephroma; frequency of scapular involvement. Cancer 1989; 64: 1429–31

becomes continuous and unrelenting. Most metastatic lesions are painful, although some may be asymptomatic and are detected only by investigations. Additional characteristics are related to the specific sites involved. Shoulder girdle metastases, which are not uncommon in kidney cancer, often present as a frozen shoulder, whereas thoracic and vertebral body involvement may cause referred pain to the chest wall and the lower extremities. Lumbar vertebral disease

a poor prognosis. One theory regarding the infrequency of metastatic involvement of these parts of the skeleton is the relative paucity of red marrow in these bones, given that haematogenous spread is the most likely cause of metastatic disease [13].

FEATURES AND GENERAL CONSIDERATIONS OF BONE METASTASES SECONDARY TO KIDNEY CANCER

Bone metastases from kidney cancer are most frequently the result of haematogenous spread and are usually multifocal rather than solitary. Solitary lesions may be present in 30% of patients with metastatic disease [8,14]. Bone that is invaded by metastatic cancer typically exhibits three patterns: osteolytic, osteoblastic and, less commonly, mixed. A given patient may demonstrate a combination of patterns. Kidney cancer's radiographic appearance is invariably lytic, often with large expansile lesions (Figure 43.1).

Clinical Characteristics

The hallmark of skeletal metastases, irrespective of histology, is localised pain. The pain pattern is initially intermittent and unrelated to activity but eventually

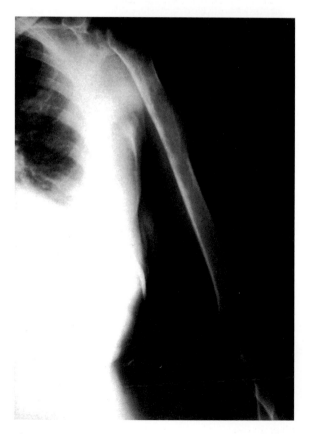

Figure 43.1.

often presents as low back pain, sciatica or both. The most serious complication of vertebral metastases is secondary epidural compression of the spinal cord and cauda equina [15].

Laboratory Evaluation

Laboratory evaluation for the detection of renal skeletal disease includes CBC, serum calcium, serum phosphorus and alkaline phosphatase levels. These tests are not specific for bony metastases. Although hypercalcaemia is not directly related to the extent of bony disease, patients with bony metastases often have high serum calcium levels.

DETECTION OF BONE METASTASES

Plain Radiographs

Plain radiographs are one of the first investigations conducted in evaluation of skeletal metastases.

Biopsy

A confirmatory pathological evaluation is often performed by simple needle biopsy under radiographic control, if clinically indicated.

Bone Scintigraphy

Bone scans have traditionally been part of the metastatic work-up in earlier stage disease, due to the importance of detecting spread before surgery, as the prognosis is not improved by radical nephrectomy in this setting [16]. With increased sensitivity over plain films and the potential for earlier detection of disease, nuclear bone scans would seem a valuable investigation, not only in the metastatic setting but also for screening. However, in the absence of bone pain or an elevated alkaline phosphatase level, bone scans provide a low yield [17]. They are, on the other hand, useful for confirming clinically or radiographically detected metastases and to determine the extent of osseous metastases in patients with renal cell carcinoma. While ordinary radiological techniques require a change in bone mineralisation of as much as 30% before a lesion becomes visible, bone scans can pick up disease much earlier. Bone scan findings correlated well with alkaline phosphatase levels and bone pain symptoms (Table 43.3).

Table 43.3. Bone scan findings correlated with alkaline phosphatase levels and bone pain

Pathological stage	Number of scans	Elevated alkaline phosphatase levels ($n=115$)	Bone pain	Abnormal bone scan
I	17	3	10	0
II	3	3	3	0
III	10	5	3	–
IV	20	13	16	15

From Benson et al. [16] Staging renal carcinoma. Arch Surg 1989; 124: 71–3

Blacher and colleagues reported on a comparison between the findings on bone scan and clinical status at presentation of patients with renal cell carcinoma. Of 29 patients with proven osseous metastases at the time of their initial evaluation, 27 had abnormal bone scans (sensitivity of 93%). Of the remaining 56 patients without metastatic disease, 48 had normal bone scans for a specificity of 86% (Table 43.4). Also, in this report, in all patients whose abnormal bone scans indicated metastatic disease, there were either clinical signs (bone pain), laboratory findings (elevated alkaline phosphatase) or routine radiographic procedures (chest X-ray, intravenous pyelogram, or angiogram) suggesting disease metastatic to bone [18]. Most reports, therefore, indicate that routine bone scans are not warranted and should be reserved for patients in whom spread is suggested on chemical or clinical grounds.

Bone scanning can also be used to follow metastases and their response to treatments. In a report by Grob and colleagues, quantitative bone scintigraphy permitted the development of several coefficients, which can be utilised as objective criteria for assessment of treatment and also development of bone metastasis during therapy [19]. The first coefficient, global ratio (GR) is the fraction of injected tracer radioactivity that is retained in the skeleton. $GR=$total activity at 3 h/total activity at 5 min. The second coefficient, $R1$,

Table 43.4. Comparison between clinical findings and bone scan interpretation

Osseous metastasis evident at presentation	Interpretation of bone scan	
	Abnormal	Normal
Yes	27	2
No	8	48

From Blacher et al. [18] Value of routine radionuclide bone scans in renal cell carcinoma. Urology 1985; 26(5): 432–4

represents the ratio of tracer activity in a region of interest and activity, in the reference zone. It ensures reproducibility of scans obtained on different occasions and under varied conditions: $R1$ =activity in region of interest/activity in reference zone. The third coefficient, $R2$, is the product of GR and $R1$ and constitutes the final, corrected measure of quantified tracer activity in metastatic sites: $R2 = (GR) \times (R1)$. The use of GR, $R1$ and $R2$ allowed patients to be followed during treatment and to evaluate the results of treatment. Coefficients were calculated before treatment and usually about every 3 months after treatment began. Patients could be divided into three groups:

1. Those with better results; coefficients were lower than before treatment.
2. Those whose coefficients did not change much during treatment.
3. Those whose coefficients increased in spite of treatment, indicating progressive disease (Table 43.5).

Computed Tomography

CT scanning has proved useful in evaluating hot spots to confirm the presence of metastatic disease. This may be especially important in solitary lesions. In addition, CT is also helpful in assessing the extent of the metastatic lesion. Hypernephromas, unlike other carcinomas, are often associated with a large extraosseous component. Therefore, before any surgical intervention, CT is recommended.

Magnetic Resonance Imaging

MRI is more sensitive than CT scanning for detection of bone marrow involvement and can be used for early detection of cancellous bone involvement by tumour [20]. MRI in the sagittal plane also allows visualisation of the entire spine and can be used for the primary investigation of epidural cord or nerve root compression, as can myelography.

Angiography

One significant surgical consideration of metastatic hypernephromas is that they are extremely vascular. Life-threatening haemorrhage can easily occur from a small incision. Therefore, before any surgical intervention, angiography is recommended. If biopsy is

Table 43.5. Normalisation of $R2$ in six treated patients with bone metastases

Patients located	Initial	3 Months	6 Months	9 Months	12 Months
1	Cervical=0.2	–	2.5	–	–
	Thoracic=8.3	–	5.4	–	–
	Lumbar=5.6	–	3.4	–	–
2	Cervical=8.5	8.5	2.6	1.5	–
	Thoracic=11.3	11.3	5.7	4.4	–
	Pelvic=6.1	6.1	3.0	2.5	–
3	Cervical=20.2	–	5.1	–	–
	Thoracic=15.2	–	4.9	–	–
	Pelvic=8.8	–	4.9	–	–
4	Cervical=13.4	3.7	5.6	2.5	2.2
	Thoracic=34.0	10.5	9.5	5.3	4.0
	Lumbar=23.7	8.9	7.3	4.7	3.2
	Pelvic=22.6	8.2	6.9	5.5	4.2
5	Thoracic=10.8	9.2	5.3	–	–
	Pelvic=7.3	7.1	5.7	–	–
6	Thoracic=17.6	–	3.8	–	–
	Lumbar=14.2	–	5.0	–	–
	Pelvic=13.2	–	4.0	–	–

From Grob et al. [19] Quantitative bone scintigraphy in the survey of bone-seeking cancers. In Bollack CG, Jacqmin D (eds), Basic Research and Treatment of Renal Cell Carcinoma Metastasis. EORTC Genitourinary Group Monograph 1990; 9: 187–94

required, needle biopsy is recommended. If an open biopsy is needed, pre-operative embolisation should be considered. The need for surgery is indicated by large lesions, progressive bony destruction, instability or impending fracture. Cryosurgery has been used as a surgical adjuvant in decreasing bleeding and in increasing local tumour control [21]. Palliative embolisation alone, without surgery, has been shown to effect good pain relief [22]. This may be especially useful in large pelvic metastases.

MANAGEMENT OF PATIENTS WITH BONE METASTASES

Radiation therapy is the mainstay for relieving the symptoms of metastatic bone lesions, although surgery, chemotherapy and immunotherapy have all been tried.

External Beam Radiotherapy

External beam radiation therapy used for palliation of symptomatic metastases has been reported to yield responses in one-half to two-thirds of patients [23]. Many radiation oncologists believe that pain from renal cell carcinoma metastatic to bone is difficult to palliate [24]. However, many feel this relative radio-resistance can be overcome by sufficiently high doses of radiation. In a report by Onufrey and Mohiuddin, the optimal dose, time and fractionation needed to achieve maximal palliative benefit in this disease was assessed [1]. Doses varied from 2000–6000 cGy. The most commonly used regimen was 3000 cGy in 10 fractions. To compare various fractionation schemes, all courses were converted to time-dose fractionation (TDF) values, using the method of Orton and Ellis. Response to treatment was evaluated on the basis of relief of symptoms, either complete, partial or no change. A significantly higher response rate of 65% was observed for total doses equal to or greater than a TDF of 70, compared to 25% for doses lower than a TDF of 70, which is equivalent to a dose of approximately 45 Gy at 180–200 cGy fractions. No difference in response was observed for either bone or soft tissue metastasis or visceral disease. The conclusions from this review suggested that metastatic bone lesions from carcinoma of the kidney should be treated to higher doses to obtain maximum response rates. Bostel and colleagues supported similar results. In 52 patients treated with palliative intent for bone metastases, it was found that success, although obtained in terms of palliation, was retarded and appeared often after a dose of more than 30 Gy [25]. Similar results have been reported by others in the literature, that tumours generally considered to be "radiation-resistant" require higher doses for pain relief (Table 43.6).

Table 43.6. Clinical reports of dose–response for local-field therapy

Author	Endpoint	Dose	Improved (%)	Failed (%)
Vikram and Chu (base of skull)	Improvement of symptoms	24 Gy	57	22 overall
		30 Gy	79	
		36 Gy	57	
Onufrey and Mohiuddin (renal cell)	Response	< 70 Gy TDF	30	Not stated
		> 70 Gy TDF	67	
		Dose range: 20–60 Gy		
Rate et al. (melanoma)	Pain relief	< 30 Gy	69	Not stated
		< 30 Gy	92	
Archangeli et al.	Complete pain relief	< 40 Gy	51	19 overall
		> 40 Gy	70	
Adamietz et al. (myeloma)	Complete pain relief	29.5 Gy + CTb	80	20 overall
		32 Gy	40	
Weber et al.	Decreased pain and disability	30 Gy	81	19
		40 Gy	88	12
Methal et al. (retreatment)	Complete or partial response	8–10 Gy	74	Not stated
		26–30 Gy	91	

TDF, time-dose factor; CT, chemotherapy.
A Even in these and other studies, 8–30% of patients failed to get any pain relief.
B Concurrent chemotherapy increased dose–response.
From Perez CA [53] Updates Principles Pract Radiat Oncol 2000; 1(1)

Table 43.7.   Results of radiation therapy: response of symptoms vs. dose

TDF equivalent	Pain (36 sites)		Mass (14 sites)		CNS metastasis (10 sites)	
	With response	Without response	With response	Without response	With response	Without response
< 45	3	1	–	–	–	1
45–65	11	3	5	1	2	4
66–85	9	2	2	2	1	2
86–100	5	2	–	1	–	–
> 100	–	–	2	1	–	–
Total	28	8	9	5	3	7
	(77%)	(23%)	(64%)	(36%)	(30%)	(70%)

From Varm et al. [22] Therapeutic embolization of pelvic metastases of renal cell carcinoma. Cancer 1983; 51: 614–17

Halperin and Harisiadis, however, presented data that did not show a dose–response relationship in metastatic renal cell carcinoma [23]. Bone pain responded at 77% of the treated sites, but the spinal cord compression response rate was only 30%. No correlation between TDF equivalent dose of radiation administered and frequency of palliative response or duration of response was found (Tables 43.7 and 43.8). Doses with TDF equivalents of 45–65 (30–40 Gy in normal fractionation) produced a frequency and duration of pain response equal to higher doses. In those sites where a response of bone pain to radiation was observed, 86% of the responses lasted the remainder of the patient's life. Objective radiographic responses occurred in 50% of patients. The conclusions from this paper suggested that radiation may be a useful palliative tool for bone pain and mass effect from metastatic renal cell carcinoma. Inordinately high doses need not be used to achieve the desired effect [23]. However, to provide structural stability for weight-bearing bones, such as the femur, a TDF equivalent of 75–85 Gy (55–60 Gy) was recommended.

Similar results, without a correlation with dose equivalence, were demonstrated by Cutuli et al. [26]. On average, this group of patients received an equivalent dose of 42 Gy. The effectiveness on pain was considered good in 39%, moderate in 18%, poor in 21% and unknown in 25% of cases.

Although conflicting results have been demonstrated in the literature to date, most feel that renal cell carcinoma is a radioresistant cancer. Controversy continues regarding the need for dose escalation to overcome the inherent resistance of these tumours when they metastasise. A recent report by DiBiase and associates used the linear quadratic model as a paradigm to assess the biologically effective dose of radiotherapy. This review included 150 patients with

Table 43.8.   Duration of bone pain control from irradiation vs. dose at 28 initially responding sites

TDF equivalent	Initial responders	Duration of response/number of sites at risk during months:			
		1–3	4–6	7–12	13+
< 45	3	1/1	1/1	1/1	–
45–65	11	6/6	1/1	2/2	1/2
66–85	9	3/3	2/2	1/1	1/3
86–100	5	1/1	–	1/1	2/3
Total	28	11/11	4/4	5/5	4/8

From Varm et al. [22] Therapeutic embolization of pelvic metastases of renal cell carcinoma. Cancer 1983; 51: 614–17

metastatic renal cell cancer. Of these, 89 had bone metastases. A biologically effective dose using an α-β of 10 was calculated. Overall, 86% of patients derived a palliative response after treatment with RT, of which 49% showed a complete palliative response. The median duration of palliation (CR and PR) was 6 months. Performance status was prognostic, with 55% achieving a CR if KPS was 70 or higher, compared to 31% if KPS was less than 70. A biologically effective dose of 50 Gy or greater vs. < 50 Gy resulted in higher response rates of 59% and 39%, respectively, a result which was statistically significant ($p=0.001$). Therefore, despite the prevailing concept that renal cell cancer is resistant to radiation, the majority of patients can be adequately palliated. A complete palliative response is more likely to occur with higher biologically effective doses of 50 Gy or higher and in patients with a higher KPS of 70 or more [27].

We recommend such a dose at our institution, especially in patients whose disease burden is minimal. These patients tend to be generally well, with good performance status. Many have long disease-free intervals between initial diagnosis and subsequent development of metastases and overall survival in these patients is also, often, appreciably prolonged. Our practice is to use a higher dose per fraction of 250 cGy to a total dose of 50 Gy. There is evidence that tumours that are felt to be radioresistant, such as melanomas and renal cell cancers, may benefit from a higher dose per fraction.

Nephrectomy and Resection of Metastases

Nephrectomy is not infrequently performed in patients with metastatic renal cell carcinoma, particularly to alleviate pain, haemorrhage, malaise, hypercalcaemia, erythrocytosis or hypertension. Removal of the primary tumour may improve some or all of these abnormalities [28]. However, there does not appear to be a benefit to nephrectomy in the metastatic setting in terms of survival. Although there are isolated reports of regression of metastatic renal cell carcinoma after removal of the primary tumour, only 4/474 patients ($< 1\%$) in nine series who underwent nephrectomy experienced regression of their metastatic foci [29,30]. Therefore, adjuvant nephrectomy is not recommended for the purpose of inducing spontaneous regression of metastatic lesions.

Resection of metastatic foci is also a surgical option that can be considered. Of the 30% of patients with metastatic renal cell carcinoma who present with metastases, less than 5% have solitary metastasis [31]. Patients with a solitary metastasis synchronous with a primary lesion have decreased survival compared to patients who develop metastasis after the primary tumour is removed [29]. Surgical resection is appropriate in selected patients. Five year survival rates of 23–34% may result after resection of a solitary metastasis which has presented in a synchronous fashion after resection of the primary tumour [32]. Resection of the primary tumour and solitary metastasis should be considered if the presentation is synchronous with the primary tumour or metachronous, as this treatment can produce some long-term survivors.

Surgery of metastatic foci may also be considered for orthopaedic palliation. The need for surgery is indicated by large lesions, progressive bony destruction, severe uncontrollable pain, instability or impending fracture. Prophylactic internal fixation is advised for long weight-bearing bones if 50% or more of the diaphysis is involved, 50% or more of the cortex is destroyed or the lesion is more than 2.5 cm in the femoral neck, sub- or intertrochanteric region or in the supracondylar region. Smith and colleagues reported on 20 palliative orthopaedic procedures of which 85% resulted in significant functional improvement and 90% resulted in significant relief of pain [33]. Average survival after the palliative procedure was 22 months. As the majority of patients will survive long enough to benefit from palliative orthopaedic procedures, this treatment option is effective and should not be overlooked. At least 2 months of survival should be expected for surgery to be indicated [14]. The use of local cryotherapy, using liquid nitrogen, at the time of surgery, or polymethyl methacrylate, can also be considered. There is a suggestion that the number of viable tumour cells may be reduced by the heat generated by polymethyl methacrylate, thereby decreasing the chance of local recurrence [13].

Hypernephromas and their bone metastases are extremely vascular tumours. Surgical treatment of hypervascular bone lesions can result in excessive operative blood loss. Pre-operative transcatheter embolisation can successfully reduce the amount of blood loss [34]. Embolisation alone may, on occasion, without simultaneous surgical intervention, result in good pain control [22,35]. O'Reilly reported on four patients with a solitary vertebral metastasis resulting in acute spinal cord compression or nerve root compression. Embolisation reduced the venous blood pool within the tumours, resulting in progressive neurological improvement often lasting for 12 weeks or more. Although none of the patients recovered completely, there was significant improvement in their neurological dysfunction. Embolisation is potentially effective in pelvic metastases, which are often quite large with an extensive soft tissue component. Embolisation of such metastases produced good pain palliation and objective recalcification in 4/5 patients [36]. In patients who have not responded to radiation therapy and in whom surgical intervention is being considered, this procedure can be tried to make surgery more manageable or in place of surgery in those who are not surgical candidates.

Cryosurgery

Cryosurgery is the use of liquid nitrogen as a surgical adjunct to freeze any residual tumour to enhance local control. This technique has been utilised by Marcove at Memorial Sloan-Kettering and is useful for tumours that have recurred despite radiation therapy and in the treatment of renal cell carcinoma [21].

Chemotherapy

Carcinoma of the kidney is considered to be a chemo-resistant tumour. There is no conventionally accepted active cytotoxic chemotherapy regimen for advanced renal cell carcinoma. A review of literature evaluating Phase II trials between 1983 and 1989 showed an overall objective response rate of less than 9%, which was also of short duration [37]. This drug refractoriness is felt to be due to expression of the multidrug resistance gene product, p-glycoprotein. Over the years, initially monotherapies and, subsequently, combination chemotherapy regimens were tried but, unfortunately, response rates have been in the 10–20% range. Anthracyclines and cisplatinum also did not improve on these results (Table 43.9).

Only four cytotoxic agents, vinblastine, CCNU, hydroxyurea and ifosfamide have resulted in a consistent effect of 10–20% response rate in metastatic renal cell cancer. Vinblastine and CCNU are the best-investigated substances and should be favoured in the treatment of metastatic renal cell cancer.

Rini and colleagues recently reported on weekly gemcitabine with continuous infusion of 5-fluorouracil (5-FU) as an active combination in patients with metastatic RCC. Gemcitabine and 5-FU resistance is not thought to be related to p-glycoprotein over-expression, which may be the cause of chemoresistance in this disease. These two agents may, therefore, be more effective than other agents in achieving adequate intracellular concentrations. Of 39 assessable patients, there were no complete responses but seven partial responses for an objective response rate of 17%. There was an improvement in progression-free survival, with the test group surviving for 28.7 weeks vs. 8 weeks for a similar historical cohort. The regimen was well tolerated, with fatigue, mucositis, nausea, vomiting and grade 2 haematological toxicities being the most common side-effects [38].

Intra-arterial chemotherapy can facilitate the delivery of cytotoxic agents into tumour-bearing regions to produce a greater differential exposure between tumours and the normal sensitive host tissues, and can allow intravascular occlusion and infusion therapy by means of selective catheterisation of the arterial supply of the neoplasm [39].

Hormonal Therapy

Medroxyprogesterone acetate has been used in the past for treatment of metastatic renal cell carcinoma. However, this practice has been questioned. The reason for this is that oestrogen and progesterone receptors have not been detected in significant numbers to give a sound basis for the introduction of hormone therapy in these patients [40]. This review did find glucocorticoid receptors in significant amounts in about half of the renal cell carcinoma specimens, as well as dihydrotestosterone receptors. The value of medroxyprogesterone therapy has been reviewed critically by Kjaer, who has concluded that, irrespective of dose and schedule, human renal cell carcinoma is neither hormone-dependent nor hormone-responsive

Table 43.9. Results of combination chemotherapy in patients with metastatic renal cancer (1979–1986)

Drug	Reference	Number of patients treated	Response (CR + PR)	
			(n)	(%)
Cyclophosphamide + VBL + hydroxyurea + MPA + prednisone	Talley et al. [2]	42	8	18
MTX-CF + VCR + bleomycin + cyclophosphamide (vs. peptichemio)	Baumgartner et al. [11]	12	2	17
VCR + ifosfamide (sequential)	Konig and Hartwich [12]	30	4	13
CCNU + cyclophosphamide + megoestrol acetate	Puckett et al. [13]	37	7	19
VBL + cyclophosphamide + 5-fluorouracil	Halpern et al. [14]	10	–	–
CCNU + cyclophosphamide + hydroxyurea	Engelholm et al. [15]	25	2	8
VBL + methylglyoxal-BG	Todd et al. [16]	15	–	–
High-dose MTX-CF + VBL + bleomycin (± tamoxifen)	Bell et al. [17]	34	10	29
Cyclophosphamide + misonidazole	Glover et al. [18]	30	1	3

VBL, vinblastine; MTX, methotrexate; BG, bis-guanylhydrazone; VCR, vincristine; CF, citrovorum factor rescue; MPA, medroxyprogesterone acetate.
From Grob et al. [19] Quantitative bone scintigraphy in the survey of bone-seeking cancers. In Bollack CG, Jacqmin D (eds), Basic Research and Treatment of Renal Cell Carcinoma Metastasis. EORTC Genitourinary Group Monograph 1990; 9: 187–94

[41]. Minervini et al., however, have presented a case of regression of disseminated skeletal metastases from a hypernephroma by long-term treatment with medroxyprogesterone acetate 1000 mg daily for 30 days, followed by 500 mg twice weekly [42].

Biological Therapy

Cytotoxic chemotherapy and hormonal therapy are ineffective treatments for advanced RCC. This has resulted in an interest in biological response modifiers. Extensive Phase II trials with interferon (IFN) preparations, IFNα and IFNβ, have shown response rates in the 15–20% range, with median response durations in the range 6–10 months [43]. Dose of 5–10 million IU/m^2 i.m. or s.c. daily or 3–5 times/week has been used most often. Responses correlate with good performance status, previous nephrectomy and lung-predominant disease. Patients with non-resected primary tumours, bulky visceral metastatic disease or bony metastatic disease are less likely to respond, although responses at all sites have been reported [44]. A Phase III trial of vinblastine plus IFNα2a vs. vinblastine alone in patients with advanced or metastatic renal cell carcinoma showed the combination to be superior to vinblastine alone in terms of median survival, which was 67.6 weeks vs. 37.8 weeks, and also in terms of overall response rates, being 16.5% vs. 2.5% for vinblastine alone [45]. However, response to vinblastine alone was lower than usual. Neither response nor survival improved with the combination of 13-cis-retinoic acid and IFNα2a [46].

Interleukin-2 (IL-2) has also been used in metastatic renal cell carcinoma to bone. Response rates with high-dose IL-2 in metastatic renal cell carcinoma, whether administered as a single agent by bolus or continuous infusion or in combination with LAK cells or IFNα are in the range 15–20%. Patients with higher performance status are likely to experience higher response rates [47–49].

The option of switching to the other cytokine after failure on one was assessed. This was felt to be a poor strategy, with only 5/113 patients showing a partial response to the alternative cytokine [50].

Other Therapies

Because of the highly vascular nature of RCC, antiangiogenesis therapy may prove to be useful. A Phase II study done on 33 patients with the fumigillin analogue, TNP 470, at a dose of 60 mg/m^2 infused over 1 h 3 times/week, showed the therapy to be well tolerated. There was only one partial response with an overall response rate of 3% [51].

PROGNOSIS

The relationship between pretreatment clinical features and survival is important to predict survival in metastatic renal cell cancer. A review by Motzer and colleagues showed the median survival time to be 10 months; 5 year survival is less than 9%. Pretreatment features associated with a shorter survival were low Karnofsky performance status (< 80%), high serum lactate dehydrogenase (> 1.5 times upper limit of normal), low haemoglobin (< lower limit of normal), high corrected serum calcium (> 10 mg/dl) and absence of prior nephrectomy. These were used as risk factors to categorise patients into three different groups. The median time to death in the favourable risk patients (0 risk factors) was 20 months. One or two risk factors resulted in intermediate risk with a median survival time of 10 months. Patients with three or more risk factors had a median survival time of 4 months. These risk categories can be used in patient management [52].

REFERENCES

1. Onufrey MD, Mohiuddin M. Radiation therapy in the treatment of metastatic renal cell carcinoma. Int J Radiat Oncol Biol Phys 1985; 11: 2007–9.
2. Guiliami L, Giberti C, Martorana G et al. Radical extensive surgery for renal cell carcinoma: long-term results and prognostic factors. J Urol 1990; 143: 468.
3. Selli C, Hinshaw WM, Woodard BH et al. Stratification of risk factors in renal cell carcinoma. Cancer 1983; 53: 899.
4. Maldazys JD, deKernion JB. Prognostic factors in metastatic renal cell carcinoma. J Urol 1986; 136: 376.
5. Saitoh H. Distant metastasis of renal adenocarcinoma. Cancer 1981; 48: 1487–91.
6. Swanson DA, Orovan WL, Johnson DE, Giacco G. Osseous metastases secondary to renal cell carcinoma. Urology 1981; 18: 556.
7. Powers WE, Ratanatharathorn V. Palliation of bone metastases. In Perez CA, Brady LW (eds), Principles and Practice of Radiation Oncology, 3rd edn. Lippincott-Raven: Philadelphia, PA, 1998: 2199–217.
8. Swanson D, Orovan W, Johnson D, Giacco G. Osseous metastases secondary to renal cell carcinoma. Urology 1981; 18: 556–61.
9. Ritchie AWS, Chisholm GD. The natural history of renal carcinoma. Semin Oncol 1983; 10: 390–400.
10. Gurney H, Larcos G, McKay M et al. Bone metastases in hypernephroma; frequency of scapular involvement. Cancer 1989; 64: 1429–31.

11. Davis RA, Milloy FJ, Anson BT. Lumbar, renal and associated parietal and visceral veins based upon a study of 100 specimens. Surg Gynecol Obstet 1958; 107: 1–22.

12. Gardner E, Gray DJ, O'Rahilly R. A Regional Study of Human Structure. WB Saunders: Philadelphia, PA, 1975: 116.

13. Goldman FD, Dayton PD, Hanson CJ. Renal cell carcinoma and osseous metastases. J Am Pediatr Med Assoc 1989. 79(12).

14. Grant T, DeKernion J. Treatment of skeletal metastases from urologic malignancies. Urology 1978; 11(6): 563–7.

15. DeVita VT, Hellman S, Rosenberg S. Principles Pract Oncol 1993; 4: 2226.

16. Benson M, Haaga J, Resnick M. Staging renal carcinoma. Arch Surg 1989; 124: 71–3.

17. Lindner A, Goldman D, deKernion J. Cost effective analysis of prenephrectomy radioisotope scans in renal cell carcinoma. Urology 1983; 22: 127–9.

18. Blacher E, Johnson DE, Thomas HP. Value of routine radionuclide bone scans in renal cell carcinoma. Urology 1985; 26(5): 432–4.

19. Grob JC, Lallot C, Methlin G, Bollack C. Quantitative bone scintigraphy in the survey of bone-seeking cancers. In Bollack CG, Jacqmin D (eds), Basic Research and Treatment of Renal Cell Carcinoma Metastasis. EORTC Genitourinary Group Monograph 1990; 9: 187–94.

20. Wetzel LH, Smalley SR, Robertson EF et al. Use of MR imaging for comprehensive staging of spine metastases: impact on radiation therapy treatment planning. Presented at 79th Scientific Assembly and Annual Meeting of the Radiological Society of North America Meeting, Chicago, IL, December 1993.

21. Marcove RC, Sadrieh J, Huvos AG et al. Cryosurgery in the treatment of solitary or multiple bone metastases from renal cell carcinoma. J Urol 1972; 108: 540.

22. Varm J, Huben RP, Wajsman Z, Pontes JE. Therapeutic embolization of pelvic metastases of renal cell carcinoma. Cancer 1983; 51: 614–17.

23. Halperin EC, Harisiadis L. The role of radiation therapy in the management of metastatic renal cell carcinoma. Cancer 1983; 51: 614–17.

24. Archangeli G, Micheli A et al. The responsiveness of bone metastases to radiotherapy. The effect of site, histology and radiation dose on pain relief. Radiother Oncol 1989; 14: 95–101.

25. Bostel F, Kuhne-velte HJ, Wollgens PS. Value of radiotherapy in metastases of hypernephroid carcinoma. Strahlentherapie 1983; 159(7): 404–11.

26. Cutuli BF, Methlin A, Teissier E et al. Radiation therapy in the treatment of metastatic renal cell carcinoma. In Basic Research and Treatment of Renal Cell Carcinoma Metastasis. 1990: 179–86.

27. DiBiase SJ, Valicenti RK, Schutz D et al. Palliative irradiation for focally symptomatic metastatic renal cell carcinoma: support for dose escalation based on a biological model. J Urol 1997; 158(3,1): 746–9.

28. Freed SZ. Nephrectomy for renal cell carcinoma with metastases. Urology 1977; 9: 613.

29. DeKernion JB, Ramming KP, Smith RB. The natural history of metastatic renal cell carcinoma. A computer analysis. J Urol 1978; 120: 148–52.

30. Middleton RG. Surgery for metastatic renal cell carcinoma. J Urol 1967; 97: 973–7.

31. Tolla BM, Whitmore WF. Solitary metastasis from renal cell carcinoma. J Urol 1975; 114: 836–8.

32. O'Dea MJ, Zincke J, Utz DC. The treatment of renal cell carcinoma with solitary metastasis. J Urol 1978; 120: 540–2.

33. Smith EM, Kursh ED, Makley J, Resnick MI. Treatment of osseous metastases secondary to renal cell carcinoma. J Urol 1992; 148: 784–7.

34. Bowers TA, Murray JA, Charnsangavej C et al. Bone metastases from renal carcinoma; the preoperative use of transcatheter arterial occlusion. J Bone Joint Surg 1982; 64: 749.

35. O'Reilly GV, Kleefield J, Klein LA et al. Embolization of solitary spinal metastases from renal cell carcinoma: alternative therapy for spinal cord or nerve root compression. Surg Neurol 1989; 31: 268–71.

36. Varma J, Huben RP, Wajsman Z, Pontes J. Therapeutic embolization of pelvic metastases of renal cell carcinoma. J Urol 1984; 131(4): 647–9.

37. Yagoda A. Chemotherapy for renal cell carcinoma. Semin Urol 1989; 7: 199–206.

38. Rini BI, Vogelzang NJ, Dumas MC et al. Phase II trial of weekly intravenous gemcitabine with continuous infusion fluorouracil in patients with metastatic renal cell cancer. J Clin Oncol 2000; 18(12): 2419–27.

39. Wallace S. Interventional radiology: intra-arterial therapy. J Radiol 1984; 65: 499.

40. Jakse G, Muller-Holzner E. Hormone receptors in renal cancer: an overview. Semin Surg Oncol 1988; 4: 161–4.

41. Kjaer M. The role of medroxyprogesterone acetate in the treatment of renal adenocarcinoma. Cancer Treat Rev 1988; 15: 195–209.

42. Minervini R, Florentini L, Carlino F et al. Scintigraphic evidence for the regression of skeletal metastases from a hypernephroma following long-term treatment with medroxyprogesterone acetate. J Nucl Med Allied Sci 1982; 26: 55.

43. Krown SE. Interferon treatment of renal cell carcinoma: current status and future prospects. Cancer 1987; 59: 647.

44. Muss MB. Renal cell carcinoma, in interferons clinical applications. In Devita VT, Hellman S, Rosenberg SA (eds), Biological Therapy of Cancer. Lippincott-Raven, Hagerstown, MD, USA, 1993: 298–310.

45. Pyrhonen S, Salminen E, Ruutu M et al. Prospective randomized trial of interferon α-2a plus vinblastine vs. vinblastine alone in patients with advanced renal cell cancer. J Clin Oncol 1999; 17(9): 2859.

46. Motzer RJ, Murphy BA, Bacik J et al. Phase III trial of interferon α-2a with or without 13-cis-retinoic acid for patients with advanced renal cell carcinoma. J Clin Oncol 2000; 18(16): 2972–80.

47. Rosenberg SA, Lotze MT, Muul LM. Observations on the systemic administration of autologous lymphokine-activated killer cells and recombinant interleukin-2 to patients with metastatic cancer. N Engl J Med 1985; 313: 1485–92.

48. Atkins MB, Sparano J, Fisher RI. Randomized phase II trial of high dose IL-2 either alone or in combination with interferon α-2 in advanced renal cell carcinoma. Proc Am Soc Clin Oncol 1991: 166.

49. Weiss GR, Margolin KA, Aronson FR. A randomized phase II trial of continuous infusion interleukin-2 or bolus injection IL-2 plus lymphokine-activated killer cells for advanced renal cell carcinoma. J Clin Oncol 1992; 10: 275–81.

50. Escudier B, Chevreau C, Lasset C et al. Cytokines in metastatic renal cell carcinoma. Is it useful to switch to interleukin-2 or interferon after failure of a first treatment? J Clin Oncol 1999; 17(7): 2039.

51. Stadler WM, Kuzel T, Shapiro C et al. Multi-institutional study of the angiogenesis inhibitor TNP-470 in metastatic renal carcinoma. J Clin Oncol 1999; 17(8): 2541.

52. Motzer RJ, Mazumdar M, Bacik J et al. Survival and prognostic stratification of 670 patients with advanced renal cell carcinoma. J Clin Oncol 1999; 17: 2530.

53. Perez CA. Updates Principles Pract Radiat Oncol 2000; 1(1).

44

Evaluation of the Patient with Bone Metastases at Presentation

Peter J. Hoskin

Mount Vernon Hospital, Northwood, UK

INTRODUCTION

Whilst in many cases bone metastases arise following identification and treatment of a primary tumour, in some instances they may be the presenting feature. When this is the case, it is likely to be because of presentation with one of the clinical complications of bone metastasis, including pain, pathological fracture, spinal cord or peripheral nerve compression or hypercalcaemia. Only rarely will bone metastasis be diagnosed as an incidental finding, usually in the setting of an X-ray diagnosis during investigations performed to assess other symptoms. Having identified bone metastasis as the cause of a presenting symptom, the next important step is to obtain a definitive tissue diagnosis and, where possible, define the site of the primary tumour. The known distribution of bone metastases will guide further investigations, the most common sites being lung, in women breast cancer and in men prostate cancer. Kidney and thyroid are the other two important sites not to be ignored but bone metastases have been reported from almost all primary sites. Overall, breast cancer is responsible for around 70% of bone metastases in women and prostate cancer for around 60% of all bone metastases in men [1].

Having identified the likely site of origin, appropriate management may then be instigated with the aims of both relieving presenting symptoms and achieving optimal control of the underlying malignant process.

The following sections will deal with the various presenting symptoms and subsequent management, an overview of which is shown in Figure 44.1

PAIN

Bone metastasis may present with bone pain or neuropathic pain secondary to nerve root involvement. Bone pain is typically a dull, aching pain, persistent and exacerbated by movement or weight-bearing, with associated local tenderness over the site of tumour involvement. It may worsen over time or may become associated with different spatial patterns, from a single persistent site of pain to scattered pain moving from site to site on a day-to-day basis. Local tenderness is typical and occasionally deformity of the bone or an associated soft tissue mass can be identified. Vascular tumours may have an audible overlying bruit, classically described with renal cancer metastases. Involvement of the vertebral bodies may result in neuropathic pain, typically paraesthesia and hyperalgesia within the affected dermatome of the spinal nerve root. Rarely metastasis involving the base of skull may present with a temporal neuralgia-type syndrome.

The differential diagnosis of pain of this type will be that of benign bone and joint disorders. It is not unusual for a patient to volunteer a history of trauma bringing the pain to notice. Whilst this is of no aetiological significance, it may initially be difficult to distinguish clinically between local tissue trauma and

Textbook of Bone Metastases. Edited by C. Jasmin, R. E. Coleman, L. R. Coia, R. Capanna and G. Saillant
© 2005 John Wiley & Sons Ltd: ISBN 0 471 87742 5

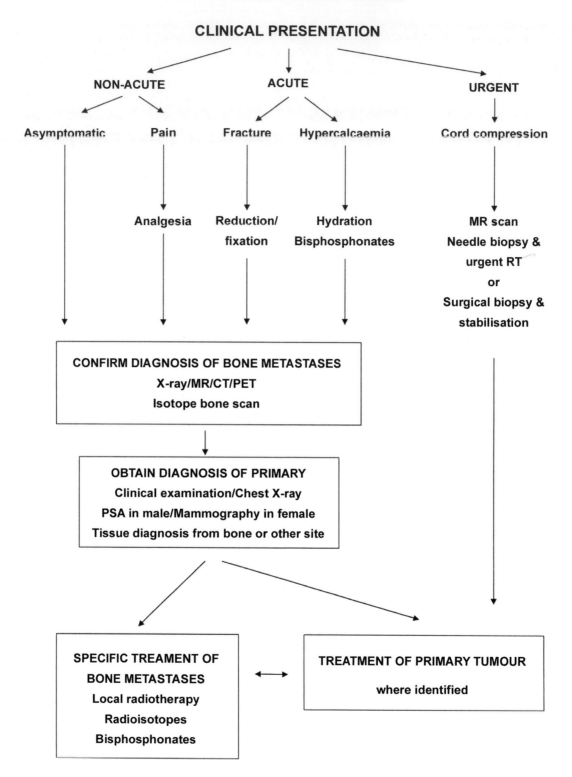

Figure 44.1. Overview of the management of a patient presenting with suspected bone metastases

the effects of bone metastasis. It is usually possible to identify degenerative joint disease by the association with pain on movement, joint stiffness and local joint tenderness and deformity. Metastases rarely if ever affect joint surfaces. Within the vertebral column, disorders of the intravertebral discs and osteoporosis are other important differential diagnoses to consider. Paraneoplastic syndromes may also cause bone pain in the absence of bone metastases, of which the commonest is hypertrophic pulmonary osteoarthropathy (HPOA), usually characterised by cortical thickening on plain X-ray (see below).

PATHOLOGICAL FRACTURE

Patients who present with a fracture in the setting of minimal trauma should be carefully evaluated to exclude an underlying bone metastasis. This will include pathological fracture of a long bone, unexplained rib fractures and vertebral collapse, together with the rarer fractures of pelvic or shoulder girdle bones. The overall incidence of pathological fracture is around 10% of patients with bone metastases and Table 44.1 shows the distribution of fracture site related to primary tumour seen in one large study [2]. Differential diagnoses in this situation include a primary bone tumour or benign bone tumours such as a chondroma, osteoma or bone cyst.

SPINAL CORD COMPRESSION

Patients presenting with the clinical symptoms and signs of spinal cord and cauda equina compression require urgent evaluation. Bilateral motor deficits, sensory changes (particularly when associated with a sensory level) and sphincter disturbances all require immediate investigation. The differential diagnosis will

Table 44.1. Distribution of primary tumour type presenting with pathological fracture

Primary tumour site	Pathological fracture (%)
Breast	53
Kidney	11
Lung	8
Thyroid	4
Lymphoma	4
Prostate	3
Others	17

include other causes of spinal canal intrusion, including a prolapsed intravertebral disc, primary CNS tumour or vascular malformation. Other medical causes of cord damage should also be considered, including demyelination and subacute combined degeneration of the cord. Radiological investigations are required as a matter of urgency. Magnetic resonance imaging (MRI) of the entire spine will usually define an anatomical diagnosis. Malignant spinal canal compression will be due to extradural tumour in 75% of cases and in the remaining 25% it will be associated with an adjacent vertebral metastasis, with or without vertebral collapse [3], as shown in Figure 44.2. In the absence of other known pathology, where a radiological metastasis is seen a needle biopsy or open operative procedure is required to obtain tissue.

HYPERCALCAEMIA

Hypercalcaemia is typically a presentation of advanced malignancy and heralds a poor prognosis, with a mean survival of around 3–4 months. The common symptoms of confusion, dehydration, polyuria and constipation should trigger an urgent estimation of the corrected serum calcium. The most common cause of hypercalcaemia is that of underlying malignancy. Initial treatment of the hypercalcaemia with fluids and bisphosphonate infusions should be followed by urgent investigations to evaluate the underlying cause.

OTHER SYMPTOMS

Bone metastasis may present with other manifestations, of which the most common is bone marrow failure, resulting in pancytopenia. More usually, patients with widespread bone metastases will run a low-grade anaemia and possibly mild thrombocytopenia. This is usually a normocytic or occasionally macrocytic anaemia with possibly a leukoerythroblastic blood film. Cranial nerve palsies may occur due to skull base infiltration, typically seen in carcinoma of the prostate.

INVESTIGATIONS

Patients presenting with the above symptoms will require further investigations to confirm a diagnosis of bone metastasis.

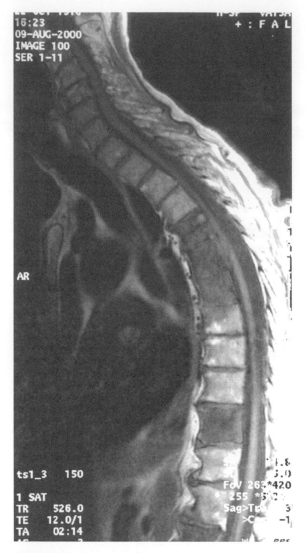

Figure 44.2. MR scan demonstrating multiple vertebral metastases and involvement of spinal canal in the dorsal region, due to direct extension from bone metastases

Plain Radiographs

Good quality X-ray films will in many instances be sufficient once symptoms have occurred. However, it is well established that quite extensive bone destruction is required before a lesion may be visible on a plain radiograph, with a 30–50% change in bone density required [4]. Whilst it may therefore be reasonable to perform X-rays of a painful site or obvious site of fracture as a screening tool, they are largely superseded

by those that follow. The one exception to this is in multiple myeloma where an X-ray skeletal survey remains an important component of the staging investigations.

The appearances on X-ray will mirror the underlying pathophysiology, with typically a mixture of osteoblastic and osteoclastic activity resulting in sclerotic or lytic lesions, often mixed, on the plain film. Pure lytic lesions may point towards a diagnosis of renal cell carcinoma or multiple myeloma, and predominantly sclerotic lesions are characteristic of prostate cancer, shown in Figure 44.3, but exceptions to these generalisations are well recognised.

Isotope Bone Scan

Bone scintigraphy is an important investigation when assessing a patient with probable bone metastasis. Bone scans will define areas of osteoblastic activity using the radioisotope tracer technetium (^{99m}Tc) linked to a diphosphonate compound, which is then preferentially absorbed into the hydroxyapatite crystal at sites of remineralisation. It may therefore be positive not only in sites of bone metastasis but also other areas of

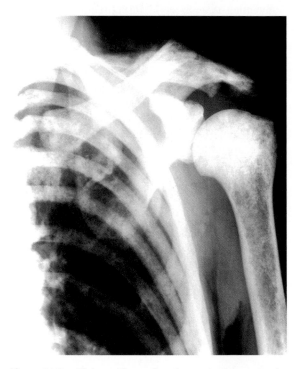

Figure 44.3. Plain radiographs demonstrating extensive sclerotic bone metastases typical of prostatic cancer

reactive bone formation, common sources of confusion being recent trauma, degenerative disease and healing fractures. Vertebral hotspots may be particularly difficult to evaluate where there is already known degenerative disease, and in this situation magnetic resonance imaging (MRI) is required. In an elderly population, where degenerative spinal disease is universal, metastases may be particularly difficult to distinguish on isotope studies alone. Another relatively common cause of marked osteoblastic activity and increased uptake on bone scan is Paget's disease, shown in Figure 44.4, which will usually be distinguished on plain X-ray. Other rare causes of confusion include primary bone tumours and osteomyelitis. Pure lytic lesions with little osteoblastic activity associated with them may not show significant uptake of the tracer, and it is recognised that both multiple myeloma and renal cell carcinoma may, despite other radiological evidence

of widespread metastasis, be associated with a normal bone scan. Gamma camera pictures will provide a whole body distribution of the isotope. Characteristic patterns of bone metastasis are described, with diffuse irregular uptake in the axial skeleton and ribs. Solitary sites of positivity are due to metastasis in around 50% of cases [5,6], one example of which is demonstrated in Figure 44.5. If bone metastases are very extensive, individual sites of uptake may not be seen, giving the features of the so-called "super scan" seen in Figure 44.6. HPOA produces a typical appearance of "tram-line" uptake along the cortical margin of long bones, giving rise to the "parallel stripe" sign.

More sophisticated forms of radionuclide imaging are now available, of which positron emission tomography (PET) is perhaps the most useful. The use of alternative tracers, such as fluorodeoxyglucose (FDG), enable metabolically active tissues to be identified, with a high correlation between these hotspots and malignant tissue. The precise role of PET scanning in patients with malignancy is still being defined. It may, however, be extremely useful in distinguishing equivocal sites of bone damage or radiologically normal sites of increased uptake on a technetium bone scan, when a positive PET scan will strongly support the diagnosis of bone metastasis also.

Where a differentiated thyroid malignancy is suspected, ^{131}I or ^{125}I scanning will confirm metabolically active thyroid metastases following thyroid ablation and *m*-iodobenzylguanidine (MIBG) scans will be helpful if a neuroendocrine tumour is suspected.

CT and MRI

MRI will give the most accurate pictures of bone morphology. It is now the investigation of choice in patients presenting with spinal cord compression and is of value in patients with unexplained bone pain despite normal scintigraphy and plain X-ray appearances. It is able to distinguish benign vertebral pathology and intravertebral disc pathology from malignant change. Metastatic infiltration of the bone marrow can also be diagnosed by MRI. Bone metastases are best defined using a T1-weighted spin-echo image, with which tumour within bone gives an abnormal low signal compared to surrounding bone. T2-weighted images will give high signal from tumour and may show sclerotic areas as low signal within this. More complex 'STIR' sequences, which suppress normal signal from fat, may give more dramatic visual images, tumour having a bright high signal intensity. With the development of MRI, CT scanning has become less

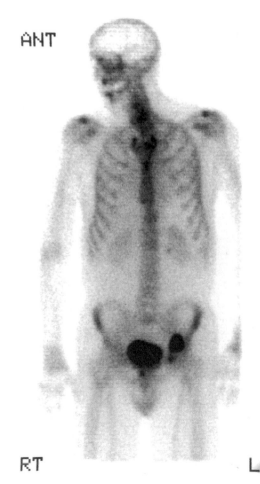

Figure 44.4. Solitary uptake on bone scan in the pelvis, subsequently shown to be Paget's disease

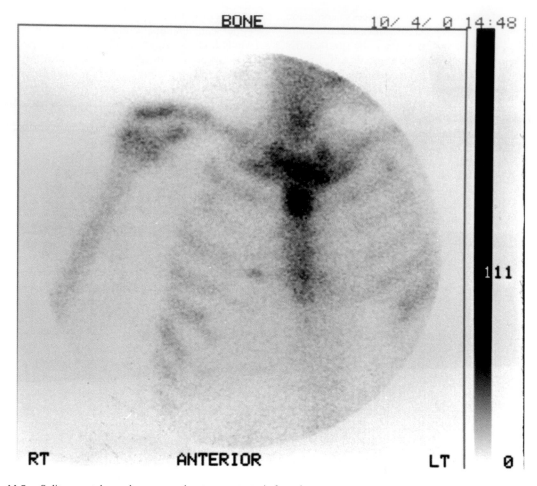

Figure 44.5.   Solitary uptake on bone scan, due to a metastasis from breast cancer

popular for the evaluation of possible bone metastasis. It does, however, have definite roles in the patient with contraindications to MRI, e.g. those with ferromagnetic prostheses, shrapnel wounds, tattoos or cardiac pacemakers. There is also some evidence to suggest that for flat bones such as the pelvis and scapulae, better definition can be determined with CT rather than MRI [7]. CT also has a major role in enabling image-guided biopsies to be taken (see below).

DEFINITIVE DIAGNOSIS

The patient, having presented with clinical symptoms and undergone radiological investigations to demonstrate the presence of bone metastasis, must then be considered for a formal tissue diagnosis to confirm malignant disease. Exceptions to this would be a male presenting with bone metastasis who has a raised PSA level within the range associated with metastatic disease, typically above 50 ng/ml. A presumptive diagnosis of multiple myeloma may be made on the finding of a paraprotein on electrophoresis, but a bone marrow examination will still be required to confirm plasma cell excess. All other patients will require a biopsy of either an accessible area of bone metastasis or a primary site subsequently identified. A reasonable management plan to lead to a definitive diagnosis will therefore be as follows, taking into account the known primary sites associated with bone metastasis:

1. Confirmation of bone metastasis on radiology, at least plain X-ray with confirmatory isotope bone scan or MRI.

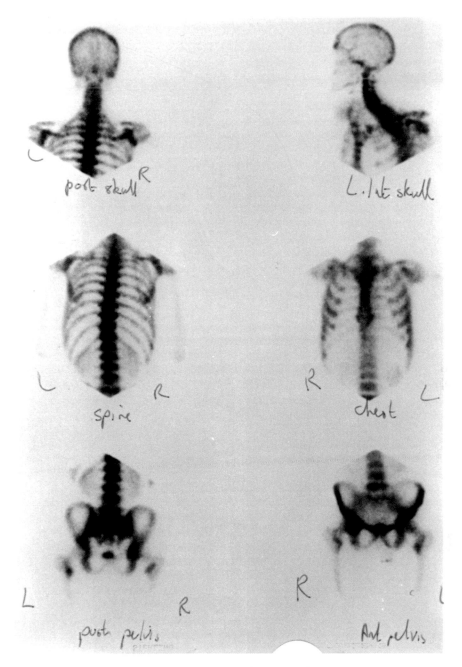

Figure 44.6. "Superscan" in a patient with widespread metastases from prostatic cancer

2. A rectal examination in males and a full breast examination in females should be included in the clinical evaluation, together with clinical assessment of the thyroid gland and careful palpation of the abdomen for a renal mass. Urine should be checked for blood and protein and urine microscopy for cytological examination. Blood in the urine should prompt further investigations into the renal tract to exclude in particular renal or bladder cancer, and proteinuria may be due to Bence-Jones protein and

be followed by a myeloma screen. A chest X-ray should be performed as a matter of course to exclude a radiologically apparent lung cancer.

3. If the above reveals an obvious primary tumour, then a biopsy from the appropriate site should be undertaken.

4. Where there is no obvious primary site, then subsequent steps will depend upon the urgency of the clinical presentation:

   (a) Patients presenting with spinal cord compression require urgent needle biopsy of the spinal mass under CT control, as shown in Figure 44.7. This will be followed by appropriate radiotherapy or, for sensitive tumours, chemotherapy. The only exceptions to this are those patients where it is considered that surgery is the best treatment for their spinal cord compression, at which time histology will be obtained. Indications for surgery include spinal instability and a relatively radioresistant tumour, such as a soft tissue sarcoma or melanoma.

   (b) Patients presenting with pathological fracture who require internal fixation, e.g. fracture of a femur, will at that time have biopsy material obtained.

   (c) Patients with lesions falling into the category of "high risk" for pathological fracture will also require referral to an orthopaedic surgeon for prophylactic surgery, at which time a biopsy of the abnormal bone can be obtained. This will include lytic lesions, such as that shown in Figure 44.8, with > 50% cortical erosion, painful lytic lesions > 3 cm in diameter and diffuse lytic infiltration of a long bone [8].

   (d) Needle biopsy or, if necessary, open bone biopsy will be indicated for the remaining patients in whom there is no other soft tissue lesion to aim for. An alternative may be a bone marrow examination, particularly in those patients with a low-grade anaemia or leuko-erythroblastic blood film, or in those where MRI demonstrates bone marrow infiltration.

TREATMENT STRATEGIES

Initial treatment will be defined by two parameters, the clinical presentation and the underlying primary site.

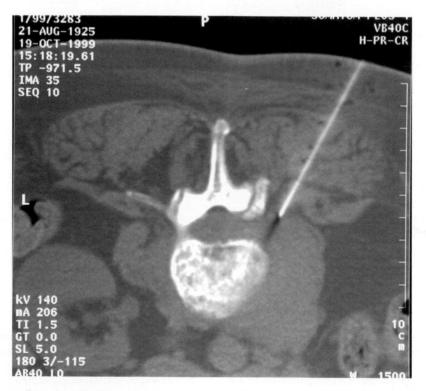

Figure 44.7. CT scan-directed needle biopsy in a patient presenting with features of spinal canal compression

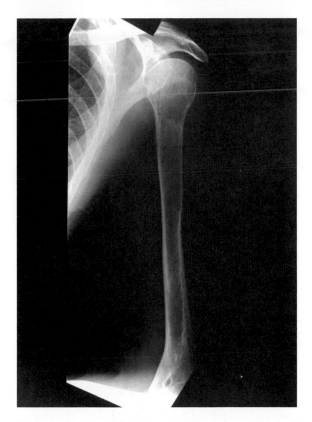

Figure 44.8. High-risk lytic lesion in the humerus in a patient with multiple myeloma, which subsequently fractured spontaneously prior to surgical fixation

- *Pain* should be dealt with initially with appropriate analgesics. Metastatic bone pain often responds poorly to opioids but conventional approaches to the use of analgesics, using the three- or four-step WHO-based analgesic ladder, should be initiated [9]. Often non-steroidal antiinflammatory drugs are the most effective and should be used amongst the first-line analgesic approaches. Where neuropathic pain is predominant, other adjuvant analgesics, such as amitryptilline or carbamazepine should be considered also.
- *Spinal cord compression* requires urgent treatment before neurological damage is allowed to become established. Initial treatment will be high-dose corticosteroids, e.g. dexamethasone 16 mg daily. Where there is spinal instability, this may require operative surgery and spinal stabilisation. Where the spine is stable, then urgent radiotherapy should be undertaken, provided that a histological diagnosis is available and that first-line chemotherapy

is not thought appropriate [10]. Chemotherapy should be considered in germ cell tumours, lymphomas and small cell lung cancer.

- *Pathological fracture* should be dealt with according to standard orthopaedic principles, including reduction and immobilisation of the fracture with, if necessary, internal fixation. Where there is proven malignancy at the site of fracture, however, local radiotherapy or systemic treatment for the malignancy should also be considered an important feature in the management.
- *Hypercalcaemia* will require urgent treatment with intravenous fluids and bisphosphonate drugs. Thereafter, appropriate treatment of the primary tumour should be considered, depending upon the site of origin.

PRINCIPLES OF FURTHER MANAGEMENT FOR METASTATIC BONE PAIN

The management of bone pain will often depend upon the underlying primary site. Where prostate cancer is diagnosed, symptomatic disease warrants early introduction of antiandrogen therapy [11]. Other sites, e.g. breast cancer, small cell lung cancer and multiple myeloma, should also be considered for systemic chemotherapy or, in the case of breast cancer, hormone therapy. Alongside this, for breast cancer and lung cancer consideration may need to be given to appropriate management of the primary site with either local excision of a breast cancer or palliative radiotherapy to a lung cancer.

Where a chemosensitive or hormone-sensitive tumour has not been identified, or where pain persists despite the introduction of systemic therapy, then local radiotherapy to sites of bone metastases is invaluable. Where there is scattered bone pain, systemic radio-isotope therapy using ^{89}Sr [12] or ^{153}Sm-EDTMP [13] should be considered if there is adequate bone marrow reserve, no renal failure or urinary incontinence, and where the expected life span is > 3 months. An alternative to this is sequential hemi-body radiotherapy.

SUMMARY

Patients presenting with bone metastases may do so with the uncomplicated picture of painful bones or the consequences of bone metastases causing spinal cord compression, pathological fracture or hypercalcaemia. Immediate management demands confirmation of a malignant metastatic process within the bone and in the case of spinal cord compression urgent treatment will be required. Radiological confirmation and evaluation of the extent of disease should then be undertaken, with isotope bone scanning supported by MRI or CT. A histological diagnosis should be attempted for all patients except those with obvious metastatic prostate cancer, evidence by a high PSA. Management will take the form of dealing with urgent complications, in particular spinal cord compression with surgery or radiotherapy, pathological fracture with immobilisation, reduction and internal fixation where appropriate, and hypercalcaemia with fluids and bisphosphonates. Subsequent management will depend upon systemic treatment for the underlying malignancy and local treatment to the bones, using radiotherapy where systemic analgesia is ineffective.

REFERENCES

1. Rubens RD. Bone metastases—incidence and complications. In Rubens RD, Mundy GR (eds), Cancer and the Skeleton. Martin Dunitz: London, 2000.
2. Higinbotham NL, Marcove RC. The management of pathological fractures. J Trauma 1965; 5: 792–8.
3. Pigott KH, Baddeley H, Maher EJ. Pattern of disease in spinal cord compression on MRI scan and implications for treatment. Clin Oncol 1994; 6: 7–10.
4. Edelstyn GA, Gillespie PJ, Grebell FS. The radiological demonstration of osseous metastases: experimental observations. Clin Radiol 1967; 18: 158–62.
5. Baxter AD, Coakley FV, Finlay DB et al. The aetiology of solitary hot spots in the ribs on planar bone scans. Nucl Med Commun 1995; 16: 834–7.
6. Coakley FV, Jones AR, Finlay DB et al. The aetiology and distinguishing features of solitary hot spots on planar bone scans. Clin Radiol 1995; 50: 327–30.
7. Zimmer DW, Berquist TH, McLeod RA et al. Bone tumors: magnetic resonance imaging vs. computed tomography. Radiology 1985; 155: 709–18
8. Hipp JA, Springfield DS, Hayes WC. Predicting pathologic fracture risk in the management of metastatic bone defects. Clin Orthop 1995; 312: 120–35.
9. Hoskin PJ, Hanks GW. Cancer pain and its relief. In Souhami RL, Tannock I, Bergasel DE et al. (eds), Oxford Textbook of Oncology, 2nd edn. Oxford University Press, Oxford, 2002; 1017–1034.
10. Findlay CFG. Adverse effects on the management of spinal cord compression. J Neurol Neurosurg Psychiat 1984; 47: 139–44.
11. Medical Research Council Prostate Cancer Working Party Investigators Working Group. Immediate vs. deferred treatment for advanced prostatic cancer: initial results of the Medical Research Council trial. Br J Urol 1997; 79: 235–46.
12. Quilty PM, Kirk D, Bolger JJ et al. A comparison of the palliative effects of strontium-89 and external beam radiotherapy in metastatic prostate cancer. Radiother Oncol 1994; 31: 33–40.
13. Serafini AN, Houston SJ, Resche I et al. Palliation of pain associated with metastatic bone cancer using samarium-153 lexidronam: a double-blind placebo-controlled clinical trial. J Clin Oncol 1998; 16: 1574–81.

Index

Note: page numbers in *italics* refer to figures and tables